FOURTH EDITION

General Surgery
Board Review

Editors

Larry A. Scher, M.D.

Professor of Clinical Surgery
Albert Einstein College of Medicine/Montefiore Medical Center
Bronx, New York

Gerard Weinberg, M.D.

Professor of Clinical Surgery and Pediatrics
Albert Einstein College of Medicine/Montefiore Medical Center
Bronx, New York

Wolters Kluwer | Lippincott Williams & Wilkins
Health

Philadelphia · Baltimore · New York · London
Buenos Aires · Hong Kong · Sydney · Tokyo

Acquisitions Editor: Brian Brown
Product Manager: Nicole Dernoski
Production Manager: Bridgett Dougherty
Senior Manufacturing Manager: Benjamin Rivera
Marketing Manager: Lisa Lawrence
Design Coordinator: Theresa Mallon
Production Service: Aptara, Inc.

© **2012 by LIPPINCOTT WILLIAMS & WILKINS, a WOLTERS KLUWER business**
Two Commerce Square
2001 Market Street
Philadelphia, PA 19103 USA
LWW.com

Printed in China

Library of Congress Cataloging-in-Publication Data

General surgery board review / editors, Larry A. Scher, Gerard Weinberg.
– 4th ed.
  p. ; cm.
Includes bibliographical references and index.
ISBN 978-1-60547-066-5 (pbk.)
I. Scher, Larry A. II. Weinberg, Gerard.
[DNLM: 1. Surgical Procedures, Operative–Examination Questions. WO 18.2]
LC classification not assigned
617.0076–dc23
                                    2011031695

Care has been taken to confirm the accuracy of the information presented and to describe generally accepted practices. However, the authors, editors, and publisher are not responsible for errors or omissions or for any consequences from application of the information in this book and make no warranty, expressed or implied, with respect to the currency, completeness, or accuracy of the contents of the publication. Application of the information in a particular situation remains the professional responsibility of the practitioner.

The authors, editors, and publisher have exerted every effort to ensure that drug selection and dosage set forth in this text are in accordance with current recommendations and practice at the time of publication. However, in view of ongoing research, changes in government regulations, and the constant flow of information relating to drug therapy and drug reactions, the reader is urged to check the package insert for each drug for any change in indications and dosage and for added warnings and precautions. This is particularly important when the recommended agent is a new or infrequently employed drug.

Some drugs and medical devices presented in the publication have Food and Drug Administration (FDA) clearance for limited use in restricted research settings. It is the responsibility of the health care provider to ascertain the FDA status of each drug or device planned for use in their clinical practice.

To purchase additional copies of this book, call our customer service department at (800) 638-3030 or fax orders to (301) 223-2320. International customers should call (301) 223-2300.

Visit Lippincott Williams & Wilkins on the Internet: at LWW.com. Lippincott Williams & Wilkins customer service representatives are available from 8:30 am to 6 pm, EST.

10 9 8 7 6 5 4 3 2 1

CCS1011

CONTRIBUTORS

Salman Ahmad, MD
Department of Surgery
New York University School of Medicine
New York, New York

Maria Amodio-Groton, PharmD
North Shore University Hospital
Division of Infectious Diseases
Manhasset, New York

Matthew Ashbach, MD
Department of Otolaryngology/Head and Neck Surgery
Albert Einstein College of Medicine/Montefiore Medical
    Center
Bronx, New York

Lillian Harvey Banchik, MD
Clinical Assistant Professor of Surgery
North Shore-LIJ Health System
Hofstra University School of Medicine
Manhasset, New York

Alexandra Bastien, MD
Assistant Professor of Anesthesia
Albert Einstein College of Medicine/Montefiore Medical
    Center
Bronx, New York

Steven Blau, MD
Department of Surgery
Hackensack Medical Center
Hackensack, New Jersey

Philip F. Caushaj, MD
Professor of Surgery
Albert Einstein College of Medicine/Montefiore Medical
    Center
Bronx, New York

Jacob Clendenon, MD
Department of Surgery
Albert Einstein College of Medicine/Montefiore Medical
    Center
Bronx, New York

Marcia E. Epstein, MD
Assistant Professor NYU School of Medicine
North Shore University Hospital
Division of Infectious Diseases
Manhasset, New York

Taynet T. Febles, MD
North Shore University Hospital
Division of Infectious Diseases
Manhassset, New York

Evan S. Garfein, MD
Assistant Professor
Department of Surgery and Department of
    Otorhinolaryngology
Albert Einstein College of Medicine/Montefiore Medical
    Center
Bronx, New York

Nicholas J. Gargiulo, MD
Associate Professor of Clinical Surgery
Albert Einstein College of Medicine/Montefiore Medical
    Center
Bronx, New York

Robert D. Goldstein, MD
Clinical Associate Professor of Surgery
Division of Plastic Surgery
Albert Einstein College of Medicine/Montefiore Medical
    Center
Bronx, New York

James Tait-Goodrich, MD
Director and Professor Division of Pediatric Neurosurgery
Albert Einstein College of Medicine/Montefiore Medical
    Center
Bronx, New York

Stuart Greenstein, MD
Professor of Clinical Surgery
Albert Einstein College of Medicine/Montefiore Medical
    Center
Bronx, New York

Daniel S. Gingold, MD
Department of Surgery
Albert Einstein College of Medicine/Montefiore Medical
    Center
Bronx, New York

Daniel Glicklich, MD
Professor of Clinical Medicine
Albert Einstein College of Medicine/Montefiore Medical
    Center
Bronx, New York

Ari Hakimi, MD
Department of Urology
Albert Einstein College of Medicine/Montefiore Medical
    Center
Bronx, New York

Paul T. Haynes, MD
Department of Orthopedics
Albert Einstein College of Medicine/Montefiore Medical
    Center
Bronx, New York

David Kaye, MD
Department of Orthopedics
Albert Einstein College of Medicine/Montefiore Medical
    Center
Bronx, New York

Steven M. Keller, MD
Director of Thoracic Surgery Weiler Hospital of the
    Montefiore Medical Center
Clinical Professor of Cardiothoracic Surgery
Albert Einstein College of Medicine/Montefiore Medical
    Center
Bronx, New York

Angela C. Kim, MD
North Shore University Hospital
Division of Infectious Diseases
Manhasset, New York

Ronald N. Kaleya, MD
Department of Surgery
Westchester Medical Center
Valhalla, New York

Milan Kinkhabwala, MD
Chief, Division of Transplant Surgery
Professor of Surgery
Albert Einstein College of Medicine/Montefiore Medical
    Center
Bronx, New York

David A. Koslovsky, DDS
Assistant Professor of Surgery
Department of Oral and Maxillofacial Surgery
Columbia University
New York, New York

Sam Lan, MD
Associate Professor of Clinical Surgery
Albert Einstein College of Medicine/Montefiore Medical
    Center
Bronx, New York

Mark D. Levie, MD
Director of Obstetrics and Gynecology
Moses Division of Montefiore Medical Center
Associate Professor of Obstetrics and Gynecology
Albert Einstein College of Medicine/Montefiore Medical
    Center
Bronx, New York

Amy Lu, MD
Professor of Surgery
Loyola University Stritch School of Medicine
Chicago, Illinois

Lloyd S. Minsky, MD
Assistant Professor of Urology
Department of Urology
Albert Einstein College of Medicine/Montefiore Medical
    Center
Bronx, New York

Randall P. Owen, MD
Assistant Professor of Surgery,
Mt. Sinai School of Medicine
New York, New York

W. Pizarro Patton, MD
Department of Surgery
Albert Einstein College of Medicine/Montefiore Medical
    Center
Bronx, New York

Sagar Reddy, MD
Department of Surgery
Albert Einstein College of Medicine/Montefiore Medical
    Center
Bronx, New York

Aksim Rivera, MD
Department of Surgery
Albert Einstein College of Medicine/Montefiore Medical
    Center
Bronx, New York

Russell H. Samson, MD
Clinical Associate Professor of Surgery (Vascular)
Florida State University Medical School
Sarasota, Florida

Gil Hauer Santos, MD
Department of Thoracic Surgery
Jacobi Medical Center
Bronx, New York

Larry A. Scher, MD
Professor of Clinical Surgery
Albert Einstein College of Medicine/Montefiore Medical
    Center
Bronx, New York

Peter Shamamian, MD
Chief, Division of General Surgery
Professor of Surgery
Albert Einstein College of Medicine/Montefiore Medical
  Center
Bronx, New York

Alok D. Sharan, MD
Assistant Professor
Department of Orthopedics
Albert Einstein College of Medicine/Montefiore Medical
  Center
Bronx, New York

Alexandre M. Scheer, MD
Department of Neurosurgery
Albert Einstein College of Medicine/Montefiore Medical
  Center
Bronx, New York

Richard S. Schechner, MD
Department of Surgery
Albert Einstein College of Medicine/Montefiore Medical
  Center
Bronx, New York

Joyce J. Shin, MD
Department of Surgery
Albert Einstein College of Medicine/Montefiore Medical
  Center
Bronx, New York

Josef A. Shehebar, MD
Department of Surgery
Albert Einstein College of Medicine/Montefiore Medical
  Center
Bronx, New York

Ronald J. Simon, MD
Professor of Surgery
New York University School of Medicine
New York, New York

Prashanth Sreeramoju, MD
Assistant Professor of Surgery
Albert Einstein College of Medicine/Montefiore Medical
  Center
Bronx, New York

Jennifer Stableford, MD
Assistant Professor of Surgery
Albert Einstein College of Medicine/Montefiore Medical
  Center
Bronx, New York

Alex Stone, MD
Professor of Surgery
New York University Medical Center
New York, New York

Melvin Stone, Jr., MD
Associate Professor of Clinical Surgery
Albert Einstein College of Medicine/Jacobi Medical Center
Bronx, New York

Peter L. Stone, MD
Assistant Clinical Professor of Urology
Department of Urology
Albert Einstein College of Medicine/Montefiore Medical
  Center
Bronx, New York

Vivian A. Tellis, MB, BS
Professor of Surgery
Albert Einstein College of Medicine/Montefiore Medical
  Center
Bronx, New York

Gerard Weinberg, MD
Professor of Clinical Surgery and Pediatrics
Albert Einstein College of Medicine/Montefiore Medical
  Center
Bronx, New York

B. Paul White, MD
General and Minimally Invasive Surgery
Northern Westchester Hospital
Mt Kisco, New York

Barbara Weinstein, PA
Department of Surgery
Albert Einstein College of Medicine/Montefiore Medical
  Center
Bronx, New York

Gila Weinstein, MD
Department of Surgery
Division of Plastic Surgery
Albert Einstein College of Medicine/Montefiore Medical
  Center
Bronx, New York

Jane Yang, MD
Department of Surgery
Albert Einstein College of Medicine/Montefiore Medical
  Center
Bronx, New York

Deborah Yu, MD
Department of Surgery
Albert Einstein College of Medicine/Montefiore Medical
  Center
Bronx, New York

It has been more than a decade since the publication of the third edition of General Surgery Board Review. Significant advances have occurred in many areas of general surgery and many surgical subspecialties. Bariatric surgery, endovascular aneurysm repair, and many other areas are now well-established surgical fields, but were considered new and exciting surgical advances when the previous edition was published. As these developments have become commonplace in today's surgical practice, they have also become important and more frequent sources of questions for examinations for general surgery certification and recertification. This fourth edition of our book incorporates this new material and updates previous chapters in all areas of general surgery and surgical specialties. The popular format used for the previous editions has been maintained. In addition to updating factual material and references, questions have again been included for self-assessment.

The editors hope that this edition of General Surgery Board Review will be as well received as the previous editions and will continue to help readers succeed in passing their qualifying, certifying, or recertification examination.

Larry A. Scher, MD
Gerard Weinberg, MD

ACKNOWLEDGMENTS

The editors are indebted to the many individuals who were invaluable in making this text a reality. Most of the material in this book derives from the Annual General Surgery Board Review Course, sponsored by the Montefiore Medical Center Office of Continuing Medical Education. The professionals who have organized and run this course for the past 45 years have made it into one of the premier courses of its kind in the country. We especially thank Dean Victor Hatcher, Director of Continuing Medical Education and his outstanding staff, with special recognition to Nada Piacentino and Marilyn Sasso.

Their dedication, hard work, and organizational skills have made our involvement in this course over so many years an enriching and highly rewarding experience.

A book is only as good as the people who contribute to it. Thankfully we have been fortunate in having had an outstanding cadre of authors who give of their time, knowledge, and specialized skills in making this project a reality. Without them there would not have been this book.

Our publisher, Lippincott Williams & Wilkins/ Wolters Kluwer Health, has been most cooperative and supportive. Kudos to Nicole Dernoski, Senior Product Manager at Lippincott. She encouraged us through a challenging gestation until the very end. We owe her a sincere debt of gratitude.

CONTENTS

Diseases of the Esophagus

ANATOMY

The esophagus is situated in three anatomic regions—cervical, thoracic, and abdominal—each with its specific blood supply. The cervical esophagus receives branches of the inferior thyroid artery. The upper thoracic esophageal blood supply is derived from bronchial arteries, and the inferior thoracic esophagus obtains blood from segmental branches of the aorta. The left gastric and splenic arteries supply blood to the abdominal segment of the esophagus. For descriptive purposes, the esophagus can be divided into three: upper, middle, and lower, each measuring an average of 8 cm.

The esophagus is a muscular organ limited by an upper esophageal sphincter (UES) and a lower esophageal sphincter. The UES is composed of the cricopharyngeus and is well defined. The lower esophageal sphincter (LES) is not well defined anatomically but physiologically is identified as a high-pressure zone (HPZ). A sling of gastric muscle fiber known as the "collar of Helvetius" is occasionally found at the esophagogastric junction. The esophagus extends about 4 to 5 cm below the diaphragm before it blends into the stomach. Attached to the esophagus as it crosses the diaphragm is the phrenoesophageal ligament, which is a continuation of the transversalis fascia and peritoneum fused with the endothoracic fascia and pleura. The esophagus is lined by squamous epithelium throughout its length, but it changes to columnar epithelium 1 to 2 cm proximal to the esophagogastric junction.

The upper esophageal muscularis externa is composed of striated longitudinal and circular layers. The striated muscle is replaced by smooth muscle at the distal three-fifths of the esophagus.

PHYSIOLOGY

The resting pressure of the UES ensures that it remains closed when not swallowing, but it falls to zero during glutination. When fluid is injected into the upper esophagus, UES pressure increases. UES pressures are asymmetric, with posterior measurements greater than those obtained anteriorly or laterally. Measured pressures differ within the sphincter, which averages 4 cm in length. Swallowing relaxes the UES, enabling contraction of the lower pharyngeal muscles together with the "pump" action of the tongue to push food into the upper esophagus. Relaxation of the UES must precede the rise in pressure in the lower pharynx produced by the contraction of the inferior constrictor of the pharynx. Once the bolus enters the upper esophagus, a propulsive wave, the primary peristaltic wave, brings it down to enter the stomach, which is made possible by the relaxation of the lower esophageal sphincter. Secondary peristaltic waves originate from distension of the esophageal wall produced by contents inside the esophagus. Cold food decreases peristaltic amplitude and frequency; warm food has the opposite effect. Nonpropulsive (tertiary) contractions, when present, may have high amplitude and duration.

The HPZ found at the LES has a resting pressure that in normal individuals varies from 6 mm Hg to 24 mm Hg and is responsible for preventing gastroesophageal (GE) reflux. When abnormal relaxation is present, gastric contents reflux into the lower esophagus, damaging the esophageal mucosa. Duodenogastric reflux consisting of alkaline contents, such as bile salts and pancreatic enzymes, can also reflux into the esophagus.

There is no consensus on a precise definition of normal esophageal pH, though most authors consider an esophageal pH below 4 to be indicative of reflux. Individuals with normal function have an acidic pH in the lower esophagus no more than 6% of time, or 1.5 hours per 24 hours. Almost 90% of physiologic reflux occurs during and after meals. Alkaline reflux may interfere with evaluation of reflux based exclusively on pH monitoring.

The length of the abdominal esophagus subject to positive intraabdominal pressure is an important factor in the prevention of reflux. Reflux more frequently occurs when the total length of the LES is less than 2 cm or when the length of the intraabdominal LES is less than 1 cm. The simultaneous presence of LES pressure less than 6 mm Hg, total length of LES less than 2 cm, and intraabdominal LES less than 1 cm almost guarantees the presence of reflex. Other less important features in controlling reflux are the oblique angle of entry of the esophagus into the stomach, the mucosal folds at the LES, and the tightness of the diaphragmatic crura.

Acid regurgitated into the lower esophagus is cleared by the peristaltic activity of the esophagus. During waking time one peristaltic wave takes place each minute, whereas during sleep the frequency of peristalsis decreases to four waves per hour. Esophageal emptying is also facilitated by gravity during daytime, and acid is neutralized by more abundant production of saliva. Regulation of LES pressure is under neurologic control, mainly through the vagus. Transection of the vagi below the atrial level does not affect the LES tone, as there is a rich network of intramural nerve plexi. α-Adrenergic receptors localized within the wall cause esophageal constriction, whereas β-receptors mediate relaxation. The LES is also under hormonal influence. Gastrin has been shown, in vitro, to double the LES pressure, although the effect may not be physiologically important. Other substances that increase the LES pressure are vasopressin, α-adrenergic drugs, cholinergic drugs, anticholinesterase, a protein meal, and gastric alkalinization. Some of the substances that decrease the LES tone are secretin, vasoactive intestinal polypeptide, nitroglycerin, cholecystokinin, glucagon, progestational agents, α-adrenergic antagonists, β-adrenergic drugs, anticholinergics, prostaglandin E, nicotine, a fat meal, chocolate, and gastric acidification.

Several tests are used to test the functional integrity of the esophagus.

1. *Manometry:* The pressure of the sphincters and the body of the esophagus, at rest and during deglutition, are measured via catheters placed at different levels and during withdrawal from the stomach as it passes through the HPZ.
2. *pH reflux:* A 300-mL dose of 0.1 N HCl is injected into the stomach after a pH electrode has been positioned 5 cm above the GE junction. If the esophageal pH drops to 4 or less, GE reflux is assumed to be present.
3. *Acid clearing test:* This test measures the ability of the esophagus to clear regurgitated acid.
4. *Acid perfusion test (Bernstein):* Acid is introduced into the lower esophagus. The occurrence of symptoms is considered a positive test result. This test has a high incidence of false positives and false negatives.
5. *pH monitoring (24 hours):* A pH probe is left in the lower esophagus. A continuous recording is made of the number of reflux episodes when the pH falls below 4, and the amount of time it takes for the esophagus to clear the regurgitated acid. The value of the test may be obscured when duodenogastric reflux brings alkaline contents into the esophagus. In this situation, a normal pH between 4 and 6 can be found even though significant reflux may be taking place. Daytime reflux in excess of 90 minutes is suggestive of gastroesophageal reflux disease (GERD). Nighttime reflux is more damaging to the esophagus because of diminished protective mechanisms (gravity, saliva production, and peristaltic activity).

MOTILITY DISORDERS OF THE ESOPHAGUS

Normal food progression from the lower pharynx to the stomach requires perfect coordination of the esophageal sphincters and the muscles of the esophageal body. The inferior constrictor of the pharynx together with the "pump" action of the tongue propel food through an already relaxed cricopharyngeus. On entering the esophagus, the food is actively transported by peristaltic activity. The LES relaxes in anticipation of the arrival of the peristaltic wave, permitting food to enter the stomach. Passage of the bolus from the pharynx to the stomach takes an average of 6 seconds. Dysphagia occurs when there is lack of coordination of this normal sequence at any level.

Transfer Dysphagia
Cricopharyngeal Dysphagia
Cricopharyngeal dysphagia occurs when there is delayed and/or incomplete relaxation of the UES.

The peak pressure produced in the lower pharynx by muscular contraction does not find a relaxed cricopharyngeus, and so the food has difficulty entering the esophagus. An HPZ is generated between the inferior constrictor and the cricopharyngeus in a region with attenuated muscles, described by anatomists as "Killian's triangle." Swallowing difficulties at this level were sometimes diagnosed as "globus hystericus" and considered to be of psychogenic origin. Radiographic studies may demonstrate the delay of contrast passing through the UES into the esophagus. With this radiologic finding and in the presence of significant symptoms, cricopharyngeal myotomy is indicated.

Zenker's Diverticulum

The motility disturbance of Zenker's diverticulum is the same as that of cricopharyngeal dysphagia. The pressure generated between the oblique fibers of the inferior constrictor of the pharynx and the transverse fibers of the cricopharyngeus push out the mucosa between the two muscles at or near Killian's triangle, producing a diverticulum whose size depends on the length of time since the condition started as well as the degree of dysfunction. As food particles and liquid accumulate inside the diverticulum, symptoms are produced, including regurgitation, bad odor, and aspiration.

Zenker's diverticula are seen more frequently in older patients. The etiology is unclear, though it is possible that spasm of the cricopharyngeus is the result of mucosal irritation secondary to GE reflux. Treatment includes myotomy and diverticulectomy. Myotomy alone may be sufficient for smaller 3- to 4-mm diverticulum. Elderly and high-risk patients may be treated with diverticulopexy in which the diverticulum is suspended posterior to the pharynx. Internal (transoral) pharyngoesophageal myotomy with elimination of the diverticulum utilizing an endostapling device has gained popularity. Postoperative complications such as wound infection and fistula are more frequent following diverticulectomy.

Transport Dysphagia

Diffuse Esophageal Spasm

Diffuse esophageal spasm is manifested by retrosternal pain that radiates to the neck and upper extremities, mimicking angina. Adding to the possible diagnostic confusion is the fact that the pain can be relieved by nitroglycerin. Manometry may detect the presence of a large number of high-amplitude tertiary (nonpropulsive) contractions. A contrast study during episodes of pain may demonstrate the presence of a typical "corkscrew" esophagus. Antispasmodics and calcium channel blockers comprise the first line of treatment. Surgery is rarely indicated.

High-Amplitude Peristaltic Contractions

High-amplitude peristaltic contractions, or hyperperistalsis, also known as "nutcracker esophagus," is produced by peristaltic contractions that in some cases reach 400 mm Hg (normal average 75 mm Hg). Painful swallowing is the most common symptom. The treatment for both diffuse esophageal spasm and high-amplitude peristaltic contraction is conservative. Surgery is indicated only when symptoms do not respond to medication and supportive care. Extended esophagomyotomy, sparing the upper and lower esophageal sphincters, is the procedure of choice. The results are not encouraging, however, with frequent recurrences reported.

Delivery Dysphagia

Achalasia

Achalasia, a clearly defined motility disturbance, is recognized by the presence of three main components.

1. Aperistalsis. High-amplitude or low-amplitude tertiary (nonpropulsive) contractions.
2. Increased LES resting pressure. This pressure may be more than double the normal values.
3. Incomplete LES relaxation. Only about 30% of relaxation of the original resting pressure is achieved.

Histologically, there is a decrease in the number of ganglion cells in Auerbach's plexus at all esophageal levels. Neurotropic viruses may be responsible for their destruction, similar to the destruction of these cells due to *Trypanosoma cruzi,* observed in Chagas' disease.

Patients with achalasia complain of progressive dysphagia associated with regurgitation of undigested food, particularly in the supine position. Esophageal carcinoma develops in 2% to 4% of patients with untreated achalasia.

Achalasia is diagnosed by esophagography, which demonstrates obstruction at the GE junction and a dilated esophageal body. The severity of the radiologic changes correlate with disease progression. Early in the course of the disease, before dilatation has occurred, the obstruction at the GE junction may be difficult to distinguish radiologically from a carcinoma. Manometry reveals the resting LES pressure to be two to three times the normal values, as well as decreased or absent LES relaxation. Peristalsis is absent even though sporadic tertiary nonpropulsive waves can be identified. In the variant of achalasia known as "vigorous achalasia," nonperistaltic high-amplitude contractions are present, sometimes in great numbers.

There are two options for the treatment of achalasia. "Conservative" treatment consists of LES dilatation with a pneumatic balloon until the sphincter muscles rupture. Frequently, more than one dilatation is necessary. The most serious complication of dilatation is esophageal perforation, which usually requires urgent repair. A myotomy should be performed on the side opposite the rupture.

Heller myotomy is an alternative to dilatation and is recommended for children and patients with vigorous achalasia. A serious complication of myotomy is reflux, which occurs in 3% of patients. There is no consensus on whether an antireflux procedure should be routinely performed. The proponents of myotomy alone advocate minimal dissection of the GE junction with muscle division not extending more than 1 cm onto the stomach. When performed properly, the resting pressure of the sphincter decreases an average of 15 mm Hg. The proponents of more extensive myotomy recommend extending it as much as 2 cm into the stomach and adding an associated antireflux procedure. However, the barrier introduced by the antireflux procedure can interfere with proper emptying of an esophagus already impaired by decreased peristaltic activity.

Intramural botulinum toxin injection has also been used as treatment for achalasia. Injections are made above the HPZ in four quadrants for a total dose of 80 units. Botulinum toxin type A acts by preventing the release of acetylcholine from peripheral nerve endings, thereby reducing the LES pressure.

Epiphrenic Diverticulum

Epiphrenic diverticula are better visualized by contrast studies than by endoscopy. They are situated just above the diaphragm and are often associated with motility disturbances such as achalasia or diffuse esophageal spasm. Therefore, a motility study is necessary prior to surgery, which consists of diverticulectomy. If achalasia is present, a Heller esophagomyotomy is added.

Traction diverticula are located in the midesophagus and are produced by inflammatory changes in the mediastinum. Because all layers of the esophagus are present, they are not true diverticula but rather a localized region of esophageal retraction. When asymptomatic, treatment is not indicated.

Gastroesophageal Reflux Disease

GE reflux is a normal event that occurs occasionally during the day, mostly associated with swallowing. GERD results from a hypotensive LES that permits excessive reflux of gastrointestinal contents. Esophageal injury correlates with esophageal exposure to pH below 4 or above 7. Two mechanisms are responsible for the production of esophageal mucosal damage (esophagitis), and both are based on the action of proteolytic enzymes. The better known, more extensively studied mechanism, is that associated with the acid pepsin. The less well-known mechanism is related to alkaline pancreatic enzymes and bile salts. Pepsinogen is secreted by chief cells at the gastric fundus and is activated to pepsin by gastric acid. Animal experiments have demonstrated that esophageal mucosal injury does not occur when the esophagus is perfused with HCl alone and that pepsin is required. Similarly, the presence of acid is necessary for injury to occur when the esophagus is exposed to bile salts. This explains the beneficial effects of reducing the acid content in patients with bile-associated reflux esophagitis. In adults, a hiatus hernia is responsible for hypotensive LES in almost 90% of cases.

Diagnosis

The initial diagnostic tests for patients with symptoms suggestive of reflux are an upper GI series followed by endoscopy. Histologic examination is performed to rule out severe dysplasia when fungal or viral esophagitis is suspected. Pain provocation techniques are not always informative. The presence of bile in the esophagus is diagnostic of duodenogastric reflux.

When the diagnosis is in doubt, a motility study can be a valuable tool. pH monitoring can provide additional information even though it may not detect reflux when alkaline reflux predominates. In uncomplicated situations, 24-hour pH monitoring may demonstrate increased esophageal exposure to refluxed acid (pH ≤ 4 for more than 6% of the time, 1.5 hours). The Los Angeles classification is the most widely utilized system for categorizing esophagitis (Table 1.1).

Treatment

Esophagitis is treated medically with the objective of decreasing the acidity of gastric contents and optimizing

TABLE 1.1	Los Angeles Classification of Esophagitis
Grade A	One (or more) mucosal break not <5 mm that does not extend between the tops of the two mucosal folds
Grade B	One (or more) mucosal break >5 mm that does not extend between the tops of the two mucosal folds
Grade C	One (or more) mucosal break that is continuous between the tops of two or more mucosal folds but that involves <75% of the circumference
Grade D	One (or more) mucosal break that involves >75% of the esophageal circumference

Lundell L, Dent J, Bennett JR, et al. Endoscopic assessment of esophagitis: clinical and functional correlates and further validation of the Los Angeles classification. *Gut* 1999;45:172–180.

the reflux-preventing function of the LES. Foods that decrease the LES resting pressure (alcohol, chocolate, coffee) should be avoided. Weight loss and smoking cessation should be strongly encouraged. At nighttime, the head of the bed is elevated to help clear the regurgitated acid. Proton pump inhibitors at standard doses will successfully treat esophagitis in more than 90% of patients with Los Angeles grades A and B esophagitis. Patients with grades C and D esophagitis require higher dosages, and the relapse rate is greater. The presence of underlying anatomic abnormalities generally mandates lifetime therapy.

Surgical treatment is indicated when medical therapy fails. Several procedures have been developed to reposition the distal few centimeters of the esophagus within the positive-pressure environment of the abdomen and simultaneously reinforce the LES. If stricture is present, dilation is necessary prior to surgery. Common operations include the Nissen procedure, represented by a 360-degree transabdominal fundoplication. A 240-degree anterior fundoplication, the Belsey Mark IV, is done transthoracically. The Hill procedure consists of a posterior gastropexy in which the gastroesophageal junction is attached to the median arcuate ligament. According to some anatomists this "ligament" is in reality the lateral border of the right crus of the diaphragm. The Toupet and Dor partial wraps are other surgical options. The antireflux procedures' repairs are readily accomplished laparoscopically.

The goal of the antireflux procedures is to obtain a resting pressure in the LES sufficient to prevent reflux while preserving a pliable GE junction that does not prevent food from entering the stomach. The crura should be closed to ensure that a segment of esophagus remains within the abdomen. When it is not possible to restore the esophagus to an intraabdominal position because the esophagus is short, it can be "elongated" by performing a gastric fundoplasty as described by Collis. When the problem is duodenogastric reflux, surgery (Roux-en-Y) is directed to prevent the alkaline substances from entering the stomach and into the esophagus. Antireflux procedures may fail for a variety of reasons: mismanagement of the short esophagus, incorrect closure of the hiatus (too tight or too loose), poorly performed fundoplication, the presence of an undiagnosed motility disorder, and impaired gastric emptying.

Barrett's Esophagus

Reflux results in replacement of the damaged squamous epithelium with a metaplastic columnar lining in 7% to 33% of patients. The resulting columnar-lined esophagus is known as "Barrett's esophagus" and is not a simple columnar epithelium but a specialized epithelium with a villous appearance composed of mucin-containing columnar gastric cells interspersed with intestinal goblet cells. Patients with Barrett's esophagus have more episodes of alkaline reflux than patients with simple esophagitis.

Complications associated with Barrett's esophagus are stricture, ulcers, and cancer, and occur 30 to 125 times more often than in the general population. Strictures have been reported in as many as 50% of patients with Barrett's esophagus.

Regression of the columnar epithelium does not occur with sufficient regularity following antireflux operation to justify surgery for that reason alone. Among 249 cases collected in the literature, 6.4% had partial regression and 2% had complete regression. Considering the difficulties encountered by endoscopists when defining exactly what they saw before and after surgery, it is not surprising that even these low numbers must be questioned.

The incidence of Barrett's esophagus–related carcinoma in the U.S. population is 1.5 per 100,000, or almost 4,000 per year. The optimal surveillance schedule for patients with Barrett's esophagus is unknown. However, once metaplasia is documented, four-quadrant biopsy every 1 to 3 years is indicated. The interval is decreased if dysplasia is identified.

Among patients with Barrett's esophagus followed for 10 years, the prevalence of carcinoma is 1% to 2%. Carcinoma occurs mostly in the setting of extensive segments of high-grade dysplasia (30% to 50% of resected specimens). Current indications for resection of Barrett's esophagus are the presence of a nondilatable stricture, malignancy including high-grade metaplasia, severe symptoms not responsive to conservative treatment, bleeding, or perforated ulcers.

Secondary Motility Disorders

Several central nervous system diseases can produce dysphagia due to interference with normal swallowing mechanisms: for example, stroke, cerebral palsy, and Parkinson's disease. Similarly, muscular diseases such as myasthenia gravis and myotonic dystrophy may cause swallowing difficulties. Scleroderma, a multisystem disease, causes a decrease in the lower esophageal resting pressure associated with a decrease or even absent esophageal peristalsis. The resulting GE reflux into an esophagus devoid of peristaltic activity causes esophagitis.

Chemical Burns of the Esophagus

Chemical burns of the esophagus result from the accidental or voluntary ingestion of strong acids or alkalis. The local caustic action on the esophageal mucosa, when severe, may result in a deep necrosis. Alkalis produce liquefaction necrosis, which predisposes to extensive penetration, whereas acids produce a type of coagulation necrosis with more limited penetration into the esophageal wall. Healing of a circumferential burn may cause a stricture. The alkali usually implicated is NaOH (lye), which is found in a variety of household products. Acids produce more damage to the stomach. Sulfuric acid, which was once an easily obtainable component of car batteries, is frequently responsible.

Symptoms are variable, depending on the nature, amount, and concentration of the substance ingested. The oropharynx, esophagus, and stomach are all at risk of injury. When large amounts have been ingested, esophageal or gastric perforation with shock can occur, requiring immediate surgery as a life-saving measure. When early perforation does not occur, esophagoscopy during the initial 24 to 48 hours is indicated to evaluate the extent of the burn. This initial evaluation cannot change the subsequent course of events but is helpful for documenting the extent of the damage. A brief inspection of the oropharynx, observing how patients handle their saliva and how they breathe and phonate, is a reliable way to evaluate the extent of the oropharyngeal injury. The early insertion of a prosthetic stent to avoid the stricture produced by contraction of the burn scar has not been uniformly successful. Steroids have not helped decrease scar formation. Antibiotics are indicated to prevent bacterial colonization of the injured mucosa, which would increase the extent and depth of the injury.

Once stricture develops, peroral dilatation beginning 2 to 3 weeks after the original injury is recommended. When protracted treatment is anticipated, a gastrostomy facilitates retrograde passage of the dilators. Weekly or even biweekly dilatation sessions for several months may be necessary. If results are good and the lumen remains open, this process should continue until a satisfactory lumen is obtained.

If after 3 to 4 months of dilatation there is no permanent lumen, surgery is indicated. A colonic bypass in a retrosternal position is preferred, with anastomosis of the proximal colon to the divided proximal cervical esophagus. The divided distal cervical esophagus is sutured and left in place. Esophagectomy is not necessary, but proper esophageal drainage should be maintained by preserving esophagogastric continuity. The risk of malignant transformation has been reported only in the functioning esophagus, not in the bypassed esophagus and reaches 4% to 6% after 40 years.

Benign chemical burns occur with ingestion of certain medications, such as potassium chloride, and some antibiotics, such as doxycycline and tetracycline. The mucosal injuries produced by these medications usually heal within 2 to 3 weeks without specific treatment after discontinuing the use of the noxious agent. Localized burns and even perforations have been reported after accidental ingestion of coin-sized batteries.

Rupture of the Esophagus

Spontaneous rupture of the esophagus after forceful vomiting was first described by Boerhaave, and the syndrome carries his name. The usual location of the rupture is at the distal esophagus just above the diaphragm. Symptoms consist of acute retrosternal pain after an episode of vomiting, soon followed by fever and later by circulatory collapse. The symptoms may be mistaken for a myocardial infarction if the clinical history does not reveal the vomiting episode preceding the pain.

Physical examination reveals the presence of Hamman's sign resulting from mediastinal emphysema. A chest radiograph confirms the presence of mediastinal air. If the mediastinal pleura has ruptured, pleural effusion and pneumothorax are also seen. A contrast swallow is necessary to clarify the location of the perforation. Bacteria, enzymes, chemical substances, and food particles are introduced into the mediastinum under high pressure.

Treatment requires prompt surgical repair after debridement of necrotic tissue and removal of all particulate and liquid material from the mediastinum. Inspection of the area of rupture will frequently reveal that the mucosal tear is more extensive than the muscular tear. The surgeon must identify the proximal and distal limits of the mucosal tear in order to accomplish a thorough repair, which is usually performed with interrupted absorbable sutures over a Bougie. Interrupted silk is utilized to close the muscular layer. A pleural flap is used to reinforce the closure and a chest tube is placed in proximity. Parenteral hydration and broad-spectrum antibiotics are given pre- and postoperatively.

Reported mortality from esophageal rupture ranges from 5% to 40% and is influenced by comorbidities and the interval between the event and repair. Although repair more than 24 hours following rupture was once thought contraindicated, it has now become standard practice to attempt repair whenever technically feasible. If dehiscence occurs following repair, some have recommended exclusion of the esophagus with a proximal diverting cervical esophagostomy and tying the esophagus distal to the tear to prevent gastric reflux. An operation of such magnitude on a very sick patient is apt to be associated with major complications and high mortality rates. If the patient survives, later reconstruction is also difficult. A less morbid, but not rigorously evaluated procedure is placement of a covered stent.

Another option is irrigation of the mediastinum and pleura via a nasogastric tube that is placed proximal to the rupture. A chest tube positioned in the mediastinum near the esophagus drains the irrigating solution.

Perforation of the Esophagus

Instrumental perforation is the most common type of esophageal perforation and occurs with both rigid and flexible esophagoscopy. The most frequent sites of esophageal perforation are proximal to the cricopharyngeus, followed by the level of the aortic arch and

proximal to the diaphragm. Perforations may also occur proximal to an area of pathology such as a stricture. A computed tomography (CT) scan with contrast will demonstrate free air in the mediastinum and often the exact location of rupture.

Small localized esophageal perforations in either the neck or chest can be treated by antibiotics alone. However, the patient must be monitored closely for signs of sepsis. Indications for surgery include fever, continuing pain, and leukocytosis.

Mallory-Weiss Syndrome

Mallory-Weiss syndrome is defined as bleeding from a mucosal tear in the fundus of the stomach or, more rarely, in the distal esophagus as a result of retching. Approximately 5% to 17% of upper gastrointestinal bleeding is caused by Mallory-Weiss tears and is associated with alcohol ingestion in about 30% of cases. Most of the tears occur only in the region of the gastric cardia. Only 10% to 25% extend to the esophagus. Endoscopic evaluation is the most accurate method for establishing the diagnosis, and it provides access for hemostasis by cautery, heat probe, or sclerosing agents.

Most patients stop bleeding spontaneously. When bleeding persists, it frequently responds to intravenous administration of vasopressin. Balloon tamponade should be reserved for the rare patient who is not a candidate for surgery and does not respond to more conservative treatment. Transabdominal transgastric suture of the tears is occasionally necessary.

ESOPHAGEAL TUMORS

Benign Tumors

Leiomyoma

Leiomyoma, the most common benign tumor of the esophagus, arises from the smooth muscle of the esophageal wall. Usually solitary and occurring in the lower half of the esophagus, these may grow into the esophageal lumen in a polypoid-like manner, or embrace the lumen circumferentially. Dysphagia and a sense of fullness are the most frequent symptoms. A contrast radiograph shows a filling defect with an intact mucosa. Endoscopy is useful for confirming the diagnosis. Treatment is surgical, and the tumor can usually be removed without entering the esophageal lumen.

Lipomas and hemangiomas are other rare benign tumors.

Duplication Cysts

Duplication cysts are the second most common benign masses of the esophagus. Most occur near the tracheal bifurcation and are within the esophageal wall. Large cysts in infants may produce severe respiratory symptoms that require urgent surgery. The cyst wall contains smooth muscle, and the lining is composed of columnar or, more rarely, squamous epithelium. The cysts may communicate with the esophageal lumen. The diagnosis can usually be firmly established with CT scan. Treatment of symptomatic or enlarging cysts consists of enucleation and is accomplished by spreading the muscle fibers while avoiding entering the esophageal lumen. Controversy persists regarding the treatment of asymptomatic cysts.

Malignant Tumors

The number of newly diagnosed cases of esophageal cancer in the United States in 2008 was estimated to be 16,470 with 14,280 deaths. Worldwide, squamous cell cancer within the body of the esophagus is the most common histology. However, in the United States and other Western countries, the incidence of squamous cell cancer is decreasing and adenocarcinoma located at or near the GE junction is the most common histology. In fact, adenocarcinoma of the esophagus represents the solid tumor with the most rapidly increasing incidence in white males. Adenocarcinomas may originate at the junctional epithelium normally found in this location, or they may be gastric cancers that grow proximal into the esophagus. Adenocarcinomas may develop within Barrett's columnar-lined esophagus. There is a strong correlation between excessive hard liquor ingestion and esophageal squamous cell cancer. Achalasia, chemical burns of the esophagus, and Barrett's esophagus are considered premalignant lesions. Other malignant tumors of the esophagus are rare and include sarcomas, mucoepidermoid carcinoma, adenoid cystic carcinoma, and small-cell carcinoma.

Esophageal cancer spreads via local invasion and regional lymphatic and hematogenous dissemination. Liver, lung, and bones are common metastatic sites.

Diagnosis and Staging

Symptoms appear late in the course of the disease, often only when distant metastasis and invasion of local structures have already taken place. Anorexia, weight loss, and progressive dysphagia are common complaints. Early stage tumors are usually identified during screening in endemic areas or during surveillance of patients with known Barrett's esophagus. The diagnosis is suggested by radiographic studies and confirmed by biopsy. When the tumor is at or above the carina, bronchoscopy is indicated to detect possible airway invasion. CT scans are informative but fail to provide definitive information regarding invasion of neighboring structures and are even less accurate for evaluating GE junction tumors. Endoscopic ultrasonography (EUS) has been utilized to determine the depth of invasion in the esophageal wall and is more accurate than CT scans. EUS is useful for detecting lymph node invasion and can differentiate N0 from N1 lesions. However, EUS cannot be utilized if the lumen is obstructed by tumor.

The TNM system is utilized for clinical and pathologic staging (Tables 1.2–1.4). Approximately 50% of patients present with distant metastases. Curative resection is possible in fewer than 60% of patients with locoregional disease due to invasion of adjacent structures or extensive lymph node metastases. The majority of resected specimens contain regional nodal metastases.

Treatment

The National Comprehensive Cancer Network has established clinical practice guidelines that reflect the results of current phase II and phase III trials. Treatment is dependent on stage and the patient's ability to undergo the proposed therapy. Superior results are obtained in high-volume centers. Patients should be evaluated for concomitant cardiac or pulmonary disease. Weight loss of more than 10% of normal body weight is a poor prognostic indicator.

Patients with stages I to III tumors are potential surgical candidates. Esophagectomy and reconstruction can be accomplished with a variety of approaches. The Ivor Lewis procedure entails a right thoracotomy and laparotomy with anastomosis at or near the azygous vein. Transhiatal resection requires a laparotomy and neck incision with anastomosis outside the thorax. A third option, a contiguous left thoracoabdominal incision, is rarely employed. The stomach (based on the gastroepiploic and right gastric arteries) is the conduit of choice, though colon interposition is preferred by some surgeons. The left colon's blood supply is via the left colic artery, the transverse colon pedicle is based on the middle colic artery, and the ascending colon is nourished by the right colic artery. Minimally invasive esophagogastrectomy involves combined thoracoscopic and

TABLE 1.2	Esophagus Cancer TNM Staging Definitions American Joint Committee on Cancer (AJCC) 7th Edition

Primary Tumor (T)
TX   Primary tumor cannot be assessed
T0   No evidence of primary tumor
Tis   High grade dysplasia
T1   Tumor invades lamina propria, muscularis mucosa, or submucosa
T1a   Tumor invades lamina propria or muscularis mucosa
T1b   Tumor invades submucosa
T2   Tumor invades muscularis propria
T3   Tumor invades adventitia
T4   Tumor invades adjacent structures
T4a   Resectable tumor invading pleura, pericardium, or diaphragm
T4b   Unresectable tumor invading other adjacent structures, such as aorta, vertebral body, trachea, etc.

Regional Lymph Nodes (N)
NX   Regional lymph nodes cannot be assessed
N0   No regional lymph node metastasis
N1   Metastases in 1–2 regional lymph nodes
N2   Metastases in 3–6 regional lymph nodes
N3   Metastases in seven or more regional lymph nodes

Distant Metastases (M)
M0   No distant metastasis
M1   Distant metastasis

Histologic Grade (G)
GX   Grade cannot be assessed- stage grouping as G1
G1   Well differentiated
G2   Moderately differentiated
G3   Poorly differentiated
G4   Undifferentiated – stage grouping as G3 squamous

TABLE 1.3	Stage Grouping - Squamous Cell Carcinoma AJCC 7th Edition

Stage	T	N	M	Grade	Tumor Location
0	Tis	N0	M0	1, X	Any
IA	T1	N0	M0	1, X	Any
IB	T1	N0	M0	2–3	Any
	T2–3	N0	M0	1, X	Lower, X
IIA	T2–3	N0	M0	1, X	Upper, middle
	T2–3	N0	M0	2–3	Lower, X
IIB	T2–3	N0	M0	2–3	Upper, middle
	T1–2	N1	M0	Any	Any
IIIA	T1–2	N2	M0	Any	Any
	T3	N1	M0	Any	Any
	T4a	N0	M0	Any	Any
IIIB	T3	N2	M0	Any	Any
IIIC	T4a	N1–2	M0	Any	Any
	T4b	Any	M0	Any	Any
	Any	N3	M0	Any	Any
IV	Any	Any	M1	Any	Any

19% reduction in the overall hazard of death, which translates into a 2-year survival benefit of 13%. Postoperative chemoradiotherapy has also demonstrated a modest survival improvement.

Definitive chemoradiotherapy has been compared with chemoradiotherapy followed by surgery in two randomized clinical trials. The majority of patients had

TABLE 1.4	Stage Grouping - Adenocarcinoma AJCC 7th Edition

Stage	T	N	M	Grade
0	Tis	N0	M0	1, X
IA	T1	N0	M0	1–2, X
IB	T1	N0	M0	3
	T2	N0	M0	1–2, X
IIA	T2	N0	M0	3
IIB	T3	N0	M0	Any
	T1–2	N1	M0	Any
IIIA	T1–2	N2	M0	Any
	T3	N1	M0	Any
	T4a	N0	M0	Any
IIIB	T3	N2	M0	Any
IIIC	T4a	N1–2	M0	Any
	T4b	Any	M0	Any
	Any	N3	M0	Any
IV	Any	Any	M1	Any

laparoscopic procedures. Although currently limited to relatively few centers, more surgeons are gaining experience with this technique. Nodal resection is an integral part of any procedure. Five-year survival rates with surgery alone range from 14% to 22%.

Neoadjuvant therapy has been employed to improve long-term survival. The results of phase III trials comparing surgery alone to chemotherapy followed by surgery have been contradictory, though meta-analyses have shown an absolute improvement of 4% in 5-year survival rates. Preoperative radiation alone has not produced any survival benefit. Combined neoadjuvant chemoradiotherapy produces a 21% to 28% complete pathologic response. Meta-analysis of 10 randomized trials has demonstrated a squamous cell cancer and locally advanced disease (T3–4, N0–1). No survival benefit for the addition of surgery was demonstrated. However, patients treated with chemoradiotherapy alone required more palliative interventions to alleviate swallowing difficulties.

Stage Ia tumors (involves mucosa, but not submucosa) may be treated with endoscopic mucosal resection or ablation utilizing photodynamic therapy.

CANDIDIASIS

Candidiasis is the most frequent inflammatory lesion of the esophagus and is found in patients who have been treated with antibiotics and immunosuppressants. The presenting symptom is odynophagia or painful swallowing. Contrast esophagography demonstrates a typical cobblestone picture. Treatment consists of oral administration of nystatin and discontinuation of the offending agent whenever possible. Other inflammatory lesions of the esophagus are produced by herpes simplex virus and cytomegalovirus.

HIATAL HERNIAS

There are two main types of hiatal hernia with different etiologies and different symptoms.

Sliding Hiatus Hernia

Normally, the distal 3 to 4 cm of esophagus is within the abdomen, where it is exposed to positive intraabdominal pressure. This pressure in conjunction with the HPZ at the GE junction is enough to prevent abnormal GE reflux. A loose esophageal hiatus and stretched phrenoesophageal ligament permits cephalad migration of the GE junction and, less frequently, migration of segments of the lesser and greater curvatures. This may result in GERD, already described in the discussion on motility disturbances.

Paraesophageal Hiatal Hernia

Paraesophageal hiatal hernia results from an asymmetric defect in the muscles comprising the crus of the diaphragm, making it possible for the phrenoesophageal ligament together with the peritoneum to stretch upward into the chest between the esophagus and the diaphragmatic hiatus. Here it forms a

true hernial sac into which the stomach can enter. The GE junction remains under the diaphragm. The consequences of herniation may be gastric torsion, gastric volvulus with obstruction, and strangulation. Repair can often be accomplished via laparoscopy.

Treatment for this type of hernia is surgical and consists of closing the patent hiatus after delivering the stomach back to the abdominal cavity. Occasionally, a paraesophageal hiatal hernia has a sliding component as well and the GE junction is found to be above the diaphragm.

QUESTIONS

Select one answer.

1. The three findings in achalasia are:
   a. Increased LES resting pressure, decreased LES relaxation, increased esophageal peristaltic activity.
   b. Decreased LES resting pressure, increased LES relaxation, decreased esophageal peristaltic activity.
   c. Increased LES resting pressure, decreased LES relaxation, decreased esophageal peristaltic activity.
   d. Decreased LES resting pressure, increased LES relaxation, increased esophageal peristaltic activity.

2. Esophageal precancerous conditions are:
   a. Cricopharyngeal dysphagia, epiphrenic diverticulum, achalasia.
   b. Achalasia, hiatus hernia, Zenker's diverticulum.
   c. Chemical burns of the esophagus, achalasia, Barrett's esophagus.
   d. Barrett's esophagus, hiatus hernia, achalasia.

3. Acidic pH in the lower esophagus should not exceed:
   a. 1 hour daily.
   b. 2 hours daily.
   c. 1.5 hours daily.
   d. 2.5 hours daily.

4. An antireflux procedure may be unsuccessful because of:
   a. Gastric outlet obstruction not previously identified.

b. Well-dilated previous stricture.

c. Decreased saliva production.

d. Transthoracic fundoplasty.

5. The most common etiology of esophageal perforations is:
   a. Spontaneous rupture (Boerhaave's syndrome).
   b. Instrumental perforation.
   c. Foreign bodies in esophagus.
   d. Barrett's esophagus.

6. Esophageal carcinoma confined to the esophagus is best treated by:
   a. Laser debulking.
   b. Prosthetic tube insertion.
   c. Local resection.
   d. Subtotal esophagectomy.

7. Middle-third esophageal carcinoma confined to the esophagus may be approached via:
   a. Left chest.
   b. Right chest.
   c. Abdomen and right chest.
   d. Abdomen and neck.
   e. Both c and d.

8. Cricopharyngeal dysphagia is associated with all but:
   a. Lack of coordination between contraction of the inferior constrictor of the pharynx and relaxation of the cricopharyngeus.
   b. GE reflux.
   c. Development of Zenker's diverticulum.
   d. Decreased primary peristaltic waves.

9. Esophageal tertiary waves are prevalent in:
   a. Esophageal carcinoma.
   b. Hiatus hernia.
   c. Diffuse esophageal spasm.
   d. Scleroderma.

SELECTED REFERENCES

Edge SB, Byrd DR, Compton CC, Fritz AG, Greene FL, eds. *AJCC cancer staging manual,* 7th ed. New York, NY: Springer, 2010.

Juergens RA, Forastiere A. Combined modality therapy of esophageal cancer. *J Nat Comp Canc Netw* 2008;6:851–860.

Patterson GA, Cooper JD, Deslauriers J, et al., eds. *Pearson's thoracic and esophageal surgery,* 3rd ed. Philadelphia, PA: Churchill Livingstone Elsevier, 2008.

Selke FW, del Nido PJ, Swanson SJ, eds. *Sabiston & Spencer surgery of the chest,* 7th ed. Philadelphia, PA: Elsevier Saunders, 2010.

Stomach and Duodenum

ANATOMY

Stomach

The stomach lies in the left upper quadrant of the abdomen and occupies a region bounded anteriorly by the abdominal wall, superiorly by the diaphragm, and inferiorly by the superior abdominal viscera. The stomach is divided into five functional regions: cardia, fundus, body, antrum, and pylorus. The cardia and fundus encompass the proximal stomach, near the gastroesophageal (GE) junction. Progressing distally is the body or corpus. The body is separated from the antrum more distally by the incisura angularis. At the distal end of the stomach lies the muscle-lined pylorus, the opening of the stomach into the duodenum.

The stomach can be further subdivided into two secretory regions: the oxyntic gland area and the pyloric gland area. The oxynitic gland area, comprising the body and fundus, contains hydrochloride (HCl)- and intrinsic factor-secreting parietal, pepsinogen-secreting chief cells, and histamine-secreting mast cells. The pyloric gland area, comprising the antrum and the pylorus, contains gastrin-secreting G cells, mucus-secreting pyloric glands, and somatostatin-secreting delta cells. Throughout the stomach are located mucus-secreting goblet cells and extracellular fluid-secreting epithelial cells.

The stomach is composed of four layers. The outer layer, the serosa, is derived from the peritoneum and covers the entire stomach except along the greater and lesser curvature where the greater and lesser omenta are attached and at the posterior stomach close to the cardiac orifice. The next layer is the muscularis, which consists of longitudinal, circular, and oblique smooth muscle fibers. The following layer is the submucosa, which contains loose connective tissue and a plexus of arteries, veins, lymphatics,

and nerves. The innermost layer is the mucosa. The stomach is connected to surrounding structures by the gastrohepatic, gastrocolic, and splenogastric ligaments.

There are six arterial sources that supply the stomach, all of which originate from the celiac axis. The lesser curvature is supplied by the left and right gastric arteries and the greater curvature by the left and right gastroepiploic arteries. The stomach is also supplied by the short gastric arteries from the splenic artery and the gastroduodenal artery. The lymphatic supply follows the distribution of the blood vessels.

The primary nerve supply to the stomach is from the vagus nerve. It is parasympathetic in nature and also provides branches to the liver, antropyloric complex, celiac plexus, and small bowel. The vagus nerve can stimulate or inhibit gastrin release and can stimulate pepsinogen and acid secretion.

Duodenum

The duodenum is traditionally divided into four portions. The first (superior) portion comprises the pylorus and the duodenal bulb. The second (descending) portion contains the ampulla of Vater. The third (transverse) portion is crossed by the superior mesenteric artery (SMA). Finally, the fourth (ascending) portion is suspended by the ligament of Treitz, which separates the duodenum from the jejunum. The majority of the duodenum lies in the retroperitoneum, except for the proximal 2 cm and the distal 3 cm. The estimated entire length of the duodenum is approximately 20 cm. The duodenum secretes many important gastrointestinal hormones.

The duodenum contains the same four layers that exist in the stomach: serosa, muscularis, submucosa, and mucosa. The outer layer, the serosa, consists of visceral peritoneum and covers only the duodenum anteriorly. The muscularis is composed of two layers of smooth muscle, a thin outer longitudinal one and a thicker inner circular one. Ganglion cells from the myenteric (Auerbach's) plexus are in the muscularis layer. Like the stomach, the submucosa is a layer of connective tissue with blood vessels, lymphatics, nerves, and ganglion cells (Meissner's plexus). The mucosa can be further subdivided into the muscularis mucosae, the lamina propria, and the epithelium. The muscularis mucosae separate the mucosa from the submucosa. The lamina propria is a connective tissue layer in the middle, which contains a diverse set of cells, including macrophages, smooth muscle cells, and lymphocytes.

There are three arterial sources that supply the duodenum. The pylorus is supplied by the gastroduodenal artery. The first and second portions of the duodenum are supplied by the superior pancreaticoduodenal artery from the gastroduodenal artery. The third and fourth portions of the duodenum are supplied by the inferior pancreaticoduodenal artery, from the SMA. The innervation to the duodenum comes from both parasympathetic and sympathetic parts of the autonomic nervous system. The vagus nerve provides the parasympathetic fibers. The sympathetic fibers come from the splanchnic nerves, whose ganglion cells lie in a plexus near the base of the SMA.

PHYSIOLOGY

Stomach

The stomach functions as a storage organ, preparing ingested food for digestion and absorption. In the stomach, initial digestion occurs, metabolizing a typical meal into fats, proteins, and carbohydrates. Starches are further broken down by amylase.

There are several peptides produced by the stomach: gastrin, somatostatin, gastrin-releasing peptide, histamine, and ghrelin. The G cells of the stomach produce gastrin, which is the major regulator hormone of the gastric phase of acid secretion on ingestion of a meal. The D cells of the stomach produce somatostatin, which inhibits parietal cell acid secretion directly. Acidification of the antrum is the primary stimulus for somatostatin release. Inhibition of somatostatin release is via acetylcholine from vagal fibers. Gastrin-releasing peptide stimulates gastrin and somatostatin release by binding to receptors on the

G and D cells in the antral mucosa. Inhibition of gastrin-releasing peptide is unaffected by vagotomy and involves the sympathetic nervous system. Histamine is involved in parietal cell stimulation. Histamine release is stimulated by gastrin, acetylcholine, and epinephrine. Somatostatin inhibits histamine release. Administration of H_2 blockers inhibits gastric acid secretion stimulated by gastrin and acetylcholine. Ghrelin stimulates growth hormone release. Exogenous administration of ghrelin results in an increase in prolactin, adrenocorticotropin hormone, cortisol, and aldosterone and a reduction in insulin secretion. Ghrelin also enhances appetite and food intake. Eighty percent of circulating ghrelin can be eliminated by removal of the acid-producing portion of the stomach. Gastric acid is secreted by the parietal cells and is modulated by three stimuli: acetylcholine, gastrin, and histamine. Somatostatin inhibits the release of gastric acid. The stomach is also responsible for secreting intrinsic factor, pepsinogen, mucus, and bicarbonate. Parietal cells secrete intrinsic factor, essential for terminal ileum absorption of vitamin B_{12}. There are two types of pepsinogens, group 1 and group 2. Group 1 pepsinogens are secreted by chief cells and group 2 pepsinogens are secreted by surface epithelial cells in the acid-secreting part of the stomach, the antrum, and the duodenum. Mucus and bicarbonate are secreted by mucus neck cells and surface mucus cells in the acid-secreting portion of the stomach and the antrum.

Gastric motility is stimulated by myogenic as well as neurogenic controls. Extrinsic neural control of motility is via the vagus (parasympathetic) and the sympathetic pathways. Intrinsic neural control of gastric motility is via the myenteric (Auerbach's) and submucosal (Meissner's) plexuses of enteric nervous system. In the greater curvature of the stomach are pacemaker cells that are depolarized during gastric motility. During the fasting state, the stomach undergoes a pattern of electrical activity, known as the myoelectric migrating complex (MMC), each cycle of which is 90 to 120 minutes in length. There are four phases of MMC activity. The initial phase (I) is the quiescent or resting phase in which there are no action potentials and only slow waves. This phase is characterized by an increase in gastric tone but no contraction. In phase II, there is a combination of motor spikes along with the slow waves, resulting in occasional gastric contraction. In phase III, each slow wave is coupled with a motor spike with an end result of gastric contractions every 15 to

20 seconds. This phase enables the stomach to clear large undigestible food particles. Phase IV is the recovery phase prior to commencement to the next MMC cycle.

Duodenum

The duodenum and proximal small intestine are the central locations for digestion of a meal after the initial processing by the stomach. In the duodenum, pancreatic enzymes, bile, and brush border enzymes continue the digestive process. The small bowel is the principal site for absorption of ingested foods. Peristalsis in the duodenum occurs at a rate of 1 to 2 cm per second. Pacesetter potentials, which are felt to originate in the duodenum, stimulate the series of contractions to propel the food down the small intestine. In the fasting phase, the bowel undergoes contractions controlled by the MMC.

There are several hormones that are produced specifically by the duodenum: gastrin, cholecystokinin, secretin, somatostatin, gastric inhibitory polypeptide, and motilin. Gastrin, as discussed previously, stimulates gastric acid and pepsinogen secretion. Cholecystokinin stimulates pancreatic enzyme secretion and gallbladder contraction, relaxes the sphincter of Oddi, and inhibits gastric emptying. Secretin stimulates release of water and bicarbonate from pancreatic ductal cells. Secretin also stimulates flow and alkalinity of bile and inhibits gastric acid secretion, motility, and gastrin release. Somatostatin is the primary inhibitory hormone, which blocks release of gastrointestinal hormones, gastric secretion, small intestine water, and electrolyte secretion and secretion of pancreatic hormones. Gastric inhibitory polypeptide inhibits gastric acid and pepsin secretion and stimulates pancreatic insulin release. Motilin stimulates the upper gastrointestinal tract motility, possibly also initiating the MMC.

DISEASES

Acid-Peptic Disease

The lifetime risk for peptic ulcer disease is approximately 10%. Only 40% of cases of peptic ulcer disease are associated with elevated acid levels. Nonsteroidal anti-inflammatory drugs (NSAIDs), alcohol, and smoking are major risk factors in peptic ulcer disease. Chronic pancreatitis, cirrhosis, chronic obstructive pulmonary disease, and alpha-1 antitrypsin deficiency are also associated with peptic ulcer disease. Eighty percent of peptic ulcer disease is associated with *Helicobacter pylori*, a gram-negative urease-producing bacillus. Fifty percent of the general population has *H. pylori*. If the infection is not adequately treated, there is a 50% to 80% chance of ulcer recurrence. The effect of *H. pylori* is probably synergistic with NSAID use. The presence of *H. pylori* is strongly linked to gastric cancer and may be associated with mucosa-associated lymphoid tissue lymphoma and Barrett's esophagus. The second most common cause of peptic ulcer disease is NSAID ingestion. NSAID-induced ulcers are found usually in the stomach, in contrast to *H. pylori* ulcers, which are located more often in the duodenum. Chronic gastritis is usually associated with *H. pylori* ulcers and less so with NSAID ulcers.

Patients with gastric ulcers do not have an increase in mean parietal cell number, but patients with duodenal ulcers do have an increase. There are four types of gastric ulcers; type I, II, III, and IV. Type I gastric ulcers usually have low to normal acid output and do not have accompanying duodenal, pyloric, or prepyloric mucosal abnormalities. These ulcers are usually located in the transition zone mucosa between the fundus and the antrum. Type II gastric ulcers, in contrast, usually involved in increased acid secretion. These ulcers are located in the body of the stomach and are associated with a duodenal ulcer. Type III ulcers also involve an increased secretion of acid and are located in the prepyloric region of the stomach. Type IV gastric ulcers are not associated with increased acid secretion and are located on the lesser curvature of the stomach near the GE junction. Duodenal ulcers are most commonly caused by secretory abnormalities, such as decreased bicarbonate secretion, increased nocturnal acid secretion, and increased duodenal acid load, the three most common.

Based on history and physical examination alone, it is difficult to differentiate between gastric and duodenal ulcers. A gastrin level can be obtained in patients refractory to medical management. Peptic ulcers can be diagnosed via upper gastrointestinal series or endoscopy. *H. pylori* testing should be performed as well.

Management of peptic ulcer disease is initially medical. There are various medications that can heal ulcers by treatment of *H. pylori* infection, neutralization of acid secretion, or inhibition of acid secretion. If NSAID use is involved, discontinuation of such medications is recommended. Patients should also be advised to stop smoking and avoid consumption of caffeine and alcohol. The treatment for *H. pylori* infection is a 2-week regimen, which involves a proton-pump inhibitor plus antibiotics. Neutralization medications are also known as antacids, which combine with hydrochloric acid to form salt and water. H_2-receptor antagonists, which eliminate acid secretion in response to gastrin and acetylcholine, result in duodenal ulcer healing rates up to 90% after 8 weeks of therapy. Sucralfate can also be given and serves to coat the stomach and particularly binds to the exposed protein in ulcers.

There are four indications for operation on patients with peptic ulcer disease: intractability, hemorrhage, perforation, and obstruction. Surgery for intractability is becoming increasingly rare and is typically limited to those patients in whom *H. pylori* infection cannot be eliminated or in patients who must remain on NSAID therapy. Bleeding from peptic ulcer disease can initially be treated with endoscopic intervention, but certain findings predict likelihood of rebleeding: visible vessel on endoscopy, oozing of bright red blood, or fresh/old blood clot at the base of the ulcer. Hemorrhage requiring massive transfusion is usually an indication for surgery. Ideally, surgery for peptic ulcer disease should reduce or prevent gastric acid secretion.

There are four categories of acid-reducing peptic ulcer disease surgery: truncal vagotomy, highly selective vagotomy (parietal cell vagotomy), truncal vagotomy and antrectomy, and subtotal gastrectomy. Truncal vagotomy involves division of both vagus nerves above the hepatic and celiac branches, superior to the GE junction. This surgery is the most frequently performed surgery for duodenal ulcer disease. Pyloroplasty is typically done simultaneously as a drainage procedure, but a gastroduodenostomy or a gastrojejunostomy can also be performed. Side effects of the drainage procedures are dumping and, specifically, diarrhea more commonly with pyloroplasty and bile reflux more commonly with gastroduodenostomy. It is a quicker procedure making this a good option for patients with bleeding duodenal ulcers, who are hemodynamically unstable. The highly selective vagotomy was introduced after a truncal vagotomy was noted to affect the pyloric antral pump function. In the highly selective vagotomy, only

the vagus nerves supplying the corpus and the fundus of the stomach, the acid-producing portion, are divided. Because the antrum is not affected by this more selective procedure, a drainage procedure is not needed. This procedure has been associated with higher recurrence with prepyloric ulcers, compared with duodenal ulcers, and is not the procedure of choice for prepyloric ulcers. The highly selective vagotomy can be performed in conjunction with a patch procedure and treatment of *H. pylori* in the case of perforated duodenal ulcers. Finally, truncal vagotomy and antrectomy is more successful in acid reduction than either of the two previously mentioned procedures. The recurrence rate for ulcers is less than 5%. Resection of the distal stomach or antrectomy requires restoring the continuity of the gastrointestinal tract via either a gastroduodenostomy (Billroth I) or a gastrojejunostomy (Billroth II). The Billroth I is typically chosen in the setting of benign disease because it prevents duodenal stump leak, afferent loop obstruction, and retained antrum syndrome. Subtotal gastrectomy is usually performed in patients with malignancies or recurrent ulcer disease in the setting of previous truncal vagotomy and antrectomy. Many of these procedures can also be done laparoscopically.

For an intractable type I gastric ulcer, a distal gastrectomy with Billroth I is typically performed. For an intractable type II or III gastric ulcer, a distal gastrectomy is performed in conjunction with a truncal vagotomy. For a bleeding gastric ulcer, the same operations are performed for the types I, II, and III ulcers. For a perforated type I gastric ulcer in a stable patient, a distal gastrectomy with Billroth I is performed. For a type I perforated gastric ulcer in an unstable patient, a biopsy is done with an omental patch, or closure of the ulcer, and the patient is treated for *H. pylori*. In the patient with a perforated type II or II ulcer, patch closure is done with accompanying *H. pylori* treatment. In a patient with obstruction as a complication of a gastric ulcer, a malignancy workup must be done along with an antrectomy and vagotomy. Type IV gastric ulcer operations are dependent on ulcer size, distance from the GE junction, and degree of surrounding inflammation.

For an intractable duodenal ulcer, surgical treatment involves a highly selective vagotomy. Truncal vagotomy with pyloroplasty and oversewing of the bleeding vessel is performed in patients with bleeding duodenal ulcers that are refractory to endoscopic and medical management. Perforated duodenal ulcers are treated with patch closure, treatment of *H. pylori* infection, and possibly a highly selective vagotomy. Treatment of an obstruction from a duodenal ulcer also warrants a malignancy workup and a highly selective vagotomy with gastrojejunostomy.

There are several postgastrectomy syndromes that can result from the above operations. Afferent loop syndrome is when there is a partial obstruction of the afferent limb of a gastrojejunostomy. This can result from kinking and angulation of the afferent limb, internal hernias, stenosis of the gastrojejunal anastomosis, volvulus, or adhesions. There are acute and chronic forms of afferent loop syndrome, but both are treated surgically. An efferent limb obstruction can also occur, but this complication is rare and usually the result of an internal herniation. Diagnosis is confirmed by a contrast barium study of the stomach. Treatment is almost always surgical, involving reduction of the retroanastomotic hernia and closing the hernia defect. Alkaline reflux gastritis can occur after gastrectomy. This complication can result in epigastric pain with vomiting at any point during the day or night. HIDA scans are diagnostic with biliary secretion seen into the stomach and even in the esophagus in some cases. Medical therapy for alkaline reflux gastritis is not typically helpful, and surgery is recommended in those patients with intractable alkaline reflux gastritis (conversion of Billroth II anastomosis to a Roux-en-Y gastrojejunostomy with a lengthened Roux limb). In some cases, retained antrum syndrome can occur since antral mucosa can extend beyond the pylorus for 0.5 cm. This syndrome can be diagnosed in patients who develop a recurrent ulcer after previous gastrectomy for ulcer disease with a technetium scan. On the scan, there is increased uptake of the tracer. These patients can be treated with H_2-receptor antagonists or proton-pump inhibitors. If the ulcers are refractory to medical management, a conversion of the Billroth II procedure to a Billroth I can be performed or excision of the retained antrum can be performed.

There are also complications as a result of vagotomy. Of the approximately 30% or more of patients who develop diarrhea after gastric surgery, most no longer experience diarrhea after the first 3 or 4 months. The diarrhea can be part of dumping syndrome, but vagotomy alone is also associated with stool frequency. Postvagotomy diarrhea usually resolves by itself and treatment should be sympto-matic. Patients can be treated with cholestyramine, an anionic exchange resin that will absorb bile salts and diminish the severity of the diarrhea. In select refractory cases, operative intervention is required for postvagotomy diarrhea. In these cases, the ideal operation is an interposition of a reversed jejunal segment 70 to 100 cm from the ligament of Treitz, which results in relief of the diarrhea. Gastric emptying can be delayed in both truncal and selective vagotomies, but typically not after highly selective vagotomy. With truncal vagotomy, antral pump function is lost, and patients have a decrease in their ability to empty solid foods. Emptying of liquids is increased because a loss of relaxation takes place in the proximal stomach, the regulator of liquid emptying. Some postvagotomy patients have persistent gastric stasis to the point of a functional gastric outlet obstruction. Initially, functional gastric outlet obstruction, in combination with documented gastroparesis, is treated with pharmacotherapy. The medications most commonly used are prokinetic agents, such as erythromycin and metoclopramide. Usually one of the two agents is enough to combat gastric atony and increase gastric emptying.

Stress Gastritis

Stress gastritis is characterized by the presence of multiple, superficial erosions that begin proximally in the stomach and progress distally. The lesions can occur in combination with central nervous system disease (Cushing's ulcer) or with burn injury (Curling's ulcer). Although the lesions are typically superficial, they can erode into the submucosa, resulting in hemorrhage. Etiology of stress gastritis appears to be multifactorial but involves the presence of acid. Treatment of hemorrhage from stress gastritis is similar to that from peptic ulcer disease. High-risk patients are treated prophylactically because of the high mortality of hemorrhagic complications from stress gastritis. Antacids can be used for prophylaxis with efficacy rates as high as 96%. H_2 blockers and sucralfate can also be used as well. In the case of intractable bleeding, total gastrectomy is usually needed.

GASTRIC NEOPLASMS

Benign

Two to 3% of gastroscopic evaluations yield the incidental finding of a gastric polyp. The most commonly found polyp is a fundic gland polyp. Hyperplastic polyps are the most commonly seen polyps, comprising 28% to 75% of all gastric polyps. Because adenocarcinoma is found in 2% of hyperplastic polyps, endoscopic polypectomy is always indicated. Adenomatous polyps account for 10% of all gastric polyps and have a risk for malignancy. Treatment for such polyps is endoscopic polypectomy. Polypectomy is sufficient in these cases provided the entire polyp is excised and there is no invasive cancer.

Malignant

There are three main types of malignant gastric tumors: adenocarcinoma, gastric lymphoma, and gastric sarcomas. Gastric cancer exhibits great geographically variation, with higher rates in Japan and parts of South America and lower rates in the United States and Western Europe. Adenocarcinoma cases have been rising steadily, especially in white men and may be potentially linked to a history of smoking or heavy alcohol use. Studies have shown that diet plays a role in gastric cancer, especially ingestion of high levels of nitrates or *H. pylori* in drinking water.

The majority of malignant gastric neoplasms are adenocarcinomas, as high as 95%. The Borrmann classification system has been used to differentiate gastric cancer into five types based on the lesion's appearance macroscopically. Borrmann type 1 includes polypoid or fungating lesions; type 2, ulcerating lesions with surrounding elevated borders; type 3, ulcerating lesions with gastric wall infiltration; type 4, diffusely infiltrating lesions; and type 5, other lesions. When type 4 carcinoma encompasses the entire stomach, the carcinoma is called *linitis plastica*. There are few specific symptoms early in gastric adenocarcinoma with most symptoms resembling those of gastritis. The pain is usually not relieved with food, nonradiating, and constant. More advanced disease is accompanied with systemic symptoms, such as anorexia, fatigue, and weight loss. At that time, physical signs become apparent. Findings on physical examination can include a palpable abdominal mass, palpable periumbilical (Sister Mary Joseph's) or supraclavicular (Virchow's) lymph nodes, palpable peritoneal metastasis on rectal examination (Blumer's shelf), or palpable ovarian metastasis (Krukenberg's tumor). The diagnosis is confirmed by endoscopic biopsy. Endoscopic ultrasonography can be used to help stage the disease. Staging is according to the TNM system (Table 2.1). In localized disease, surgical resection is the treatment of choice. A 6-cm margin is necessary from the tumor margin to ensure a low rate of anastomotic recurrence. For the 20% to 30% of patients who present with advanced disease (Stage IV) palliative treatment is chosen, which may include a bypass procedure. There is little data to support adjuvant chemotherapy or radiation therapy in the treatment of gastric adenocarcinoma.

Gastric lymphomas are another important class of gastric tumors. While relatively uncommon, primary gastric lymphoma is the most common of the gastrointestinal lymphomas. There are similar symptoms to those in gastric adenocarcinoma. The majority of patients present with anemia. The most

TABLE 2.1	TMN Clinical Classification of Gastric Carcinoma	
Primary tumor (T)	Tx	Primary tumor cannot be assessed
	T0	No evidence of primary tumor
	Tis	Carcinoma in situ: no invasion of lamina propria
	T1	Tumor invades lamina propria or submucosa
	T2	Tumor invades muscularis propria or submucisa
	T3	Tumor penetrates serosa without invasion of adjacent structures
	T4	Tumor invades adjacent structures
Regional lymph nodes (N)	NX	Regional lymph nodes cannot be assessed
	N0	No regional lymph node metastasis
	N1	Metastasis in 1–6 regional lymph nodes
	N2	Metastasis in 7–15 regional lymph nodes
	N3	Metastasis in >15 regional lymph nodes
Distant metastasis (M)	MX	Distant metastasis cannot be assessed
	M0	No distant metastasis
	M1	Distant metastasis

common subtype of lymphoma found in the stomach is diffuse large B-cell lymphoma. Mass lesions are rare on endoscopic examination. Endoscopic ultrasonography can be helpful in diagnosing tumor wall invasion. Unlike with gastric adenocarcinoma, gastric lymphoma has a multimodal approach to treatment. Many, if not most, patients are treated with chemoradiation alone.

Gastric sarcomas make up approximately 3% of all gastric malignant tumors and arise from the mesenchymal components of the stomach wall. The most common type of mesenchymal tumors in the gastrointestinal tract is the gastrointestinal stromal tumors (GISTs). GISTs are found most commonly in the stomach. GISTs are known to express the Kit protein, a transmembrane tyrosine kinase receptor. GISTs most commonly present with bleeding and pain. The tumor is best seen using computed tomographic scan. In about 50% of cases, endoscopic biopsy can provide the diagnosis. Surgical treatment is the mainstay for control of such tumors. Until the discovery of imatinib mesylate (Gleevac), an inhibitor of tyrosine kinases, there was no good adjuvant therapy for GISTs.

Mallory-Weiss Tear

Mallory-Weiss tears are disruptions of gastric mucosa at the proximal end of the stomach, near the GE junction. They occur as the result of straining, coughing, retching, or vomiting. Although they are rarely associated with massive bleeding, 3% to 4% of cases can result in mortality. These patients can be endoscopically treated with electrocoagulation, heater-probe, injection of epinephrine, band ligation, or hemoclipping. Angiography and embolization can be utilized in select cases. As a last resort, surgery can be used to treat such tears by oversewing the bleeding site.

Gastric Varices

Isolated gastric varices can be subdivided into two types depending on location of the varices. Type 1 varices can be found in the fundus of the stomach and type 2 varices are found anywhere in the stomach. Portal hypertension and splenic vein thrombosis are the usual causes of gastric varices. Splenectomy can treat gastric varices due to splenic vein thrombosis. For gastric varices caused by portal hypertension, treatment is similar to that of esophageal varices. Endoscopy can be

used for diagnosis and treatment. Hemorrhage from gastric varices can be controlled with transjugular intrahepatic portosystemic shunting.

Gastric Volvulus

There are two ways that the stomach can twist upon itself: along the longitudinal axis (organoaxial) or the vertical axis (mesenteroaxial). The more common gastric volvulus occurs along the organoaxial axis. An acute gastric volvulus can present with obstructive symptoms of distention, vomiting, chest or abdominal pain, and hemorrhage. The combination of sudden-onset abdominal pain, retching with little emesis, and the inability to pass a nasogastric tube is Borchardt's triad and characteristic of a gastric volvulus. An acute volvulus is treated with surgery through a transabdominal approach. The stomach is reduced, and the diaphragmatic defect closed. If there is no associated diaphragmatic defect, the volvulus is reduced and fixed via gastropexy or tube gastrostomy.

Duodenal Diverticula

After the colon, the duodenum is the most common site for formation of diverticula. Unlike in the colon, duodenal diverticula are usually asymptomatic and found incidentally on endoscopy. As a consequence, these lesions should be treated conservatively. If a diverticulum becomes symptomatic, then resection of the diverticulum is the treatment of choice. In extreme cases of diverticular perforation, the perforated diverticulum is excised and the defect closed with a jejunal loop serosal patch. A small intestinal bypass may be necessary if the surrounding inflammation is severe.

Duodenal Compression by the SMA

The SMA can compress the third portion of the duodenum in a condition called the SMA syndrome or Wilkie's syndrome. Symptoms that patients will report are nausea and vomiting, abdominal distention, weight loss, and epigastric pain after meals. The syndrome is usually precipitated by weight loss. Women are affected more than men. Other predisposing factors include supine immobilization, scoliosis, and body cast placement. The surgical treatment is duodenojejunostomy.

QUESTIONS

Select one answer.

1. Which of the following is the primary stimulus for gatric somatostatin release
   a. Distension of the stomach
   b. Release of acetylcholine by the vagus
   c. Acidification of the antrum
   d. Release of cholecystokinin
   e. Cephalic phase of digestion

2. Which of the following does *not* stimulate histamine release by the stomach
   a. Gastrin
   b. Acetylcholine
   c. Epinephine
   d. Somatostatin
   e. Caffeine

3. Which of the following hormones are produced by the duodenum
   a. Gastrin
   b. Cholecystokinin
   c. Secretin
   d. Somatostatin
   e. All the above

4. Which of the following statements is *not* true
   a. Type I gastric ulcers are associated with normal acid output
   b. Type II gastric ulcers are associated with increased acid output
   c. Type III ulcers are located in the prepyloric region of the stomach
   d. Type IV ulcers are located on the greater curvature of the stomach close to the antrum
   e. Duodenal ulcers are often associated with increased nocturnal acid production

5. The operation most appropriate for severe stress ulcer bleeding is
   a. Vagotomy and pyloroplasty
   b. Highly selective vagotomy
   c. Near-total or total gastrectomy
   d. Ligation of the bleeding sites
   e. Antrectomy with Billroth II reconstruction

6. The most appropriate operation of a 30-year old patient with a history of peptic ulcer disease who presents with a perforated duodenal ulcer is
   a. Patch closure with a highly selective vagotomy

   b. Gastrectomy with a Billroth I reconstruction
   c. Gastrectomy with a Billroth II reconstruction
   d. Vagotomy and pyloroplasty
   e. Gastrojejunostomy and Omeprazol

7. Which of the following is true regarding post-vagotomy diarrhea
   a. It is a common condition occurring about 30% of cases
   b. Most cases of the diarrhea is self-limiting and resolves in 4-6 months
   c. Cholestyramine can be effective in severe cases
   d. Severe, refractory diarrhea can be treated by a jejunal interposition
   e. All the above

8. Which of the following modalities is *not* indicated in the treatment of a bleeding Mallory-Weiss tear
   a. Band ligation
   b. Heater-probe application
   c. Angiography and embolization
   d. Injection of epinephrine
   e. Near-total gastrectomy

9. Which of the following is *not* true regarding alkaline reflux gastritis following gastrectomy
   a. It usually does not respond to medical therapy
   b. It is uncommon following a Billroth II reconstruction
   c. HIDA scan can be diagnostic
   d. It may require a Roux-en-Y gastrojejunostomy
   e. The vomiting may occur day or night

10. Which of the following is true regarding GISTS (gastrointestinal stromal tumors)
    a. Surgery is the mainstay of treatment
    b. Most GISTS are found in the stomach
    c. GISTS respond well to imatinib mesylate (Gleevec)
    d. GISTS usually present with upper gastrointestinal bleeding
    e. All the above

SELECTED REFERENCES

De Franchis R. Emerging strategies in the management of upper gastrointestinal bleeding: *Digestion* 60 (suppl 3):17, 1999.

Hohenberger P, Gretschel S. Gastric cancer. *Lancet* 362:305, 2003.

Corless CL, Fletcher JA, Heinrich MC, Biology of gastrointestinal stromal tumors. *J Clin Oncol* 22: 3813, 2004.

Feliciano DV. Do perforated duodenal ulcers need an acid-decreasing surgical procedure now that omeprazole is available? *Surg Clin North Am* 72:369, 1992.

Kauffman GL Jr. Duodenal ulcers disease: treatment by surgery, antibiotics, or both. *Adv Surg* 34:121, 2000.

Savides TJ, Jensen DM. Therapeutic endoscopy for nonvariceal upper gastrointestinal bleeding. *Gastroenterol Clin North Am* 29:465, 2000.

Sugawa C, Benishek D, Walt AJ. Mallory-Weiss syndrome: a study of 224 patients. *Am J Surg* 145:30, 1983.

Josef A. Shehebar
Deborah Yu
B. Paul White

CHAPTER 3

Diseases of the Small Bowel

ANATOMY

The small intestine, a tubular viscus about 3-m long *in vivo*, is divided into three segments: duodenum, jejunum, and ileum. The duodenum is 20-cm long and largely retroperitoneal, lying immediately adjacent to the head and inferior border of the pancreas. This portion and operations on it are described in another chapter 2. The jejunoileal segment begins at the ligament of Treitz and ends at the ileocecal valve. It is intraperitoneal and tethered to the retroperitoneum by a broad based. There is no distinct landmark demarcating the jejunum from the ileum; the proximal 40% (100 cm) of the jejunoileal segment is arbitrarily defined as the jejunum and the distal 60% (150 cm) as the ileum.

The small intestine forms during the fourth week of fetal development. The duodenum arises from the foregut, and the jejunum and ileum derive from the fetal midgut. The endoderm forms the absorptive epithelium and the secretory glands. The splanchnic mesoderm gives rise to the rest of the intestinal wall, including the musculature and the serosa. During the fifth week of fetal development, the intestine herniates through the umbilicus, rotating 90 degrees around the axis of the vitelline duct and the superior mesenteric artery (SMA). By the 10th week, the intestine returns to the abdominal cavity and rotates another 180 degrees. This rotation places the ligament of Treitz in the left upper quadrant and the cecum into the right upper quadrant. Around the fourth month, the cecum descends to the right lower quadrant.

The wall of the small intestine is made up of four concentric layers: serosa, muscularis propria, submucosa, and mucosa. Circular folds of mucosa and submucosa called plicae circulares or valvulae conniventes are present throughout but decrease in number and prominence distally in the ileum. These folds are also visible radiographically to help distinguish between small intestine and colon. Gross examination of the small bowel mucosa also reveals aggregates of lymphoid follicles most prominent in the ileum, in which they are designated Peyer patches.

At the mesenteric aspect of the small bowel, the leaves of the mesentery split and encircle the bowel to form the visceral peritoneum. Blood vessels, nerves, and lymphatics run within the two peritoneal layers of the mesentery to enter and exit the intestine. Most of the duodenum derives its arterial blood from branches of both the celiac and SMAs. The distal duodenum, jejunum, and ileum derive their arterial supply from the SMA. Venous drainage is through the superior mesenteric vein into the portal vein. Lymph drainage occurs through lymphatic vessels that accompany the mesenteric arteries and drain through mesenteric lymph nodes to the subdiaphragmatic cisterna chyli, which empties into the thoracic duct and ultimately into the left subclavian vein. Both divisions of the autonomic nervous system innervate the small bowel. The parasympathetics are carried by the celiac division of the posterior trunk of the vagus nerve. The sympathetics reach the bowel through the celiac and superior mesenteric ganglia. Sympathetic afferent fibers detect luminal distention, which is perceived as pain in the periumbilical region.

PHYSIOLOGY

The principal functions of the small intestine are to propel the gastric chyme it receives forward, continue its digestion, and absorb into the blood and lymphatics the water, electrolytes, minerals, and nutrients released by digestion.

Gastric effluent is hypertonic and acidic. It is neutralized in the duodenum with bicarbonate and rendered isotonic with secretions. Although daily oral ingestion amounts to only 1.0 to 1.5 L of fluid, the salivary, gastric, pancreatic, biliary, and intestinal secretions add another 8 to 9 L. Most of this fluid is absorbed by the time it reaches the ileocecal valve, which leaves approximately 1.0 to 1.5 L for colonic absorption. The maximum daily capacity for small bowel fluid absorption is estimated to be 12 L.

Carbohydrate digestion occurs in the mouth, stomach, duodenal lumen, and brush border of the small intestine. Pancreatic amylase is the major enzyme of starch digestion, with salivary amylase initiating the process and brush border disaccharidases completing the process. Carbohydrate absorption begins in the duodenum and is completed in the jejunum.

Protein digestion begins in the stomach with pepsin, but the gastric contribution is small and nonessential under normal circumstances. Digestion continues in the duodenum with the actions of a variety of pancreatic peptidases, which hydrolyze proteins to small peptides and free amino acids. Additional digestion occurs through the actions of peptidases that exist in the enterocyte brush border and cytoplasm. Peptide absorption occurs in the jejunum and accounts for most of the protein assimilation. Amino acid absorption occurs predominantly in the ileum, and absorbed amino acids and peptides then enter the portal venous circulation. Of all amino acids, glutamine appears to be a unique and major source of energy for enterocytes.

Although lipolysis of triglycerides to form fatty acids and monoglycerides is initiated in the stomach by gastric lipase, fat digestion and absorption occurs rapidly in the duodenum by pancreatic lipases and is completed in the proximal jejunum. Bile salts are required to solubilize the products of fat digestion in the form of mixed micelles before absorption can occur. Within the enterocytes, long-chain triglycerides are resynthesized and incorporated into chylomicrons that are secreted into the intestinal lymphatics and ultimately enter the thoracic duct. Medium-chain triglycerides contain fatty acids with 6 to 12 carbon atoms that are water-soluble and are processed differently than the more common long-chain triglycerides, which make up 90% of dietary fat. Medium-chain triglycerides can be absorbed intact without pancreatic lipase or micellar transport. Hydrolysis of these triglycerides within the enterocyte releases the medium-chain fatty acids, which can enter the portal circulation directly and thereby bypass the lymphatic channels. Clinical applications include the use of medium-chain triglycerides in patients with pancreatic insufficiency (fat maldigestion), chylous effusions from lymphatic leaks (chylous ascites, chylothorax), and short-bowel syndrome (SBS) (deficient bile salt pool and fat malabsorption).

After participating in lipid absorption, 95% of the bile salts are actively absorbed in the distal ileum. They then return to the liver to be recycled into bile to complete the enterohepatic circulation of these substances.

Most water-soluble vitamins are absorbed in the jejunum with the exception of vitamin B_{12}, which binds the gastric intrinsic factor to facilitate absorption in the distal ileum. Vitamin B_{12} (cobalamin) malabsorption can result from a variety of surgical manipulations. The vitamin is initially bound by saliva-derived R protein. In the duodenum, R protein is hydrolyzed by pancreatic enzymes, allowing free vitamin B_{12} to bind to gastric parietal cell-derived intrinsic factor. The vitamin B_{12}—intrinsic factor complex—is able to escape hydrolysis by pancreatic enzymes, allowing it to reach the terminal ileum, which expresses specific receptors for intrinsic factor, facilitating vitamin B_{12} absorption. Because each of these steps is necessary for vitamin B_{12} assimilation, gastric resection, gastric bypass, and ileal resection can each result in vitamin B_{12} insufficiency. The fat-soluble vitamins (A, D, E, and K) are solubilized by the mixed micelles and are absorbed with fat in the proximal jejunum. Calcium and magnesium absorption occurs throughout the small bowel, although most takes place in the ileum. Iron absorption occurs in the duodenum and proximal jejunum.

The endocrine function of the upper gastrointestinal (GI) tract is regulated by neural, hormonal (both autocrine and paracrine), and anatomic mechanisms.

- **Cholecystokinin** is produced by duodenal and jejunal I cells and enteric nerves in response to intraluminal amino acids and fats. It induces gallbladder contraction, pancreatic enzyme secretion, and relaxation of the sphincter of Oddi.
- **Enteroglucagon** from ileal and colonic L cells is produced in response to intraluminal fat and bile acids. Of note, inflammatory processes, such as Crohn's disease and celiac sprue, can dramatically increase enteroglucagon secretion.
- **Gastric inhibitory peptide**, secreted by duodenal and jejunal K cells in response to active transport of monosaccharides, long-chain fatty acids, and amino

acids, inhibits gastric acid and pepsinogen secretion and gastric emptying but stimulates insulin release.

- Duodenal G cells secrete **gastrin** in response to vagal stimulation and intraluminal peptides. Gastrin stimulates acid secretion by the gastric fundus and body and increases gastric mucosal blood flow.
- **Motilin** is produced by duodenal and jejunal M cells in response to duodenal acid, vagal stimulation, and gastrin-releasing peptide. Motilin initiates phase III of the migrating motor complex during the fasting state. Erythromycin is useful as a promotility agent due to its action as a motilin agonist.
- Duodenal and jejunal S cells release **secretin** in response to acid, bile salts, and fatty acids in the duodenum. Secretin increases bicarbonate and water secretion from pancreatic ducts. It inhibits gastric acid secretion and gastric motility.
- **Somatostatin** broadly inhibits gut exocrine and endocrine function. Somatostatin and its analog, **octreotide**, are often used to decrease the volume of intestinal secretions in patients with enterocutaneous fistulas. Intestinal D cells and enteric neurons secrete somatostatin in response to intraluminal fat, protein, and acid.
- **Vasoactive intestinal peptide** is secreted throughout the small intestine in response to vagal stimulation. It increases mesenteric blood flow, intestinal motility, and pancreatic and intestinal secretions.

DISEASES OF THE SMALL INTESTINE

Crohn's Disease

Presentation and Pathophysiology

Crohn's disease is a chronic transmural inflammatory disease that affects any part of the GI tract from the mouth to the anus. Most commonly the disease affects the terminal ileum with or without colonic involvement. In some patients, the disease is limited to the colon and rectum. The distal ileum is the single most frequently affected site, being diseased at some time in 75% of patients with Crohn's disease. The small bowel alone is affected in 15% to 30% of patients, both the ileum and colon are affected in 40% to 60% of patients, and the colon alone is affected in 20% to 30% of patients. Isolated perineal and anorectal disease occurs in 5% to 10% of affected patients. Crohn's disease limited to the colon is considered in a subsequent chapter.

Crohn's disease is characterized by progression and frequent recurrence. Its cause is unknown. Medical and surgical therapy is palliative not curative.

Both sexes are affected equally. The disease tends to run in families, but no clear mode of transmission has been established. Various hypotheses on the roles of environmental factors, including infectious agents, and derangements in immune regulation have been proposed. Specific genetic defects associated with Crohn's disease in human patients are beginning to be defined. In the United States, Crohn's disease occurs two to three times more often among Jews than among non-Jews. The median age at which patients are diagnosed with Crohn's disease is approximately 30 years; however, age of diagnosis can range from early childhood through the entire life span.

The bowel wall is thickened by fibrosis and edema, which ultimately narrows the lumen in advanced cases and converts the involved segment to a rigid stenotic tube. Although the disease is transmural, the submucosa shows some of the most striking changes in terms of fibrosis and edema. Noncaseating granulomas with Langerhans giant cells are found in 60% to 70% of the diseased intestines, primarily in the submucosal layer, and may also be found in apparently normal intestine. The intestinal wall is infiltrated transmurally with inflammatory cells, but lymphoid aggregates tend to concentrate in the submucosa. The mucosa is usually ulcerated. Early aphthous ulcers are small, superficial, and discontinuous. They are thought to arise from a microabscess in an underlying lymphoid follicle. With more advanced disease, deep longitudinal ulcers and transverse fissures give the mucosa a cobblestone appearance with edematous mucosal islands situated between the ulcers.

Inflammation in Crohn's disease can occasionally (25%) affect discontinuous portions of intestine: so-called skip lesions that are separated by intervening normal-appearing intestine. With advanced disease, inflammation can be transmural. Serosal involvement results in adhesion of the inflamed bowel to other loops of bowel or other adjacent organs, such as the bladder. Transmural inflammation also can result in fibrosis, with stricture formation, intra-abdominal abscesses, fistulas, and, rarely, free perforation. The mesentery can appear inflamed, thickened, and shortened, often with enlarged lymph nodes with noncaseating granulomas. The mesenteric fat tends to creep onto the serosal aspect of the involved small bowel, a feature of Crohn's disease that is grossly evident and helpful in identifying affected segments of intestine during surgery. Penetration into the mesentery or retroperitoneum can lead to abscess formation.

Perianal manifestations of the disease include fistulas, fissures, ulcers, and abscesses. They are encountered in up to 30% of the patients with small bowel Crohn's disease and in up to 50% of those with colonic involvement. Rectal bleeding is uncommon in small bowel Crohn's disease, occurring in 10% of these patients. This symptom occurs more frequently in those with colonic involvement. Massive bleeding is rare.

The abdominal pain is intermittent and crampy when caused by partial obstruction. It is persistent when caused by an abscess or tender mass of inflamed intestine encountered during an acute exacerbation of the disease.

Clinical presentation can be that of an acutely developing disorder that mimics appendicitis. More frequently, the early symptoms are vague and nonspecific. They include episodic mild abdominal discomfort and diarrhea. Patients are often diagnosed as having irritable bowel syndrome until an acute exacerbation delineates the true nature of the disorder. During this interval of misdiagnosis, which lasts on average 2 to 3 years, the patient may experience malaise, weight loss, periods of unexplained fever, or even growth retardation in children.

The diarrhea is usually nonbloody and worse at night. Causes include partial small bowel obstruction (SBO), impaired bile salt absorption from extensive ileal disease, bacterial proliferation proximal to a partial obstruction, ileosigmoid fistula formation, and extension of the disease to the colon. Steatorrhea may complicate the picture when extensive segments of small bowel are involved.

With progression of the disease, increasing fibrosis may result in signs and symptoms of SBO in more than one-third of patients. The ureters may become encased by retroperitoneal inflammation that results in hydroureter and hydronephrosis.

Free perforation is rare, occurring in 1% to 2% of the patients. More common is the development of fistulas and intra-abdominal abscesses. Most fistulas are associated with sepsis to a variable extent. Enteroenteral fistulas may be asymptomatic unless associated with an abscess. Enterovesical fistulas cause dysuria, pyuria, hematuria, and occasionally pneumaturia and fecaluria. Ileosigmoid fistulas may present as sepsis or an exacerbation of the diarrhea. Enterocutaneous fistulas usually occur through old abdominal scars from an appendectomy or bowel resection. The source of the fistula is frequently recurrent disease at an ileocolic anastomosis following bowel resection. External drainage of an intra-abdominal abscess may result in a residual enterocutaneous fistula. Spontaneous fistulas are uncommon and result from the discharge of purulent material from an underlying abscess. Intra-abdominal abscesses occur in 20% of the patients and develop when a perforation is walled off by surrounding loops of bowel, omentum, mesentery, and parietal peritoneum.

There is an increased incidence (60- to 300-fold increased risk) of small bowel adenocarcinoma in patients with Crohn's disease of the small intestine. The adenocarcinomas tend to occur in the ileum. The symptoms of carcinoma are similar to those of Crohn's ileitis. As a result, delayed recognition has led to a poor prognosis with cure rates less than 10% (vs. 20% to 30% in those with small bowel adenocarcinoma unassociated with Crohn's disease). Crohn's colitis is associated with a 4- to 20-fold increased risk of colon cancer. However, many patients require resection before a carcinoma can develop.

Extraintestinal manifestations may precede overt bowel disease, including polyarthritis, ankylosing spondylitis, iritis, uveitis, erythema nodosum, and pyoderma gangrenosum. Patients with ileal involvement have an increased incidence of gallstone formation due to failure to reabsorb bile salts.

Inadequate protein–calorie intake is primarily responsible for the nutritional complications of this disease. Patients are reluctant to eat because food aggravates the abdominal pain. In addition, bacterial proliferation proximal to partially obstructed bowel (blind loop syndrome) or as a consequence of small to large bowel fistula formation can result in fat, protein, carbohydrate, and vitamin malabsorption. A variety of anemias are encountered, including iron-deficiency anemia secondary to occult blood loss and megaloblastic anemia secondary to vitamin B_{12} malabsorption from the diseased or resected terminal ileum.

Diagnostic Workup

The diagnostic evaluation of a patient with suspected Crohn's disease should begin with a complete history and physical examination, which includes a careful rectal examination. Perianal disease can appear before symptomatic intestinal disease. The perianal lesions are relatively painless except for an abscess. Fissures are often wide, multiple, painless, and in atypical locations. Anal canal ulcers can also occur, which may give rise to pain on defecation. Fistulas may be single and simple or multiple and complex. They tend to be asymptomatic.

The colon should be evaluated with either colonoscopy or double-contrast barium enema. Colonoscopy has the advantage of obtaining material for histologic examination, and the presence of noncaseating granulomas in a rectal or colonic biopsy is helpful for diagnosing Crohn's disease. Studies have questioned the value of a routine rectal valve biopsy in the absence of proctocolitis. Barium enema has the advantage of demonstrating transmural disease, where extravasation of barium into an abscess cavity or into a neighboring viscus would differentiate Crohn's disease from ulcerative colitis.

An upper GI series with small bowel follow-through should be performed in all patients after the colorectal evaluation. The presence of small bowel lesions in a patient with colitis supports the diagnosis of Crohn's disease. Small bowel lesions seen on contrast evaluation include thickened blunted valvulae conniventes, cobblestoned mucosa, strictures, skip areas, and fistulas. In addition, a computed tomography (CT) scan or ultrasonography is helpful for identifying abscess formation and directing percutaneous drainage.

Treatment

Treatment of Crohn's disease includes medical management to achieve temporary remission of an acute exacerbation, palliate symptoms, reduce bowel inflammation, and to correct nutritional disturbances. In patients with severe disease, steroid therapy should be initiated after active infection or abscess has been excluded. Prednisone, with initial daily doses of 40 to 60 mg orally, is a common outpatient treatment for acute flares; inpatients may receive hydrocortisone 50 to 100 mg intravenously every 6 hours. Response to therapy should become evident within 7 days. Their role in disease isolated to the colon is less certain. Steroids should be withdrawn once remission is achieved, as they do not prevent recurrent disease. Patients whose disease relapses as steroids are tapered may benefit from maintenance steroids to control their disease. Oral aminosalicylates (sulfasalazine, mesalamine) that contain the anti-inflammatory salicylate moiety can be effective in patients with Crohn's colitis or ileocolitis but has little effect on isolated ileitis. As with steroids, sulfasalazine as a prophylactic agent has not been shown to prevent recurrent disease. The immunosuppressant azathioprine or its metabolite mercaptopurine can be combined with steroids or sulfasalazine to control active disease. These immunosuppressants have an unusual ability to cause fistulas

to close and have also permitted the decrease or elimination of steroid therapy in many instances. Recent data have shown that infusions of infliximab (Remicade), a monoclonal antibody against tumor necrosis factor, are effective for Crohn's flares and even Crohn's fistulas. Before receiving infliximab, the patient must have no active source of infection and be purified protein derivative negative. Infliximab is of particular use in poor surgical candidates who have otherwise failed medical management and is generally tolerated well. For colonic and perianal Crohn's disease, the antibiotic metronidazole, which is bactericidal to intestinal anaerobes, has shown some benefit.

Antidiarrheals, cholestyramine, and a low-fat diet may be required to provide satisfactory bowel function. Antibiotics effective against enteric aerobes and anaerobes are used to combat septic complications. Nutritional support with elemental diets and total parenteral nutrition (TPN) may help bring active disease into remission when combined with other existing medical therapy. TPN has been used for operative preparation of nutritionally depleted patients in an attempt to reduce postoperative morbidity and mortality.

Although a well-planned nonoperative approach can successfully treat most acute exacerbations and complications as they develop, 70% to 80% of patients with Crohn's disease will ultimately require surgical therapy due to unresponsiveness to aggressive medical therapy or complications of their disease. However, not all complications are absolute indications for surgery, with the exception of undrained intra-abdominal abscesses, free perforation of the intestine, and uncontrolled intestinal hemorrhage, the latter two being less commonly seen. As with medical management, surgical intervention cannot cure Crohn's disease, but a remission can be achieved for a variable length of time. Postoperative recurrence rates are 60% by 5 years and 94% by 15 years. Most recurrences occur in the region of the anastomosis at the neoterminal ileum. Neither the amount of grossly normal bowel removed proximal and distal to the lesion, the presence or absence of microscopic disease at the resection margins, nor any combination of drugs can prevent a recurrence after resection. Therefore, the surgeon should be conservative: the goal is to treat a specific complication, and every attempt is made to preserve as much bowel as possible to prevent SBS.

Acute SBO in Crohn's patients can usually be managed successfully without surgical intervention, as the obstruction is usually partial and responds to intravenous fluids, bowel rest, nasogastric (NG) suction, and steroids. Mural fibrosis occurs with chronic disease, and the bowel has a diminished capacity to recover. The patient experiences recurrent attacks, persistent obstructive symptoms, or both, which are best managed with an operation. Intestinal obstruction is the most common indication for surgery in small bowel Crohn's disease.

When the obstructing lesion is in the terminal ileum, resection of the involved ileum and cecum with anastomosis of the neoterminal ileum to the ascending colon is the operation of choice. The proximal margin should be free of gross disease. Because the mucosa of the ileocecal valve is almost always involved, the distal margin should be placed in the ascending colon just above the cecum or distal to any colonic disease in cases of ileocolitis. Strictureplasty is useful for proximal skip areas and cases of diffuse jejunoileitis with multiple strictures. This technique allows for preservation of intestinal surface area and is especially well suited to patients with extensive disease and fibrotic strictures who may have undergone previous resection and are at risk for developing SBS. The Heineke-Mikulicz technique can be used for short-segment strictures and the Finney technique for long-segment strictures. Strictureplasty sites should be marked with metallic clips to facilitate their identification on radiographs and during subsequent operations. Strictureplasty is associated with recurrence rates that are no different from those associated with segmental resection. Bypass of diseased segments is avoided. Future problems with the bypassed segment include closed loop obstruction, blind loop syndrome, free perforation, and carcinoma.

The distinction between an inflammatory mass or phlegmon and an abscess is difficult but has important clinical implications. Both present as a right lower quadrant tender mass (in ileitis or ileocolitis) with associated fever and leukocytosis indicative of a suppurative process caused by transmural penetration of fissures. A phlegmon is treated conservatively with bowel rest, intravenous fluids, and systemic antibiotics. This suppurative process has a capacity for resolution without surgical intervention. However, if the suppurative process extends and pus loculates, an abscess forms; drainage then frequently becomes necessary if the patient does not respond promptly to antibiotic therapy. Steroids may increase the morbidity of these suppurative processes. A CT scan may define the pathology. If a frank abscess is present, CT-guided percutaneous drainage may be effective for resolving the sepsis. A residual enterocutaneous fistula may occur. This approach would then necessitate subsequent resection to treat the fistula. Clinical deterioration from an undrained abscess or persistent phlegmon and signs of spreading peritonitis from abscess rupture or free perforation are indications for immediate operation. Primary resection plus drainage is effective. Surgical judgment must be used to determine if an anastomosis can be safely performed. Otherwise an end-ileostomy and mucous fistula can be constructed, as most perforations and abscesses originate from the ileum rather than the jejunum.

Because many fistulas are associated with sepsis to a variable extent, antibiotics are generally indicated; steroids are generally contraindicated. Enterovesical fistulas should be treated surgically to prevent repeated urinary tract infections. At operation, the fistula is disconnected, the diseased bowel is resected, and the bladder is closed. Catheter drainage of the bladder is maintained for 7 to 10 days to ensure healing.

An enteroenteral fistula is not an absolute indication for surgery unless other surgical problems such as obstruction or abscess are present. Ileosigmoid fistulas can lead to severe diarrhea and are managed surgically in that instance. Fistulas are common between adjacent loops of ileum or between the ileum and cecum or ascending colon and have no physiologic consequence in the absence of sepsis. Many remain clinically unrecognized until a contrast evaluation demonstrates their presence. In fact, the process of fistulization may have resolved a remote episode of sepsis as an abscess decompressed into an adjacent loop of bowel. When such a fistula is associated with sepsis, surgery is indicated to drain the abscess and resect the fistulous intestine. The extent of Crohn's disease in both segments of intestine involved in the fistulization should be assessed. If both are diseased, two resections are performed. With ileosigmoid fistulization, in most instances, the sigmoid is passively involved, as Crohn's disease does not spread into that viscus. Therefore, the treatment is takedown of the fistula and ileocecal resection with debridement and closure of the sigmoid.

Enterocutaneous fistulas are managed operatively for the most part. Although a regimen of TPN, bowel rest, and immunosuppressants can close these fistulas, they usually reopen with resumption of oral intake. The fistula is taken down and the diseased bowel resected. Patients with early postoperative enterocutaneous fistulas arising from apparently normal bowel after resection of diseased bowel have been successfully managed with TPN, provided there has been no distal obstruction or undrained septic focus.

If acute ileitis is encountered on exploration for appendicitis, the terminal ileum should not be resected because many of these patients recover spontaneously and do not have other attacks. Specific etiologic agents (e.g., *Yersinia* sp.) have been identified in some of these cases. Even if the patient was known or suspected to have Crohn's disease prior to laparotomy, resection of uncomplicated ileitis is not indicated. If the cecum is soft, pliable, and otherwise normal, appendectomy is performed (unless the cecum is inflamed, increasing the potential morbidity of this procedure) to prevent future diagnostic dilemmas, particularly in those patients with Crohn's disease who may be destined to have recurring symptoms.

Excision of the appendix if the cecum is involved may lead to a postoperative colocutaneous fistula. When enterocutaneous fistulas occur after appendectomy and the cecum is uninvolved, the origin of the fistula is almost always the diseased ileum, not the appendiceal stump.

Operations for growth retardation are being performed less frequently with modern nutritional support. Provision of adequate protein and calories (with TPN if necessary) restores growth in many children. Most patients with Crohn's disease require only one or two operations over the entire course of their disease and are able to lead normal productive lives.

SHORT-BOWEL SYNDROME

Short-bowel syndrome (SBS) is defined as malabsorption resulting from anatomical or functional loss of a significant length of the small intestine. This causes insufficient intestinal absorptive capacity, which results in the clinical manifestations of diarrhea (>2 L/d of fluid and electrolyte losses), dehydration, and malnutrition. This occurs most commonly after bowel resection in the newborn period (i.e., secondary to malrotation with midgut volvulus, intestinal atresias, necrotizing enterocolitis) or conditions seen later in life (i.e., Crohn's disease, acute mesenteric ischemia). The amount of bowel that must be lost to produce malabsorption is variable and depends on whether the ileocecal valve is preserved and which portions of the small bowel are left in situ. The normal length of small intestine is approximately 300 to 850 cm for an adult, 200 to 250 cm for an infant older than 35 weeks' gestation, and approximately 100 to 120 cm for a premature infant younger than 30 weeks' gestation. Loss of greater than 80% of the small bowel is associated with increased requirement for parenteral nutrition support and decreased overall survival.

When the duodenum and/or jejunum are resected, the ileum can largely adapt to perform their absorptive functions. However, the duodenum and jejunum cannot adapt to perform the functions of the ileum. Because transport of bile salts, vitamin B_{12}, and cholesterol is localized to ileum, resection of this region is poorly tolerated and steatorrhea and diarrhea are more pronounced if the ileocecal valve is removed. Thus, resection of the duodenum or jejunum is generally much better tolerated than resection of the ileum. The ileocecal valve is the main barrier between the small and large intestine. It helps regulate the exit of fluid and malabsorbed nutrients from the small bowel. It also helps keep bacteria from the large bowel from refluxing into the small bowel. Resection of the ileocecal valve results in decreased fluid and nutrient absorption and increased bacterial overgrowth in the small bowel. The resulting bacterial contamination of the small intestine mandates more small intestines for tolerance of oral/enteral feeding. Moreover, an intact ileocecal valve is believed to be associated with decreased malabsorption and delays transit of chyme from the small intestine into the colon, thereby prolonging the contact time between nutrients and the small-intestinal absorptive mucosa.

In addition, malabsorption in patients who have undergone massive small-bowel resection is exacerbated by a characteristic hypergastrinemia-associated gastric acid hypersecretion that persists for 1 to 2 years postoperatively. The increased acid load delivered to the duodenum inhibits absorption by a variety of mechanisms, including the inhibition of digestive enzymes, most of which function optimally under alkaline conditions.

Also during the first 1 to 2 years following massive small-bowel resection, the remaining intestine undergoes compensatory adaptation, whereby there is a reduction in volume and frequency of bowel movements, an increase in the capacity for enteral nutrient assimilation, and a reduction in TPN requirements. Understanding the mechanisms mediating intestinal adaptation may suggest strategies for enhancing adaptation in patients with SBS who are unable to achieve independence from TPN. To date, the phenomenon of intestinal adaptation in human patients remains poorly understood.

Medical Therapy

In the early period after intestinal loss, attention is directed toward keeping the fluids and electrolytes in the body within normal limits. TPN is started, and excessive secretions, which are lost through stomas or diarrhea, must be replaced. Aggressive electrolyte repletion and supplementation of vitamins and minerals must also be instituted.

As soon as GI function has returned, intestinal feeds are introduced gradually. Infants and young children must be fed at least in part orally, however, to establish their ability to suck and eat. Because adaptation begins early after loss of intestine, small amounts of feeds are started early to stimulate adaption of the intestine. Small volumes of liquid feedings are introduced first. A trial-and-error method maximizes the results. High-dose histamine-2 receptor antagonists or proton pump inhibitors should be administered to reduce gastric acid secretion. Antimotility agents, such as loperamide or diphenoxylate, may be administered to delay small-intestinal transit. Octreotide can be administered to reduce the volume of GI secretions, although its use is associated with an inhibition of intestinal adaptation in animal models. Patients who remain dependent on TPN face substantial TPN-associated morbidities, including catheter sepsis, venous thrombosis, liver and kidney failure, and osteoporosis.

Use of elemental diets has become increasingly popular to feed patients with SBS because they have the advantage of being better absorbed. However, more complex diets are more trophic (promoting growth) to the GI tract and help increase adaptation. The decision to use one formula over the other depends on each individual patient.

Nontransplant Surgical Therapy

Surgical therapy for SBS aims to slow down the transit time of food through the residual bowel or to increase the mucosal surface area for improved absorption. These surgical techniques include segmental reversal of the small bowel, interposition of a segment of colon between segments of small bowel, construction of small-intestinal valves, and electrical pacing of the small intestine—all operations designed to slow down intestinal transit. Reported experience with these procedures is limited to case reports or series of a few cases. Objective evidence of increased absorption is lacking; furthermore, these procedures are frequently associated with intestinal obstruction.

Two methods are now available to lengthen the intestine. Bianchi originally described longitudinal intestinal lengthening and tailoring procedure in 1980. The procedure entails separation of the dual vasculature of the small intestine, followed by longitudinal division of the bowel with subsequent isoperistaltic end-to-end anastomosis. Therefore, the enlarged (dilated) small intestine can be split into two parallel portions, each with its own blood supply with the potential to double the length of small intestine to which it is applied. This procedure has generally been used for pediatric patients with dilated residual small bowel.

More recently, the serial transverse enteroplasty procedure has been described in the pediatric short-bowel population. This procedure is designed to accomplish lengthening of dilated small intestine by employing serial transverse applications of a GIA stapler, from opposite directions, to create an accordion-like or zig zag channel, thereby drastically amplifying its length. An advantage to this procedure is that there is no need for separating the dual vasculature of the bowel as in the Bianchi method, and preliminary studies lack any evidence of postprocedure obstruction. Initial experimental and clinical experience with this procedure has been promising; however, its long-term efficacy needs to be determined. This procedure may be a safe and facile alternative for intestinal lengthening in children with SBS.

Intestinal Transplantation

Approximately 100 intestinal transplants are performed in the United States annually, with most of these procedures applied to patients with SBS. The currently accepted indication for intestinal transplantation is the presence of life-threatening complications attributable to intestinal failure and/or long-term TPN therapy; specifically complications for which intestinal transplantation is indicated include impending or overt liver failure, thrombosis of major central veins, frequent episodes of catheter-related sepsis, and frequent episodes of severe dehydration.

Currently, approximately 45% of transplants involving the small intestine are performed as isolated intestinal transplants, 40% are performed as combined intestine/liver transplants, and 15% are performed as multivisceral transplants. Isolated intestinal transplantation is used for patients with intestinal failure who have no significant liver disease or other organ failure. Combined intestine/liver transplantation is used for patients with both intestinal and liver failure.

Multivisceral transplantation has been used for patients with giant desmoid tumors involving the vascular supply of the liver and pancreas, as well as that of the intestine, for diffuse GI motility disturbances and for diffuse splanchnic thrombosis.

Improved immunosuppressive medications, which include tacrolimus and CellCept, as well as a better means of identifying rejection of the intestine, have improved survival. Nearly 80% of survivors have full intestinal graft function with no need for TPN at 1 year as per the most recent UNOS cohort evaluated. More specifically, the 1-year patient and graft survival rates for isolated intestine recipients were 79% and 64%, respectively, and 50% and 49%, respectively, for intestine/liver recipients. Five-year patient and graft survival rates for isolated intestine recipients were 50% and 38%, respectively, and for intestine/liver recipients, 37% and 36%, respectively.

However, rejection is a major issue in small intestine failure and morbidities associated with intestinal transplantation are substantial including CMV infection and posttransplant lymphoproliferative disease. Differentiating between infection and rejection can be difficult. Utilization of endoscopy to both visualize and selectively biopsy an intestinal allograft has become the standard for early recognition and treatment of intestinal allograft rejection.

Prognosis

Approximately 50% to 70% of patients with SBS who initially require TPN are ultimately able to achieve independence from TPN. Prognosis for achieving enteral autonomy is better among pediatric patients than among adults.

The results of small intestine transplant are improving, and when indicated, this procedure offers an acceptable option. The most promising approach for the future is the use of growth factors to stimulate growth of the intestinal cells and to improve their ability to absorb nutrients. Because most SBS patients adapt within 2 years after resection, ample time should be allowed for adaptation to occur before small intestine transplant is considered.

SMALL BOWEL OBSTRUCTION

Mechanical small bowel obstruction (SBO) is a common problem confronting surgeons. The usual cause in adults is adhesions following surgery. Congenital

and postinflammatory adhesions are occasionally responsible. Hernias are the second most common cause. Abdominal wall hernias, including inguinal, femoral, umbilical, and incisional, account for most cases of obstruction from hernias. Rarer forms exist. Internal hernias are related to abnormalities of intestinal rotation and fixation or are caused by mesenteric defects or internal traps created following bowel resection and gastric bypass procedures. Primary benign and malignant or metastatic malignant neoplasms are the third most common cause. Adhesions, hernias, and neoplasms account for 90% of the cases of SBO. Gallstones, Crohn's disease, and many other etiologies account for the rest.

Simple obstruction implies an adequate blood supply to the obstructed segment. Strangulation obstruction implies vascular compromise. Closed loop obstruction indicates occlusion at both ends of an obstructed segment with no possibility of antegrade or retrograde decompression. Partial obstruction indicates a residual narrowed lumen through which intestinal contents can pass. Complete obstruction indicates total occlusion of the lumen.

When the bowel lumen becomes occluded, the proximal bowel distends with fluid and swallowed air. The fluid is initially derived from the normal daily 8-L output of salivary, gastric, pancreatic, and biliary secretions. As the luminal pressure rises proximally, intestinal absorption decreases followed by an increase in intestinal secretion. Because intestinal fluid has a tonicity and electrolyte composition similar to that of extracellular fluid, electrolyte and acid–base abnormalities are not remarkable initially unless there is a proximal SBO (duodenum, proximal jejunum) with copious vomiting. Here, gastric losses of H^+, Cl^-, and K^+ lead to a hypochloremic, hypokalemic metabolic alkalosis. As the extracellular fluid compartment shrinks from losses into the bowel (third space) or externally (vomiting), oliguria follows. Attempts by the kidneys to conserve Na^+ (elevated aldosterone) aggravate the tendency toward hypokalemia in the setting of copious vomiting. With distal obstructions and little vomiting, the tendency is toward a metabolic acidosis because of starvation, ketosis, and loss of pancreatic secretions in the intestinal lumen.

With closed loop obstructions, there is no possibility for antegrade or retrograde decompression. The bowel becomes markedly distended and a vicious circle is established: distension increases secretion, which further increases distension leading to a rise in intraluminal pressures to 40 mm Hg or more, and diminished intestinal blood flow. At first, there is venous obstruction with vascular engorgement and bowel wall edema, followed by arterial vasospasm and local tissue anoxia. Capillary integrity is lost, and intramural hemorrhage can occur. A strangulation obstruction can occurred and, if unrelieved, results in necrosis of tissue and proliferation of bacteria in the affected segment. Eventually, bacteria and endotoxin escape transmurally into the free peritoneal cavity even before free perforation has occurred. A dark blood-tinged peritoneal fluid is produced. Sepsis, cardiovascular collapse, and death follow if the infarcted segment is not resected.

Patients classically present with crampy abdominal pain, nausea and vomiting, abdominal distension, and obstipation. One or more of these characteristics may be missing depending on the anatomic level of obstruction (proximal or distal), degree of occlusion (partial or complete), and presence or absence of strangulation. Patients with proximal obstruction present with pain and vomiting on the first day and are less likely to experience distension and obstipation. Patients with distal obstruction present with pain for a couple of days followed by distension, vomiting, and obstipation once the distal unobstructed segment empties. With late established obstructions, as bacteria proliferate in the stagnant contents of the obstructed loops, the vomitus can turn feculent. On physical examination, borborygmi correlate with abdominal cramps. In neglected cases, bowel motility diminishes, and the abdomen becomes distended, silent, and tender. Patients with partial obstruction may continue to pass flatus and have explosive bouts of diarrhea with sudden relief of the pain. Patients with strangulation obstruction ultimately develop continuous pain and signs of peritonitis.

Unfortunately, the clinical picture does not allow one to distinguish reliably between simple and strangulation obstruction. The distinction is important, as mortality rates for simple obstruction range from 0% to 6%, whereas for strangulation obstruction the rates range from 15% to 30%. Patients with simple obstruction may have a low-grade fever, mild tachycardia, and mild generalized tenderness related to compression of distended loops of bowel. Patients in extremis with diffuse peritonitis and septic shock likely have advanced gangrene of the bowel. The goal that has been so elusive is to recognize the early reversible ischemia of strangulation. No combination of clinical criteria or laboratory data has reliably met that goal. In this era of NG intubation and intestinal

decompression as initial primary therapy, there is always the possibility of delaying treatment of potentially reversible ischemia.

Recognizing the above limitations, many authorities recommend immediate operation after resuscitation for patients with feculent vomiting or NG aspirate, marked leukocytosis ($>18,000/mm^3$), peritoneal signs, absent bowel sounds, high fever, and marked tachycardia. Some patients with simple obstruction have one or more of the above; however, some patients with strangulation obstruction will have none. A more aggressive approach is taken in elderly patients in whom the physical findings accompanying peritonitis may be unimpressive.

Abdominal radiographs confirm the diagnosis 85% of the time and allow differentiation of small bowel and large bowel obstruction. False-negative abdominal films occur when there is no intestinal dilatation, as is occasionally seen with early or very proximal SBO. False-negative films also occur when the bowel loops are filled with fluid rather than air.

Contrast studies with barium (small bowel series or enteroclysis study) can be helpful if the diagnosis of SBO is unclear from the plain films or if an attempt at nonoperative therapy is chosen. CT scanning is reported to have a sensitivity of 90% or higher in detecting complete or high-grade SBO. It can also provide information as to the cause of the obstruction and the severity of bowel injury. The CT scan may reveal a whirling pattern in the mesentery of patients with a volvulus and closed loop obstruction as well as raise the suspicion of intestinal ischemia by documenting thickening and edema of the bowel wall or, in late cases, intramural air.

The management of all cases of SBO begins with fluid resuscitation, electrolyte replacement, and NG tube decompression. A Foley catheter is required, and central venous pressure monitoring should be considered if the patient is oliguric. Patients with complete SBO (i.e., whose abdominal films show dilated proximal loops with empty distal small bowel, colon, and rectum) and those with suspected strangulation should be given prophylactic antibiotics and taken promptly to surgery once resuscitation is complete. Patients with prior abdominal surgery and partial SBO (i.e., whose abdominal films show some colonic gas and feces or in whom intermittent episodes of diarrhea persist) thought to be secondary to adhesions may benefit from continued nonoperative management if they show improvement over the initial 24 hours. Unfortunately, abdominal films cannot reliably differentiate partial from complete SBO. Patients with early complete SBO have residual colon gas and feces until it is expelled and obstipation becomes complete. Nonoperative therapy is successful in only a few patients with complete SBO (15% to 25%) but helps in most patients with partial SBO (65%) caused by adhesions. Contrast studies can differentiate between the two entities.

There are other circumstances in which nonoperative therapy is a reasonable alternative to immediate operation. Incomplete obstruction, postoperative obstruction, a history of numerous previous operations for obstruction, radiation enteritis, inflammatory bowel disease, and abdominal carcinomatosis are situations demanding mature judgment, and judicious nonoperative management may be in the patient's best interests. Failure to resolve any obstruction nonoperatively makes operative therapy mandatory.

Incarcerated abdominal wall hernias frequently represent a closed loop obstruction of bowel with the potential for strangulation. Therefore, all such hernias should be considered surgical emergencies. Patients without prior abdominal surgery or an incarcerated abdominal wall hernia should also be promptly operated once resuscitation is complete, as the obstruction requires surgical relief in most instances. Operative treatment involves lysis of adhesions, reduction of hernias with obliteration of the defect, repair of intestinal injuries, and resection of nonviable bowel.

NEOPLASMS OF THE SMALL INTESTINE

Neoplasms of the small intestine occur frequently. Although the small bowel contains 90% of the mucosal surface area of the alimentary tract, only 5% of all GI neoplasms and 2% of all GI malignancies arise from the small bowel. Approximately 85% of patients are older than 40 years. There is a high correlation of small bowel tumors with primary neoplasms elsewhere.

Benign tumors of the small bowel are frequently asymptomatic and are found incidentally at the time of laparotomy or autopsy. The most common benign tumors include adenoma (adenomatous polyp and villous adenoma), leiomyoma, lipoma, and hemangioma. These tumors occur 20% of the time in the duodenum, 30% in the jejunum, and 50% in the ileum. If symptomatic, it is because the lesions have caused bleeding or obstruction. Evidence suggests an adenoma-to-adenocarcinoma sequence, as has been proposed for the colon: large sessile villous adenomas are particularly worrisome in this regard.

When found incidentally at the time of laparotomy, a small bowel tumor should be assessed for evidence of malignancy (i.e., hard consistency, invasion, or lymphatic metastasis). If none of these features is present and the tumor is small, intraluminal, and presumably epithelial in origin (i.e., adenoma), an enterotomy, submucosal excision, frozen section examination if doubt remains, and transverse closure should be performed. Wide resection would be appropriate for intermediate-size benign lesions and those involving the submucosa (i.e., hemangioma). Large benign lesions involving much of the bowel circumference, especially leiomyomas, should be managed with segmental resection of the bowel with an end-to-end anastomosis.

When a benign small bowel tumor causes an obstruction, the preoperative evaluation frequently identifies only the obstruction, not the etiology, although it is easily discernible at laparotomy. Adult patients without prior abdominal surgery, incarcerated abdominal wall hernias, or evidence of gallstone ileus who present with SBO have an increased incidence of obstructing small bowel tumors. This obstruction can result from intussusception or, rarely, a mass effect. Unlike childhood intussusception, adult intussusception in most instances has some obvious etiologic factor, which is usually a benign small bowel tumor acting as the lead point. Adult intussusception is frequently relapsing and intermittent with spontaneous reduction and pain relief until incarceration occurs. A patient who gives a history of intermittent postprandial crampy abdominal pain with a variable degree of bloating and occasional vomiting should be evaluated for an SBO. Small bowel series and especially enteroclysis studies are helpful for demonstrating small bowel tumors.

At laparotomy, an intussusception is reduced by milking the intussusceptum backward. Traction is never used on intussuscepted bowel. After manual reduction, resection of the small bowel lesion is performed. If the bowel is necrotic or the intussusception cannot be reduced, en bloc resection of the intussusceptum and intussuscipiens is performed.

Benign small bowel tumors can cause chronic slow blood loss with iron-deficiency anemia and intermittent melena or, rarely, acute brisk blood loss with blood expelled per rectum. Leiomyomas and hemangiomas are more apt to bleed. The diagnostic workup for occult GI bleeding after gastroduodenal and colonic sources are ruled out includes a bleeding scan, angiography, enteroclysis, and small bowel enteroscopy. Surgical exploration, combined with intraoperative enteroscopy if necessary, can be both diagnostic and therapeutic. Small, soft polyps should not be missed when using this approach.

The tumors of the Peutz–Jeghers syndrome are hamartomas that are found throughout the GI tract but tend to concentrate in the jejunum and ileum, where they can cause intussusception and bleeding. This syndrome is inherited as an autosomal dominant trait and has the additional feature of mucocutaneous melanotic pigmentation. The malignant potential of these polyps is very small. Operation is indicated only for symptoms (e.g., obstruction, bleeding), at which time all polyps greater than about 1 cm should be removed. Because there is widespread involvement, extensive resections are not indicated and treatment should be limited to the segment responsible for the complication. A combined surgical and endoscopic approach is the best strategy.

Malignant tumors of the small bowel include adenocarcinoma (the most common), carcinoid tumor, leiomyosarcoma, lymphoma, small bowel gastrointestinal stromal tumors (GIST), and metastasis. Adenocarcinomas have been found alone, within villous adenomas, and in association with Crohn's disease. Most of these tumors occur in the duodenum, especially in the periampullary region, and in the proximal 100 cm of jejunum. Duodenal malignancies, especially periampullary tumors, are closely associated with familial adenomatous polyposis (familial polyposis coli, Gardner's syndrome) also characterized by multiple intestinal and colonic polyps, osteomas, and subcutaneous cysts or fibromas. These are discussed elsewhere in this text. Ileal lesions are less frequent except when associated with Crohn's disease. These lesions infiltrate the intestinal wall, metastasize to regional lymph nodes, and spread to the liver and peritoneal surfaces.

There is no specific symptom complex. Patients may experience abdominal pain, anemia, weight loss, obstruction, bleeding, and rarely perforation. A palpable mass is present one-third of the time. Barium studies may identify an apple-core defect with mucosal ulceration, but a correct preoperative diagnosis is made only one-third of the time. Most cases are diagnosed at laparotomy for intestinal obstruction.

Jejunoileal carcinomas are removed by segmental resection with an approximately 10-cm margin on either side and a wedge of continuous mesentery. The proximal extent of the lymphadenectomy is limited by the SMA. Tumors of the terminal ileum require right colectomy. Five-year survival rates are poor (25%) because of the late clinical presentation of advanced disease where metastases can be present in 80% of cases at the time of operation.

Carcinoid tumors develop from the enterochromaffin cells situated in the crypts of Lieberkühn. They are slow-growing yellow-gray submucosal neoplasms that have the capacity to invade locally and to metastasize. Malignant potential depends on the location of the tumor and its size. The appendix is the most common site of a carcinoid tumor, but the malignant potential here is low. The small bowel is the next most common site, and most of these tumors are located in the ileum with about 10 times as many originating within 2 ft of the ileocecal valve as compared with the jejunum. The malignant potential for small bowel carcinoids is high. Lesions less than 1 cm in diameter rarely metastasize. Lesions between 1 and 2 cm have a 50% incidence of metastasis, and lesions larger than 2 cm have an 80% incidence of metastasis. Altogether, 75% of the lesions are less than 1 cm in diameter, 20% are 1 to 2 cm, and 5% are larger than 2 cm. Carcinoids of the small bowel are multiple in 40% of cases. Carcinoids tend to occur in patients 25 to 45 years of age. Neoplasms of other organs—most commonly the colon, lung, stomach, or breast—are present in 15% of patients. Carcinoids may be associated with multiple endocrine neoplasia (MEN) type 1 and type 2, although rare familial clustering not associated with MEN has also been reported.

Most small bowel carcinoids are asymptomatic and are found incidentally at laparotomy or autopsy. When symptomatic, a carcinoid frequently has metastasized. Symptoms are usually obstructive in nature secondary to an extensive desmoplastic reaction around the tumor or its mesenteric metastases, which leads to kinking and matting of intestinal loops with constriction and partial obstruction. Intussusception and bleeding are unusual. Additional symptoms of metastatic disease in general (anorexia, weight loss, fatigue) may be present. Small bowel series may show partial obstruction with thickening of the bowel wall, tethering of its folds, and kinking of loops. This picture can resemble Crohn's disease or other inflammatory conditions. Unlike the carcinoid syndrome, urinary levels of 5-hydroxyindoleacetic acid (5-HIAA) are normal.

Local excision is adequate for small lesions less than 1 cm in diameter with no evidence of metastatic disease encountered incidentally at laparotomy. For lesions more than 1 cm in diameter, a standard cancer operation is indicated. When the tumors are in the distal ileum, a right hemicolectomy is indicated to include the node-bearing tissue in the resection. Otherwise a segmental resection with en bloc removal of adjacent mesentery suffices. With advanced disease and hepatic metastases, the primary tumor should be resected if possible to avoid future complications (e.g., obstruction). Nonanatomic resection of liver metastases (tumorectomy) is performed whenever feasible. Five-year survival rates following curative resection approach 70%. Twenty percent of those with liver metastases live 5 years. Patients are followed up postoperatively with CT and octreotide scans.

The carcinoid syndrome is usually caused by metastatic liver disease and is related to a variety of vasoactive substances produced by the tumor: serotonin, histamine, bradykinin, and others. About 5% to 10% of the patients with small bowel carcinoids develop this syndrome. For the syndrome to occur, sufficient disease must be present in the liver to overwhelm the normal detoxifying mechanisms. The symptoms include episodic cutaneous flushing of the head and upper trunk, watery diarrhea, and bronchospasm. Symptoms can occur spontaneously or can be precipitated by foods, alcohol, emotional stress, or defecation.

A life-threatening carcinoid crisis consisting of intense flushing, severe diarrhea, tachycardia, arrhythmias, and vascular collapse has been described. Permanent manifestations include endocardial fibrosis (carcinoid plaques), which most commonly affects the right side of the heart and leads to tricuspid insufficiency and pulmonary stenosis with subsequent right-side heart failure. The cutaneous lesions of pellagra may appear, as functioning tumors divert most of the essential amino acid tryptophan into the serotonin pathway, leaving less available for niacin production.

Diagnosis is made by finding increased 24-hour urinary excretion of 5-HIAA, which is the major metabolite of serotonin. Rare patients have normal 5-HIAA levels. A CT scan can demonstrate metastatic liver disease, which is usually massive once the syndrome manifests.

Treatment of carcinoid syndrome is palliative. Surgical debulking and hepatic artery embolization have been tried with some success, but the responses are frequently short-lived. A somatostatin analog, such as octreotide, can be used to suppress tumor growth and control the symptoms of carcinoid syndrome. Octreotide inhibits release of GI hormones; in carcinoid syndrome, it relieves flushing, wheezing, and severe diarrhea refractory to other measures. In addition, chemotherapy with streptozotocin, 5-fluorouracil, and doxorubicin has yielded some palliation as well.

Jejunoileal leiomyosarcomas arise from smooth muscle cells in the muscularis propria and grow extrinsically away from the bowel lumen to reach a large size before causing symptoms. Most tumors are larger than 5 cm in diameter when discovered. Spread is by direct extension to adjacent structures and hematogenous dissemination. Intermittent abdominal pain with weight loss and a palpable abdominal mass is a common clinical presentation. There is a high incidence (50% in some series) of bleeding because these tumors have a tendency to outgrow their blood supplies and develop central necrosis and mucosal ulceration. Perforation occurs in 10% of patients. Obstruction can occur and is often caused by external compression rather than intrinsic circumferential growth or intussusception.

Small bowel series demonstrate a large extraluminal mass effect causing obstruction with pooling of barium in the necrotic center of a cavitating lesion. A CT scan frequently shows a large mass with a central lucent area that represents necrosis. In patients who present with GI bleeding, mesenteric angiography shows irregular tumor vessels, a tumor blush, or pooling of contrast in the mass.

Surgical treatment consists in wide resection with associated mesentery. Lymphatic involvement with leiomyosarcomas is not common, and the mesenteric resection is performed more or less to achieve clear margins. Leiomyosarcomas are radioresistant, but combination chemotherapy using doxorubicin, cyclophosphamide, and vincristine has shown some activity against advanced disease.

Small bowel metastases are found in 50% of patients dying of malignant melanoma. Carcinomas of the cervix, kidney, breast, lung, etc, may also spread to bowel. Obstruction or hemorrhage may require operation if life expectancy is reasonably good. Significant palliation may be achieved, particularly in patients with solitary metastatic lesions.

Gastrointestinal Stromal Tumors

Gastrointestinal stromal tumors (GISTs) are mesenchymal tumors of the GI tract (80% of all mesenchymal tumors) and affect an estimated 5,000 to

10,000 new people each year in the United States; however, they represent only 0.2% of all GI tumors. Approximately 25% of GIST arise in the small bowel, with 50% gastric, 15% rectal, and 10% colonic in origin.

These tumors thought to start in specialized cells found in the wall of the GI tract, called the *interstitial cells of Cajal*, the pacemaker cell of the GI tract. Intercalated between the intramural neurons and the smooth muscle cells, GISTs are characterized by the presence of activating c-kit mutations, a transmembrane receptor tyrosine kinase involved in the regulation of cellular proliferation, apoptosis, and differentiation.

More than 95% of GISTs express kit (CD117) mutations. This molecular marker allows for the distinction of GISTs from other histologically similar mesenchymal tumors of the small bowel including leiomyomas, leiomyosarcoma, schwannomas, and others. This feature has led to reclassification of up to 70% small bowel tumors as GISTs that had previously been classified as a variety of other mesenchymal tumors. Those GISTs that do not express c-kit mutations may express a mutation in another tyrosine kinase receptor, the platelet-derived growth factor receptor alpha. Present in approximately 5% to 7% of GISTs, these activating mutations also result in abnormal cellular proliferation.

Like other primary small bowel tumors, GISTs are characterized by vague abdominal pain, weight loss, and occult GI bleeding. Diagnostic strategies are the same as for other tumors of the small bowel, although acute hemorrhage, perforation, or obstruction may lead to an emergency presentation. Given the tendency of GIST to grow to a large size with characteristic compression of adjacent organs away from the expanding mass, a CT scan is most likely to be the initial positive test. A typical finding is the presence of a large space-occupying mass, occasionally with calcification and hypervascularity and often with evidence of central necrosis.

All GISTs should be considered to be malignant, with malignant potential based on two major criteria: size of the tumor and mitotic rate observed in the tumor. Biologically aggressive tumors are large lesions with a high mitotic index, whereas tumors with benign features are small and exhibit a low mitotic index. Tumors are thus stratified within a range from *very low* to *high-risk* lesions for malignant potential, a classification that has prognostic significance.

Treatment

Surgery is the primary therapeutic option with the goal being complete resection. At operation, wide local excision of the primary tumor with in continuity resection of adherent organs is appropriate to attain curative resection. Lymph node metastasis is rare, negating the need for wide mesenteric resection.

Imatinib mesylate is a small molecule that occupies the adenosine triphosphate binding pocket of the kit-kinase domain, blocking phosphorylation of the receptor and intracellular signaling. This binding arrests cellular proliferation and survival signaling. Clinical use of imatinib is now routine in the management of GISTs. This oral agent is well tolerated and highly effective for patients with metastatic GISTs. Although complete regression of tumor is rare, partial regression of disease and arrest of progression of disease can be achieved for durable intervals with continuous treatment in up to 80% of patients.

With greater clinical experience with imatinib, resistant clones have been identified with eventual progression of disease. For these patients, a newer receptor tyrosine kinase inhibitor SU11248 has recently been introduced for clinical trials. This inhibitor has a broader spectrum of activity than imatinib and has shown early promise in patients with progression of disease on imatinib or in those relatively few patients who cannot tolerate imatinib.

Use of imatinib in the neoadjuvant setting for unresectable or locally aggressive tumors is currently being evaluated in cooperative group clinical trials. The efficacy of imatinib in the adjuvant setting for high risk or partially resected tumors is also being evaluated in ongoing trials. Given the favorable risk profile of the agent, such applications may prove useful in these settings as well, although definitive survival data are not yet available.

INTESTINAL ISCHEMIA

The small intestine is susceptible to interruption of its normal circulation resulting in ischemia, which if left untreated can result in catastrophic consequences to the patient. Four types of mesenteric ischemic syndromes have been recognized, each having a different etiology, clinical picture, and treatment.

1. *Acute mesenteric arterial embolism.* Most emboli to the SMA originate from thrombi in the left atrium

or the left ventricle. Often these thrombi have been there for some time and are suddenly dislodged by an arrhythmia, such as sudden onset of atrial fibrillation, or an episode of hypokinesia of the heart following an acute myocardial infarction. Twenty percent of emboli to the SMA are associated with emboli to other arterial beds. Most of the emboli lodge in the SMA just beyond the origin of the middle colic artery; about 15% lodge in the proximal SMA.

2. *Acute mesenteric arterial thrombosis.* Thrombosis of the SMA occurs in a vessel that has become progressively more diseased, often over a period of time. The vessel is usually narrowed or filled with plaque. A sudden episode of low flow, as can occur during an intercurrent illness or a bout of sepsis, can aggravate a critical stenosis resulting in complete thrombosis. Often these patients have had symptoms of chronic mesenteric ischemia for years. The symptoms include postprandial abdominal pain, early satiety, or weight loss. Unlike emboli, most thromboses of the SMA occur in its proximal portion just beyond its takeoff.

3. *Nonocclusive mesenteric ischemia* (NOMI). This condition is less well understood than the first two and has a different set of symptoms, making the diagnosis much more difficult. Patients with NOMI have decreased mesenteric perfusion without specific vessel blockage. The poor blood flow is often associated with cardiac failure or sepsis or is found in patients taking digitalis. Digitalis has been found sometimes to cause contraction of the smooth muscle in both the mesenteric arterial and venous mesenteric vessels resulting in poor flow and symptoms of ischemia.

4. *Acute mesenteric venous thrombosis.* These patients often have a hypercoagulable state such as portal hypertension, protein S or C, or antithrombin III deficiency or they are on oral contraceptives. Other conditions predisposing patients to venous thrombosis include trauma to the abdomen and malignancies.

Clinical Presentation

Acute mesenteric ischemia usually presents with sudden, severe abdominal pain. Ischemia due to arterial embolization tends to be the most precipitous with exquisite abdominal pain accompanied by nausea and vomiting. Often a cardiac arrhythmia is present as well.

Mesenteric ischemia due to thrombosis, nonocclusive ischemia, or mesenteric venous thrombosis presents in a less dramatic fashion, with pain increasing in nature over several days. The pain is associated with nausea, vomiting, and progressive abdominal distension. Most patients have guaiac-positive stools. As the ischemia progresses, the entire thickness of the bowel wall necroses, and the abdominal examination reveals classic signs of peritonitis, with rebound and guarding. Laboratory findings include nonspecific elevation and the white blood cell count; elevated levels of amylase, lactate dehydrogenase, and creatine phosphokinase; and an increasing base deficit.

Radiographs are often nonspecific, with 25% of them reported as normal. Some specific findings in patients with intestinal ischemia include adynamic ileus with bowel wall thickening. Duplex ultrasonography can detect poor or absent blood flow in the celiac axis or SMA, but these tests are highly operator dependent. Large air-filled loops of overlying bowel may make accurate ultrasonography difficult.

The CT scan has proved somewhat helpful in diagnosing embolic occlusion to the SMA, but the definitive study is still the mesenteric angiogram, obtaining both anteroposterior and lateral views of the SMA and, if needed, of the celiac axis. As mentioned earlier, most SMA emboli are lodged 3 to 10 cm from the origin of the SMA, whereas most thrombi are found near the origin of the SMA.

NOMI usually is associated with narrowed, irregular branches of the SMA, whereas the vessel itself is patent. With mesenteric venous thrombosis, the arterial phase is prolonged. The venous phase shows filling defects within the superior mesenteric view or in the protal vein itself.

Treatment

Initial treatment of patients suspected of having acute mesenteric ischemia is fluid resuscitation, correction of acidosis, and administration of antibiotics. Anticoagulation with intravenous heparin should be part of the regimen. A Foley catheter is placed to monitor urine output, and a NG tube is placed on suction to decompress the stomach.

The key to treatment is obtaining the appropriate imaging studies. Emergency angiography must be done in an expedient fashion. In selected patients in whom the angiogram shows an SMA embolus and in whom there are no signs of peritonitis and symptoms have been present for 8 hours or less, thrombolytic therapy through the SMA catheter can be instituted. If there is no response within 4 hours of beginning therapy or if peritonitis appears, surgical exploration is warranted. The abdomen is opened and the SMA is exposed by elevating the root of the transverse mesocolon and mobilizing the duodenum all the way to the ligament of Treitz. A transverse arteriotomy is made over the SMA, a Foley catheter is inserted and the embolus is extracted. Care is needed to make sure that no fragments of clot are passed into the distal vessel. Once blood flow is restored, the bowel is examined and any obviously necrotic bowel is resected. Marginally viable areas should be resected unless they are extensive, in which case they can be left in place and a second-look operation planned for 24 hours later.

Patients with an SMA thrombosis have a more complex problem. Thrombectomy is unlikely to maintain long-term patency in the circulation, and most of these patients require some sort of aortomesenteric artery bypass surgery.

The treatment of NOMI is usually nonoperative, involving the use of intra-arterial vasodilators, such as papaverine, in conjunction with anticoagulation with heparin. Patients who develop signs of peritonitis must undergo surgical exploration while continuing the intraarterial infusion of papaverine. Any obviously necrotic bowel is resected. Marginally viable bowel is left in place, and a second-look operation is planned for 24 hours later.

The treatment of patients with mesenteric venous thrombosis is surgical. The long-term results of venous thrombectomy have been poor, with recurrent thrombus appearing more often than not. These patients should be explored and all nonviable bowel resected. The bowel that is marginally viable can be resected if the segment removed is not too long or left in place and then reexamined 24 hours later at a second-look operation.

Patients with mesenteric ischemia comprise a group of high-risk patients. Their ultimate prognosis depends on the speed with which the diagnosis is made and how quickly and appropriately the treatment can be started.

QUESTIONS

Select one answer.

1. Which of the following does not contribute to the digestion of the fats in the small intestine?
   a. Brush border enzymes.
   b. Pancreatic lipases.
   c. Bile salts.
   d. Lacteals.

2. Which of the following is not characteristic of Crohn's disease?
   a. Perianal disease.
   b. Rectal bleeding.
   c. Diarrhea.
   d. Abdominal pain.

3. Which of the following complications of Crohn's disease is least common?
   a. Enteroenteral fistulas.
   b. Enterocutaneous fistulas.
   c. Free perforation.
   d. Strictures.

4. What percentage of patients with Crohn's disease eventually needs surgery?
   a. 20%
   b. 50%
   c. 75%
   d. 90%

5. A patient is taken to the operating room for appendicitis and is found to have ileitis. What is the correct management?
   a. Biopsy of ileum.
   b. Heal resection with ileocolic anastomosis.
   c. Appendectomy.
   d. Ileostomy.

6. Which of the following can most reliably distinguish simple from strangulation small intestinal obstruction?
   a. High nasogastric output.
   b. Fever over 101°F.
   c. Tachycardia.
   d. None of the above.

7. Which of the following is true of nonoperative management of patients with small bowel obstruction (SBO)?
   a. It is most likely to be successful in patients who have SBO from adhesions.
   b. Long-tube decompression is superior to nasogastric tube decompression.
   c. It is most useful for the younger patient.
   d. It is successful in cases of complete SBO.

8. Which is the most likely cause of
    intussusception in a 20-year-old man?
    a. Idiopathic.
    b. Lymphoma of the small bowel.
    c. Carcinoid.
    d. Adhesions.

9. Which is true of the lesions responsible for the
    symptoms in patients with Peutz–Jeghers
    syndrome?
    a. They are sessile adenomas.
    b. They tend to cluster in the duodenum.
    c. They are hamartomas.
    d. The syndrome is inherited as an autosomal
        recessive trait.

10. A patient is found to have a small bowel
    carcinoma 2 cm in diameter in the distal ileum.

Which of the following is the operation of
choice?
a. Wedge resection with 2-cm margins.
b. Biopsy and chemotherapy.
c. Right hemicolectomy.
d. Wedge resection with 5-cm margins.

SELECTED REFERENCES

Bizer LS, Liebling RW, Delany HM, Gliedman ML. Small
bowel obstruction. *Surgery* 1981;89:407–413.

Cameron JL. *Current surgical therapy.* 4th ed. St. Louis, MO:
Mosby Year Book, 1992.

Moody FG. *Surgical treatment of digestive disease.* 2nd ed.
Chicago, IL: Year Book Medical Publishers, 1990.

Scott HW, Sawyers JL. *Surgery of the stomach, duodenum and
small intestine.* Boston, MA: Blackwell Science, 1987.

Ziudema GD. *Shackelford's surgery of the alimentary tract.* 3rd ed.
Philadelphia, PA: WB Saunders, 1991.

Colon, Rectum, and Anus

ANATOMY

The colon, rectum, and anus measure approximately 1.5 m in length. The colon is divided into four parts— the ascending, transverse, descending, and sigmoid. The colon diameter is greatest at the cecum (8 cm) and narrowest at the distal descending colon (2.5 cm). These variations in diameter are important in the colon's ability to tolerate distension in the setting of distal obstruction, as the cecum will more likely perforate than other areas of the colon at equal pressures secondary to the higher tensions that develop as calculated by Laplace's law. Patients with extra loops of colon, resulting in a longer length, have a redundant colon. Rarely, this may lead to a volvulus resulting in obstruction that may require decompression via sigmoidoscopy.

The rectum is divided into three parts, the lower third extending approximately 3 to 6 cm from the anal verge, the mid rectum from 5–6 to 8–10 cm, and the upper third of the rectum from 8–10 to 12–15 cm. There are variations, but the determination of the boundary between the sigmoid colon and rectum is important to defining adjuvant therapy for cancers, to define operative treatment for diverticular disease, and in the stabilizing point for volvulus.

Fecal continence is a multifactorial process that occurs through the function of sphincter control, nervous innervation, and the preservation of the normal muscular anatomy, which creates an anorectal angle or puborectalis sling. The pelvic floor is composed of the levator ani muscles, which separate the pelvis from the perineum and ischiorectal fossa. The urethra, vagina, and anus pass through the levators, and this violation of the levator ani musculature may ultimately lead to the development of pelvic floor syndromes.

The colon is composed of four layers (mucosa, submucosa, muscularis, and the serosa). The outer longitudinal layer of smooth muscle is incomplete and converges in three teniae coli that are ultimately confluent at the base of the appendix. The teniae coli are shorter than the colon, causing sacculation of the colonic wall thus forming outpouchings that are the haustra coli. Semilunar folds between adjacent haustra are the plicae semilunares. In the rectum, the teniae spread to form a continuous longitudinal coat of muscle while there is no serosal layer.

Arterial blood flow to the colon is supplied by the superior and inferior mesenteric arteries (SMA and IMA, respectively). The branches of the SMA and the IMA form an anastomotic vessel located along the mesenteric border of the colon wall known as the marginal artery of Drummond. Incomplete development of this marginal artery may be present at the splenic flexure (Griffith's point) in 43% of humans (1) and between the last sigmoid branch of IMA and the superior rectal artery (Sudeck's point) in 4.7% of humans (2). The IMA gives rise to the superior hemorrhoidal artery, which supplies the upper rectum, and the internal iliac artery gives rise to the middle and inferior hemorrhoidal arteries that supply the lower rectum and the anorectum. Venous drainage of the colon usually mirrors arterial supply, with the inferior mesenteric vein draining into the splenic vein, and the superior mesenteric vein joining the splenic vein to form the portal venous system. Lymphatic drainage for the colon and proximal two-thirds of the rectum is through the para-aortic nodes to the cisterna chyli. The distal rectum and anus can alternatively follow the same route or drain via the internal iliac and superficial inguinal nodes.

Innervation of the colon is provided by the thoracolumbar (sympathetic), vagal, and sacral (parasympathetic) nerve fibers. The parasympathetic fibers synapse with the ganglia of the myenteric plexus of Auerbach and Meissner's plexus. Parasympathetic stimulation promotes peristalsis and internal relaxation, whereas sympathetic stimulation has the opposite effect. Bowel activity can continue with disruption of parasympathetic and sympathetic innervation, as much of it is reflexive, dependent upon the intramural nerve plexuses of Meissner and Auerbach.

The primary function of the colon is to provide absorption, storage, digestion, and propulsion of food and food by-products. The colon absorbs up to 200 mEq/day of sodium and chloride via a Na/K ATPase pump with water passively following the active ion. Chloride is actively absorbed for bicarbonate within the colon. Urea is secreted, metabolized by bacteria into ammonia, and then reabsorbed passively in its nonionized form or excreted directly via feces. Potassium is actively secreted in mucus. Therefore, hypochloremic, hypokalemic metabolic alkalosis is associated with a secreting villous adenoma of the rectum. Conjugated bile acids are absorbed through the ileal and colon cells, but deconjugation by colonic bacteria interferes with sodium and water absorption and may be responsible for diarrheal states.

Giant migrating complexes (GMC) in the proximal colon and distal colon are coupled with mass movement of feces and defecation, respectively. An increase in frequency of GMCs can result in diarrheal states. Enteric neural control of GMCs is unclear at present, but they increase in frequency during inflammatory states, including enteric infections, and exposure to ionizing radiation (3).

Defecation begins with the movement of gas, liquid, or stool contents into the rectum. Distention of the rectum leads to stimulation of pressure receptors located on the puborectalis muscle and in the pelvic floor muscles, which in turn stimulate the rectoanal inhibitory reflex (RAIR). The loss of the RAIR is of clinical significance in Hirschsprung's disease and can be impaired in patients following a low anterior resection (LAR) (4), total mesorectal excision (5), and restorative proctocolectomy (6) for cancer. In addition, the loss of the volume compliance in the rectum associated with altered states such as fibrosis, Crohn's disease, or radiation can lead to the presence of tenesmus even though the RAIR is intact. When satisfactory conditions are met for defecation, the abdominal pressure will increase. The puborectalis consequently will relax, resulting in straightening of the anorectal angle, and the pelvic floor descends slightly. The external anal sphincter relaxes and the internal anal sphincter will relax after accommodation. Then the rectal contents are evacuated in a socially acceptable manner (7).

Trauma

The colon is susceptible to injury following blunt or penetrating abdominal or pelvic trauma. The colon is the second most commonly injured organ in penetrating trauma, but blunt trauma rarely causes injury to the colon although the mesentery can often be injured by this mechanism (2% to 5%). Rectal injuries are more common in blunt trauma, especially when associated with pelvic fracture injuries (8). In cases of penetrating trauma, multiorgan system injury occurs in approximately 80% to 91% of the cases (5% in blunt trauma).

The evaluation of the injured patient always begins with the primary survey. Following this, the secondary survey will include physical evaluation for colorectal injuries. The colon may be injured by blunt and penetrating forces. Blunt forces can be associated with shearing injuries to the colon or mesentery. Penetrating injuries are more easily diagnosed at the time of celiotomy. Patients with colon injuries often present with peritoneal signs. A careful history and physical examination in association with the mechanism of injury will help establish the appropriate differential diagnosis. Radiological evaluation for suspected colonic injuries is frequently done by computed tomographic (CT) scan. Colonic injury is suggested by free extraluminal air, intraperitoneal or retroperitoneal free fluid, focal thickening of the bowel wall, bowel wall hematoma, or intramural air. CT scans should be reviewed through both abdominal and "lung" windows to evaluate for free air. The overall accuracy of computed tomography for diagnosing bowel injury is 82%, with sensitivity of 64% and specificity of 97%. There is little current evidence to recommend the use of oral or rectal contrast for evaluation of colonic injuries. Simple upright chest x-ray film can reveal free abdominal air, but is not pathognomic for colonic injury. In blunt trauma, 13% of colonic injuries are missed by CT scan initially, so close clinical monitoring should be recommended especially in mechanism of injury that would require admission to a level-one trauma center.

Historically, most colon wounds in the civilian population were managed by exteriorization of the wound or proximal colostomy due to the fear of a high rate of breakdown. In the past 20 years, there has been an increasing trend toward primary repair. The advantages of primary repair are the avoidance of colostomy, with the subsequent reduction in the morbidity of the colostomy closure and the additional cost associated with colostomy care and the subsequent hospitalization for closure. Potential drawbacks of primary repair are the morbidity and mortality associated with failure of repair. Current recommendations are for primary repair of colon injuries secondary to penetrating trauma involving less than 50% of the undervascularized bowel wall in the absence of peritonitis and resection and primary anastomosis of colon injuries involving more than 50% of bowel wall or devascularized segment in the absence of hemodynamic instability, significant underlying disease, minimal associated injuries, minimal fecal contamination, and/or peritonitis (9). Otherwise, patients with colonic injuries should be managed with resection and colostomy.

Reversal of colostomy following colorectal trauma can be performed within several months if contrast enema reveals distal colon healing. In patients with nonhealing bowel injury, unresolved wound sepsis, or who remain unstable secondary to multiorgan failure or other associated injuries the stoma can be left as long as clinically necessary. Prior to colostomy closure, it had been recommended in the past that a barium study was necessary. However, there is no level-one evidence to support this behavior and consequently it is unnecessary to obtain this study prior to colostomy closure in patients who are not at risk for colon cancer or other colon problems, that is, Crohn's disease and/or polyps.

Technically, primary closure of the colon may be accomplished in many ways. The use of single layer, multiple layer, or stapled closure has adherents; however, none has been conclusively demonstrated to be superior. Exteriorization of the colonic injury has many fans in the literature; however, it is of limited applicability and may be technically difficult to perform in contradistinction to a simple Hartmann procedure. Colostomies should completely divert the fecal stream and be matured if possible. Following treatment of the colon injury the peritoneal cavity should probably be copiously irrigated with saline and suctioned dry. However, there is a growing respect for the peritoneal surface including the much beloved macrophage. Abdominal closure should leave the skin and subcutaneous tissue open for either delayed primary closure (4 to 7 days) or healing by secondary intention.

All patients with penetrating wounds to the pelvis, perineum, buttock, or upper thigh should be evaluated for rectal injury. Initial physical examination should include a digital rectal examination and rigid proctoscopy. Careful inspection of the penile meatus for blood may be a harbinger of other injuries including a rectal injury. In the event of an injury to the rectum, wounds located in the anterior and lateral upper two-thirds of the rectum are technically intraperitoneal and should be managed like colonic injuries. The posterior upper two-thirds and lower third of the rectum do not have serosa, and these injuries should be classified as extraperitoneal and be managed according to a different protocol. After resuscitation and administration of antibiotics, the abdomen should be explored and a completely diverting sigmoid colostomy should be created. Extraperitoneal wounds usually can be explored and sutured primarily. Wounds that are unreachable can be managed with proximal fecal diversion and presacral drainage, although evidence suggests that it does not lessen morbidity (10). Any procedure to repair rectal injuries often involves removal of all fecal content, although studies have not borne out a reduction in morbidity.

Iatrogenic Injury

Colorectal injuries secondary to diagnostic or therapeutic procedures such as sigmoidoscopy, colonoscopy, and enemas are exceedingly rare (11). Patients with prior surgery and associated adhesions may be at a higher risk for perforation with endoscopy due to these adhesions causing a fixation of the colon, especially in the sigmoid colon. There are also sporadic reports of colorectal trauma caused by insertion of foreign objects. The issues that occur with colonic and rectal injuries secondary to colonoscopy are important.

Once recognized, these injuries can be treated in a similar manner to traumatic wounds detailed above. However, in the case of patients with injuries secondary to endoscopy, they tend to have had mechanical bowel preparation and oral antibiotics. If their injuries are nondestructive, they can often be closed with a primary closure. There is growing experience with intraluminal clipping of these iatrogenic injuries in the gastrointestinal (GI) literature. At present these injuries secondary to perforation following polypectomy or thermal injury following polypectomy often include antibiotic therapy. In the case of significant injuries that cannot be treated conservatively, resection and reanastomosis is the preferred course. Significantly, more of these injuries are being repaired laparoscopically.

Conservative management of iatrogenic injury to the colon (bowel rest, antibiotics, observation) is recommended for high-risk patients or for small perforation after colonoscopy in a well-prepared colon with minimal or no symptoms. It is clear that not all colonic injuries are the same and not every injury requires a colostomy or repair.

Appendix

The appendix vermiformis is a thin tubular organ that is located at the inferior part of the cecum. It varies in length from 4 to 12 cm and has no fixed position. It originates 1.7 to 2.5 cm below the terminal ileum in a dorsomedial location (most common) from the cecal fundus, directly beside the ileal orifice, or as a funnel-shaped opening (2% to 3% of patients). The appendix has a retroperitoneal location in 65% of patients and may descend into the iliac fossa in 31%.

It is part of the gut-associated lymphoid tissue and secretes immunoglobulins. Appendicitis, or inflammation of the appendix, is often caused by the occlusion of the appendiceal lumen by an appendicolith or fecalith, has a lifetime incidence of 7%, and most often occurs in people 15 to 30 years of age. The history and physical findings of appendicitis vary, but the cardinal signs of appendicitis are anorexia and periumbilical pain followed by nausea and radiation of the pain to the right lower quadrant (RLQ). Migration of pain from the periumbilical area to the RLQ is the most significant feature of the patient's history, with a sensitivity and specificity of approximately 80%. Nausea and anorexia generally follow pain. Fever and leukocytosis are common. Often the parents will offer that the child is uncomfortable walking or felt discomfort when the car hit a bump driving to the hospital. This is a sign of peritoneal irritation.

Clinical diagnosis is more difficult in female patients, among whom 50% may have gynecologic pathology when appendicitis is not found at operation. Associated conditions that can mock the presentation of appendicitis are salpingitis, tuboovarian abscess, mittelschmerz syndrome, ovarian torsion, ruptured ovarian follicle, endometriosis, or ectopic pregnancy.

Radiological diagnosis is often established by ultrasound or CT scan. CT scan has a higher sensitivity and specificity (12) but is more expensive and exposes patients to higher levels of radiation. Studies reveal ultrasound sensitivity of 76% and CT sensitivity of 96%, with ultrasound accuracy of 83% compared with the CT accuracy of 94% (12).

The subset of patients who present several days after onset of symptoms, with long histories of abdominal pain and in those whose CT scans reveal phlegmon or abscess can be treated conservatively with bowel rest, antibiotics, and close observation in an attempt to mitigate the possibility of needing to remove part of the colon when performing the appendectomy. This situation often occurs in children. Interval appendectomy can be performed several weeks later once symptoms have resolved, although this practice is controversial, and conservative therapy may be sufficient (13,14). There is controversy in the literature regarding the rate of recurrent appendicitis following conservative therapy.

Appendectomy can be performed via open or laparoscopic techniques. There is controversy regarding the best technique. The data would support that in nonperforated appendicitis, laparoscopic appendectomy is associated with fewer wound complications. On the other hand, the data would also support that in perforated appendicitis there may be a higher incidence of pelvic abscesses. Clearly, the advocates of laparoscopy express the visibility and ability to examine the entire pelvis and run the small bowel in cases of an error in diagnosis. The advocates of open appendectomy also state cost and length of stay issues in this regard. The common practice would appear to favor laparoscopic appendectomy at present. Neither approach has been found to be superior in any parameter except quality of life at 2 weeks (15), so the decision on how to proceed should be based on the surgeon's and the patient's preference. There is evidence that if the appendix is not removed to the base of the appendix close to the cecum the recurrent appendicitis may and can occur.

Tumors of the appendix are uncommon. They are usually found after routine appendectomy. Carcinoid tumors are the most common, and appendectomy may be sufficient if the tumor is less than 2 cm and is found within the mucosa. However, if a carcinoid tumor spreads beyond these parameters, right hemicolectomy is indicated. Mucoceles can result from obstruction of the appendiceal lumen without sufficient distal bacterial flora to produce appendicitis and can be treated with an appendectomy. Adenocarcinoma of the appendix is treated in a manner similar to an adenocarcinoma of the right colon.

Inflammatory Bowel Disease

Granulomatous colitis (Crohn's disease) and chronic ulcerative colitis (CUC) are the most common generalized chronic inflammatory diseases of the colon and the rectum. The etiology of these diseases is still under investigation; however, susceptibility to inflammatory bowel disease (IBD) may be of genetic origin. Several genes have been characterized as permissive, with mutations associated with the disease (*CARD15 IBD1* 5q31, 6p21, and 19p). First-degree relatives have a 5- to 20-fold increased risk of developing IBD compared with patients from unaffected families. IBD is generally diagnosed in young adults, with equal prevalence in male and female populations and four to five times more prevalent in Ashkenazi Jews. Whatever the precipitating cause, activation of the immune system leads to acute and chronic inflammation of the intestinal tract, with increased lymphocyte activation, increased TNF, IL-1 levels, tissue macrophages, and circulating antibodies to colonic mucosal cells.

Crohn's disease and CUC differ in their pathological manifestations. Crohn's pathological features include transmural inflammation, serositis with segmental involvement, thickened mesentery, granulomas, and enlarged lymph nodes. Perineal abscesses, fissures, and/or fistulae occur in 10% to 25% of Crohn's disease and in 10% of cases may be the first sign of disease. Anorectal disease is not improved by resection of proximally involved small bowel or colon in most cases. Abdominal wall or internal fistulas are common. CUC is limited to the colonic mucosa and submucosa, with initial involvement of the rectum in 90% to 95% of cases. Perineal disease and fistulae are uncommon, and resection of the colon and rectum can be curative.

IBD has extraintestinal manifestations. Systemic diseases such as iritis, uveitis, arthritis, erythema nodosum, vasculitis, sclerosing cholangitis, retroperitoneal fibrosis, hepatic cirrhosis, and pyoderma gangrenosum are associated with both diseases but more commonly in CUC (one-third of cases). Colectomy in CUC patients can prompt an improvement in extraintestinal symptoms of the disease; however, sclerosing cholangitis and axial arthritis may be the least likely to improve. Patients with IBD can be in a hypercoagulable state, leading to strokes, pulmonary emboli, and retinal thrombi. Anemia is common, either from chronic blood loss or anemia of chronic disease. Cholelithiasis can be seen in Crohn's disease and can be treated with cholecystectomy. Patients with CUC have an increased risk of colorectal cancer, approximately 0.5% to 1.0% per year 8 to 10 years after diagnosis. Those with Crohn's disease are at similar risk if the entire colon is involved. Surveillance

colonoscopy every 2 years after 8 years of disease is recommended, more frequently if areas of pathological concern are evident. Stricture of the colon in a patient with CUC is a malignancy until proved benign.

Both conditions can be treated medically with aminosalicylates, steroids, immunomodulators like 6MP or azathioprine, or infliximab.

The pathological variation of Crohn's disease and CUC dictate surgical management. The surgical treatment of CUC is curative by removing the colon, rectum, and anus by either a proctocolectomy or a restorative ileal pouch procedure. The surgical treatment for Crohn's disease is to treat the complications of the disease only. Primarily the complications for the patient with Crohn's disease are obstruction, fistula, abscess, bleeding, cancer, perforation, and intractability. Surgical intervention for CUC is indicated in patients for whom medical management is insufficient to control symptoms or produces adverse effects, premalignant or malignant lesions detected on colonoscopy, toxic megacolon, hemorrhage, colonic strictures, or if symptoms create a poor quality of life. Surgical management of Crohn's disease is not curative, and interventions are intended to treat complications. With the associated high rate of recurrence following surgery, care must be taken to remove as little bowel as possible, thus avoiding short gut syndrome. Segmental resection of affected bowel or stricturoplasty is a common operation for the treatment of Crohn's disease. Strictureplasty preserves bowel length.

The treatment of anorectal disease requires an understanding of the underlying condition. Perianal Crohn's disease should be treated by draining the underlying abscess and minimizing any direct insult to the sphincter mechanism. The advent of infliximab in combination with metronidazole has been very useful in directly treating fistulous disease in patients with Crohn's disease. The role for draining setons and cutting setons is established for the surgical management of these different disorders.

Toxic Megacolon

Toxic megacolon presents with abdominal pain, tenderness, distention, fever, dehydration, bloody diarrhea, elevated white blood count, and signs of sepsis. Radiographic features include dilatation of the colon, the classic finding being a transverse colon of more than 6 cm. It also occurs as a complication of other primary diseases (IBD, Hirschsprung's, *Salmonella*, *Shigella*, and cholera infections; Chagas' disease; and ischemic and pseudomembranous colitis), with no known etiology. It has been suggested that its development can be hastened with opiates, antidiarrheal agents, barium enemas, and rapid discontinuation of medications such as sulfasalazine and steroids.

The goals of initial management of patients presenting with toxic megacolon are to reduce colonic distention, treat underlying conditions, and correct fluid and electrolyte imbalances. This includes nasogastric decompression, fluid resuscitation, broad-spectrum antibiotics, and sigmoidoscopy. Opiates and barium enemas should be avoided as these medications impact colonic activity. Cyclosporine has been suggested for use in CUC patients with toxic megacolon. Surgical management is controversial, with the old philosophy being an early operation (within 24 hours) leads to the best outcome. This could be due to a five-fold increase in mortality after perforation. Subtotal colectomy, total proctocolectomy, or the less traumatic Turnbull procedure (loop ileostomy and blowhole transverse or sigmoid colostomy, or both) is the option, although the value of the Turnbull has not been demonstrated and has been abandoned by many colorectal surgeons. Conservative management is also an option, necessitating close observation for peritonitis, hemorrhage, free intraperitoneal air, or subserosal air in the colon. Such might require immediate surgical management.

Whether to perform a total proctocolectomy or subtotal colectomy with the rectal remnant remaining is controversial. The preference is to perform a subtotal colectomy because (a) the patient usually is very ill and not lengthening the operation is prudent if at all possible, (b) it preserves the possibility for an ileal pouch anal anastomosis, and (c) approximately 50% of patients with Crohn's disease have minimal or no involvement of the rectum. Performance of a total proctocolectomy in a patient who is acutely ill, exposed to toxicity and on high-dose steroids would increase the risk of complications, morbidity, and likely mortality. The incidence of perineal fistula is also increased following these procedures.

Diverticular Disease

Diverticula of the colon can be classified as true or false. The relatively rare true diverticula involve the mucosa, submucosa, and muscularis of the colon, are congenital, and usually solitary. The classic true diverticulum is a jejunal diverticulum. The more common false diverticula involve the mucosa and submucosa and emanate from weaknesses in the colonic wall where mesenteric vessels penetrate the circular muscle wall. False diverticula are responsible for most diverticular diseases. Diverticular disease of the colon includes both diverticulosis and diverticulitis. Diverticulosis refers to the presence of symptomatic or asymptomatic diverticula and diverticulitis refers to inflammation of these diverticula. Diverticulosis is a disease of Western and affluent nations, whose increased consumption of refined food and decrease in fiber intake have resulted in a high prevalence of this condition. It is estimated that two-thirds of people 80 years of age and older have this condition, and with the aging population will increase its prevalence. Theoretically, diverticula form from increased intraluminal pressure and decreased strength of the muscle wall. High-pressure zones at the site of penetrating blood vessels will lead to mucosal and submucosal outpouchings. Recent evidence dispels the notion that nuts, popcorn, and corn can lead to higher rates of diverticular disease (16). It has also been suggested that the causes are related to neuromuscular dysfunction with a genetic basis (17).

Sixty-five percent of patients with diverticulosis have disease limited to the sigmoid colon. Thirty-five percent of patients with disease have involvement in other parts of the colon. Only 1% to 4% of patients with the disease do not have sigmoid involvement (18).

Most patients with colonic diverticula are asymptomatic. Patients can have abdominal pain with diverticulosis, but this is generally from excessive pressure by segmentation of the colon. Abdominal pain in patients with known diverticula (seen on colonoscopy, barium enema, CT scan) should have other diagnoses excluded, including chronic constipation, diverticulitis, irritable bowel syndrome, IBD, adenocarcinoma of the colon, or appendicitis.

Treatment of diverticulosis includes a high-residue diet with or without stool softeners to decrease transit time of stool in the colon and decrease intraluminal pressures. The efficacy of bulk laxatives or fiber supplementation to treat pain associated with diverticulosis is controversial.

Diverticular bleeding is a common complication of diverticulosis and accounts for 60% of lower GI bleeding in adults (19). Patients often present with painless bright red blood per rectum in varying volumes. The cause of this bleeding appears to be the thinning of the vasa recta within the diverticulum. Patients with diverticular bleeding tend to be treated conservatively, with close observation, serial hematocrits, and transfusions as necessary. Most bleeds resolve spontaneously (70% to 80%), though recurrence is common (20% to 40%) (20). Diverticular bleeds originate throughout the colon. Localization of bleeds can be ascertained through digital rectal examinations, bleeding scans, angiography, and colonoscopy. Digital examinations with an anoscope can diagnose an anorectal source; isotope scanning with intravenously tagged red blood cells can generally localize bleeds as low as 0.5 mL/min and angiography more accurately at 1 to 2 mL/min. All patients with GI bleeds should have a gastric lavage performed to rule out a gastroduodenal source.

Treatment of persistent bleeds includes direct therapy with colonoscopy with various endoscopic methods to control hemorrhage, angiography with identification of the bleeding vessels and selective injection of vasopressin or embolization with cellulose or gelatins, or segmental resection of identified regions of bleeding or subtotal colectomy.

Acute diverticulitis can be a catastrophic situation. This process leads to inflammation that is peridiverticular and leads to focal necrosis and perforation. This often occurs in the sigmoid colon, where intraluminal pressures are at their greatest (21). Patients present with lower abdominal pain, fever, and elevated white blood counts. A tender mass may be palpable in the left lower quadrant or on rectal or pelvic examination. Radiographic diagnosis is generally carried out by CT scan, which can identify the diverticula, thickened colonic wall, pericolic stranding, and presence of collections.

The modified Hinchey classification divides the presentation of diverticulitis into four stages. Stage IA indicates confined pericolic inflammation or phlegmon, Stage IB confined pericolic abscess, Stage II a pelvic, distant intra-abdominal or retroperitoneal abscess, Stage III generalized purulent peritonitis, and Stage IV fecal peritonitis. Stage IA and IB cases are often treated conservatively, with bowel rest, intravenous fluids, and intravenous antibiotics. Stage II disease can also be treated conservatively but often requires percutaneous drainage. These cases can lead to fecal fistulae but often resolve spontaneously once the inflammation has resolved.

The more complicated Stage III and IV presentations, and recalcitrant uncomplicated case, require operative intervention. The procedure of choice is surgical/radiological drainage of the purulent and/or fecal contents within the abdomen, the resection of the diseased sigmoid colon with proximal and distal colostomy, or proximal sigmoid colostomy and distal rectosigmoid closure. These operations may be performed at the original stage of diagnosis or in staged procedures. This approach removes the source of contamination, and patients are generally reversed several months later. In cases in which the inflammation obscures the pelvic anatomy, drainage and a diverting proximal colostomy are less desirable but often necessary options. Diverticulitis can lead to partial or complete obstruction due to edema, fibrosis, muscle thickening, and spasm. Lack of resolution on conservative therapy indicates the need for colonic resection with proximal colostomy and distal mucous fistula or rectosigmoid closure. If technically impossible, an alternative is an initial transverse colostomy (or descending colon colostomy) and then a sigmoid resection as a second-stage procedure 2 to 3 weeks later.

Traditional thinking has been that patients should have an elective colectomy after two episodes of diverticulitis. However, recent data have determined that past episodes are an imperfect predictor of future perforation, and that future research should focus on which patients are more likely to perforate. The data also recognize that the addition of dietary fiber may also have a significant impact on the outcome of treatment algorithms. The new data point to deter most elective operative management until after the fourth or more attacks. There is also evidence regarding lower mortality and wound infections with resection with primary anastomosis than with a two-stage procedure in selected series (17).

POLYPS AND CANCER OF THE COLORECTUM

Colorectal Polyps

Polyps of the colorectum are in many cases associated with carcinoma, or carcinoma may arise from the polyp itself. The transition from polyp to cancer mostly develops over 5 to 10 years or longer. This transition involves the loss or mutation of tumor-suppressor genes on chromosomes 5, 17, or 18; activation of an oncogene (K-ras, myc, or src); or mutations on chromosomes 2, 3, or 7 that interfere with maintenance of DNA fidelity during replication. This is generally true with large adenomatous (tubular) polyps (>1 cm), villous adenomas, mixed villoadenomatous (villoglandular) polyps, and adenomatous polyps associated with genetically determined syndromes (familial polyposis, Gardner syndrome, Turcot syndrome, and Lynch syndromes I and II [hereditary nonpolyposis colorectal cancer syndromes]).

Adenomatous (tubular) polyps occur most frequently in the rectum and sigmoid but are common throughout the colon. They are frequently multiple. Ninety percent of polyps are less than 1 cm and malignant change is uncommon (1% to 2%). The remaining 10% are greater than 1 cm and carry an approximately 10% chance of containing cancer. The risk of progression from polyp to carcinoma is related to the size and the histology of the adenoma. Adenomas greater than 1 cm and that contain a substantial (>25%) villous component, or have high-grade dysplasia, are often referred to as advanced neoplasia and carry an increased cancer risk (22).

Villous adenomas commonly occur in the rectum, are generally larger (>2 cm), and have a nonpedunculated, cauliflower-like appearance. They can cause hypersecretory syndromes and harbor cancer in 20% to 30% of cases. These polyps should be removed at endoscopy, and if incomplete, should be resected surgically with its segment of colon. Villoglandular polyps have an amalgamated appearance and malignant potential between that of adenomatous and villous polyps.

Familial adenomatous polyposis is an autosomal dominant condition caused by a germ line mutation of the APC gene, and the most common *adenomatous polyposis syndrome*. Other APC-related colonic polyposis disorders include Gardner syndrome (dental abnormalities, osteomas, and soft tissue tumors) and Turcot syndrome (medulloblastoma). It is characterized by the onset of hundreds to thousands of *adenomatous polyps* throughout the colon in the affected individuals' midteens and if left untreated, all patients with this syndrome develop colon cancer between the ages of 35 and 40 years. Patients generally present with diarrhea, bloody stools, and abdominal cramping, although many are asymptomatic. Diagnosis is confirmed by sigmoidoscopy, colonoscopy, or barium air-contrast enema. The National Comprehensive Cancer Network recommends anyone at risk for familial adenomatous polyposis with unknown or positive APC mutation status to have sigmoidoscopy or colonoscopy annually beginning ages 10 to 15 years.

Surgical therapy is indicated because of the diffuse nature of the polyposis and the inevitability of colorectal cancer. A definitive operation should be performed prior to the typical onset of cancer. Approaches include total abdominal colectomy with ileorectal anastomosis, total proctocolectomy with ileal pouch anal anastomosis, total proctocolectomy with end ileostomy, and total proctocolectomy with continent ileostomy. The choice of operation depends upon rectal polyp burden, presence of cancer, age, symptoms, continence, genotype, and patient compliance (23).

Benign polyps include pseudopolyps of ulcerative colitis and granulomatous colitis, inflammatory or lymphoid polyps, the hamartomatous polyps of children (juvenile polyps), Cronkhite-Canada and Peutz-Jehgers syndromes, and hyperplastic polyps of the colorectum (usually <0.5 cm in size). Fecal occult blood testing remains the screening test of choice among patients at low risk for colorectal polyps or cancer, but sensitivity is low and specificity is poor (patient who eat raw meat, beets, iron, radishes, vitamin C, and aspirin before testing can have false-positives). Cumulative mortality reduction from colon cancer has been demonstrated with the use of yearly fecal occult blood testing in patients 50 years or older.

Colorectal Cancer

Colorectal cancer is the second most common cancer in the United States, diagnosed in 150,000 patients annually and results in 60,000 deaths. It occurs equally in both sexes. It is classified by location, right-sided lesions being supplied by the superior mesenteric artery including the splenic flexure, and left-sided lesions, which are supplied by the inferior mesenteric artery and includes the descending colon, sigmoid colon, and upper rectum. The final group is rectal lesions, with no serosal covering. The TNM system has become the internationally accepted system for staging colorectal cancer. Current recommendations for average-risk individuals include annual fecal occult blood testing and flexible sigmoidoscopy every 5 years. Colonoscopy is recommended every 10 years (24).

Carcinoembryonic antigen, a marker for colorectal cancer, is obtained preoperatively. While not a good screening tool, suspicion for recurrence should be raised if levels decrease postoperatively and rise at a later date. Carcinoembryonic antigen has been shown to be most useful for the early detection of liver metastases (25).

Surgical excision is accepted as the primary therapy for colorectal cancer. Operative strategy should be to achieve an en bloc resection with adequate oncologic margins, lateral margins if the tumor has directly extended to surround tissues, and to remove regional lymph nodes. Synchronous polyps occur in 25% to 30% of patients with colorectal carcinoma and synchronous tumors occur in approximately 6% of patients. Preoperative colonoscopy and detection of the lesions lead to an alternate operative plan in 20% of patients.

Perioperative blood transfusions have been shown to have a detrimental effect on the recurrence of curable colorectal cancers, so such should be restricted as much as possible (26). However, a causal relationship has yet to be determined. Preoperative mechanical bowel preparation has and still is a common practice, but its role in reducing anastomotic leaks and wound infection has not been shown to be necessary in a number of prospective randomized trials. Perioperative antibiotics have been shown to reduce wound infections, which in elective colorectal resections have been reported as high as 26%, though there is a wide range of opinion upon what defines a wound infection (27). Nasogastric tubes, once the mainstay of postoperative care, have been demonstrated to be unnecessary in the majority of cases. Chewing gum has been shown to improve return of GI function.

Lesions within the intraperitoneal colon and upper third of rectum should be treated with resection and anastomosis. Patients presenting with colonic obstruction or perforation should be approached with resection and possible diverting ostomy, although lesions in the right colon can be treated with right hemicolectomy and ileocolic anastomosis in most cases. Right colon perforations can be approached usually with resection and anastomosis. If the perforation is in the right colon with a left colon mass, subtotal colectomy is usually the preferred approach. In lesions confined to the upper third of the rectum, sometimes an anterior resection is indicated. The advent of laparoscopic approaches to colorectal operations has offered an alternative to laparotomy that has been shown to reduce wound infections (28) and has been shown to be equivalent to traditional open approaches (24).

Lesions in the lower third of rectum (5 to 8 cm from anal verge) can be treated with abdominoperineal resection (APR). APR involves wide excision of the rectum to include surrounding attachments and pelvic rectal mesocolon total mesorectal excision (TME) with the creation of a colostomy. Lesions in the mid-dle third (8 to 12 cm from anal verge) can be treated with APR, but other alternatives exist with similar outcomes. LAR involving resection of the middle rectum and use of an end-to-end anastomosis stapler can avoid the need for colostomy and spares the anal sphincter. End-to-end or end-to-side hand-sewn anastomosis can also be used, and a diverting colostomy or loop ileostomy can be created for temporary protection of the anastomosis. Coloanal anastomosis has been utilized to maintain bowel continuity, though increased stool frequency, urgency, and incontinence may necessitate the need for a colonic J-pouch.

Less radical approaches to rectal cancer have been employed to preserve sphincter function and avoid the morbidity of APR and LAR. Originally, local excision, ablation, electrocoagulation, and irradiation were reserved for patients who could not tolerate a large operation or had advanced disease. Recently, local excision of tumors less than 4 cm in diameter and 10 cm or less from the dentate line (T2 patients receiving postoperative chemoradiation) has been shown to have similar rates of local recurrence and survival, though more detailed prospective data are unavailable. Poor surgical candidates can also be treated locally with transanal electric fulguration, endocavitary irradiation, and laser ablation.

In combination with surgical therapy, radiotherapy has been shown to decrease local recurrence in Stage IIA and III rectal lesions, with increased overall survival as well as actual 5-year survival (24). There does not appear to be any survival advantage to preoperative versus postoperative radiotherapy, but patients receiving preoperative therapy have lower rates of recurrence and fewer side effects. The role of chemotherapy has been established by the National Comprehensive Cancer Network. Patients with node- positive colon cancer should be treated with adjuvant chemotherapy, most commonly 5-FU and leucovorin, and 5-FU, leucovorin and Oxaliplatin. The same applies to Stage IIA and III rectal cancer.

Bilateral oophorectomy may be necessary in selected colorectal carcinoma patients—women (especially when perimenopausal or postmenopausal). The ovaries are involved with microscopic metastases in about 3% to 5% of cases, and oophorectomy eliminates the development of primary ovarian carcinoma or large colonic metastases that may require resection at a later date. Unfortunately, oophorectomy does not increase the 5-year disease-free survival of those with colorectal cancer.

Liver metastases from colorectal cancer may be surgically resectable, which results in long-term survival if there is no extrahepatic recurrence, can be resected with at least 1-cm margins, are less than 3, and have no medical contraindications to surgery, and then 5-year survival rate can be 25% to 30%. Intraoperative ultrasound improves detection of additional liver metastases, as also may immunoscintigraphy using labeled monoclonal antibodies that demonstrate undiagnosed extrahepatic metastasis. Patients with unresectable liver metastases confined to that organ have been treated with hepatic intra-arterial chemotherapy with fluorouracil derivatives, which has been shown to have improved survival to systemic chemotherapy.

Ischemic Colitis

Ischemic colitis, usually seen in elderly and debilitated patients, usually results from small-vessel vascular disease in or near the colonic wall. Patients at higher risk include those on dialysis, hypertension, cardiovascular disease, and/or on vasoactive medication. It usually presents with rectal bleeding, vague abdominal pain, and diarrhea. Severity is correlated with the degree of ischemia and the extent of the colon involved. The disease may vary from mild mucosal edema with healing, to circumferential mucosal sloughing and subsequent stricture, and to full-thickness bowel wall necrosis and perforation. Etiologies include "low flow" states like vasopressor use or shock, embolic disease, blunt abdominal trauma, irradiation, vasculitis, or in some cases from the iatrogenic ligation of the inferior mesenteric artery. Diagnosis is best made by colonoscopy, though abdominal x-ray, CT scan, barium enema, and angiography can be helpful. Most patients will recover with bowel rest, intravenous fluids, and broad-spectrum antibiotics. Operative management is reserved for those who have failed conservative therapy and have signs of colonic gangrene, perforation, or obstruction.

Colonic Pseudoobstruction

Also known as *Ogilvie's syndrome*, the acute obstruction of the colon without identifiable mechanical cause generally occurs in elderly, bedridden, hospitalized patients. They frequently are on narcotics or anticholinergic medications, or have pneumonia, renal failure, sepsis, pancreatitis, or spinal or pelvic trauma. The usual presentation is painless abdominal distention and obstipation. The major risk is cecal perforation.

Initial therapy includes conservative measures such as nasogastric suction, bowel rest, intravenous fluids, and correction of electrolyte abnormalities. Colonoscopy is both diagnostic and therapeutic and should be performed if conservative measures fail. Failure of colonoscopy can lead to colostomy, and if patient shows signs of perforation or peritonitis, immediate operative intervention should be carried out to resect the perforated portion of bowel. Mortality can exceed 40% to 50% in these cases.

Volvulus

Volvulus of the colon occurs when a mobile portion of the colon twists on itself, producing a closed-loop obstruction. Occurring most frequently in the sigmoid colon (75% to 85%), elderly patients, those with neglected bowel habits and afflicted with neurological disease are the most affected. Those who take medications that decrease colonic motility are at higher risk. Sigmoid volvulus tends to occur in patients with a long, redundant sigmoid loop with or without a narrow attachment at the base of the sigmoid mesentery. Interestingly, if the patient's ileocecal valve is competent, a sigmoid volvulus results in two closed-loop obstructions within the colon.

Patients present with abdominal pain, distension, and obstipation. Vomiting generally occurs late in presentation, if at all. There may be a history of prior episodes with spontaneous resolution. If the loop becomes gangrenous, signs of peritoneal irritation with fever appear and the white blood cell is elevated, although in some elderly patients the white blood cell count remains normal or low with a "left shift."

Supine and upright abdominal films reveal a large, distended colonic loop with its apex frequently in the right upper quadrant ("bent inner tube" or "omega" signs). If there are no signs of peritonitis, sigmoidoscopy or colonoscopy may be diagnostic and is therapeutic in 85% to 90% of cases. Barium enema may be necessary to establish the diagnosis if sigmoidoscopy is not diagnostic. A "bird's beak" deformity is seen on barium enema and points to the site of obstruction.

If the sigmoidoscopy is successful in releasing the obstruction, and no signs of gangrene are observed in the sigmoid loop, a rectal tube is left in place for several days. Elective sigmoid resection should be performed as recurrence is 50% to 90%. In cases in which signs of strangulation or gangrene are present, urgent laparotomy is indicated. Resection of the sigmoid loop should be carried out with sigmoid colostomy and either the creation of a distal mucous fistula, or oversewing or stapling of the distal sigmoid.

In cases of cecal or ascending colon, the cause is usually because of a congenital lack of fixation or failure of the right colon to descend into the RLQ of the abdomen. This usually occurs in a younger age group.

Adhesions developing to the right colon from previous operations may be indicated in the development of a volvulus. Sometimes a true volvulus does not develop; rather, a mobile cecum folds superiorly and lies on the ascending colon (cecal bascule). The clinical picture suggests a distal small intestinal obstruction, and previous episodes with spontaneous resolution are common.

Diagnosis of right colon volvulus is frequently made with abdominal x-ray films, with a large, distended cecum seen along with numerous loops of dilated small intestine. If necessary, the diagnosis is confirmed with a barium enema. Detorsion is often not possible without an operation. Past approaches (cecostomy or cecopexy) have not shown to have satisfactory outcomes and resection of the involved segment is recommended. There has been a limited experience with laparoscopic approaches.

Rectal Prolapse

Rectal prolapse is a disease in which some or all of the layers of the rectal wall prolapse externally. It occurs six times more commonly in women than in men. Historically, this entity has been divided into three categories. Type I is prolapse only of the rectal mucosa through the anus and frequently associated with internal hemorrhoids that enlarge and push the mucosa ahead of them in radial folds. Type II denotes a protrusion of all layers of the rectal wall through the anus (rectal intussusceptions) without an associated hernia of the pelvic cul-de-sac. Type III is a full-thickness prolapse with a perineal sliding hernia of the pelvic cul-de-sac. There is a large defect in the pelvic diaphragm, and the cul-de-sac hernia invaginates through the anterior rectal wall, producing the intussusceptions. Other descriptions usually involve incomplete and complete prolapse with or without fecal incontinence associated with the disease. These are more clear definitions of the patient's problem. The patient with rectal prolapse should have a fecal incontinence score preferably the Wexner score. The development of a Type II or III prolapse is associated with loss of adherence of the rectum to the sacral curve, with elongation, straightening, and eventually a lax, dilated external sphincter and loss of continence and mucus discharge. These symptoms are often preceded by a long history of severe constipation and frequent tenesmus or anterior rectal ulceration. Eventually, the rectal mucosa constantly prolapses in concentric folds outside the anal canal with persistent soilage, odor, and mucosal excoriation with bleeding from minor trauma. Many patients with Type II or III prolapse are elderly and have multiple chronic medical conditions. Incontinence reaches 50%, the apparent result of pressure and stretching of the internal and external anal sphincters. A solitary rectal ulcer can develop from a prolapse that does not present externally. The etiology of a complete prolapse is unclear.

Numerous operative procedures have been devised for this disease. Type I mucosal prolapse can be treated with any form of fixation surgery. DeLorme may also be considered, as has the recent application of the Stapled Trans-Anal Rectal Resection (STARR) technique. Complete prolapse is most frequently managed by a transabdominal operation that mobilizes the rectum and fixes it to the presacral fascia. The Goldberg-Frykmann resection and rectopexy has been supplanted mostly by a laparoscopic rectopexy. Some consider the addition of a resection important in younger patients. An outlet perirectal circular suture (Thiersch) may be used alone to palliate the problem in poor-risk patients but frequently results in fecal impaction. Alternatively, perineal rectosigmoidectomy (Altemeier) may be performed more definitely as the procedure of choice in elderly patients with or without levatorplasty.

Radiation Proctitis

The deleterious effects of radiation on the rectum and other areas of the intestinal tract are roughly dose-dependent (rarely occurs if the tissue dose is <40 Gy). The effect is also determined by the method of fractionation and the rapidity with which the total dosage is delivered. Rapidly proliferating intestinal epithelium is highly sensitive to the effects of ionizing radiation. When used for long-term, progressive vasculitis with subintimal foam cells leads to arteriolar occlusion and thrombosis that is worsened in patients who are elderly, diabetic, or severely atherosclerotic or who have fixed bowel.

The rectum is most frequently injured when radiotherapy is used to treat malignancies of the uterus, bladder, or prostate. The true incidence is unknown. Early proctitis is frequently medically treated with oral

5-ASA and metronidazole and rectal therapies including 5-ASA, hydrocortisone, formalin, and sucralfate. There is some evidence that hyperbaric therapy can stem refractory radiation-induced hemorrhage, but more studies need to be performed (29).

Late symptoms include chronic proctitis, rectal ulcers, rectovaginal fistulae, strictures, or perforation. The lesions are usually 4 to 8 cm above the dentate line and are worse on the anterior rectal wall.

Up to 50% of patients with severe chronic radiation enteropathy require surgical intervention. Operative management must include rectal or vaginal biopsies to exclude the possibility of residual cancer. End-sigmoid colostomy is usually safe and effective. Localized lesions in the rectum may be resected but should be protected by a proximal colostomy until satisfactory healing is ensured. Nonirradiated colon is used to replace the resected radiation-damaged rectum.

Anorectal Diseases

Hemorrhoids

Hemorrhoids are varicosities of the submucosal veins with or without arteriovenous communications of the area. Everyone has hemorrhoids. They seem to be part of the normal defecatory process and allow us to differentiate between flatus and stool. The hemorrhoids may allow complete closure of anal canal and prevent weeping. The hemorrhoid becomes pathological under certain conditions like straining to pass hard stools, pregnancy, and increased resting anal pressure (internal sphincter). Internal and external hemorrhoids are different entities. The internal hemorrhoid has no nervous innervation and may be treated with various methods in the office since there is no pain associated with treatment. The external hemorrhoid requires anesthesia to treat as it has nervous innervation. Internal hemorrhoids may bleed but are otherwise asymptomatic except in cases of prolapse and thrombosis. Bleeding may be severe enough to produce anemia. It is important to exclude other sources of bleeding from the colorectum by sigmoidoscopy or colonoscopy.

Bleeding internal hemorrhoids may be treated by sclerotherapy, laser, or rubber band ligation. These methods are appropriate if the hemorrhoids are not prolapsed. Following treatment the patient is best managed with a high-fiber diet and stool softeners to produce soft bowel movements that do not require excessive straining for evacuation. Injection sclerotherapy is contraindicated in the presence of concomitant fissure, abscess, or fistula in ano.

Large internal hemorrhoids that prolapsed with defecation or exertion may not retract because of sphincter spasm. They then thrombose, and the overlying mucosa becomes gangrenous. If the patient is seen early (<24 hours), an emergency closed hemorrhoidectomy is beneficial, but usually the patient presents at a later time when associated edema, gangrene, and infection are more appropriately treated with bed rest, stool softeners, and analgesia. Surgical hemorrhoidectomy may be necessary after resolution of the above symptoms.

External Hemorrhoids

External hemorrhoids may rupture or thrombose from straining, and the initial pain is produced by separation of the anal skin from the underlying soft tissues. If the patient is seen during the first 24 to 48 hours, evacuation of the clot (using local anesthesia) is helpful. Later, the overlying anal skin frequently becomes inflamed and necrotic, and it sloughs. The conservative treatment described for strangulated internal hemorrhoids is then appropriate.

Anorectal abscess and Fistula in Ano

Anorectal abscesses and fistula in ano are usually secondary to the infection of the 4 to 10 anal glands that line the space between the external and internal sphincters of the rectal wall. Delay in diagnosis and prompt incision and drainage can result in extensive tissue destruction. In patients with poor resistance to infection (diabetic patients, immunocompromised patients, and steroid users) this may be a serious problem. This infection may spread to perianal, ischiorectal, intersphincteric, and supralevator spaces. Occasionally the infection can track up the rectal wall to rupture back into the rectal lumen. When satisfactory external drainage is performed without fistulotomy, the patient frequently develops a fistula in ano or a recurrent abscess (50% to 60% of the time); anal function disturbances are infrequent. When healing occurs without the development of a fistula in ano, it is probably because the involved anal crypt and its glands have been destroyed by the intense inflammation or because of a concomitant fistulotomy at the time the perirectal abscess is drained.

Fistulas in ano usually represent sequelae of a perirectal abscess that is spontaneously or surgically drained but the cavity does not heal completely. An inflammatory tract forms between an internal opening in the anal crypt and an external opening in the perianal skin. More common in men than women, they are frequently intersphincteric but may be transsphincteric or suprasphincteric. Goodsall's rule generally predicts the path between the external and internal openings—curved with a posterior external opening and straight with an anterior external opening. Patients sometimes present with multiple tracts, and this should raise a suspicion of Crohn's disease. Operative management includes unroofing the fistula, eliminating the internal opening, and establishing adequate drainage. Granulation tissue in the tract should be curetted or cauterized along with the anal crypt of origin. All fistulae should be biopsied to rule out Crohn's disease or cancer. Transection of the internal and external sphincter muscle in the posterior half does not always lead to anal incontinence in young patients. In older patients and women, transection of the external sphincter muscle risks incontinence. In cases in which sphincter transection appears likely, the use of a seton, loosely tied through the fistula, will allow drainage. Six to eight weeks after application, the seton is removed and fistulotomy or curettage of the epithelialized tissue with closure of the internal opening and fibrin glue application to the tract may be performed. The anal advancement flap is another modality, where after drainage and infection have resolved, a U-shaped flap of mucosa is advanced and the distal strip with the internal opening is excised. The introduction of the anal fistula plug, fabricated from porcine collagen, stimulates tissue remodeling and full closure of fistulous tract has had promising results (30). Tight setons, whose pressure would slowly cut through the sphincter and create fibrosis, are no longer usually recommended as their use led to incontinence.

Anal fistulae associated with Crohn's disease should be treated medically, as these patients heal very poorly after surgical intervention. Metronidazole and ciprofloxacin have been shown to be beneficial, as has infliximab.

Anal Fissure
Primary fissure in ano most frequently occurs in the posterior midline where the anal skin is overstretched from passage of hard stool and where the least striated muscular support is present. It can also occur in the anterior midline, as is seen in 20% of women with the disease. Secondary fissure is also associated with IBD with diarrhea and cryptitis. In this situation the fissure may occur laterally or be multiple. Once the anal skin is torn there is associated edema, inflammation, and spasm of the underlying internal and external

sphincters. Rarely a subcutaneous abscess forms in the area. The patient often avoids having bowel movements, which produce severe pain and a small amount of blood on the stool or toilet paper. The diagnosis is generally made on physical examination, where spreading of the buttocks reveals fissures from the anal skin to within a millimeter of the dentate line. There may be an associated hypertrophied anal papillae and sentinel pile associated with acute fissure. Resting anal pressures have shown to be higher in these patients, and Doppler studies have revealed low flow at fissure sites, the resulting ischemia causing their inability to heal. When the acute anal fissure has not healed following the acute injury, it becomes chronic in nature. Conservative management involves a high-fiber diet, stool softeners, nitric oxide, and topical anesthetic ointments. Most will heal in 6 weeks. Chronic anal fissures can be treated with topical nitroglycerin, diltiazem, and nifedipine, and there is some evidence that botulinum toxin A into the internal sphincter may improve fissure healing. The mainstay of surgical therapy for anal fissures is the lateral internal sphincterotomy. Success has been reported up to 94% (31), but fecal incontinence can occur.

Anal Cancer
For the purpose of discussing anal cancer and because the clinical courses and responses to therapy are similar, the pathologic variants of squamous carcinoma are considered together (cloacogenic, basaloid, mucoepidermoid, transitional cell). These tumors tend to invade sphincter muscles early and, like esophageal epidermoid carcinoma, may extend submucosally upward into the rectal wall. They are frequently related to human papilloma virus infection. The closer the primary lesion to the dentate line, the more likely it is that lymphatic spread will occur superiorly into mesenteric or internal iliac lymph nodes. Patients tend to present with pain and mild bleeding, often attributed to benign disease and thus diagnosis is often delayed.

Unlike that for colorectal adenocarcinoma, prognosis is related to the size of the primary lesion. Treatment of these cancers used to be primarily surgical by APR, but the success of the Nigro protocol, first described in 1972, has led to chemoradiation being the primary modality. The combination of 5-FU, mitomycin C, and pelvic radiation therapy saw that 5-year survival rates surpass those reported for surgical treatment. Nodal disease is covered by radiotherapists targeting pelvic lymph nodes. APR continues to play a role for patients with recurrent or residual local disease.

Anorectal melanoma is rare, encompassing less than 1% of all anal malignancies and generally occurs at the epidermoid lining of the anal canal. Patients present with rectal bleeding, and can be detected on physical examination, though 50% of lesions are amelanotic. They are often misdiagnosed as polyps or squamous cell carcinomas. These melanomas spread submucosally to the rectum, and one-third of patients will have metastases to the mesenteric nodes on initial diagnosis. Anal melanomas are resistant to radiotherapy, chemotherapy, and immunotherapy and APR has not shown any survival benefit. Wide local excision can be performed if the procedure is sphincter-sparing. Basal cell carcinoma, Bowen's disease, and Paget's disease can also be treated with local excision.

QUESTIONS

Select one answer.

1. Which of the following is NOT true of colonic diverticular bleeding.
   a. Most bleeding stops spontaneously
   b. Recurrent bleeding is very common
   c. Few patients will need a colon resection
   d. Angiography is the most sensitive test to localize rectal bleeding
   e. Patients who bleed often need blood transfusions

2. Which of the following is true regarding adenomatous colonic polyps.
   a. Polyps less than 1 cm in diameter are unlikely to be malignant
   b. Villous adenomas most commonly occur in the cecum
   c. FAP (familial adenomatous polyposis) is an autosomal recessive condition
   d. Hamartomatous polyps have a high incidence of malignant transformation
   e. Fecal occult blood testing has not changed the mortality from colon cancer

3. Patients who have suffered a penetrating colon injury involving more than 50% of the rectal wall should undergo which of the following:
   a. A diverting colostomy
   b. Exteriorization of the injured segment
   c. Primary repair of the injury

   d. Segmental resection and anastomosis
   e. A Hartmann's procedure and drainage

4. Which of the following may be appropriate initial therapy for a 4cm anal cancer involving the internal sphincter
   a. Abdominoperineal resection
   b. Wide local excision
   c. Radiotherapy and chemotherapy
   d. Interstitial radiotherapy
   e. Wide local excision with bilateral groin dissection

5. The extraintestinal manifestation of ulcerative colitis *least* likely to improve after total proctocolectomy is
   a. uveitis
   b. Sclerosing cholangitis
   c. Pyoderma gangrenosum
   d. Erythema nodosum
   e. Iritis

6. A patient with longstanding Crohn's disease develops a colonic stricture. Which of the following is the best treatment option.
   a. A short course of infliximab
   b. Segmental resection and primary anastomosis
   c. Bowel rest
   d. A proximal diverting colostomy and mucous fistula
   e. Stricturoplasty

7. Which of the following is the most important determinant of survival after treatment of colorectal cancer.
   a. Lymph node involvement
   b. Transmural extension
   c. Tumor size
   d. Histologic differentiation
   e. DNA content

8. An 80-year old patient undergoes an elective colonoscopic polypectomy. Six hours later he is noted to be distended and is found to have a pneumo-peritoneum. Which is of the following is the best treatment plan.
   a. Colonic resection and primary anastomosis
   b. Exteriorization of the injury
   c. Simple repair of the injury
   d. Bowel rest, observation and antibiotics
   e. Colostomy with mucous fistula

9. Treatment of toxic megacolon should all of the following *except*
   a. Steroid administration
   b. Antibiotics
   c. Nasogastric intubation
   d. Early colectomy
   e. Opiates

10. A sixty-old patient with two bouts of Hinchey Stage II diverticular disease should be treated with
   a. Sigmoid colectomy and anastomosis
   b. Transverse colostomy
   c. Sigmoid resection, end colostomy and mucous fistula
   d. Bowel rest, IV antibiotics
   e. Total abdominal colectomy

REFERENCES

1. Meyers MA. Griffiths' point: critical anastomosis at the splenic flexure. Significance in ischemia of the colon. *Am J Roentgen* 1976;126(1):77–94.
2. Van Tonder JJ, Boon JM, Becker JHR, van Schoor A-N. Anatomical considerations on Sudeck's critical point and its relevance to colorectal surgery. *Clin Anat* 2006;20(4): 424–427.
3. Koch T. *Colonic diseases*. Totowa, NJ: Humana Press, 2003;30–31.
4. O'Riordain MG, Molloy RG, Gillen P, Horgan A, Kirwan WO. Rectoanal inhibitory reflex following low stapled anterior resection of the rectum. *Dis Colon Rectum* 1992;35(9): 874–878.
5. Van Duijvendijk P, Slors F, Taat CW, Heisterkamp SH, Obertop H, Boeckxstaens GE. A prospective evaluation of anorectal function after total mesorectal excision in patients with a rectal carcinoma. *Surgery* 2003;133:56–65.
6. Saigusa N, Belin BM, Choi HJ, et al. Recovery of the rectoanal inhibitory reflex after restorative proctocolectomy; does it correlate with nocturnal continence? *Dis Colon Rectum* 2003;46(2):168–172.
7. Wolff BG. *The ASCRS textbook of colon and rectal surgery*. New York, NY: Springer, 2006;36–37.
8. Brohi K. Injury to the colon and rectum. Trauma.org. Accessed July 8, 2003.
9. Cayten CG, Fabian TC, Garcia VF, et al. *EAST practice parameter workgroup for penetrating colon injury management. Patient management guidelines for penetrating intraperitoneal colon injuries.* Chicago, IL: Eastern Association for the Surgery of Trauma, 1998.
10. Wiley W. Souba. *ACS surgery: principles and practice*, 6th ed. Philadelphia, PA: Decker Publishing Inc.
11. Nelson RL, Abcarian H, Prasad ML. Iatrogenic perforation of the colon and rectum. *Dis Colon Rectum* 1982;25(4): 305–308.
12. Balthazar EJ. Acute appendicitis: CT and US correlation in 100 patients. *Radiology* 1994;190:31–35.
13. Willemsen PJ. The need for interval appendectomy after resolution of an appendiceal mass questioned. *Dig Surg* 2002;19(3):216–220.
14. Kaminski A, Liu IL, Applebaum H, Lee SL, Haigh PI. Routine interval appendectomy is not justified after initial nonoperative treatment of acute appendicitis. *Arch Surg* 2005;140:897–901.
15. Katkhouda N. Laparoscopic versus open appendectomy: a prospective randomized double-blind study. *Ann Surg* 2005;242(3):439–450.
16. Strate LL, Liu YL, Syngal S, Aldoori WH, Giovannucci EL. Nut, corn, and popcorn consumption and the incidence of diverticular disease. *JAMA* 2008;300(8):907–914.
17. Flume D. Diverticulitis: changing paradigms of therapy. Montefiore, University of Washington, 2009.
18. Otterson MF, Korus GB. Diverticular disease. In: Mullholland MW, Lillemoe KD, Doherty GM, et al, eds. *Greenfield's surgery: scientific principles & practice*, 4th ed. Philadelphia: Lippincott Williams & Wilkins, 2006;1130–1137.
19. Vernava AM, Longo WE, Virgo KS. A nationwide study of the incidence and etiology of lower gastrointestinal bleeding. *Surg Res Commun* 1996;18:113–120.
20. Kim KE. *Acute gastrointestinal bleeding: diagnosis and treatment.* Totowa, NJ: Human Press, 2003;163.
21. Greenberger N, Blumberg R, Burakoff R. *Current diagnosis and treatment in gastroenterology, hepatology and endoscopy.* New York: McGraw-Hill, 2009;247.
22. Enders GH and El-Deiry WS. Colonic Polyps. http://emedicine.medscape.com/article/172674-overview. Updated December 15, 2009.
23. Dietz DW. Familial Adenomatous Polyposis. http://www.fascrs.org/physicians/education/core_subjects/2006/fap/.
24. Chang AE, Morris AM. Colorectal cancer. In: Mullholland MW, Lillemoe KD, Doherty GM, et al, eds. *Greenfield's surgery: scientific principles & practice,* 4th ed. Philadelphia: Lippincott Williams & Wilkins, 2006;1115.
25. Duffy MJ. Carcinoembryonic antigen as a marker for colorectal cancer: is it really useful? *Clin Chem* 2001;47:624–630.
26. Amato A, Pescatori M. Perioperative blood transfusions for the recurrence of colorectal cancer. *Cochrane Database Syst Rev* 2006;1:CD005033.
27. Smith RL, Bohl JK, McElearney ST, et al. Wound infection after elective colorectal resection. *Ann Surg* 2004;239(5): 599–607.
28. Nakamura T, Mitomi H, Ihara A, et al. Risk factors for wound infection after surgery for colorectal cancer. *World J Surg* 2008;32(6):1138–1141.
29. Girnius S, Cersonsky N, Gesell L, et al. Treatment of refractory radiation-induced hemorrhagic proctitis with hyperbaric oxygen therapy. *Am J Clin Oncol* 2006;29(6):588–592.
30. Van Koperen PJ, Bemelman WA, Bossuyt PM, et al. The anal fistula plug versus the mucosal advancement flap for the treatment of the Anorectal Fistula (PLUG trial). *BMC Surg* 2008;8:11. http://www.medscape.com/viewarticle/583440.
31. Hyman N. Incontinence after lateral internal sphincterotomy: a prospective study and quality of life assessment. *Dis Colon Rectum* 2004;47(1):35–38.

CHAPTER 5

Prashanth Sreeramoju
Peter Shamamian

Diseases of the Biliary Tract

ANATOMY

Biliary tract anatomy is perhaps the most variable in the abdominal cavity. The development of the liver and biliary tree, including the gallbladder and ventral pancreas is from the hepatic diverticulum, which appears on the ventral portion of the primitive gut during the 4th week of human embryo development (Ando).

Within the liver the proximal bile ducts drain into one main channel. The final common pathway for the left lobe is always a single trunk. The right lobe drains in one of two ways: In 75% of patients, the right anterior and right posterior ducts join to form a single right hepatic duct; in 25% there are two right segmental ducts, each of which joins with the left hepatic duct. About 2 to 4 mm of the left and right hepatic ducts are usually external to the liver. The length of the common hepatic duct is dictated by the entrance point of the cystic duct. The average diameter of the common hepatic and common bile duct (CBD) is 8 mm with a normal range of 4 to 15 mm. The size increases slowly with age and does so slightly following a cholecystectomy.

Ducts that, in the past, were termed "accessory ducts" are now thought to represent a nonjoined right hepatic duct, producing three ducts that drain from the liver. When they are recognized, caution must be taken to protect them from inadvertent injury and not to assume that these ducts are aberrant or accessory ducts.

In 0.5% of a large series of autopsies, the cystic duct entered the right hepatic duct, presenting a potential for right hepatic duct injury during cholecystectomy. Cholecystohepatic ducts are probably not congenital but acquired, resulting from large stones eroding through the gallbladder wall into the hepatic parenchyma. Subvesical ducts are slender (1 to 2 mm) ducts that occasionally emerge from the liver in the gallbladder fossa, pass toward the hilum, and join with the right hepatic or common hepatic duct. Ligation of these small ducts presents no problem, although division without ligation may result in short-term bile leak.

The gallbladder lies in a fossa in a line with the vena cava, separating the anatomic right and left hepatic lobes. The infundibulum is located at the point where the gallbladder leaves the fossa. The cystic duct exits from the infundibular segment of the gallbladder and has an average diameter of 2 to 3 mm. In 80% of patients, the cystic duct joins the common hepatic duct on the right lateral side of the hepatoduodenal ligament. The triangle bounded by the cystic duct, common hepatic duct, and inferior border of the liver forms the triangle of Calot. An absent cystic duct probably represents effacement by a stone in Hartman's pouch and is rarely congenital. In 80% of patients the cystic artery is single and arises from the right hepatic artery posterior to the cystic duct; 20% originate from the left or common hepatic artery, and a small number originate directly from the superior mesenteric artery. Venous drainage of the gallbladder is directly to the liver via small venous plexuses.

The CBD lies to the right of the hepatic artery and anterior to the portal vein. The arterial supply is via small vessels from the surrounding arteries, and venous drainage is via small tributaries to the portal vein. Lymphatics drain toward lymph ducts around the celiac axis. The CBD runs behind the duodenum and enters a groove in the dorsal portion of the head of the pancreas. A symmetric narrowing at the distal intrapancreatic bile duct is normal. The bile duct then joins the main pancreatic duct (Wirsung) in a short common channel and enters the ampulla of Vater. The bile duct is posterior and to the right of the pancreatic duct in 80% of patients. The ampulla of Vater is on the medial or posteromedial side of the duodenum, usually in the mid or distal half of the descending duodenum. The most common error when performing a duodenotomy for surgical access to the ampulla is making the incision too proximal on the duodenum.

Anomalies of the gallbladder are common, with some variation occurring as frequently as 50% in autopsy series. Rarely, the gallbladder is absent (0.02%), and when this occurs it is often associated with other congenital anomalies. Double or, rarely, triple gallbladders have been reported as well. Left-sided gallbladders have been reported with and without situs inversus. A partially intrahepatic gallbladder is common, but one that is totally intrahepatic is rare.

PHYSIOLOGY

The liver secretes about 500 to 1,000 mL of bile continuously each day. Major constituents of bile include water, bile acids, cholesterol, phospholipids, and bile pigments, among which bile acids/salts are most abundantly present. The bile acids are synthesized from cholesterol and consist mainly of cholic and chenodeoxycholic acids. Cholesterol is maintained in a solution by forming a mixed micelle and aggregates with lecithin. Bile enters the gallbladder in between the digestion period and gets concentrated by 6 to 10 times. When secreted, these substances are activated by pancreatic lipase in the duodenum.

Bilirubin is a waste product of hemoglobin, and conjugated bilirubin is actively secreted into the bile. The daily hepatic excretion of bilirubin is approximately 300 mg, most of which is excreted in the feces. Bile acids are reabsorbed, primarily in the terminal ileum, returning to the liver via the portal vein. Therefore, the liver secretes 20 to 30 g of bile per day from a total bile acid pool of 3 to 5 g recycled 4 to 12 times a day. Hepatic bile acid synthesis is controlled via a negative feedback mechanism. Serum levels of bile acids are low. Less than 5% of total bile acids are excreted in the feces, approximately 500 to 600 mg/day. The process of reabsorption of bile acids from the intestine and their secretion from the liver is known as the enterohepatic circulation.

Biliary tract pain is related to distension. The rapidity of the distension directly correlates with the degree of pain. The nerve supply consists of splanchnic nerves via the celiac ganglion from T7 to T10, branches of the right phrenic nerve from C3 to C5, and the intercostal nerves from T8 to T10. Biliary colic is probably not true colic but is caused by sudden stretching or distension. Gradual distension is usually painless.

The gallbladder functions to concentrate bile by reabsorption of water and electrolytes. The release of cholecystokinin (CCK) is stimulated within 10 minutes of the appearance of food in the duodenum, resulting in contraction of the gallbladder and relaxation of the sphincter of Oddi. The duodenal muscle contracts and relaxes with the sphincter, and contraction generally concludes in 30 minutes. Truncal vagotomy doubles the resting volume of the gallbladder, but the significance of this in the etiology of stone formation is unclear. Normal resting pressure in the sphincter of Oddi is 8 to 15 cm H_2O.

The incidence and significance of biliary pancreatic reflux in normal subjects are not clearly known. Using intraoperative and postoperative cholangiography, the incidence has been variously reported as 7% to 46%. However, reflux is probably rare at normal physiologic pressure.

DIAGNOSTIC PROCEDURES

Abdominal Radiography

A plain abdominal film may reveal significant diagnostic information. Approximately 15% of gallstones contain sufficient calcium to be radiopaque and are visualized on a plain film. Other helpful information, such as the presence of air in the biliary tree or a calcified gallbladder, may also be apparent. Air in the biliary tree is present in 75% of patients with a cholecystoenteric fistula in conjunction with a gallstone ileus, rarely with a choledochoduodenal fistula from stones, or more commonly with a duodenal ulcer. Demonstration of air in the biliary tree along with a small bowel obstructive pattern and stone in the distal ileum on KUB constitutes Rigler's triad.

Ultrasonography

Ultrasonography is 95% accurate for demonstrating the presence gallstones greater than 2 to 5 mm. It should be the primary screening test for the initial evaluation of the patient presumed to have biliary tract disease, gallbladder disease, or obstructive jaundice. Choledocholithiasis, when present, is demonstrated in 50% of patients. Although ultrasound is less accurate than computed tomography (CT), masses in the head of the pancreas larger than 3 cm in diameter may be visualized.

Ultrasonography is now generally accepted as the initial diagnostic test to confirm the presence of gallstones, biliary tract dilatation, and pancreatic pathology. Ultrasonography occasionally shows tiny stones or sludge after an oral study has produced normal results. Because ultrasonography only rarely gives false-positive results (<1%), there seems to be little reason to follow a positive sonogram routinely with an oral cholecystogram (OCG).

One important indication for obtaining an OCG following a normal sonogram is unexplained biliary tract pain secondary to cholesterolosis or dysfunctional emptying. In these patients, the delayed emptying, seen as opacification of the gallbladder beyond 36 hours, is highly suggestive of biliary dyskinesia, and improvement with cholecystectomy can be expected in 75% to 90% of cases.

Oral Cholecystography

The incidence of false-positive and false-negative results on OCGs is each less than 5%. Contraindications for an OCG include significant hepatic or renal failure, vomiting, a bilirubin level of greater than 2 mg/dL, or a known sensitivity (rare) to iopanoic acid. Reasons for nonvisualization include significant gallbladder disease due to an inability to concentrate the dye or cystic duct obstruction. Vomiting or failure to take pills, gastric outlet obstruction, subclinical jaundice, previous cholecystectomy, or acute pancreatitis can also result in nonvisualization. This test is rarely used because of the availability and accuracy of ultrasonography as an initial diagnostic tool.

Computed Tomography Scan

CT scans are less sensitive (75%) than ultrasound in evaluating stones in the biliary tract. The limited role of CT scan can be explained by the high cholesterol content in gallstones and CBD stones, making them isodense to bile and radiolucent. Most of the CT scans obtained are for the evaluation of complications associated with gallstones such as emphysematous gallbladder, pancreatitis, etc. CT cholangiography is a new technique, which improves the sensitivity of detecting choledocholithiasis by 96%. Limitations include high incidence of nausea and less accuracy in jaundiced patients. CT scan when used as an imaging modality for evaluation of cholangiocarcinoma (CCA) lesions has a sensitivity of approximately 70% to 90%.

Magnetic Resonance Cholangiopancreatography

Magnetic resonance cholangiopancreatography (MRCP) is widely used for the evaluation of gallstone-associated complications, such as choledocholithiasis and also for biliary tree tumors. Gallstones are visualized in T2-weighted images as signal voids against the bright bile. MRCP is highly sensitive in the evaluation of CCA with near 100% sensitivity in diagnosing biliary obstruction, 98% accuracy in identifying the level of lesion, and 88% to 95% accuracy in diagnosing the cause of obstruction. Since MRCP sensitivity is limited in the evaluation of CCA spread by inflammation either from infection or procedural trauma, imaging should be obtained before any planned procedures.

Endoscopic Ultrasound

Endoscopic ultrasound (EUS) is most sensitive for the evaluation of lesions less than 2 mm, making it useful for the evaluation of distal biliary tree abnormalities. It is more accurate (91%) than magnetic resonance imaging (MRI) in the assessment of regional lymph node spread and vascular involvement of CCA. EUS-guided fine needle aspiration (FNA) may give an additional benefit in the evaluation of primary lesions and regional lymph nodes.

Hepatoiminodiacetic Acid Scanning

Scanning with hepatoiminodiacetic acid (HIDA) is the procedure of choice for the diagnosis of acute cholecystitis. It is also useful for documenting the patency of any biliary–enteric anastomosis or for demonstrating the presence of a biliary fistula or emptying of the afferent limb in a gastroenterostomy. Nonvisualization of the gallbladder at 2 hours after injection is a reliable evidence of cystic duct obstruction, although in about 5% of patients gallbladders not visualized at this point may be visualized at 4 hours. Delayed visualization is indicative of chronic cholelithiasis and cholecystitis in 80% of patients. There are virtually no contraindications, and side effects are almost unknown. An HIDA scan followed by CCK administration is helpful for documenting biliary dyskinesia when gallbladder contraction accompanies typical biliary tract pain in patients without evidence of stones. Following infusion of CCK, measurements of the gallbladder ejection fraction (GBEF) (normal is >35%), gallbladder ejection period (GBEP) (normal is 8 to 12 minutes), gall-bladder latent period (GBLP) (normal is <3.0 minutes), and gallbladder ejection rate (GBER) (normal is 3.5% per minute) are performed. Abnormal values in association with reproduced pain suggest a high likelihood of symptomatic relief from cholecystectomy.

Cholangiography: Endoscopic Retrograde Cholangiopancreatography and Percutaneous Transhepatic Cholangiography

Cholangiography has remained the gold standard for diagnosis of biliary tree obstructive diseases. Endoscopic retrograde cholangiopancreatography (ERCP) is indicated for suspected obstructing lesions of the distal bile duct or the head of the pancreas. Many endoscopists believe that ERCP is the preferred procedure following ultrasonography when dilated ducts have been demonstrated. Others think that ERCP should follow ultrasonography regardless of ductal dilatation. When choledocholithiasis is suspected, ERCP followed by endoscopic papillotomy may be indicated. Contraindications include sensitivity to oral contrast and pyloric obstruction. Data suggest that Billroth II gastrectomy, acute pancreatitis, pancreatic pseudocyst, or known hepatitis antigen do not represent contraindications for ERCP.

Although it is safe in experienced hands, the incidence of complications with ERCP, especially when combined with papillotomy, is still significant. Acute pancreatitis is the most notable complication of ERCP and is seen in approximately 5% of the cases. Hyperamylasemia follows ERCP in 25% of patients, although it is usually of no clinical significance.

Percutaneous transhepatic cholangiography (PTC) is indicated in patients when endoscopic retrograde cholangiography (ERC) is not successful or the biliary tree proximal to a stricture was not adequately filled. In addition to its diagnostic value, PTC can be followed by placement of transhepatic catheters to assist in therapy, such as decompression of the biliary system, to provide guidance during surgical reconstruction, and to provide access for nonoperative dilation.

Intraoperative Cholangiography

Mirrizi reported the first series of intraoperative cholangiography (IOC) in the 1930s. The technique evolved from a painstaking and time-consuming procedure to a faster and more efficient procedure with the introduction of C-arm and fluoroscopy. IOC can be successfully preformed laparoscopically in 92% to 97% cases, adding only about 15 minutes to the original procedure. IOC has almost equal sensitivity and specificity rates of 80% to 98% for the detection of choledocholithiasis. These rates are comparable to the ERCP without the risk of pancreatitis. IOC is recommended for patients presenting with intermediate risk of having choledocholithiasis. Recent studies show that use of IOC along with laparoscopic cholecystectomy in these patients can decrease the length of stay and hospital expenses. An observed rate of 8% to 12% of CBD stones on IOC after ERCP (either due to false-negative rates of ERCP or passage of stone during the manipulation) further supports these recommendations.

GALLSTONE DISEASE AND MANAGEMENT

Gallstone disease is the most common biliary tract problem in the United Stated and is seen in 20 to 25 million Americans representing 10% to 15% of the adult population. Gallstones are classified by their composition varying from pure cholesterol, mixed cholesterol stones to black and brown pigmented stones. Cholesterol and black pigmented stones are formed in the gallbladder unlike brown pigmented stones, which are primary CBD stones formed due to infection, inflammation, and cholestasis. Most patients with cholesterol stones can be shown to have supersaturated bile. The relative proportion of cholesterol, phospholipids, and bile acids determines whether cholesterol is maintained in micellar solution or precipitates and forms the nidus for stone formation.

Asymptomatic Gallstones

About 50% to 70% of gallstones are asymptomatic when they are diagnosed. They have a benign natural history and a relatively low percentage (10% to 25%) progress to symptomatic cholelithiasis. The annual risk of developing biliary colic is insignificantly low (1% to 4%) when compared with symptomatic cholelithiasis with a risk of developing biliary colic as high as 50% annually. Development of life-threatening complications such as pancreatitis and cholangitis is very rare before the development of biliary pain in the first 5 years. It is now generally accepted that asymptomatic gallstones do not require treatment. Selective cholecystectomy is recommended in a subgroup of patients who are at higher risk for the development of symptoms, including transplant patients, patients with chronic hemolytic conditions, porcelain gallbladder, gallstones associated with a polyp of greater than 1 cm, and in certain ethnic groups (American Indians, Mexican Americans) who are at increased risk for the development of gallbladder cancer (Sakorafas et al.).

Laparoscopic Cholecystectomy

Laparoscopic cholecystectomy is a method of removing the gallbladder using laparoscopic techniques. In 1987, Phillip Mouret in France removed a diseased gallbladder during a laparoscopic gynecologic procedure. Indications are the same as for the open cholecystectomy and include symptomatic gallstones, gallstone pancreatitis, symptomatic gallbladder polyps, acute cholecystitis, and a calcified gallbladder wall.

Laparoscopic cholecystectomy has become the gold standard for the surgical management of gallstone disease. The ongoing quest for less invasive surgical management has evolved from traditional laparoscopic surgery into single incision (single incisions laparoscopic surgery [SILS]) and no incision (natural orifice transluminal endoscopic surgery [NOTES]) procedures (Chamberlain and Sakpal).

The basic principles are the same as for the open procedure. Limitations are a two-dimensional view, a field of vision limited to the view through the endoscope, and an abdomen that cannot be explored manually. Equipment includes a high-resolution camera, two video monitors, a high-intensity light source, a high-flow insufflator (6 L/min), and a cautery or laser device. Techniques of dissection use an electrosurgical hook, scissors, a spatula, a suction irrigator, and a cautery device or an Nd-YAG laser.

Absolute contraindications are portal hypertension and cirrhosis, major bleeding disorders, and sepsis with diffuse peritonitis. Relative contraindications are significant bowel distension, previous major upper abdominal surgery, obesity, and acute pancreatitis. Pregnancy was previously thought to be a contraindication, but recent reports have refuted this concept. Emphysematous cholecystitis and suspected gangrenous cholecystitis are also considered indications for open cholecystectomy.

A 5% to 10% conversion rate to open cholecystectomy usually reflects good surgical judgment. Reasons for conversion include bleeding, bile leak or bile duct injury, rupture of an empyema, instrument failure,

a thick-walled gallbladder, and an inability to correctly identify the anatomy. Open cholecystectomy represents a safety net for the surgeon and pressure to complete a laparoscopic procedure can lead to technical misadventures.

The major postoperative complications reported to require laparotomy are bleeding, CBD injury, biliary peritonitis, bowel perforation, sepsis, and subcapsular hematoma. Early large series have reported major complication rates well below 1%. Although the true incidence of bile duct injuries is not known, the incidence of complications appears to be related to the experience of the surgeon. Although initial reports from referral centers suggested a bile duct injury rate 5 to 10 times higher than that with the open technique, recent data report an injury rate equivalent to that with open cholecystectomy.

Options for management of common duct (CD) stones when found on cholangiography include (a) conversion to open CD exploration; (b) laparoscopic CD exploration via the cystic duct; (c) laparoscopic T-tube insertion, followed by closure and postoperative ERCP; and (d) close observation of small stones (<5 mm) in a nondilated duct. The appropriate choice depends on the operator's skill and experience with these procedures.

Acute cholecystitis can be managed laparoscopically. The gallbladder is decompressed with a needle for easier manipulation, and if possible a cholangiogram is obtained. Approximately one-third of patients require conversion to open cholecystectomy.

The main benefits of laparoscopic cholecystectomy are a shorter hospital stay (often ambulatory, <24 hours) and a shorter recovery. Most patients can return to normal activity by 1 week. Cosmesis is also significantly improved.

Several series comparing laser cautery have failed to show any advantage for laser dissection. In fact, operating time, costs, and perhaps rates of injury are greater with laser with a higher potential for technical misadventures.

Although we are entering an exciting new era of minimal access general surgery, it is important to remember that even with minimal access, the operations and potential for complications can be significant.

Medical Dissolution of Stones

Because cholecystectomy is a safe, effective, remarkably well-tolerated procedure, the role of medical dissolution of gallstones must be defined. Chenodeoxycholic acid and ursodeoxycholic acid have been approved for general use. The basic mechanism is to increase the bile acid pool and allow dissolution of gallstones. Criteria for treatment include (a) a functioning gallbladder, determined on an OCG; (b) nonradiopaque stones (mainly cholesterol); (c) no stones larger than 2 cm diameter; (d) no evidence of significant liver disease; (e) infrequent pain; and (f) no risk or anticipation of pregnancy during treatment.

Most patients require treatment for at least 1 year and many for 2 years. An OCG or ultrasound scan is obtained every 3 to 6 months. Lack of reduction in the size of the stones is considered treatment failure. About 8% to 10% of patients develop acute cholecystitis or other complications and require cholecystectomy while on treatment. By 5 years after termination of treatment, 50% of patients have been reported to re-form stones. Currently, oral dissolution is recommended only for patients who fulfill the above criteria and have a significant medical contraindication for cholecystectomy.

Extracorporeal Shock Wave Therapy

Acoustic energy properly focused may fragment biliary stones. Lithotripters generate longitudinal waves that are able to pass through the body and concentrate on stones. The goal is to fragment the stones into pieces small enough to proceed through the cystic duct and papilla of Vater. Oral dissoluting agents should be used as adjunctive therapy after the procedure. Repeated extracorporeal shock wave therapy (ESWL) may be necessary 4 to 6 weeks later if there are residual stones larger than 5 mm. The cost of the equipment, the need for repeated procedures, the need for dissolution agents, and the specific clinical indications and contraindications have limited the use of ESWL especially after the development of laparoscopic techniques.

Acute Cholecystitis

In 95% of patients, acute cholecystitis results from a stone obstructing the cystic duct. Acalculous cholecystitis most often accompanies conditions that result in significant inactivity of the gastrointestinal (GI) tract with biliary stasis. Bacterial contamination in cholecystitis is secondary and probably occurs via lymphatics. *Escherichia coli* is the most commonly found organism, followed by other enteric organisms, such as *Klebsiella*, *Proteus*, *Pseudomonas*, and *Streptococcus*

faecalis. Anaerobes are uncommon and usually produce mixed infections with aerobes; *Clostridium* is most common, and *Bacteroides* is rare.

Clinical resolution of acute cholecystitis can be accomplished in 85% of patients by GI rest, antibiotics, and intravenous fluid replacement. Acute free perforation occurs in 2%, most commonly diabetics. The HIDA scan is 95% accurate for demonstrating cystic duct obstruction. Ultrasonography may show ductal dilatation, stones, or thickening of the gallbladder wall, but it is not specific for cystic duct obstruction. Some degree of jaundice is noted in up to 25% of patients with acute cholecystitis. Bilirubin elevation as high as 8 mg may occur without the presence of stones in the CBD and may be due to pericholedochal edema and ampullary stasis.

Prompt cholecystectomy, within 24 to 48 hours, is generally accepted as the preferred treatment of acute cholecystitis. Diabetics should undergo surgery with more urgency. Significant sepsis with high fevers and shaking chills is rare and more suggestive of cholangitis. If a rapid response to fluids and antibiotics is not seen, surgery is performed without delay. A systemic meta-analysis review of all randomized controlled trials between early and delayed cholecystectomy showed no significant difference in complication and conversion rates (Gurusamy et al.).

Choledocholithiasis

The overall prevalence of CD stones in patients with symptomatic gallstones varies from 10% to 20% and most are secondary stones that have migrated from the gallbladder. Primary CBD stones are usually soft, ovoid, crumbling, and brown pigmented and are often associated with ampullary dysfunction, ductal parasite infections, or hemolytic disorders.

The most common predictive factors for the preoperative assessment of CD stones are age, elevated serum liver panel, and ultrasound findings. Although none are absolute, by using these predictive factors, patients can be categorized as having a low probability (5%), intermediate probability (5% to 50%), and high probability (>50%) for choledocholithiasis.

Low-probability patients are those with normal serum liver panel and normal ultrasonogram (USG) findings. These patients usually do not require any further evaluation. Patients at intermediate risk are those with age above 55 years, elevated serum liver panel, CBD dilatation, or recent history of biliary pancreatitis or acute cholecystitis. These patients should undergo further preoperative workup with MRCP or EUS followed by ERCP if positive for CD stones. Recent literature supports initial EUS evaluation for CBD stones before ERCP as it has a high accuracy rate and carries minimal risks of complications when compared with ERCP. High-risk patients for choledocholithiasis are those who present with cholangitis, CBD dilated greater than 6 mm, and ultrasound finding of CBD stone. These patients should undergo ERCP before cholecystectomy (Karakan et al.).

Indications for CBD exploration include a palpable impacted stone, ductal dilatation of more than 17 mm, a positive cholangiogram, primary choledochal stones, and clinical cholangitis. Other relative indications are multiple small calculi, elevation of bilirubin and alkaline phosphatase, and a history of jaundice. Using the above criteria, a palpable stone yields a positive exploration in 95%, a positive cholangiogram in 70%, clinical cholangitis in 70%, and dilatation of more than 17 mm in 50%. The generally reported incidence of postexploration retained stones is 5% to 10%. Several reports suggest that combining cholangiography with choledochoscopy for all duct explorations can reduce this incidence to near zero. Based on the current literature, there is no difference in mortality, morbidity, and complication rate between laparoscopic CBD exploration (LCBDE) and perioperative ERCP. In fact, it has been shown that patients who undergone cholecystectomy with LCBDE have shorter length of stay compared with patients undergoing laparoscopic cholecystectomy and perioperative ERCP (Frossard and Morel).

Choledochoduodenostomy

A CD with a diameter larger than 1.4 cm containing multiple stones is an indication for choledochoduodenostomy (CDD). In patients who meet these criteria, a CDD of at least 2.5 is safer than T-tube drainage and is associated with almost no long-term sequelae. Other indications for CDD include a benign distal stricture or a periampullary diverticulum. The morbidity and mortality of cholecystectomy are approximately doubled when CD exploration with T-tube insertion is added. Late cholangitis following CDD when the criteria for duct and stoma size are met is less than 5%. Postoperative evaluation of a CDD can be done when needed with HIDA scanning or an upper GI series.

Surgical sphincteroplasty should be reserved for an impacted distal stone in a duct smaller than 1.4 cm diameter. The complication rate is reported to be substantially higher for a sphincteroplasty than for CDD. Postoperative pancreatitis has been reported to occur in as many as 5% of cases. Failure to remove an impacted distal stone has not been shown to result in any long-term sequelae and should not be considered a contraindication for CDD.

The management of retained stones has now progressed to a point where few patients require reoperation. Flushing of T-tubes with materials ranging from chloroform to heparin solution has been tried and abandoned. Relaxation of the sphincter by local anesthetics and glucagon followed by vigorous flushing with saline may allow passage of stones up to 1 cm in size. Infusion with monoctanoin, a normal metabolic product of short-chain triglycerides may be successful, with reports indicating successful dissolution of cholesterol stones in up to 60% of cases. Infusion may be started as early as 1 week postoperatively and continued for up to 4 weeks. Side effects are minimal and can generally be controlled by reducing the rate of infusion.

After waiting a minimum of 4 weeks, mechanical extraction via the T-tube tract can be accomplished successfully via fluoroscopically controlled basket retrieval or under direct visualization with a flexible choledochoscope in 90% of patients. If unsuccessful, endoscopic papillotomy usually allows retrieval or passage. Fewer than 5% of patients with retained CD stones will ultimately require surgical removal.

Endoscopic Papillotomy

Endoscopic papillotomy is indicated in patients with postcholecystectomy choledocholithiasis or benign ampullary stenosis. Patients with symptomatic CD stones or cholangitis and with an intact gallbladder who are at poor risks for surgery have been treated with endoscopic papillotomy alone, with satisfactory results. Contraindications include hematologic disorders, stones larger than 2.5 cm in diameter, inability to locate the papilla, or a papilla located in a duodenal diverticulum. Biliary pancreatitis is not a contraindication. Although technically more difficult, patients have undergone successful papillotomy after a Billroth II gastrectomy. An international survey of a large number of patients undergoing papillotomy reported a 95% success rate, with an overall complication rate of 9%. The most frequent complication was hemorrhage, which generally is self-limited, requiring laparotomy in only 2% of cases. An overall mortality rate of approximately 1% was reported. Retroperitoneal air occurs in 10% of patients but usually does not require laparotomy. Other reported complications include cholangitis, especially after unsuccessful papillotomy, mild pancreatitis, and free perforation.

OTHER BILIARY TRACT PROBLEMS AND MANAGEMENT

Benign Biliary Strictures

Benign strictures constitute 25% of all biliary strictures; most commonly result from operative bile duct injuries. The other causes of biliary strictures are chronic pancreatitis, strictures after orthotopic liver transplant, and primary sclerosing cholangitis. The reported frequency of duct injuries varies from 1:300 to 1:500 cholecystectomies. The rate of injury during laparoscopic cholecystectomy was initially higher but is now thought to be equivalent to that seen with open surgery. Injuries most commonly result from inadequate demonstration of ductal anatomy or hazardous attempts to control bleeding without proper visualization. Bile duct anomalies are a far less common cause.

When recognized initially, management varies depending on whether the injury is circumferential or partial. Partial injuries are repaired and stented with a T-tube inserted via a separate choledochotomy using a limb of the tube as a splint. Most authors recommend leaving the tube in place for a minimum of 1 month. A circumferential injury may be managed by primary anastomosis with fine interrupted absorbable sutures, provided an adequate length can be obtained for a tension-free anastomosis. A T-tube stent through a separate choledochotomy is used and left in place for at least 4 to 6 weeks. If any doubt exists about the adequacy of a primary reanastomosis, a biliary intestinal anastomosis to a Roux-en-Y jejunal limb is undertaken. There is increasing evidence that initial management of bile duct injuries with Roux-en-Y jejunal anastomosis may yield superior results. The incidence of late stricture formation varies between 30% and 50% and usually occurs within 3 years. Late postoperative and other benign biliary strictures are usually treated endoscopically with stricture dilatation and multiple plastic stents placement (Gupta et al.).

CHOLANGITIS

Cholangitis is an acute bacterial infection within the biliary tree. Malignant strictures are considered to be the main cause of cholangitis, followed by choledocholithiasis, benign duct strictures, and sclerosing cholangitis. Biliary duct obstruction with bacterial contamination of the bile may lead to a clinical presentation known as *Charcot's triad* (fever with chills, jaundice, abdominal pain). The entire triad is found in 19% of patients. The diagnosis is based on clinical findings, an elevated white blood cell (WBC) count and liver function tests (LFTs), and ultrasonography and CT results. Endoscopic cholangiography or PTC is required in most patients to define the biliary pathology. The results of blood cultures are positive in 30% of patients with cholangitis, helping to identify the causative organism and guiding antibiotic treatment.

Traditionally, aminoglycosides can provide adequate coverage of gram-negative bacteria, with addition of ampicillin for *Enterococcus* and metronidazole or clindamycin for anaerobic pathogens such as *Bacteroides fragilis*. Endoscopic biliary decompression or transhepatic external drainage are preferable to surgical decompression and is indicated for approximately 30% of patients not responding to initial supportive therapy.

Primary Sclerosing Cholangitis

Most commonly associated with ulcerative colitis, sclerosing cholangitis may occur alone or, rarely, with other inflammatory bowel diseases. Although unproven, various bacterial or viral agents have been implicated. A characteristic pattern of diffuse ductal thickening, usually with intrahepatic and extrahepatic involvement, is evident. Surgical decompression is rarely possible. Steroids are of limited value, and antibiotics help only to control secondary bacterial cholangitis. There is some evidence that colectomy may result in alleviation of sclerosing cholangitis in patients with ulcerative colitis, but the overall prognosis is poor, with 90% undergoing progressive liver failure and death within 5 years. Liver transplant may be necessary.

Papillary Stenosis

Benign ampullary dysfunction and stenosis are associated with a dilated, often thickened CD. Typically, the patient has undergone cholecystectomy with a pain-free interval followed by the onset of right upper quadrant abdominal pain and abnormal liver chemistries. HIDA scan, ERCP, and transhepatic cholangiography are useful diagnostic tools. Endoscopic papillotomy is the initial treatment of benign papillary stenosis. If surgical treatment is required, CDD is usually performed.

Biliary Tumors

Benign biliary tumors include adenomyomatosis (also called Rokitansky–Aschoff sinuses, adenomyoma, or cholecystitis cystica), polyps, and sessile mucosal tumors (adenomas and papillomas). They are most commonly diagnosed on an ultrasound scan or by oral cholecystography. Cholecystectomy is indicated if the tumors produce biliary symptoms or are associated with gallstones or a gallbladder polyp of more than 10 mm.

At cholecystectomy, 1% to 2% of patients, usually aged 65 years or older, are found to have carcinoma of the gallbladder. About 70% to 80% of gallbladder carcinomas occur in older patients with a long history of gallstone disease (usually >10 years). It is the most common biliary tract neoplasm and the fifth most common malignancy in the digestive tract. Porcelain gallbladder (calcification of the gallbladder wall), when seen on a plain abdominal film, should be considered a premalignant state and is an indication for cholecystectomy. In patients older than 50 years with symptomatic gallstones for 10 years or more, the risk of carcinoma is as high as 6%. The female/male ratio is 3:1.

No diagnostic modality can reliably distinguish symptomatic chronic cholelithiasis from gallbladder carcinoma. Sonography and CT may suggest malignancy, but their accuracy is still questionable. Radical surgery, including wedge resection of adjacent liver and hepatic lobectomy, has been suggested but has not been proven to provide significant cure rates. The prognosis is poor: 80% of patients die within 1 year, and the 5-year survival is only 2% to 5%.

Bile Duct Carcinoma/Extrahepatic Cholangiocarcinoma

Bile duct carcinoma is a relatively rare tumor with annual incidence of 1 to 2 cases per 100,000 in the Western countries. The peak age for CCA is around the seventh decade with slight male preponderance. Different types of histological patterns have been described, among which mucin-producing adenocarcinoma type is the most common. Macroscopically they are classified as sclerosing, nodular, or papillary. About 80% of the CCAs are the sclerosing type with intense desmoplastic reaction. Risk factors for CCA include primary sclerosing cholangitis, intrahepatic biliary stones, Caroli's disease, congenital fibropolycystic disease, and liver fluke parasite infection. Chronic exposure to environmental toxins such as dioxins and consumption of alcohol can also increase the risk of CCA.

TABLE 5.1	Bismuth–Corlette Classification
Type I	Tumor involving common hepatic duct (CHD)
Type II	Tumor involving CHD and the junction of right and left hepatic duct
Type IIIa	Tumor involving confluence of the CHD with extension to the right hepatic duct
Type IIIb	Tumor involving confluence of the CHD with extension to the left hepatic duct
Type IV	Tumor involving confluence of the CHD with bilateral extension to the ducts

Based on the location and extent of distant spread, CCA are classified by Bismuth–Corlette classification (see Table 5.1) and TNM staging, respectively. Discussion about their classification is beyond the scope of this chapter. Often CCA patients present with jaundice, pruritus, weight loss, and sometimes abdominal pain. Surgery remains the mainstay treatment for patient suffering from resectable CCA. Preoperative workup includes ultrasonogram, EUS/ERCP, and MRCP to determine the respectability of the tumor. The proximal common hepatic duct, including the hilum and hepatic ducts (Klatskin's tumor), accounts for 40% to 50% of these tumors. *En bloc* resection with liver resection is occasionally possible. Palliation with some form of biliary stent, usually a T-tube, is usually required. Although survival beyond 12 to 24 months is uncommon, distant metastases are rare, and prolonged benefit may be obtained by intubation (Zografos et al.).

Tumors of the mid and distal bile ducts are less common. Mid-duct tumors can occasionally be resected with reconstruction via Roux-en-Y hepaticojejunostomy. Distal bile duct tumors require pancreaticoduodenectomy (Whipple resection), after which a 20% to 30% 5-year survival can be attained. The role of adjuvant chemotherapy and radiation therapy is still controversial, with conflicting data on survival rates. Currently there is no curative adjuvant and neoadjuvant therapy available.

Biliary Cysts

Choledochal cysts are uncommon. They are usually seen in children, although they can appear in adults. The classic symptom complex consisting of abdominal pain, jaundice, and a palpable abdominal mass is present in only 0% to 17% of cases. Among pediatric patients, the most common presenting features are cholangitis, pancreatitis, and biliary peritonitis from cyst rupture. Among adults, choledochal cysts are often incidental findings on imaging. A modified classification of choledochal cysts by Todani et al. has described five categories. Type I is a fusiform dilation of the CBD and it is the most commonly reported type. Type II is a saccular diverticulum of the CBD. Type III is cystic dilatation of the intramural portion of the CBD (choledochocele). Type IV is the second most common and represents both intrahepatic and extrahepatic dilatation of the biliary tree. Type V is also known as Caroli's disease presents with multiple intrahepatic biliary dilatations. Ultrasonography used as the primary diagnostic modality can outline the cyst in most cases. Additional information can be obtained from CT, transhepatic cholangiography, and ERCP. Complications include infection, malignant degeneration, and rarely rupture.

Bile duct malignancy in association with choledochal cysts is 20 times more common than malignancy in the general population and is almost uniformly fatal. Traditionally, only Roux-en-Y bypass was the preferred treatment when resection was considered too risky. An awareness of the increased risk of malignancy combined with better surgical techniques has led to current recommendations for resection of the cyst with Roux-en-Y reconstruction.

Biliary Fistulas

External biliary fistulas most commonly occur after biliary tract surgery. They are easily documented with HIDA scanning. Anatomic delineation should be accomplished with ERCP, transhepatic cholangiography, or fistulography. These procedures determine the presence or absence of distal obstruction. If no distal obstruction is seen, the fistulas will generally close with local control and adequate nutrition. Uncontrollable sepsis or distal obstruction (e.g., stone, stricture) require surgical intervention.

An internal bile leak following laparoscopic cholecystectomy is suspected when patients develop fever, pain, and abnormal liver chemistries, usually within 24 hours of surgery. Initial confirmation with an HIDA scan should be followed by ERCP with stenting. If a leaking cystic duct is the cause, no further intervention is indicated and additional surgery is usually not required.

Cholecystoenteric fistulas from gallstones occur to the duodenum and less commonly to the stomach, colon, or small intestine. Gallstone ileus may result from obstruction at the ligament of Treitz, terminal ileum (most common), or sigmoid colon. Most patients with cholecystoenteric fistulas have air in the biliary tree. Obstructing stones are at least 2.5 cm in diameter. In the United States, gallstone ileus comprises 2% of mechanical intestinal obstruction. It remains controversial as to whether a cholecystectomy should be undertaken at the time of laparotomy for stone extraction in the presence of gallstone ileus. There is general agreement, however, that if another large stone is present in the gallbladder, the stone must at least be removed.

Hemobilia

Hemorrhage through the biliary tract is most commonly due to blunt or penetrating trauma. Ascarides is common in the Orient but rare in Western countries. Gallstone disease, primary biliary tract malignancies, true or false intrahepatic aneurysms, or iatrogenic causes (PTC or removal of stones high in the biliary tree) are reported causes of hemobilia. The most common presenting symptom is melena followed by colicky pain, anemia, hematemesis, jaundice, shock, and fever. The diagnosis is established by endoscopic visualization of bleeding from the ampulla, and the site is best confirmed by angiography.

Treatment consists of arteriography and embolization or suture of false aneurysms or traumatic tears. Cholecystectomy should be performed when the gallbladder is found to be the source of bleeding. In most instances, hepatic artery ligation with intrahepatic suture, if needed, can control the bleeding. Hepatic resection is rarely needed.

QUESTIONS

Select one answer.
1. Which of the following is true?
   a. The cystic duct, common hepatic duct, and cystic artery form the triangle of Calot.
   b. The venous drainage of the gallbladder does not empty into the portal circulation
   c. In most cases, the hepatic artery passes cephalad within the hepatoduodenal ligament to the right of the bile duct and anterior to the portal vein.
   d. In 20% of patients the cystic artery originates from the left or common hepatic artery.
   e. All of the above

2. Acute cholecystitis is best diagnosed by which of the following imaging studies:
   a. Ultrasonography.
   b. CT scan.
   c. MRCP.
   d. HIDA scanning.
   e. Elevated direct plasma bilirubin.

3. Primary sclerosing cholangitis is most often associated with which of the following disorders:
   a. Crohn's disease.
   b. Diabetes mellitus.
   c. Rheumatoid arthritis.
   d. Ulcerative colitis.
   e. Chronic pancreatitis.

4. Which of the following are accepted indications for cholecystectomy ?
   a. Porcelain gallbladder.
   b. Gallbladder polyp measuring greater than 10 mm.
   c. Asymptomatic cholelithiasis.
   d. a and b.
   e. b and c.

5. Which of the following statements are true?
   a. In the setting of acute cholecystitis early cholecystectomy has a higher complication rate than does delayed cholecystectomy.
   b. EUS is less sensitive than ERCP for the detection of choledocholithiasis.
   c. The sensitivity of HIDA scan decreases with elevated bilirubin of greater than 7 mg/dL.
   d. None of the above.
   e. All of the above.

6. Which of the following does not stimulate bile flow?
   a. Cholecystokinin.
   b. Bile salts.
   c. Vagal stimulation.
   d. Splanchnic stimulation.
   e. Secretin.

7. Which of the following statements regarding choledochal cysts is *not* true?
   a. The most common type of cholechochal cyst is type III.
   b. Cholangiocarcinoma risk is increased in the presence of a choledochal cyst.

   c. Most adult choledochal cysts are diagnosed incidentally.
   d. The best surgical procedure for the management of choledochal cysts is resection and reconstruction with a Roux-en-Y biliary enteric anastomosis.

8. All of the following increase the risk for cholangiocarcinoma except:
   a. Choledochal cyst.
   b. Liver fluke infection.
   c. Caroli's disease.
   d. Dioxins.
   e. History of gallstones for less than 10 years.

9. Which of the following is the most common type of gallstone:
   a. Pure cholesterol stones.
   b. Mixed cholesterol stones.
   c. Brown pigment stones.
   d. Black pigment stones.

10. A 55-year-old man presents with hematemesis associated with abdominal pain and melena. His past medical history is significant for asthma, pancreatitis, and previous motor vehicle accident. Laboratory values are significant for hematocrit 23, WBC 8.0 k/UL, platelets 450.0 k/UL, total bilirubin 3.5 mg/dL, direct bilirubin 1.5 mg/dL, alkaline phosphatase 180U/L, AST 45 U/L, ALT 34 U/L. Ultrasonography revealed a distended gallbladder with sludge. The most likely diagnosis is:
   a. Acute cholecystitis.
   b. Peptic ulcer disease.
   c. Hemobilia.
   d. Portal gastropathy.
   e. Mallory–Weiss tear.

REFERENCES

Ando H. Embryology of the biliary tract. *Dig Surg* 2010;27(2): 87–89.

Chamberlain RS, Sakpal SV. A comprehensive review of single-incision laparoscopic surgery (SILS) and natural orifice transluminal endoscopic surgery (NOTES) techniques for cholecystectomy. *J Gastrointest Surg* 2009;13:1733–1740.

Frossard JL, Morel PM. Detection and management of bile duct stones. *Gastrointest Endosc* 2010;72(4):808–816.

Gupta R, Rao GV, Reddy DN. Benign biliary stricture—should they be dilated or treated surgically? *Indian J Gastroenterol* 2006:25(4):202–205.

Gurusamy K, Samraj K, Gluud C, et al. Meta-analysis of randomized controlled trials on the safety and effectiveness of early versus delayed laparoscopic cholecystectomy for acute cholecystitis. *Br J Surg* 2010;97:141–150.

Karakan T, Cindoruk M, Alagozlu H, et al. EUS versus endoscopic retrograde cholangiography for patients with intermediate probability of bile duct stones: a prospective randomized trial. *Gastrointest Endosc* 2009;69: 244–252.

Metcalfe MS, Wemyss-Holden SA, Maddern GJ. Management dilemmas with choledochal cysts. *Arch Surg* 2003;138: 333–339.

Reitz S, Slam K, Chambers LW. Biliary: pancreatic, and hepatic imaging for the general surgeon. *Surg Clin North Am* 2011;91:59–92.

Sakorafas GH, Milingos D, Peros G. Asymptomatic cholelithiasis: is cholecystectomy really indicated? A critical reappraisal 15 years after the introduction of laparoscopic cholecystectomy. *Dig Dis Sci* 2007;52:1313–1325.

Stinton LM, Myers RP, Shaffer EA. Epidemiology of gallstones. *Gastroenterol Clin North Am* 2010;39(2):157–169.

Zografos GN, Farfaras A, Zagouri F, et al. Cholangiocarcinoma: principles and current trends. *Hepatobiliary Pancreat Dis Int* 2011;10:10–20.

The Pancreas

ANATOMY AND PHYSIOLOGY

The pancreas is a centrally located, retroperitoneal organ with both endocrine and exocrine functions. The celiac and superior mesenteric arteries (SMAs) provide arterial inflow to the pancreas. The gastroduodenal artery provides the major inflow to the head of the pancreas, whereas the splenic artery is responsible for most of the inflow to the body and tail. The superior pancreaticoduodenal artery originates from the proximal SMA and provides additional inflow to the head of the pancreas. Venous drainage of the pancreas is via the portal circulation: splenic vein for the tail and the portomesenteric vein for the head.

The exocrine secretions of the pancreas are drained by two ductal systems, the main duct (MD) of Wirsung and accessory duct of Santorini. The main and accessory ducts may drain independently into the intestine or fuse to create a common channel for biliary and pancreatic secretions (ampulla of Vater). In embryonic development, the pancreas is formed from the rotation and fusion of a dorsal and ventral foregut outpouching, at approximately 7 weeks of gestation. The dorsal pancreatic forebud accounts for the majority of the pancreas (body and tail), whereas the ventral bud accounts for the uncinate (posterior portion of the pancreatic head). Failure of fusion, known as "pancreatic divisum," may result in the bulk of the pancreatic parenchyma draining through the minor duct, resulting in inadequate ductal drainage of the main body of the pancreas and recurrent pancreatitis.

The exocrine pancreas is composed of acinar cells which produce enzymes needed for digestion, dissolved in 1 to 2 L/day of bicarbonate rich fluid. Pancreatic secretion is regulated by complex neurohumoral mechanisms. There are three phases of pancreatic response to a meal: cephalic phase (mediated by the vagus nerve), gastric phase (mediated by gastrin), and the intestinal phase (induced by acidification of the duodenum). The primary humoral factors are secretin and cholecystokinin (CCK), both produced by duodenal enterocytes in response to fat and protein. Secretin induces pancreatic fluid secretion and CCK promotes release of digestive enzymes. Enzymes are released in an inactive proenzyme state to prevent autolytic digestion in the pancreas. Activation of trypsin by duodenal enteropeptidase triggers the cascade leading to activation of other proenzymes.

ACUTE PANCREATITIS

Acute pancreatitis is an inflammatory condition of the pancreas, which can range, in severity, from mild to life threatening. More than 90% of acute pancreatitis cases in the United States are caused by either gallstones or alcohol ingestion. In gallstone pancreatitis, the mechanism of injury is ductal obstruction caused by passage of stones through the ampulla of Vater. The pathogenesis of pancreatitis is thought to be related to activation of trypsinogen within the pancreas causing autolysis, either by ductal obstruction, direct toxic injury to the acinar cells, or by abnormal transport and packaging of proenzymes in the acinar cells. The exact mechanism of alcohol-induced pancreatitis is uncertain, though it has been postulated that alcohol may cause dysfunctional CCK-mediated transport of zymogen granules in pancreatic acinar cells, in addition to direct toxic effects (1).

Other known causes of pancreatitis include iatrogenic injury during endoscopic retrograde cholangiopancreatography (ERCP), hyperlipidemia, and medications. Common medications that have been associated with pancreatitis include thiazide diuretics, azathioprine, and furosemide. Infectious etiologies include viral syndromes (mumps, coxsackie, and cytomegalovirus) and parasites (Ascaris, Clonorchis).

Clinical Syndrome and Presentation

Patients typically exhibit epigastric abdominal pain radiating to the back. Symptoms range from a feeling of discomfort and "dyspepsia" to an incapacitating, unrelenting, boring pain. Mild pancreatitis is usually self-limiting and associated with pancreatic edema on imaging studies. In severe pancreatitis, widespread activation of pancreatic enzymes results in autodigestion, pancreatic necrosis, local and systemic inflammatory cytokine activation, and microcirculatory disturbances with capillary leak.

Clinical signs include leukocytosis, hypovolemia and shock, acidosis, acute respiratory distress syndrome (ARDS), and disseminated intravascular coagulation. Hypocalcemia may complicate severe pancreatitis as a result of fat necrosis and precipitation of calcium. Serum amylase and lipase levels are often elevated in acute pancreatitis but do not reflect severity. Amylase may also be elevated in parotitis, perforated viscous, and ectopic pregnancy.

Ranson et al.'s criteria (2) has been utilized to score severity at initial presentation (Table 6.1), though several more recent ICU-based scoring systems such as APACHE II are useful in predicting mortality after initial presentation (3,4). Patients with APACHE II scores greater than 8, complicated by multisystem organ failure, are at greatest risk for mortality, especially when the organ failure persists for more than 48 hours. Overall mortality of acute pancreatitis is approximately 5%, though severe pancreatitis with organ failure is associated with a mortality exceeding 30%.

Diagnosis of acute pancreatitis is based on clinical syndrome with supportive laboratory values, which should include complete blood cell count, coagulation profile, electrolytes including calcium and phosphorus, serum amylase, lipase, and liver function tests. Patients with acute epigastric pain and abnormal amylase in the setting of appropriate history (alcohol ingestion, known gallstones, recent ERCP) may be managed with simple bowel rest and intravenous fluids until symptoms resolve.

Patients with suspected pancreatitis should undergo imaging to document the presence of gallstones, to exclude choledocholithiasis (especially with abnormal liver enzymes), and to image the pancreas. Abdominal imaging is routine for most patients with abdominal pain who present to the emergency department. Although sonography is the optimal imaging study for gallstone disease, sonographic visualization of the pancreas is difficult due to overlying bowel gas, so most patients with suspected pancreatitis undergo computed tomography (CT).

Following initial resuscitation with crystalloid to restore functional extracellular fluid volume and maintain organ perfusion, patients with ongoing suspected clinical pancreatitis should be imaged with a dynamic contrast-enhanced CT scan with fine cuts through the pancreas (pancreatic protocol), to document the presence of pancreatic necrosis. Timing and rate of the iodinated contrast bolus is extremely important in obtaining high-quality pancreatic imaging, and the radiologist should be alerted to the purpose of the exam to properly protocol the study (5). In more severe pancreatitis, admission to a monitored setting is advisable for fluid resuscitation and surveillance for multiorgan dysfunction (6). Contrast-enhanced CT scan should be delayed until after restoration of hemodynamic stability and renal perfusion, to avoid contrast-induced exacerbation of pancreatitis and acute tubular necrosis. If the diagnosis of pancreatitis is uncertain and the patient is not a candidate to receive intravenous contrast due to acute renal dysfunction, an initial noncontrast CT scan may be useful in documenting pancreatic edema.

Although infection is the principal late cause of morbidity and mortality in severe pancreatitis, prophylactic antibiotic therapy has not been shown to be of value (7). Routine use of nasogastric decompression is unnecessary in mild or uncomplicated transient pancreatitis, but severe or complicated pancreatitis often requires gastric decompression because of gastric ileus. Patients with severe pancreatitis have elevated metabolic needs and are often unable to meet adequate caloric intake due to gut dysfunction. Nutritional support is generally difficult in acutely ill, unstable patients, but

TABLE 6.1	**Ranson's Criteria of Severity of Acute Pancreatitis**

Present on admission:
  Age > 55 years
  White blood cell count > 16,000/μL
  Blood glucose > 200 mg/dL
  Serum lactate dehydrogenase > 350 I.U/L
  SGOT (AST) > 250 I.U/dL
Developing during first 48 h:
  Hematocrit fall > 10%
  Blood urea nitrogen increase > 8 mg/dL
  Serum Ca^{2+} < 8 mg/dL
  Arterial PO_2 < 60 mmHg
  Base deficit < 4 mEq/L
  Estimated fluid sequestration > 600 mL

after resuscitation and hemodynamic stability is achieved, early and aggressive nutritional intervention should be a standard part of management. Nutritional intervention is best accomplished enterally, though when the enteric route is unavailable due to ileus, parenteral nutrition is an acceptable alternative (8).

Routine use of somatostatin and other inhibitors of pancreatic secretion has not been proven to be of value. Antiproteases have also been studied extensively in animal and clinical studies, though no benefit has been shown to date in altering the natural history of acute pancreatitis in humans, possibly because once clinical signs are present, the tissue damage has already happened.

In summary, aggressive support of circulation, initial bowel rest, early intervention for organ failure, surveillance and selective surgical intervention for infection, and nutritional support have emerged as consensus treatment guidelines. Early support of multisystem failure includes ventilatory support for hypoxemia or evolving ARDS and early renal replacement therapy to correct metabolic derangements and fluid overload exacerbated by renal failure.

Necrotizing Pancreatitis

Severe acute pancreatitis may be complicated by necrosis of variable portions of the pancreas. Diagnosis is based on nonvisualization of portions of the pancreas on dynamic contrast CT scan. Necrosis is associated with a dramatic increase in mortality: most deaths in patients with acute pancreatitis occur in the presence of necrotizing pancreatitis. In some cases, necrotic pancreas may become superinfected, resulting in infected pancreatic necrosis (IPN). IPN is confirmed by fine needle aspiration (FNA) of the necrotic area to assess microbiology (gram stain and culture). Clinical diagnosis of IPN may also be made without FNA confirmation and in fact may be preferable given the risks associated with needle aspiration, especially in patients already treated with empiric antibiotics.

Persistent fevers, bacteremia and clinical deterioration in the presence of known necrotizing pancreatitis, or CT evidence of air suggestive of infection are highly suggestive of infection. Early surgical intervention is unhelpful in sterile necrotizing pancreatitis; indeed, early laparotomy may increase mortality. The general trend is toward less aggressive surgical intervention, especially early in the disease process (9,10). However, in the presence of documented or suspected IPN, surgical intervention is clearly indicated. Timing of surgical intervention remains a matter of debate, with some centers advocating delayed laparotomy and initial treatment

with antibiotics even with documented IPN (11). Regardless of timing, once a decision to proceed with surgery has been made, the goals of surgical intervention are debridement of devitalized pancreatic tissue and large bore drainage of the pancreatic bed. Large bore drainage catheters are useful in that they permit evacuation of large particle debris and facilitate drainage of pancreatic fistulae, which commonly complicate debridement. Drainage alone without debridement of devitalized tissue is less successful and should be avoided.

Biliary Pancreatitis

The diagnosis of biliary pancreatitis is based on clinical findings including the presence of gallstones or common duct stones, biliary dilation, and elevated liver enzymes suggestive of biliary obstruction. A threefold increase in alanine aminotransferase 24 to 48 hours after onset of symptoms has a 95% positive predictive value for biliary pancreatitis. Most patients undergo imaging to confirm the diagnosis: initial ultrasound and in some cases magnetic resonance cholangiopancreatography (MRCP). Most cases of gallstone pancreatitis are self-limited. Cholecystectomy is indicated during the same hospitalization or soon after discharge (once pancreatitis has resolved) because there is an approximately 50% risk of recurrent pancreatitis within 3 months.

Routine preoperative ERCP is not required prior to cholecystectomy if liver enzymes have normalized, though a history of biliary pancreatitis is an indication for intraoperative cholangiography. When there is a lack of normalization of liver enzymes, jaundice, or documented choledocholithiasis on initial sonography or MRCP, preoperative ERCP is reasonable after resolution of pancreatitis (12). In severe biliary pancreatitis, suspected cholangitis, or biliary obstruction by an impacted stone (rising liver enzymes and ductal dilation), early endoscopic decompression within 24 hours of presentation may reduce morbidity (13).

PANCREATIC PSEUDOCYST AND ABSCESS

Localized peripancreatic fluid collections are common in severe acute pancreatitis. Approximately half of these fluid collections resolve spontaneously, while the remainder may become infected or evolved into pseudocysts (14). Pseudocysts lack a true epithelial lining and may be associated with disruption of the pancreatic ductal system, which must be taken into account when considering drainage. The traditional teaching that asymptomatic cysts more than 6 cm should undergo operative drainage after 6 weeks of observation is based on a study of 93 patients by Cheruvu et al. in 1979 (15): 40% of early fluid collections resolved spontaneously following an episode of acute pancreatitis. However, in patients followed for more than 12 weeks, no spontaneous resolutions were observed and the risk of complications increased dramatically. Major complications of pseudocysts include GI obstruction, bleeding, and infection, which occur in approximately 9% of patients treated with initial observation (16). Subsequent studies have suggested that resolution is also a function of cyst size, with smaller cysts (<6 cm) having a greater likelihood of resolution.

More recently, there has been a trend toward more expectant management in asymptomatic cysts following acute pancreatitis, reserving intervention for cyst growth with serial imaging or the interval development of symptoms during observation. There is also a growing experience using laparoscopic and endoscopic drainage of pseudocysts. External drainage is associated with a high failure rate and should not be considered first-line therapy unless the pseudocysts are secondarily infected before maturation. Percutaneous approaches are preferable when external drainage is required, though if the cyst is inaccessible, an open approach may be required. Bleeding into a cyst may reflect erosion of the cyst into a pseudoaneurysm, as the pancreatic enzymes in the cyst fluid dissolve the arterial wall. Mortality associated with bleeding is high, ranging from 40% to 80%. Initial treatment is rapid resuscitation and immediate angiographic evaluation and embolization.

In symptomatic or growing noninfected pseudocysts, internal drainage is the treatment of choice. Internal drainage is accomplished with anastomosis of the cyst wall to the GI tract: cyst gastrostomy, cyst enterostomy, and cyst duodenostomy are all options based on the location of the cyst. Cyst gastrostomies are ideal for large lesser sac cysts that bulge the posterior stomach wall. Cyst duodenostomies are best performed via a transduodenal approach when possible, rather than a side-to-side cyst-duodenal anastomosis, which has a higher rate of leakage. When a cyst enterostomy is appropriate, a tension-free anastomosis may require a Roux en Y limb of defunctionalized jejunum (17). There is an increasing experience with endoscopic drainage of pseudocysts via transgastric or transduodenal placement of stents. Decision-making endoscopic versus open drainage should be based on size and location of the cyst and experience of the endoscopist.

PANCREATIC FISTULAE AND ASCITES

Free rupture of a localized peripancreatic fluid collection or ductal disruption may present as ascites. Peritonitis may be present, but is not a uniform finding. The location of the disruption may influence the location of the subsequent fluid collection: posterodistal ductal disruptions may present as retroperitoneal fluid and pleural effusions rather than free ascites. Initial management of both ascites and pancreatic pleural effusions is drainage, usually percutaneous. Subsequent management of pancreatic fistulae is primarily supportive: attention to fluid and electrolyte status, initial bowel rest until there is normal GI function, and nutrition, which in some cases may require chronic parenteral nutrition. Delineation of ductal anatomy is important in management of pancreatic fistulae that fail to resolve within 2 to 4 weeks.

Ductal anatomy may be assessed noninvasively by MRCP, or through direct pancreatography via ERCP. ERCP offers the benefit of potential therapeutic intervention as well, including sphincterotomy and pancreatic duct stenting to decompress the duct and promote healing of the disruption. Octreotide may be useful in reducing the volume of pancreatic secretions, which may reduce fluid and electrolyte losses, but there is no clear evidence that octreotide shortens the time to closure of pancreatic fistulae. Failure of prolonged conservative therapy and ERCP decompression of pancreatic fistula may ultimately require operative approaches. Elective surgical options include distal pancreatectomy for ductal injuries in the body and tail and Roux en Y enteric drainage of the fistula for locations in the head (10).

CHRONIC PANCREATITIS

Inflammation associated with acute pancreatitis can sometimes lead to pancreatic fibrosis and stricture of the pancreatic duct. The exact trigger for chronic pancreatitis is uncertain, as even a single episode of acute pancreatitis can evolve into the chronic form; however, it has been postulated that additional insults (alcohol) during the recovering phase of acute pancreatitis may trigger a cascade leading to fibrosis (18). Indeed, the vast majority of chronic pancreatitis cases are associated with alcohol.

Chronic inflammatory changes seem to predominate in the pancreatic head compared with other regions and the disease process may involve local structures including the distal common bile duct, duodenum, and portal vein (PV). Distal biliary stricture may result in jaundice or pruritus, whereas duodenal stricture may result in symptoms of gastric outlet obstruction. Intractable pain, however, is the most common presenting symptom of chronic pancreatitis. The chronic pain associated with chronic pancreatitis may be severe and disabling, sometimes requiring lifelong narcotics. Pancreatic enzyme insufficiency and loss of islet function leading to diabetes are also associated signs of chronic pancreatitis.

Evaluation of CP includes contrast-enhanced cross-sectional imaging and pancreatic ductography (MRCP or ERCP) to evaluate the pattern of pancreatic ductal obstruction. More recently, endoscopic ultrasonography has also emerged as a tool to investigate and stage CP. Initial management is generally conservative, with analgesia, dietary counseling, pancreatic enzyme replacement, and abstinence from alcohol. Operation is indicated with failure of medical management, or when malignancy is suspected, which can be very difficult to differentiate in patients with head of pancreas inflammation. Patients with suspected head of pancreas cancer should undergo preoperative staging and endoscopic ultrasound (EUS) evaluation, followed by pancreaticoduodenectomy (PD) (either traditional or pylorus preserving) as the procedure of choice.

Drainage procedures to decompress the pancreatic duct through an enteric anastomosis are options in patients with proximal pancreatic ductal stenosis and dilation of the pancreatic duct in the body and tail, especially when there is minimal inflammation. Endoscopic decompression of the obstructed pancreatic duct is also possible, though open surgical drainage has been associated with better pain control (and with higher morbidity). Most gastroenterologists prefer an initial trial of endoscopic drainage, which does not preclude later surgical options, especially when there is a single-accessible obstruction with proximal dilation. Surgical options for pancreatic ductal drainage include the procedure described by Puestow in 1956, though this operation has subsequently been modified. Current drainage options include the Partingon Rochelle procedure (lateral longitudinal pancreaticojejunostomy) and the Frey procedure (addition of a partial head of pancreas resection in a Partingon Rochelle procedure).

Prior to surgical drainage procedures for chronic pancreatitis, EUS sampling of dilated pancreatic duct fluid is of value to exclude intrapancreatic papillary mucinous neoplasms (IPMNs), which can often present in a similar fashion. Distal pancreatectomy up to a subtotal resection has also been utilized for chronic pancreatitis but with variable results in improving symptoms. More recently, Sutherland and colleagues at the University of Minnesota have argued that total pancreatectomy and islet autotransplantation is a more definitive therapy for CP (18). This approach requires facilities for immediate islet isolation and infusion, and the experience is at present very limited at only a handful of centers.

PANCREATIC TUMORS

Adenocarcinoma

Adenocarcinoma of the pancreas is the fifth leading cause of cancer deaths in the United States. Overall survival of patients with pancreatic cancer is dismal, with 5-year survival of only 20% even with curative resection and uniform mortality in patients unable to undergo resection. Median survival of patients with locally advanced disease is 6 to 10 months, whereas patients with metastatic disease or carcinomatosis can expect median survival of only 3 to 6 months. Pancreatic cancer frequently recurs locally after resection, which is why there has been intense interest in neoadjuvant and adjuvant multimodality therapy (chemoradiation) in reducing local failure rates. Adjuvant therapy has been shown to prolong survival after PD and should be considered in all patients who undergo curative resection. The benefit of neoadjuvant therapy prior to resection is less certain, though there is emerging evidence that some subsets of patients may benefit with preoperative therapy.

The classical presentation of pancreatic cancer is painless jaundice, though jaundice may occur in only 50% of patients. Patients without jaundice may present with larger, more locally advanced tumors due to the lack of symptoms leading to diagnosis. Advanced tumors may be associated with pain due to neural involvement, gastric outlet obstruction, pancreatitis, exocrine insufficiency due to pancreatic ductal obstruction, and cachexia. Ascites may indicate carcinomatosis.

Evaluation of painless jaundice usually begins with sonography and serologic testing to exclude benign causes such as stone disease or liver parenchymal disease. Further evaluation requires contrast-enhanced dynamic CT scan with thin pancreaticobiliary cuts. If a mass is visualized, resectability is assessed based on CT criteria. Criteria for resectability include disease limited to the pancreas, patency of the superior mesenteric vein (SMV) and PV, and absence of involvement of the SMA or celiac axis. Abutment of the SMV/PV or hepatic artery without encasement (<180 degrees circumference) suggests a high likelihood of leaving positive margins with resection and are therefore considered borderline resectable. Patients with borderline resectable lesions should be considered for enrollment in neoadjuvant trials designed to improve rates of R0 (complete) resection. If a mass is not visualized on CT, EUS is indicated. EUS with FNA for histologic confirmation is also indicated when patients are deemed unresectable by CT criteria, or the patient fits criteria for enrollment in a neoadjuvant trial.

In patients who are not candidates for initial surgical resection, endoscopic biliary decompression is indicated. Routine biliary decompression for resectable patients is *not* considered standard of care, provided that the operation can proceed in a timely fashion. Both plastic and metal/covered stents are options when biliary decompression is required, each with their own advantages and disadvantages. When future surgery is felt to be a potential option after initial chemoradiation, plastic stents may be preferable but require regular replacement, usually every 3 months.

Operative Management of Head of Pancreas Cancer

Pancreaticoduodenectomy (PD or Whipple procedure) remains the principal curative intervention for patients with tumors involving the head of the pancreas. Overall morbidity associated with PD is approximately 30%, though operative mortality at experienced centers is less than 2%. The goal of operation is an R0 en bloc resection; consequently, the preoperative and intraoperative planning in PD is based on a stepwise approach to confirm resectability. Initial laparoscopy may be of value to exclude carcinomatosis when resectability is in question, though laparoscopy is of limited value in assessing vascular involvement. Local regional lymph node involvement is not considered a contraindication to resection, though it is a poorer prognostic sign. Extensive lymphadenectomy beyond the peripancreatic lymphatics has not been shown to prolong survival and may increase morbidity.

Initial exposure for PD can be accomplished through either a bisubcostal or midline incision, depending on body habitus. Mechanical retractors are useful in exposure. The pancreas is widely exposed through the gastrocolic omentum and by Kocher maneuver to mobilize the duodenum and uncinate process. The root of the mesentery is inspected and palpated to assess direct extension of inferior pancreatic lesions. For lesions located close to the superior pancreatic border, the hepatic artery and gastroduodenal artery are evaluated. The porta hepatis is palpated to assess adenopathy and to identify an accessory right

hepatic artery, which originates from the SMA, usually within 1 cm of the aortic origin of the SMA.

If no contraindications to resection are identified on initial survey, the common bile duct is encircled and divided after cholecystectomy. If a distal cholangiocarcinoma is suspected, the proximal bile duct margin should be sent for frozen section analysis. After division of the bile duct, the PV and hepatic artery can be exposed. If there is no direct tumor extension to the hepatic artery or PV involvement at the superior pancreatic border, the gastroduodenal artery can be exposed and divided. In mobilizing the hepatic artery, the right gastric artery is commonly sacrificed, except when pylorus-preserving technique is planned, in which case the right gastric artery should be preserved. The superior portion of the retropancreatic tunnel can now be developed. The inferior retropancreatic tunnel is developed by dissection of the mesenteric root, to expose the SMV. A careful but blind blunt dissection is performed to complete the retropancreatic tunnel, which will confirm absence of tumor involvement of the mesenteric vessels anteriorly (but not medially).

The surgeon must now make a final decision regarding resectability. If en bloc R0 resection does not seem possible based on the evaluation to this point, surgical biliary decompression with a Roux en Y hepatojejunostomy, biopsy of the mass for histologic confirmation, and possible gastrojejunostomy would be performed for palliation. If R0 resection seems achievable, the stomach is divided taking the antrum with the specimen (or distal to the pylorus for pylorus-preserving PD). The proximal jejunum is divided just distal to the ligament of Treitz. The third and fourth portions of the duodenum are then mobilized and the duodenal mesenteric arcades are divided.

The pancreas is then divided over the retropancreatic tunnel. The pancreatic duct is often visualized in dividing the pancreas, and care should be taken in preventing cautery injury to the duct. The final step in PD is separation of the uncinate process from the medial border of the SMV and SMA, after which the specimen can be removed.

After resection, reconstruction of the biliary tract, pancreatic duct, and GI tract is accomplished through a biliary enteric anastomosis, pancreatic anastomosis, and gastric anastomosis to the remaining jejunum. There are many variations in pancreaticojejunostomy techniques, based on factors such as the size of the pancreatic duct and the quality and consistency of the pancreatic parenchyma. Mucosal anastomosis and inversion of the pancreas into the intestine without duct anastomosis are both possible techniques, with or without pancreatic duct stents. Overall rates of postoperative pancreatic anastomotic leak are between 10% and 20%, with reduced morbidity with greater center experience. Octreotide prophylaxis has been extensively studied as a pharmacologic intervention to reduce pancreatic leaks after PD, though trials have been mixed in showing a benefit. In high-volume centers with low underlying leak rates after PD, routine octreotide prophylaxis is likely of no benefit (19).

Special Considerations in Pancreaticoduodenectomy

The parenchymal margin of the pancreas should routinely be sent for frozen section; if the margin is positive, additional pancreatic parenchyma should be resected until a negative margin is achieved. If a negative margin cannot be achieved despite additional parenchymal resection, total pancreatectomy is a potential option but is associated with a significant increased morbidity.

Inflammation can often mimic tumor in pancreas cancer, which can make involvement of the vessels difficult to assess. High-quality CT can often predict vascular abutment, in which case the surgeon should be prepared to perform vascular resection and reconstruction of SMV or PV if necessary to obtain negative margins. Limited hepatic artery involvement can also be addressed with resection and arterial reconstruction, though SMA involvement is considered evidence of unresectability.

Pylorus preservation rather than distal gastric resection has been suggested as a means of reducing postoperative bile reflux into the stomach, though this technique should probably be reserved for early stage ampullary cancer or pancreatic tumors, or limited distal cholangiocarcinomas. Pylorus preservation is not considered a standard of care but is an option in certain clinical settings, based on surgeon preference.

Common causes of morbidity after PD include pancreatic leak, abscess/infected fluid collections, delayed gastric emptying, and bile reflux gastritis. Less common causes of morbidity include biliary leak or stricture, hepatic ischemia, and portomesenteric venous thrombosis. Pancreatic leaks are usually self-limited and are managed conservatively by drains placed at the time of initial operation and in some cases bowel rest if the volume of drainage is high. Supportive care, maintenance of nutrition, and avoidance of closed space infections leading to sepsis are the mainstays of management. Occasionally, if the operative drains do not adequately drain leaks or infected collections, percutaneous placement of additional drains may be necessary.

Delayed gastric emptying occurs in approximately 20% to 25% of patients after PD and is characterized by a persistent gastric ileus and inability to tolerate oral diet beyond the first postoperative week. Anastomotic obstruction or extrinsic compression should be excluded: both conditions can be evaluated by CT with oral and intravenous contrast. Management is usually conservative, with promotility agents, acid suppression, gastric decompression, and parenteral nutrition. Some surgeons prefer to place routine surgical gastrostomies at the time of PD to avoid the morbidity and discomfort associated with prolonged nasogastric decompression in patients with delayed gastric emptying.

Cystic Neoplasms

Cystic neoplasms of the pancreas are rare but seem to be increasing in incidence, possibly as incidental findings on abdominal imaging. Cystic neoplasms include several categories of disease such as simple epithelial benign cysts and pseudocysts to intrapapillary mucinous neoplasms, to frank cystic carcinomas. The challenge for the pancreatic surgeon is differentiation of benign from malignant etiology and assessment of malignant potential to identify indications for surgical intervention. Stratification of malignant risk of cystic neoplasms is based on size and appearance, clinical presentation, and symptoms.

Pseudocysts, unlike cystic neoplasms, are commonly associated with a history of pancreatitis and contain thin serous fluid without mucin upon aspiration by EUS. Benign epithelial cysts lack internal septations and like pseudocysts contain serous rather than mucinous fluid. There is no single pathognomonic clinical finding indicating malignancy cystic neoplasms, but in general, larger lesions more than 3 cm have greater malignant potential, as do lesions with complex septations/loculations, solid/nodular mural components, or mucin. EUS-obtained cytology may indicate mucin-staining columnar cells, sometimes with atypia, and tumor markers such as carcinoembryonic antigen (CEA) may be elevated. Although EUS aspiration cytology lacks sensitivity in confirming malignancy, it has high specificity, especially in the context of other findings.

Indications for Operation in Cystic Neoplasms
1. Size greater than 3 cm
2. Size less than 3 cm *and* additional findings:
   i. EUS aspiration with suspicious features:
      Mucin
      Abnormal cytology
      Abnormal tumor markers (CEA)
   ii. Complex cystic appearance on CT or EUS

3. Symptomatic lesion (abdominal pain, GI obstruction, jaundice)

Intrapapillary Mucinous Neoplasms

IPMNs, also known as intrapapillary mucinous tumors, are intraductal lesions that may present as cystic dilation associated with segmental or main ductal obstruction. IPMN may represent a continuous, premalignant diffuse field abnormality of the pancreatic ductal epithelium. Abnormalities may be seen throughout the ductal system, so that resection of a lesion in one portion of the pancreas may not eliminate malignant potential in the remnant pancreas. The challenge for the surgeon is assessment of malignant risk to trigger surgical intervention. Some surgeons originally advocated total pancreatectomy, though the lifelong brittle diabetes and exocrine insufficiency have led most surgeons to prefer a more conservative approach consisting of limited resection in selected patients, as more data have emerged stratifying risk factors for malignancy based on clinical findings (20).

IPMNs are classified based on the pattern of ductal dilation, which is suggestive of the location of the underlying obstructing lesion and also serves as a guide to operative planning: diffuse MD ectasia with a duct more than 10 mm suggests a proximal duct obstruction with diffuse distal dilation (MD-IPMN), whereas segmental or branch duct (BD) ectasia suggests a more peripheral obstruction (BD-IPMN). In some cases, there may be multiple areas of obstruction with multiple cystic dilations in continuity with the pancreatic duct.

Patients with IPMN may present with pancreatitis or with vague GI complaints. Imaging with CT and MRCP demonstrates ductal dilation. ERCP is often useful to document the pattern of ductal obstruction and obtain fluid and cells for cytologic analysis. There is a consensus that MD IPMNs with duct dilation more than 10 mm and features of potential malignancy (cytology, nodularity, etc.) should be resected due to their higher rate of malignant potential. The duct margin is assessed intraoperatively for dysplasia or cancer, with additional resection performed (sometimes even total pancreatectomy) to achieve a complete resection (21). Total pancreatectomy may be indicated in the diffuse pattern of MD-IPMN, where complete resection of malignant disease may not be possible with limited resection.

There is more controversy surrounding BD-IPMN, which often occurs in the uncinate and may have a lower rate of progression to malignancy. Recent guidelines have stratified lesions more than 3 cm as high risk and therefore requiring surgery in BD-IPMN (22). Additional criteria for resection include symptoms and worrisome clinical or cytologic features. It should be recognized that even smaller lesions can still harbor cancer and should be evaluated by EUS aspiration to discriminate small benign simple cysts from potentially malignant conditions.

Criteria for Resection of Intrapapillary Mucinous Neoplasm (23)
1. MD-IPMN
2. BD-IPMN
   a. More than 3 cm
   b. Enlarging
   c. Symptomatic
3. Any lesion with suspicious aspiration findings:
   a. Mucin
   b. Abnormal tumor markers
   c. Abnormal cytology

Endocrine Tumors of the Pancreas

Endocrine tumors of the pancreas (islet cell tumors) are generally rare neoplasms that are of neuroendocrine origin. They may exhibit function or may be nonfunctional, benign or malignant, and are often indolent in nature. Endocrine tumors are classified according to their cell type, which imply associated clinical syndromes (see later). Endocrine tumors may be sporadic or exist as part of multiple endocrine neoplasia syndromes. Endocrine tumors have similar imaging characteristics on CT (solid or complex cystic arterially enhancing lesions). After initial characterization of the functional syndrome, localization and staging of endocrine tumors is approached through a combination of contrast-enhanced CT, endoscopic ultrasonography, and indium-111 octreotide nuclear scanning (OctreoScan). The sensitivity of OctreoScan is only approximately 40% due to the lack of somatostatin receptors on most islet cell tumors. More recently, functional positron emission tomography/CT may also emerge as an important diagnostic tool. Once localized, indications for intervention include palliation of symptoms and resection for cure. Surgical options, depending on cell type and pattern of disease, include enucleation, formal pancreatic resection, and transplantation of the liver in selected patients with isolated liver metastases.

Endocrine Tumor Syndromes
Insulinoma

Insulinomas are the most common type of islet cell tumor. The diagnosis is established by demonstrating inappropriately high serum insulin concentrations during a spontaneous or induced episode of hypoglycemia, followed by imaging studies to localize the lesion. Ninety percent of insulinomas are benign, which after localization are preferentially treated with enucleation when possible.

Gastrinoma

Patients with gastrinoma typically present with severe ulcer disease with elevated serum gastrin levels. Initial management is medical control of peptic ulcer disease with high-dose proton pump inhibitors. Patients with sporadic-type gastrinoma who do not have metastatic disease may be surgical candidates. Gastrinomas occurring in patients with MEN-I syndromes tend to be multifocal, with a lower chance for cure with resection. Eighty percent of gastrinomas will be found in the "gastrinoma triangle," defined by the head of the pancreas and the duodenal sweep. With a combination of careful palpation by an experienced surgeon, intraoperative sonography, and transduodenal illumination, gastrinomas can be localized in a majority of cases. Postresection, gastric secretion, and gastrin levels may remain high due to the trophic effect of chronic hypergastrinemia; therefore, most patients will require postoperative acid–suppressive therapy even after surgery.

Carcinoid (can occur anywhere in the body) (23)

Heterogenous group of tumors that release a variety of potentially active peptides. Type of peptides may depend on the origin of the carcinoid (foregut/midgut/hindgut). Carcinoid syndromes arise due to alterations in tryptophan metabolism. Classic midgut carcinoids are associated with elevated serotonin, which is a product of tryptophan metabolism. Serotonin is metabolized to 5-HIAA, which can be measured in the urine in patients with functioning carcinoid and forms the basis for diagnosis of carcinoid syndrome: Elevated 24-hour urinary excretion of 5-HIAA is 100% specific. Foregut carcinoids may produce histamine rather than serotonin. Symptoms of carcinoid syndrome include diarrhea and episodic flushing.

Rare pancreatic endocrine neoplasms: glucagonoma, somatostatinoma, VIPoma.

QUESTIONS

Select one answer.

1. All of the following are indicative of poor prognosis in acute pancreatitis except:
   a. Serum calcium less than 8.0 mg/dl
   b. Hyperglycemia
   c. Serum amylase more than five times normal on admission
   d. Arterial oxygen tension less than 60 mm Hg.
   e. Serum lactic dehydrogenase more than three times normal

2. Which of the following is *not* an indication for operation in a patient with a pancreatic cystic lesion:
   a. Abdominal pain
   b. Lesion is 2.0 cm in diameter
   c. Elevated CEA level
   d. Mucin in cyst
   e. Ultrasound showing septations

3. Infected pancreatic necrosis can be diagnosed using which of the following:
   a. Fine needle aspiration
   b. CT scan
   c. Clinical course
   d. Clinical deterioration
   e. All of the above

4. Patients who develop gallstone pancreatitis should have the following interventions prior or during cholecystectomy
   a. ERCP
   b. EUS
   c. UGI
   d. MRCP
   e. Cholangiography

5. Most patients with gallstone pancreatitis should be managed by which of the protocols
   a. Cholecystectomy with common duct exploration within 24 hours of admission
   b. Urgent ERCP followed by laparoscopic cholecystectomy
   c. Stabilization with cholecystectomy on the same admission
   d. Stabilization followed by elective cholecystectomy 6 weeks later
   e. Nonoperative therapy with cholecystectomy at a later time if symptoms recur

6. Enlarging or symptomatic pancreatic pseudocysts are best treated by which of the following modalities *except*:
   a. Cystgastrostomy
   b. Endoscopic drainage
   c. TPN and bowel rest
   d. Cystjejunostomy
   e. Cystduodenostomy

7. Which of the following is the risk factor most closely associated with increased incidence of pancreatic adenocarcinoma
   a. Chronic pancreatitis
   b. Diabetes mellitus
   c. Coffee consumption
   d. Alcohol consumption
   e. Cigarette smoking

8. Delayed gastric emptying following a pancreaticodudenectomy is best managed by
   a. Reoperation and revision of the gastrojejunostomy
   b. PEG placement
   c. Promotility agents and acid suppression
   d. Parenteral nutrition
   e. Roux-en-y gastrojejunostomy

9. Which of the following is true regarding insulinomas
   a. The vast majority are benign
   b. Diazoxide can be used to treat the severe hypoglycemia associated with this lesion
   c. Most insulomas can be treated by simple enucleation
   d. They are not associated with MEA-I syndrome
   e. All the above

10. Which of the following is true regarding pancreas divisum
    a. It may be associated with pancreatitis
    b. It is associated with intestinal malrotation
    c. It is common cause of acute pancreatitis
    d. It results from abnormal rotation of the ventral pancreas
    e. It is usually diagnosed by CT scan

REFERENCES

1. Elfar M, Gaber L, Sabek O, et al. The inflammatory cascade in acute pancreatitis: relevance to clinical disease. *Surg Clin North Am* 2007;87:1325–1340.
2. Ranson JCH, Rifkind KM, Turner JW. Prognostic signs and nonoperative peritoneal lavage in acute pancreatitis. *Surg Gynecol Obstet* 1976;143:209–219.
3. Harrison DA, D'Amico G, Singer M. The pancreatitis outcome prediction (POP) score: a new prognostic index for patients with severe acute pancreatitis. *Crit Care Med* 2007;35(7):1703–1708.
4. Bollen TL, van Santvoort HC, Besselink MG, et al. The Atlanta classification of acute pancreatitis revisited. *Br J Surg* 2008;95(1):6–21.
5. Kim D, Pickhardt P. Radiologic assessment of acute and chronic pancreatitis. *Surg Clin North Am* 2007;87:1341–1358.
6. Nathens AB, Curtis JR, Beale RJ, et al. Management of the critically ill patient with severe acute pancreatitis. *Crit Care Med* 2004;32(12):2524–2536.
7. Dellinger EP, Tellado JM, Soto NE, et al. Early antibiotic treatment for severe acute necrotizing pancreatitis: a randomized, double blind, placebo controlled study. *Ann Surg* 2007;245(5):674–683.
8. Curtis K, Kudsk K. Nutrition support in pancreatitis. *Surg Clin North Am* 2007;87:1403–1415.
9. Jamdar S, Siriwardena AK. Contemporary management of infected necrosis complicating severe acute pancreatitis. *Crit Care* 2006;10(1):101.
10. Buchler MW, Gloor B, Muller CA, et al. Acute necrotizing pancreatitis: treatment strategy according to the status of infection. *Ann Surg* 2000;232(5):619–626.
11. Haney J, Pappas T. Necrotizing pancreatitis: diagnosis and management. *Surg Clin North Am* 2007;87:1431–1446.
12. Attasaranya S, Abdel Aziz A, Lehman G. Endoscopic management of acute and chronic pancreatitis. *Surg Clin North Am* 2007;87:1379–1402.
13. Fan ST, Lai E, Mok F, et al. Early treatment of acute biliary pancreatitis by endoscopic papillotomy. *N Engl J Med* 1993;328(4):228–232.
14. Bergman S, Melvin WS. Operative and nonoperative management of pancreatic pseudocysts. *Surg Clin North Am* 2007;87:1447–1460.
15. Cheruvu CV, Clarke MG, Prentice M, et al. Conservative treatment as an option in the management of pancreatic pseudocyst. *Ann R Coll Surg Engl* 2003;85(5):313–316.
16. Vitas GJ, Sarr MG. Selected management of pancreatic pseudocysts: operative versus expectant management. *Surgery* 1992;111(2):123–130.
17. Cohen M, Prinz R. Pancreatic pseudocyst. In: Cameron, ed. *Current surgical therapy.* 7th ed. St. Louis, MO: Mosby, 2001:543–546.
18. Blondet JJ, Carlson AM, Kobayashi T, et al. The role of total pancreatectomy and islet autotransplantation for chronic pancreatitis. *Surg Clin North Am* 2007;87:1477–1501.
19. Yeo CJ, Cameron JL, Lillemoe KD, et al. Does prophylactic octreotide decrease the rates of pancreatic fistula and other complications after pancreaticodoudenectomy? Results of a prospective randomized placebo controlled trial. *Ann Surg* 2000;232(3):419–429.
20. Paye F, Sauvanet A, Terris B, et al. Intraductal papillary mucinous tumors of the pancreas: pancreatic resections guided by preoperative morphological assessment and intraoperative frozen section examination. *Surgery* 2000;127:536–544.
21. Tang RS, Weinberg B, Dawson DW, et al. Evaluation of the guidelines for management of pancreatic branch duct intraductal papillary mucinous neoplasm. *Clin Gastroenterol Hepatol* 2008;6(7):724–725.
22. Tanaka M, Chari S, Adsay V, et al. International consensus guidelines for management of intraductal papillary mucinous neoplasms and mucinous cystic neoplasms of the pancreas. *Pancreatology* 2006;6:17–32.
23. Modlin IM, Kidd M, Latich I, et al. Current status of gastrointestinal carcinoids. *Gastroenterology* 2005;128(6):1717–1751.

CHAPTER 7

Larry A. Scher
Nicholas J. Gargiulo
Russell H. Samson

Peripheral Arterial Disease

CHRONIC ARTERIAL OCCLUSIVE DISEASE OF THE LOWER EXTREMITIES

Clinical Manifestations

Atherosclerosis is the most common cause of lower extremity arterial occlusive disease. Lesions may be asymptomatic and manifest only as abnormal pulse examinations, or they may cause symptoms including claudication, ischemic rest pain, and gangrene.

Disease patterns may be segmental or diffuse and involve the aortoiliac, femoropopliteal, and tibial arteries alone or in combination. Atherosclerosis most commonly involves the superficial femoral artery in the adductor (Hunter's) canal. It is important to remember that patients with lower extremity atherosclerotic occlusive disease may also have silent or symptomatic atherosclerosis in their coronary, cerebral, or other arteries.

Claudication is the most benign symptom of chronic arterial occlusive disease. Exercise-related muscle pain usually occurs in the calf but may also be present in the thigh or buttocks. The location of the claudication is often, but not always, indicative of the level of arterial stenosis or occlusion. Claudication has been demonstrated repeatedly to be a benign symptom that improves or remains stable in most patients. Unless significant disability exists and interferes with the patient's life style, treatment is conservative.

Ischemic rest pain is a more severe manifestation of peripheral vascular disease. Typically, nocturnal pain occurs in the foot and is relieved with dependency. Dependent rubor (from peripheral vasodilatation) and elevation pallor on physical examination are findings consistent with severe arterial occlusive disease. Unlike claudication, the natural history of ischemic rest pain is more ominous. Frequent progression to ischemic ulceration and impending or frank gangrene occurs and may threaten limb viability. Therefore, interventional therapy for limb salvage is often indicated during these later stages.

Diagnosis

The history and physical examination are important when assessing patients with lower extremity arterial occlusive disease. The typical symptoms (intermittent claudication, ischemic rest pain, ulceration, gangrene) have already been described. Careful pulse examination, auscultation for bruits, and examination for signs of chronic ischemia (elevation pallor, dependent rubor, ulceration, trophic changes) are important aspects of the physical examination.

Arterial noninvasive studies including Doppler segmental pressures and pulse volume recordings, or plethysmography, may offer supportive information to the history and physical examination. Doppler pressures are measured with blood pressure cuffs on the thigh, calf, and ankle and auscultation with a Doppler stethoscope distal to the cuff (usually over the dorsalis pedis or posterior tibial artery). Because of the variation in systemic blood pressure, an ankle/brachial index (ABI) is determined by dividing the ankle pressure by the brachial pressure. The normal ABI is 1.0 or greater, and an ABI less than 0.95 is suggestive of arterial occlusive disease. Typically, patients with intermittent claudication have an ABI in the range of 0.7, and limb-threatening ischemia generally occurs only with an ABI less than 0.5. Diabetic patients may have arterial calcification that prevents cuff occlusion of major arteries and can preclude accurate measurement of ankle blood pressures. In this situation, supplemental information obtained by volume plethysmography with analysis of waveform amplitude and pattern is useful. In addition, plethys-mographic tracings obtained at the forefoot and toes may provide accurate information about distal circulation and aid in the planning of vascular reconstructive operations or amputations. In selected patients, noninvasive evaluation following exercise or reactive hyperemia may provide useful information about the etiology and significance of lower extremity symptoms. A significant reduction in ankle brachial index after exercise suggests significant arterial occlusive disease. Conversely, normal hemodynamics after exercise should prompt a search for alternative explanation for symptoms, such as spinal stenosis and neurogenic claudication.

Imaging to provide anatomic information is necessary to plan therapeutic interventions. This may be accomplished by duplex imaging, computerized tomography (CT), magnetic resonance (MR) angiography, or conventional contrast angiography. Duplex ultrasound is a noninvasive technique combining grayscale imaging and color-Doppler and provides both anatomic and physiologic information to identify lesions. Administration of iodine-based agents for CT or conventional angiography or gadolinium for MR angiography should be utilized with caution in patients with renal insufficiency. Contrast-induced nephropathy may occur with iodine-based agents and nephrogenic systemic sclerosis is a rare but devastating complication of gadolinium which can occur in patients with compromised renal function. Angiography gives anatomic information about arterial lesions but is not necessary in all patients. This invasive diagnostic technique is reserved for patients who, by history, physical examination, and noninvasive diagnostic studies, are considered candidates for interventional therapy. Ultimate decisions regarding optimal endovascular or surgical interventions can be made by visualizing the infrarenal aorta and the iliac, femoral, popliteal, and tibial arteries down to and including the foot vessels in appropriate patients.

Treatment

Initial treatment of non–limb-threatening arterial occlusive disease is conservative. Cessation of smoking and modification of diet may prevent disease progression. Graded exercise programs improve walking distances in many patients with intermittent claudication. Two medications have been approved for the treatment of intermittent claudication. Pentoxifylline is a hemorrheologic agent that alters red cell membrane deformability and has demonstrated limited effectiveness in the symptomatic treatment of intermittent claudication. Cilostazol is a phosphodiesterase inhibitor that has been shown in clinical trials to significantly increase walking distance. Cilostazol can infrequently cause diarrhea, palpitations, or headaches, necessitating reduction in dosage or discontinuation of the medication. It is also contraindicated in patients with a history of congestive heart failure.

Patients with severely disabling claudication or limb-threatening ischemia may require surgical or endovascular treatment. Appropriate therapy is selected after complete imaging of the aortoiliac and femoropopliteal arteries. Percutaneous transluminal angioplasty (PTA) and stenting are effective treatment for most hemodynamically significant iliac artery stenoses and short-segment occlusions, with results equivalent to aortofemoral surgical reconstruction. Long-term results of angioplasty and stenting of the superficial femoral, popliteal, and tibial arteries are not as well established when compared with open surgical techniques. Although less invasive with potential savings in cost, morbidity, and mortality, reinterventions are frequently necessary and continuing outcome assessment is critical. Despite being less invasive than conventional surgical techniques, these procedures should be performed only in patients with disabling claudication or critical limb ischemia. Newer endovascular techniques such as atherectomy have had encouraging early results but uncertain long-term results and the role of these procedures are not clearly established.

Despite significant advances in endovascular therapies, surgery remains a mainstay for treatment of severe lower extremity arterial occlusive disease. In patients with predominantly aortoiliac occlusive disease primary attention must be focused on the correction of these anatomic lesions. If PTA is not feasible or is unsuccessful, arterial reconstruction is required. Unilateral iliac lesions can be effectively treated with femorofemoral bypass. Patients with bilateral disease requiring operation are usually best managed with aortobifemoral or axillofemoral bypass.

Synthetic grafts made of Dacron polyester or expanded polytetrafluoroethylene (PTFE) are preferred by most surgeons. Results of aortofemoral bypass are excellent and approach 90% patency at 5 years. Occlusion of the superficial femoral artery does not appear to influence graft patency in the majority of patients in whom the deep femoral artery is patent and free of disease. In addition, correction of hemodynamically significant aortoiliac disease is successful in relieving symptoms in more than 80% of patients despite uncorrected superficial femoral artery occlusion.

Extra-anatomic bypass has assumed a controversial role in the management of selected patients with aortoiliac occlusive disease. As mentioned above, femoro-femoral bypass is an acceptable option for patients with unilateral iliac disease. In the absence of hemodynamically significant disease of the donor iliac artery, patency rates have been excellent, and arterial "steal" should not occur. Results of axillary–femoral and axillary–bifemoral bypass have been less satisfactory and should be reserved for poor-risk patients or patients with hostile abdomens in whom conventional aortoiliac reconstruction carries prohibitive risks. Extra-anatomic bypass has also been valuable for treating patients with intra-abdominal graft infections (see Aneurysms, below).

Femoropopliteal and femorotibial bypasses play a major role in the treatment of patients with infrainguinal atherosclerosis. Indications for femoropopliteal reconstruction include severely disabling claudication and limb-threatening ischemia. The autogenous saphenous vein, whether reversed or left in situ after destruction of venous valves, is the graft of choice. In the absence of suitable greater saphenous vein, alternative conduits include the lesser saphenous vein, arm veins, and prosthetic materials such as PTFE. The popliteal artery may provide suitable outflow for a vascular reconstruction even in the absence of continuous outflow into the tibial arteries. Bypasses to isolated popliteal segments have excellent patency rates and often result in alleviation of symptoms. When the popliteal artery is unsuitable for distal anastomosis, femorotibial bypass is advocated. This operation is performed only for limb salvage, and autogenous vein grafts are far superior to prosthetics. Five-year patency rates of 80% have been achieved for femoropopliteal bypass, and these rates have been approached for infrapopliteal bypass when autogenous grafts are used. If prosthetic distal bypass is necessary, adjuncts such as vein cuffs or distal arteriovenous (AV) fistulas may improve outcomes.

Selected patients with hemodynamically significant disease of the profunda femoris artery, in addition to superficial femoral artery occlusion, may benefit from profundaplasty. However, isolated profundaplasty has a limited role in the management of lower extremity ischemia due to the excellent results of femoropopliteal and femorotibial reconstructions. Profundaplasty has most commonly been utilized in conjunction with an inflow procedure (e.g., aortofemoral bypass).

Thrombolytic therapy is occasionally useful for management of patients with chronic arterial occlusive disease. The Surgery Versus Thrombolysis for Ischemia of the Lower Extremity (STILE) trial was designed to evaluate intra-arterial thrombolytic therapy for patients who require revascularization for non-embolic arterial or graft occlusion causing lower extremity ischemia of less than 6 months' duration. Surgical revascularization was more effective and safer than catheter-directed thrombolysis. A significant reduction in the complexity of planned surgical procedures was noted after thrombolysis, and a combination of the two modalities yielded the best results.

Lumbar sympathectomy has no role in the treatment of patients with lower extremity arterial occlusive disease. The major role of lumbar sympathectomy or lumbar sympathetic block appears to be in the management of patients with reflex sympathetic dystrophy.

Amputation

Major amputation is used infrequently as the primary treatment of patients with lower extremity arterial occlusive disease. It remains necessary in the presence of extensive gangrene or severe sepsis, gangrene in the presence of a dysfunctional limb, or unreconstructable occlusive disease. Minor toe or transmetatarsal amputation can be performed alone to treat infection or gangrene if hemodynamic testing reveals adequate arterial pressure to achieve wound healing (ABI >0.5). Major amputation, when required, is preferred at the below-knee level to facilitate ambulation and mobility. Above-knee amputation is required for severe peripheral vascular disease or infection only when amputation at a lower level is not feasible or when patients have dysfunctional limbs with severe contractures. Although numerous methods have been proposed to predict the level of amputation healing, clinical assessment and noninvasive laboratory testing remain the most commonly utilized modalities. Concerns have arisen that a failed vascular reconstruction may lead to a higher level of amputation than would have been necessary had no revascularization been attempted. Several studies have proved this not to be the case in most patients. Newer techniques with an immediate postoperative prosthesis and rigid plaster dressings following amputation are available and may facilitate stump healing and rehabilitation.

ACUTE ARTERIAL OCCLUSION

Acute arterial occlusion may be thrombotic or embolic in etiology. Differentiation between the two is frequently difficult because many patients with acute arterial occlusion have severe underlying chronic atherosclerotic occlusive disease. Duplex ultrasound or angiography may be useful for diagnosis. Acute ischemia can result from acute thrombosis in low flow or hypercoagulable states, trauma, compartment syndrome, and iliofemoral venous thrombosis in patients with phlegmasia cerulean dolens. The management of acute thrombotic occlusion generally involves thrombectomy or thrombolysis and angioplasty or bypass of the underlying arterial lesion if one can be identified. The management of acute embolic arterial occlusion is discussed below.

Source of Emboli

Most arterial emboli are cardiac in origin and may be related to atherosclerotic heart disease with myocardial infarction, mural thrombus, or ventricular aneurysm. Rheumatic valvular disease, atrial fibrillation, and atrial myxoma are also possible sources of cardiac emboli. Emboli can also originate from proximal atherosclerotic lesions and produce major or minor episodes of distal embolization (blue-toe syndrome). Angiographic evaluation of patients with blue-toe syndrome is mandatory to identify the source of atheroembolic lesions, as the natural history of this disease is one of the recurrent episodes of embolization. Emboli can also originate from arterial aneurysms, particularly those in the aorta and popliteal arteries. Paradoxical emboli are rare and originate in the deep venous system and enter the arterial circulation via intracardiac septal defects.

Clinical Manifestations

Clinical manifestations of acute arterial occlusion include pain, pallor, absent pulses, paresthesias, and paralysis. Progressive ischemia results from distal propagation of thrombus. Rapidly progressive ischemia may cause motor and sensory loss and can threaten limb viability within 6 hours. Most arterial emboli involve the lower extremity, with 35% at the femoral bifurcation. Other common sites include the iliac and popliteal arteries. Noninvasive testing and arteriography may help confirm the diagnosis and localize the arterial occlusion.

Treatment

Immediate heparinization helps to prevent distal propagation of thrombus. Acute arterial emboli result in a high incidence of limb loss or persistent symptoms if left untreated. Duplex ultrasound or angiography may help to localize emboli (which are frequently multiple) and plan an operative approach. Balloon catheter embolectomy can be accomplished via the femoral artery for aortic ("saddle"), iliac, or femoral emboli. The procedure is often performed under local anesthesia. Popliteal emboli may require direct exposure of the popliteal and proximal tibial arteries. Thrombolytic therapy may be considered for selected patients, but in general the urgency of the situation makes operative intervention preferable. Multicenter trials comparing thrombolysis and surgery have indicated that thrombolytic therapy is safe and effective and may reduce the requirement for complex surgery if lysis is successful.

Results

Results of treatment of acute ischemia depend on the duration and location of the occlusion. Muscle necrosis with calf tenderness or rigor may preclude a successful outcome. Complications include persistent ischemia, catheter-related complications, and metabolic derangements related to lactic acidosis and myoglobinemia. Mortality is high and is usually associated with underlying cardiac disease. Long-term anticoagulation may be beneficial in reducing the risk of recurrent embolization. The results of treatment are favorable if a noncardiac source of embolization can be identified and successfully treated.

DIABETIC FOOT INFECTIONS

Diabetic foot ulcers are typically produced by a combination of neuropathy, ischemia, and infection. Diabetic neuropathy may present as a diffuse sensory disturbance or as neuropathic pain. Neuropathy renders the foot more susceptible to trauma and infection. Degenerative arthropathy (Charcot joint) may be present. Once an ulcer has developed, local infection may occur. Infection is further promoted by the relative immunocompromised state of the diabetic patient. Infections are frequently polymicrobial and require aggressive treatment with appropriate antibiotics (usually intravenous) and debridement of infected and devitalized tissue. Hyperbaric oxygen therapy and new adjuncts in wound care including negative pressure wound therapy may be useful in selected patients.

Diabetic patients may also develop significant peripheral vascular disease. The disease is usually multisegmental, but there is a predilection for severe involvement of the infrapopliteal arteries. Evaluation of patients with diabetic foot ulcers or infections requires careful pulse examination supplemented by noninvasive hemodynamic testing. If significant disease is present, angiography and revascularization may be required to achieve healing. Although distal bypass procedures are often required, results of vascular reconstruction in diabetic patients generally parallel those in nondiabetic patients.

Perhaps the most important aspect of diabetic foot care is patient education and prevention. Careful attention to hygiene and appropriate footwear can avert many limb-threatening problems.

NONATHEROSCLEROTIC VASCULAR LESIONS

Popliteal Artery Entrapment

Developmental defects that displace the popliteal artery may cause arterial compression and stenosis or segmental occlusion. This syndrome is uncommon and occurs most often in young patients. Symptoms may include claudication or severe ischemia and may be unilateral or bilateral. With the most common variety of entrapment, the popliteal artery passes medial to the medial head of the gastrocnemius muscle and is subject to compression. Less commonly, a fibrous band of the popliteus muscle, deep to the medial head of the gastrocnemius, is the compressing structure. The diagnosis may be made by noninvasive hemodynamic studies with positional maneuvers to tense the gastrocnemius. In addition, angiography may demonstrate medial deviation of the popliteal artery or stenosis, occlusion, or aneurysm formation at the appropriate level. Treatment is aimed at removal of the compressing muscular structure plus popliteal artery reconstruction if necessary. Aggressive treatment of asymptomatic contralateral lesions may avert popliteal artery thrombosis and disabling ischemia.

Cystic Adventitial Disease of the Popliteal Artery

Rarely, cyst formation in the wall of the popliteal artery produces ischemic symptoms. Treatment consists of resection and graft replacement of the involved arterial segment.

Thromboangiitis Obliterans (Buerger's Disease)

Thromboangiitis obliterans is an occlusive disease of medium-size and small arteries affecting the distal upper and lower extremities. It is pathologically a segmental panangiitis and affects primarily young men. The cause is not known, but a striking relation to tobacco smoking has been observed. Recurrent episodes of superficial thrombophlebitis may also be present. Angiography typically reveals multiple segmental occlusions in the small arteries of the forearm, hand, leg, and foot with many fine collateral vessels, often in a corkscrew configuration. Treatment is symptomatic and must include avoidance of tobacco. Reconstructive surgery is often difficult because of the pattern of occlusive disease, and minor or major amputation is often required.

Takayasu's Arteritis

Takayasu's arteritis is an inflammatory arteritis that usually occurs in young and middle-aged women. It most frequently involves the brachiocephalic vessels, renal arteries, and abdominal aorta, and it may be associated with acute nonspecific systemic symptoms. Other symptoms include stroke, upper or lower extremity ischemia, or renovascular hypertension. Retinal vasculitis was originally described and may also be present. Active disease is treated with corticosteroids, but vascular reconstructive surgery is required in selected cases with symptomatic arterial stenosis or occlusion. Procedures may be complex and generally involve bypass from uninvolved arterial segments.

Giant Cell (Temporal) Arteritis

Temporal arteritis is an inflammatory disease of the medium and large arteries of the head and is associated with a clinical syndrome of pain and stiffness in the trunk and proximal extremities in elderly patients. Headaches may be associated with tenderness over the course of the temporal artery. Blindness may occur if the disease is untreated. Diagnosis is made by temporal artery biopsy and treatment with corticosteroids is recommended.

Raynaud's Syndrome

Raynaud's syndrome is defined as episodic attacks of vasoconstriction of the arteries and arterioles of the extremities in response to cold or emotional stimuli. It manifests clinically as sequential pallor, cyanosis, and rubor of the digits. Patients may have some identifiable associated condition, such as immunologic or connective tissue disorders (e.g., scleroderma), drug-induced syndrome (ergot, β-blockers), or obstructive arterial disease. The diagnosis can be made clinically and may be confirmed by ice water immersion testing, measuring the recovery time to normal digital temperature. Noninvasive vascular examination of the digits with analysis of the digital pulse waveform and hand arteriography may also be helpful for differentiating vasospastic and obstructive conditions.

Treatment consists of cold avoidance and discontinuation of offending drugs. In severe cases, nifedipine may be useful. Cervical sympathectomy is rarely indicated.

Persistent Sciatic Artery

This is a rare congenital vascular anomaly caused by persistence of the embryological sciatic artery often with hypoplasia of the iliofemoral arterial system. The persistent sciatic artery is prone to atheromatous degeneration and thrombosis and may present as a buttock aneurysm, ischemia, or embolic disease. Angiographic diagnosis depends on recognition of an abnormally large internal iliac artery and differentiation of a tapering superficial femoral artery from routine occlusive disease.

Thoracic Outlet Syndrome

Thoracic outlet syndrome is caused by compression of the brachial plexus, subclavian artery, and subclavian vein in the thoracic outlet. These structures may be compressed between the clavicle and the first rib or by a number of anatomic variations. Neurologic compression, the most common form of thoracic outlet syndrome, is discussed elsewhere (see Chapter 19). Vascular complications of thoracic outlet syndrome occur infrequently. Arterial complications usually result from subclavian artery compression by complete cervical ribs, which may result in poststenotic dilatation of the subclavian artery with aneurysm formation and thromboembolic complications. Treatment is aimed at decompression of the arterial stenosis combined with arterial reconstruction when necessary.

Venous complications of thoracic outlet syndrome are often related to compression of the subclavian vein by the subclavius or pectoralis minor muscle and present as acute venous thrombosis following vigorous exercise or trauma. Current recommendations for treatment of "effort thrombosis" include catheter-directed thrombolysis to restore venous patency, followed by anticoagulation and often surgical decompression of the thoracic outlet to prevent recurrence. This can be accomplished by first rib resection through a transaxillary or supraclavicular approach.

Hypercoagulable States

As our understanding of the coagulation cascade has increased, so has our ability to diagnose congenital clotting defects, which may be responsible for unexplained venous, arterial, or graft thrombosis. Antithrombin III binds thrombin and several other activated clotting factors and neutralizes their activity. Protein C is a vitamin K-dependent glycoprotein that inhibits activated factors V and VIII and enhances fibrinolytic activity. Protein S is a cofactor of protein C and potentiates the inactivation of factor V. Congenital deficiencies of any of these factors, as well as fibrinolytic deficiencies or dysfibrinogenemia, may be responsible for hypercoagulable states. Factor V Leiden is a recently discovered and relatively common hereditary disorder causing hypercoagulability through a variation of human Factor V which prevents inactivation by activated protein C. Antiphospholipid syndrome is a coagulation disorder than can cause arterial or venous thrombosis as well as pregnancy-related complications. The syndrome occurs because of the autoimmune production of antibodies against phospholipid and specifically against cardiolipin which is present in the cell membrane. The evaluation of patients with unexplained or recurrent thrombosis should include measurement of prothrombin time, partial thromboplastin time, bleeding time, and platelet count, tests for antiphospholipid syndrome including anticardiolipin antibodies and lupus anticoagulant, Factor V Leiden, genetic tests for prothrombin G20210 A mutation, and assays for antithrombin III, protein C, and protein S.

CEREBROVASCULAR DISEASE

Clinical Manifestations

Carotid artery disease may present as asymptomatic carotid bruits. Transient ischemic attacks (TIAs) are neurologic deficits that resolve within 24 hours. They are usually caused by microemboli of platelets, fibrin, and atheromatous material from carotid bifurcation plaques. Amaurosis fugax represents transient monocular blindness from embolization to the ophthalmic artery, a branch of the internal carotid artery (ICA). Atheromatous material may be visualized in the branches of the retinal artery (Hollenhorst plaques). TIAs may also present as hemispheric ischemia with symptoms such as hemiparesis and dysarthria. Reversible ischemic neurologic deficits resolve within 48 to 72 hours. Long-lasting or permanent neurologic deficits are categorized as strokes.

Diagnosis

Many techniques are available for the diagnosis of extracranial carotid artery disease. Auscultation of the cervical region for bruits is a commonly used screening technique but is not specific for significant ICA stenosis. Duplex scanning combines ultrasound imaging and Doppler spectral analysis and has replaced all previously available noninvasive techniques for evaluation of extracranial cerebrovascular disease. This technique is extremely accurate and reproducible and provides both direct visualization of carotid artery lesions and accurate hemodynamic information to quantify the degree of stenosis. In addition, transcranial Doppler techniques are available to provide information regarding blood flow in intracranial vessels. Additional imaging techniques include CT or MR angiography and conventional contrast arteriography and may provide supplemental information to plan endovascular and surgical interventions.

Prognosis

Before treatment can be recommended, the natural history of carotid artery disease must be clarified. Controversy regarding the natural history and treatment of symptomatic and asymptomatic carotid stenosis led to the initiation of several multicenter prospective randomized studies. The North American Symptomatic Carotid Endarterectomy Trial (NASCET) evaluated 659 patients from 50 centers with symptomatic high-grade stenosis (70% to 99%) of the ICA. Patients were prospectively randomized to medical (antiplatelet therapy) and surgical (carotid endarterectomy [CEA]) groups. After 2 years the cumulative risk of stroke in the medical group was nearly three times higher than in patients who underwent CEA. The authors concluded that CEA is highly beneficial in patients with recent hemispheric and retinal TIAs or nondisabling strokes and with ipsilateral high-grade stenosis.

The Asymptomatic Carotid Atherosclerosis Study (ACAS) was a prospective randomized study of 1,659 patients from 39 centers with asymptomatic high-grade stenosis (60% or more). After a median follow-up of 2.7 years, the authors concluded that patients treated with CEA have a reduced risk of ipsilateral stroke if surgery can be performed with less than 3% perioperative morbidity and mortality.

Treatment

Treatment options for the management of symptomatic and asymptomatic carotid disease can be medical, endovascular, or surgical. Although endovascular techniques have been utilized with increasing frequency, surgery remains the treatment of choice for most symptomatic patients with high-grade ipsilateral stenosis of the ICA. Prophylactic CEA for patients with asymptomatic high-grade stenosis of the ICA also appears warranted to reduce the incidence of stroke. CEA involves removal of atherosclerotic lesions localized at the carotid bifurcation. Moderate degrees of intracranial occlusive disease are not a contraindication to surgery. The technical aspects of the operation are critical for achieving good results. General or local anesthesia may be used. Adequate exposure of the carotid bifurcation while avoiding injury to adjacent structures (e.g., vagus and hypoglossal nerves) is important. The need for cerebral protection by intraluminal shunting during carotid clamping is controversial. Shunts may be used routinely or selectively on the basis of measurement of stump pressure, electroencephalographic monitoring, somatosensory-evoked potential monitoring, or neurologic evaluation with the patient under regional block anesthesia. Closure of the arteriotomy with a prosthetic or venous patch is advocated by most surgeons to decrease the incidence of recurrent stenosis. An alternative operative technique is eversion endarterectomy, which involves complete transaction of the ICA at its origin, removal of the plaque by everting the outer wall of the ICA, and reimplantation of the ICA onto the common carotid artery. Potential advantages of this technique include avoidance of prosthetic patch material, shorter operative time, effective elimination of kinks and coils in the ICA, and lower rate of restenosis. Randomized trials have demonstrated this technique to be safe and effective but no significant difference in outcome or rate of restenosis has been demonstrated.

When properly performed, serious morbidity or mortality following CEA should occur in fewer than

2% of patients. Additional complications of local nerve injury are reported in up to 10% of patients undergoing CEA and include injuries to the hypoglossal, vagus, and marginal mandibular nerves. These injuries can be minimized by the use of careful operative technique. Cerebral hyperperfusion syndrome is a potentially devastating complication of CEA. It is caused by loss of cerebral autoregulation resulting from chronic cerebral ischemia and hyperperfusion that occurs after restoration of normal cerebral blood flow. This condition is manifested by severe headaches or seizures occurring 1 to 7 days after CEA. The incidence of cerebral hyperperfusion syndrome is increased in patients who have undergone a contralateral CEA within the past 3 months. Symptomatic recurrence from neointimal fibrous hyperplasia (6 to 18 months after surgery) or recurrent atherosclerosis (2 to 20 years after surgery) occurs in 1% to 2% of patients. Up to 15% of patients may have varying degrees of asymptomatic recurrent stenosis detected by routine postoperative noninvasive surveillance.

Although CEA for transient cerebral ischemia and asymptomatic high-grade lesions is now widely accepted, controversy exists regarding the performance of this operation for chronic cerebral ischemia and stroke-in-evolution. Total carotid occlusion is generally considered a contraindication to CEA. Although some symptomatic patients benefit from extracranial-to-intracranial (superficial temporal to middle cerebral) bypass, the results of a multicenter study have shown this procedure to be ineffective in the long-term prevention of stroke in asymptomatic patients. Selected patients with internal carotid occlusion and persistent symptoms may be candidates for external CEA. This artery provides important collateral pathways to the brain in the presence of occlusion or high-grade stenosis of the ICA. Numerous reports document the efficacy of external CEA in relieving hemispheric ischemia in the presence of ipsilateral internal carotid occlusion in selected patients.

Endovascular therapy with carotid angioplasty and stenting has assumed an increasing role in the management of cerebrovascular occlusive disease. Use of cerebral protection devices placed prior to angioplasty has improved outcomes. Technical factors including anomalous aortic arch anatomy and vessel tortuosity continue to present difficult challenges. Generally accepted indications for carotid angioplasty and stenting include high-risk symptomatic patients with ICA lesions who are not candidates for surgical treatment, recurrent high-grade or symptomatic carotid stenosis following previous CEA, and symptomatic carotid stenosis in the presence of previous neck irradiation or inaccessible ICA lesions. Randomized trials including the Carotid Revascularization Endarterectomy vs Stenting Trial (CREST) have demonstrated the safety and efficacy of carotid angioplasty and stenting but its role in the management of symptomatic or asymptomatic patients who are suitable candidates for CEA remains controversial.

Vertebrobasilar Insufficiency and Subclavian Steal

Although symptoms referable to the carotid territory are far more common, vertebrobasilar symptoms occasionally require evaluation and consideration for surgical reconstruction. These symptoms include motor or sensory disturbances, diplopia, vertigo, and drop attacks. Many of these patients have associated carotid artery disease. If direct vertebral reconstruction is required, endarterectomy or bypass techniques have been utilized.

Vertebrobasilar insufficiency may also occur as a manifestation of subclavian steal syndrome. With this entity, a lesion in the innominate or subclavian artery proximal to the vertebral artery may cause upper extremity ischemia. The vertebral artery becomes an important collateral pathway to the arm and may "steal" blood from the posterior circulation through the circle of Willis.

Asymptomatic subclavian steal documented on noninvasive testing or angiography does not require treatment. Treatment of symptomatic subclavian steal is by upper extremity revascularization. Stenosis or short segment occlusion of the subclavian artery can be treated successfully with angioplasty and stent. A number of surgical techniques are available when endovascular options are not feasible or are unsuccessful. These include direct transthoracic endarterectomy or bypass, or extra-anatomic revascularization by axillary–axillary, subclavian–subclavian, or left carotid–subclavian bypass or transposition. Over 90% of the lesions causing subclavian steal occur in the left subclavian artery and carotid–subclavian bypass or transposition is the most commonly utilized surgical options.

Fibromuscular Dysplasia

Fibromuscular dysplasia of the carotid artery is an uncommon nonatherosclerotic condition that occurs primarily in women. It is frequently bilateral and may produce symptoms of transient cerebral ischemia. Although asymptomatic lesions require no special attention, symptomatic disease is best treated by operative resection or dilatation of the involved carotid artery. Associated intracranial aneurysms may be present in up to 15% of patients.

Carotid Body Tumors

Carotid body tumors (chemodectomas) often present as asymptomatic neck masses. These lesions are highly vascular tumors that occur at the carotid bifurcation. They are frequently bilateral and usually benign, and the diagnosis can be confirmed by angiography. Treatment is by surgical resection. Preoperative embolization of large tumors may minimize the vascularity and facilitate resection. The major blood supply to the tumor often emanates from the external carotid artery, and ligation and resection of this vessel is sometimes required.

Carotid Dissection

Dissection of the cervical carotid artery may be spontaneous or traumatic. Spontaneous dissection is often related to hypertension, fibromuscular dysplasia, or arteriopathies (e.g., Marfan syndrome). Traumatic dissection may be related to cervical hyperextension or blunt cervical trauma. Angiography demonstrates a tapered narrowing of the extracranial carotid artery.

Treatment is generally nonoperative and consists of anticoagulation with heparin and warfarin. Patients with persistent symptoms may require surgical intervention.

Aberrant Right Subclavian Artery

A rare congenital abnormality can occur when the right subclavian artery originates directly from the aortic arch distal to the left subclavian artery. Affecting less than 1% of the population, this condition is usually asymptomatic and requires no treatment. It is frequently associated with a nonrecurrent right laryngeal nerve. Symptoms may occur when there is aneurysmal degeneration of the origin of the aberrant subclavian artery (Kommerell's diverticulum) or when esophageal compression causes difficulty swallowing (dysphagia lusoria). Surgical treatment options for symptomatic patients include thoracotomy with aneurysm resection or supraclavicular transposition of the right subclavian artery to the right common carotid artery.

ANEURYSMS

Abdominal Aortic Aneurysms

Abdominal aortic aneurysms have traditionally been described as atherosclerotic aneurysms because of the variable finding of atherosclerosis within the aneurysm wall. It is now recognized that the finding of atherosclerosis within an aneurysm is coincidental and does not necessarily implicate it in the formation of the aneurysm. A high incidence of aortic aneurysms among many members of the same family has suggested an increasingly important genetic role in the pathogenesis of aneurysms. Alterations in the metabolism of collagen and elastin have been found in the walls of aortic aneurysms and are caused by altered gene expression. The precise cause of aneurysms remains unknown, but it likely involves a combination of altered gene expression, alterations in inflammatory response, and to a limited degree atherosclerosis. Occasionally, aneurysms are mycotic (infected) or traumatic. Aortic aneurysms appear predominantly in men, and most are infrarenal. The risk of rupture of infrarenal aortic aneurysms is significant for aneurysms larger than 5.5 cm in anteroposterior or transverse diameter, or three times the diameter of the normal proximal aorta.

Diagnosis

Most asymptomatic abdominal aortic aneurysms can be detected by palpation on routine physical examination. Only 50% of aneurysms have calcifications, allowing detection on plain abdominal radiographs. CT and ultrasonography are reliable diagnostic tools and accurately define aneurysm size. CT may be especially useful for evaluating symptomatic aortic aneurysms and is sensitive for the detection of rupture. Computed tomographic angiography is also useful in the evaluation for and planning of endovascular aneurysm repair (EVAR). Aortography is a poor test to evaluate aneurysm size (laminated thrombus may limit contrast to the vessel lumen) but may be useful in identifying associated renal, visceral, or peripheral arterial occlusive disease and in providing accurate measurements for EVAR.

Treatment

Small aneurysms may be followed by serial ultrasound examinations. Studies suggest that the average growth rate of small aneurysms is 0.3 to 0.5 cm per year, but it is extremely variable. Treatment of asymptomatic abdominal aneurysms larger than 5.5 cm in diameter in good-risk patients is recommended to prevent rupture. Results of several prospective trials evaluating the natural history of small abdominal aortic aneurysms (<5.5 cm.) have failed to demonstrate a benefit for routine intervention for smaller asymptomatic aneurysms.

EVAR has achieved an increasingly important role in the management of abdominal aortic aneurysms. Reduced morbidity and mortality in high-risk patients has been documented in several reports and a number of approved devices are available for use. These devices are constructed of polyester or expanded PTFE grafts attached to self-expanding nitinol stents. Most devices are modular, consisting of a main body, contralateral limb, and proximal and distal cuffs if needed. The components are assembled under fluoroscopic guidance, with additional cuffs placed until successful exclusion of the aneurysm is documented. Some devices have additional fixation hooks to improve fixation to the aortic wall. The devices are deployed in the infrarenal aorta through femoral artery cutdowns or more recently with a percutaneous approach. Anatomic and technical criteria important for successful EVAR include length, diameter, and tortuosity of the aortic neck and size and tortuosity of the iliac arteries. In addition, the presence of extensive calcification or thrombus may contraindicate EVAR. Patients with critical branches arising off the aneurysm such as a dominant inferior mesenteric artery in the presence of occlusive disease of the superior mesenteric and celiac vessels cannot undergo EVAR without concomitant reconstruction of these vessels. Branched endografts are under investigation to treat juxtarenal, suprarenal, and thoracoabdominal aneurysms.

Patients who undergo EVAR require surveillance with computed tomographic scan or duplex ultrasound to identify endoleaks and possible graft migration or failure. Endoleaks represent continued blood flow into the aneurysm after endovascular repair. These leaks can cause by fixation or device failure or collateral retrograde perfusion of the aneurysm sac and may cause continued pressurization of the aneurysm, leading to potential expansion and rupture. Endoleaks are classified as follows:

• Type I: proximal or distal attachment site leak due to an incomplete seal of the endograft.
• Type II: retrograde flow into the aneurysm from a patent branch within the aneurysm, most commonly lumbar or inferior mesenteric arteries.
• Type III: focal area of leak at attachment site in modular system.
• Type IV: diffuse graft porosity.

Type I endoleaks represent a failure to successfully exclude the aneurysm and generally require treatment. If identified at the conclusion of endograft deployment, additional endovascular options (cuff extension, balloon dilatation, or coil embolization) or conversion to open repair should be considered. Type II endoleaks are the most common and can occur in approximately 20% of patients. They should be managed expectantly unless aneurysm growth occurs. If aneurysm enlargement occurs, treatment is usually indicated. Treatment options include coil embolization of lumbar or inferior mesenteric branches via femoral approach, direct aneurysm sac puncture or surgical ligation of patent aortic branches. Type III endoleaks represent device failures and generally require graft extension or relining. Type IV endoleaks are usually self-limiting and seal with reversal of intraoperative anticoagulation and deposition of fibrin in the porous graft.

Aneurysmectomy and graft replacement (straight tube or bifurcation) is the standard open surgical approach when EVAR is not feasible. It may also be performed in EVAR candidates who have no comorbidities which would contraindicate open repair and who are reluctant to undergo the continued surveillance necessary following EVAR. Although selected patients require preoperative cardiac evaluation before surgical repair of abdominal aortic aneurysms, routine cardiac screening has not been productive in the absence of risk factors for coronary artery disease. Large aneurysms in poor-risk patients can be managed by a retroperitoneal approach to the aorta to avoid the cardiopulmonary complications of transperitoneal dissection.

Ruptured abdominal aortic aneurysms may present with abdominal or back pain, syncope or hemodynamic instability, and a pulsatile abdominal mass. Emergency operative intervention is required. Prompt, uncomplicated proximal aortic control is the key to successful management of this critical condition. Most infrarenal aneurysm ruptures are contained by the retroperitoneum. Intraperitoneal rupture carries an exceptionally grave prognosis. As previously mentioned, computed tomographic scan may be useful in the occasional symptomatic patient who is hemodynamically stable to identify patients who are candidates for endovascular management. Although perioperative mortality rates for ruptured aneurysms remain significant (30% to 50% in most series), improvements in outcomes for ruptured aneurysms have been achieved with the use of EVAR. Devices must be readily available in appropriate sizes and imaging must be performed to determine the suitability for endovascular repair. Temporary transfemoral balloon occlusion of the aorta may be necessary for hemodynamic stabilization of the patient during preparation for EVAR.

Aneurysms, on rare occasions, rupture into adjacent structures. An aortocaval fistula results from rupture of an aneurysm into the inferior vena cava and manifests as high-output cardiac failure, a continuous abdominal bruit, and lower extremity ischemia with venous engorgement. Rupture into the left renal vein has also been reported and may present with hematuria. Operative treatment requires control of the abdominal aorta, but dissection of hypertensive venous structures is hazardous and should be avoided. Treatment is by graft replacement of the aortic aneurysm and repair of the inferior vena cava from within the lumen of the aorta.

Aneurysms can also rupture into the gastrointestinal (GI) tract, producing GI hemorrhage. The usual site of fistula formation is the duodenum. Repair of these primary aortoenteric fistulas is by aortic graft and repair of the duodenum or involved bowel. This protocol is different from the traditional management of secondary aortoenteric fistulas resulting from a previously placed aortic graft (see later).

Complications

Although the risk of major morbidity or mortality from elective aneurysm resection is less than 5%, there are many potential complications. Bleeding, peripheral embolization, and lower extremity ischemia may occur. Impotence may result from neurologic or vasculogenic causes. Avoidance of the presacral neural plexus and maintenance of pelvic blood flow through the hypogastric arteries should minimize this complication. Paraplegia is a rare but devastating complication of abdominal aortic surgery, resulting from spinal cord ischemia. It occurs more commonly after surgery for ruptured abdominal aortic aneurysms. Colonic ischemia can be minimized by preoperative evaluation of visceral arterial anatomy and preservation of hypogastric and inferior mesenteric blood flow when feasible. Postoperative rectal bleeding mandates prompt sigmoidoscopy for inspection of colonic mucosa. Mucosal ischemia can be managed conservatively, but transmural intestinal ischemia requires aggressive operative intervention.

Aortic graft infection is an uncommon but serious complication of surgery for both aneurysmal and occlusive diseases. Prophylactic antibiotic use should minimize this complication. Graft sepsis requires removal of prosthetic material and extra-anatomic revascularization. Secondary aortoenteric fistula may be a manifestation of aortic graft infection and usually requires graft removal. This complication can occur years after aortic graft insertion and should be suspected in any patient who presents with GI bleeding following aortic surgery. Immediate upper GI endoscopy to rule out other potential causes of bleeding is required, followed by prompt exploratory laparotomy. Rupture of the ligated aortic stump remains a potential cause of mortality following graft removal. Although controversial, recent reports describe successful management of secondary aortoenteric fistulas with aggressive surgical débridement and irrigation, in situ revascularization, and long-term antibiotic therapy.

Miscellaneous Problems

Thoracoabdominal aneurysms require an approach different from that used for infrarenal aneurysm resection. Aortic graft replacement and intraluminal attachment of visceral and renal arteries, as advocated by Crawford, have produced excellent results. Paraplegia is more common with thoracoabdominal aneurysms but may be minimized by reattaching large intercostal arteries that originate from the descending aorta, where the major blood supply to the spinal cord originates. Additional techniques, such as somatosensory-evoked potentials and spinal fluid drainage to increase spinal cord perfusion pressure, may also be used. Although thoracic endografts are now available and widely utilized for treatment of descending aortic aneurysms, branched endografts for the treatment of thoracoabdominal aneurysms remain investigational.

Inflammatory abdominal aortic aneurysms may be identified on preoperative computed tomographic scan or intraoperatively by a typical dense retroperitoneal fibrosis overlying the aorta. The conduct of the operation must be modified to avoid hazardous dissection of the duodenum or other adherent structures off the aneurysm. Although partial or (rarely) complete ureteral obstruction may be present, ureterolysis is usually unnecessary because the retroperitoneal inflammation tends to subside after repair of the aneurysm.

Horseshoe kidney in association with aortic aneurysm is an uncommon but interesting problem. Because the kidney may interfere with aneurysm dissection, and blood supply to the isthmus may originate from the aneurysm, a retroperitoneal approach and revascularization or resection of the isthmus may be required.

Coincidental malignancy discovered at the time of laparotomy for aortic aneurysm may present a therapeutic dilemma. In general, a ruptured or symptomatic aneurysm requires urgent treatment. Perforated, bleeding, or obstructing GI malignancy without impending aneurysmal rupture should take precedence. If both lesions can be dealt with electively, treatment of the aneurysm is advocated because it is imminently life-threatening. Initial reports of ruptured abdominal aneurysms following laparotomy for treatment of unrelated intra-abdominal pathology have not been substantiated.

Peripheral Aneurysms

Peripheral aneurysms likely have the same etiology as those of the aorta. The most common peripheral aneurysms occur in the popliteal artery. These lesions typically occur in men, are bilateral in more than 50% of patients, and are associated with an abdominal aortic aneurysm in about one-third of patients. Although rupture of popliteal artery aneurysms is uncommon, thrombosis or distal embolization may produce limb-threatening ischemia. Most popliteal aneurysms can be treated by ligation and bypass. Thrombosis of popliteal aneurysms may result in occlusion of the distal tibial arteries. In such cases, prompt administration of thrombolytic therapy may result in restoration of patency of outflow arteries, which can be followed by surgical correction to prevent recurrent thrombosis. Endovascular approaches with placement of covered stents have been utilized to treat popliteal aneurysms. Although initial results have been encouraging, long-term data are not available.

Femoral artery aneurysms may also be bilateral, and a significant association with abdominal aortic aneurysms exists. These lesions can be visualized on ultrasonography or computed tomographic scan. Aneurysms occur rarely in the carotid, subclavian, or other arteries. Ulnar artery aneurysms have been reported following repetitive trauma (e.g., use of vibratory tools) to the hypothenar eminence of the hand. Ligation of the ulnar artery suffices in most patients, but reconstruction may be required in the absence of a complete palmar arch.

Visceral Aneurysms

Among visceral aneurysms, splenic artery aneurysms are the most common (60%). These lesions are often asso-

ciated with arterial fibrodysplasia and occur predominantly in women. They are prone to rupture during pregnancy with potentially catastrophic outcomes. These aneurysms require treatment if symptomatic, larger than 2 cm in diameter, or diagnosed in childbearing age females. Endovascular approaches with coil embolization of the splenic artery have been extremely successful in treating splenic artery aneurysms. These catheter-based procedures can be performed during pregnancy if appropriate radiation safety measures are utilized. If endovascular therapy is not feasible or unsuccessful, surgical resection is indicated for large or symptomatic aneurysms. Aneurysms in the proximal splenic artery can usually be treated with splenic preservation.

Other visceral aneurysms are rare. Hepatic aneurysms comprise 20% of this group, and their precise cause is unknown. Superior mesenteric aneurysms comprise 5.5% of the group and are usually mycotic.

Renal artery aneurysms are uncommon and may be caused by fibromuscular dysplasia. Although most are asymptomatic, these lesions may be associated with hypertension. Rupture and dissection are potential complications, and treatment of all symptomatic and asymptomatic aneurysms larger than 2 cm is indicated.

Polyarteritis nodosa is a rare necrotizing vasculitis that affects small- and medium-sized arteries and can result in multiple small visceral and renal artery aneurysms. Aneurysm regression has been seen after treatment with corticosteroids and immunosuppressive therapy.

Infected (Mycotic) Aneurysms

Infected aneurysms of the aorta should be suspected in patients with fever, pain, and a pulsatile abdominal mass. These lesions are false (pseudo) aneurysms and may occur in patients without generalized atherosclerosis. They appear as noncalcified, saccular aneurysms and may erode adjacent lumbar vertebrae. *Salmonella, Staphylococcus,* and other organisms have been described as potential pathogens. Treatment usually requires excision of infected tissue and extra-anatomic bypass.

Mycotic femoral artery aneurysms may occur in intravenous drug abusers. These false aneurysms should be treated by excision with selective vascular reconstruction. Acute limb-threatening ischemia is most common with aneurysms involving the femoral bifurcation, and revascularization is considered if control of local sepsis can be achieved.

MESENTERIC ISCHEMIA

Mesenteric ischemia may be acute or chronic. Acute mesenteric ischemia can be caused by superior mesenteric artery embolism or thrombosis, mesenteric venous thrombosis, or nonocclusive mesenteric ischemia. Accurate diagnosis requires prompt mesenteric arteriography and appropriate surgical (e.g., embolectomy) or pharmacologic (e.g., vasodilator therapy) intervention or both. Nonocclusive mesenteric ischemia is related to low flow states. Angiography demonstrates a patent superior mesenteric artery with pruning of branch vessels. Treatment involves selective catheter infusion of vasodilators into the superior mesenteric artery and improvement of cardiovascular hemodynamics. Mesenteric venous thrombosis can be identified on abdominal computed tomographic scan and is related to hypercoagulable states or inflammatory diseases such as pancreatitis. Treatment is anticoagulation and selective use of thrombolysis. Peritoneal signs suggest the presence on nonviable bowel and laparotomy is indicated. Mortality remains high for this condition, usually because of delayed recognition.

Chronic mesenteric ischemia usually requires significant disease of at least two of the three visceral arteries (superior mesenteric, inferior mesenteric, celiac). Symptoms of chronic mesenteric ischemia include postprandial abdominal pain (mesenteric angina), anorexia, weight loss, and diarrhea.

Treatment is by aortomesenteric revascularization and often utilizes prosthetic grafts to prevent graft kinking in the retroperitoneal position. Prophylactic mesenteric revascularization during surgery on the abdominal aorta has been suggested with superior mesenteric stenosis and a large, meandering mesenteric artery, but this subject remains controversial. Endovascular approaches with angioplasty and stent have also been utilized for treatment of superior mesenteric artery occlusive disease with promising results. Celiac artery compression by the median arcuate ligament is an uncommon syndrome of questionable clinical significance.

RENAL ARTERY STENOSIS

Renovascular Hypertension

Renal artery stenosis accounts for less than 3% of hypertension. Approximately two-thirds of renovascular hypertension is caused by atherosclerosis and one-third is caused by fibromuscular dysplasia. Rarely, renal artery aneurysms can cause renovascular hypertension.

Diagnosis requires a high index of suspicion in young patients or patients with recent onset of severe hypertension. Controversy exists regarding optimal screening tests to identify renovascular hypertension. Hypertensive intravenous pyelogram (evaluating renal size, contrast uptake and excretion, and ureteral notching), radionuclide renal perfusion scans, and selective renal vein renin sampling (renin output 1.5 times the output from the normal kidney) may suggest a diagnosis of renovascular hypertension. Duplex ultrasound has replaced many of these tests in screening patients for renal vascular disease. Accurate information regarding renal artery anatomy and hemodynamics can easily be obtained with this noninvasive modality.

Treatment options include medical therapy (e.g., captopril), PTA and stent, surgical revascularization, and nephrectomy. The ability of medical therapy to prevent progressive loss of renal mass and consequent renal failure has been poor. PTA and stenting has yielded excellent results and is advocated for appropriate fibromuscular and atherosclerotic lesions.

Surgical therapy by endarterectomy or bypass has excellent patency rates. Transaortic endarterectomy is effective in treating bilateral orificial lesions. Aortorenal bypass may be performed with autogenous vein or prosthetic material. Because of the potential for aneurysmal dilatation of saphenous vein grafts in children, autogenous hypogastric artery is preferred. In patients with extensive aortic disease not requiring simultaneous treatment, renal revascularization can be successfully accomplished with hepatorenal or splenorenal bypass if these arteries are free of disease. A lateral aortogram is necessary to evaluate the origin of the celiac axis prior to these procedures. Branch lesions may be treated by bench surgery and autotransplantation. Nephrectomy is reserved for end-stage disease or uncorrectable renal artery lesions. Results of renal revascularization depend on the patient's age, duration of hypertension, and kidney size.

Ischemic Nephropathy

Patients with ischemic nephropathy have severe extra-parenchymal renal artery occlusive disease and renal insufficiency. Renal excretory function may be improved with the surgical techniques described above, which are applicable to two groups of patients. In some patients with normal or slightly elevated serum creatinine and a poor or nonfunctioning kidney, the contralateral normal kidney maintains overall renal function. These individuals are often identified during a renovascular hypertension workup, and renal revascularization may salvage the dysfunctional kidney. The second group comprises azotemic or dialysis-dependent individuals with extraparenchymal renal artery occlusive disease. Significant improvements in glomerular filtration rates and reversal of renal insufficiency have been achieved with renal artery reconstruction in properly selected patients from this group.

ANGIOACCESS SURGERY

Patients with acute or chronic renal failure require vascular access for hemodialysis. Acute access can be initiated via a central venous catheter. Catheters can be cuffed for long-term use and are usually placed in the internal jugular vein. Subclavian vein catheters should be avoided to preserve future access sites in the upper extremities. Access for chronic hemodialysis is preferred via a surgically created AV fistula. This procedure was originally described as a radiocephalic AV fistula by Brescia and colleagues. Although this remains the preferred location, fistulas may also be created between the brachial artery and the cephalic vein. If a primary cephalic vein fistula is not feasible, a fistula may be created by transposition of the forearm or upper arm basilic vein into a subcutaneous position. If no superficial veins are available for primary AV fistula or transposition, prosthetic AV grafts may be placed and punctured directly for access.

Complications of angioaccess surgery include thrombosis, infection, aneurysm or pseudoaneurysm formation, venous hypertension, carpal tunnel syndrome and ischemia secondary to steal syndrome, or ischemic monomelic neuropathy. Graft infection generally requires removal of the infected prosthetic material. Thrombosis can be managed by surgical or endovascular techniques to restore patency and treat underlying etiologies. Intimal hyperplasia remains the most common problem reducing long-term patency of dialysis grafts and fistulas. Carpal tunnel syndrome can be caused by venous hypertension or amyloid deposition in the carpal tunnel.

Significant ischemic complications of AV access occur in less than 5% of patients. Complications can include ischemic monomelic neuropathy, which is acute and selective nerve ischemia. This will often necessitate ligation of the access and a search for alternative sites. Vascular steal can produce significant clinical ischemia after AV grafts or fistulas. Both conditions are more common after brachial artery–based

procedures. Treatment options for angioaccess steal syndrome include access ligation, distal arterial ligation for radiocephalic fistulas to prevent flow reversal in the distal radial artery, banding of the access to restrict flow, and distal revascularization and interval ligation procedures. This procedure involves a bypass around the fistula or graft anastomosis with ligation of the distal artery to prevent retrograde flow and has been successful in reversing ischemic symptoms.

VASCULAR TRAUMA

Etiology

Vascular injuries may be blunt or penetrating. A number of iatrogenic conditions can occur as well, including injuries secondary to angiography, umbilical catheters, indwelling arterial cannulas, intra-aortic balloon pumps, embolectomy catheters, lumbar laminectomy (iliac AV fistula), and cardiac catheterization among others.

Principles

Pathologic lesions include transection, laceration, thrombosis, or intimal flaps. In addition, a false aneurysm or AV fistula may be present. Blunt trauma frequently produces orthopedic injury and secondary vascular trauma. The diagnosis may be difficult, particularly in the absence of significant hemorrhage or pulse deficits. Noninvasive testing with duplex ultrasound is accurate and can be used liberally in the evaluation of potential vascular injuries.

Treatment

Resuscitation of the trauma patient is described in detail in Chapter 14. Specific priorities regarding vascular injury include control of bleeding, stabilization of fractures, and repair of arterial and venous injuries. Venous repair, if possible, is recommended, particularly in the popliteal area. Primary repair of arterial injuries is advocated. If it is impossible, autogenous graft material is recommended, although reports suggest that prosthetic grafts (e.g., expanded PTFE) may function satisfactorily, even in potentially contaminated wounds.

Compartment Syndrome

Muscles of the extremities are encased in fascial compartments. Swelling within the compartment may increase compartmental pressure and interfere with vascular and neurologic function, eventually causing muscle necrosis. Compartment syndromes may be caused by direct trauma (e.g., fractures), hemorrhage, or prolonged compression of an extremity (e.g., crush syndrome); or they may occur after revascularization of an acutely ischemic extremity (e.g., for arterial embolus or trauma). Upper extremity compartments may be similarly affected (e.g., Volkmann ischemic contracture), but the lower extremity is the usual site of compartment syndrome. Pressure in each of the four lower extremity compartments (anterior, lateral, superficial posterior, and deep posterior) can be measured by direct techniques. Pressure of more than 40 mmHg, or pressure within 30 mmHg of the diastolic blood pressure, may result in cessation of flow through capillaries and arterioles. In most cases, treatment of an elevated compartment pressure is by fasciotomy of all compartments via a single incision over the fibula or in combination with a second medial incision. The sequelae of an unrelieved acute compartment syndrome are muscle and nerve necrosis with resulting functional disability.

Specific Injuries

Although a discussion of all vascular injuries is beyond the scope of this review, several specific injuries warrant further consideration. Large acute *AV fistulas* are best closed early to prevent ischemic and hemodynamic complications. Small distal AV fistulas can be observed or embolized and require only selective operative intervention. *Carotid artery injuries* should be repaired if possible, even if minor neurologic deficits are present. Vascular *injuries in the thoracic inlet* are often lethal and require a thorough knowledge of anatomy to plan the operative exposure. *Popliteal artery injuries,* if unrecognized or untreated, are associated with a high incidence of limb loss. Posterior *knee dislocation* has a significant association with arterial injury, and aggressive evaluation of these patients is recommended with duplex scan or angiography to identify lesions. *Brachial artery injuries* may occur with supracondylar fracture of the humerus and if unrecognized can result in Volkmann ischemic contracture. *Intraarterial drug injection* may threaten limb viability. In general, elevation, anticoagulation, dextran, and aggressive fasciotomy can minimize tissue loss. Reference to a text devoted to vascular trauma is recommended for treatment of other injuries.

QUESTIONS

Select one answer.

1. Acute ischemia of the lower extremity:
   a. Is most often the result of femoral artery thrombosis.
   b. Can never occur as a consequence of deep venous thrombosis.
   c. Is never amenable to treatment with thrombolytic therapy.
   d. Is most often the result of a cardiac embolic event.
   e. Rarely results in limb-threatening ischemia.

2. Evaluation for hypercoagulable states should include measurement of:
   a. Antithrombin III.
   b. Protein C.
   c. Protein S.
   d. Anticardiolipin antibody.
   e. All of the above.

3. Regarding carotid endarterectomy (CEA):
   a. Eversion endarterectomy results in a higher incidence of recurrent stenosis than CEA with patch angioplasty.
   b. Routine shunting is necessary when CEA is performed under regional anesthesia.
   c. The glossopharyngeal nerve is the most frequently injured cranial nerve during the performance of CEA.
   d. It is preferable to carotid angioplasty and stent in the treatment of carotid stenosis in patients with previous neck irradiation.
   e. It is preferable to medical therapy in patients with symptomatic high-grade carotid stenosis.

4. Which of the following is true regarding diabetic foot infections?
   a. They are usually caused by infection with gram-positive organisms only.
   b. Surgical débridement is unnecessary when pedal pulses are present.
   c. Oral antibiotics are adequate treatment in most cases.
   d. Neuropathy is rarely a contributing factor in their development.
   e. Revascularization may be required even if adequate surgical débridement is done and appropriate antibiotics are used.

5. Which of the following statements regarding aneurysms is true?
   a. Inflammatory aneurysms of the aorta rarely rupture.
   b. Splenic artery aneurysms are usually atherosclerotic in origin.
   c. Thrombosis of popliteal artery aneurysms may be treated with thrombolysis only.
   d. Infected aneurysms of the aorta usually require complete excision and extra-anatomic revascularization.
   e. Aneurysms of the hepatic artery are the most common visceral aneurysms.

6. Which of the following is true?
   a. Surgery is indicated for most visceral aneurysms associated with polyarteritis nodosa.
   b. Takayasu's arteritis most commonly involves the distal arm and hand arteries in middle-aged men.
   c. Patients with fibromuscular dysplasia of the carotid artery may have associated intracranial aneurysms.
   d. Most patients with Raynaud's disease require sympathectomy.
   e. Popliteal entrapment syndrome usually results in lateral displacement of the popliteal artery.

7. Which of the following is true about patients with intermittent claudication?
   a. Lumbar sympathectomy effectively relieves symptoms in most patients.
   b. A graded exercise program improves the walking capacity of most of the patients.
   c. Arteriography should be performed as part of the initial clinical assessment.
   d. Pentoxifylline is more effective than cilostazol in improving walking distance.
   e. Amputation is required in up to one-third of patients if left untreated.

8. Which of the following is true regarding endovascular abdominal aortic aneurysm repair?
   a. Most Type I endoleaks can be safely observed without treatment.
   b. Endovascular repair should never be considered for treatment of ruptured aneurysms.
   c. Endovascular repair is indicated for treatment of aneurysms less than 5 cm in diameter.
   d. Type II endoleaks associated with aneurysm growth should be treated.
   e. Endovascular repair is suitable for most juxtarenal aneurysms.

9. Subclavian steal syndrome:
   a. May be treated with endovascular or surgical techniques.
   b. Requires treatment in asymptomatic patients.
   c. Can be diagnosed by visualizing retrograde blood flow in the subclavian artery.
   d. May cause amaurosis fugax.
   e. Is more common on the left side.

10. Ischemic complications of hemodialysis access:
    a. Rarely require access ligation for ischemic monomelic neuropathy.
    b. Are clinically manifest in up to 15% of patients.
    c. May be successfully treated with a distal revascularization and interval ligation procedure for steal syndrome.
    d. Are most frequent after radiocephalic AV fistulas.
    e. Are usually caused by intimal hyperplasia.

SELECTED REFERENCES

Baron JF, Mundler O, Bertrand M, et al. Dipyridamole-thallium scintigraphy and gated radionuclide angiography to assess cardiac risk before abdominal aortic surgery. *N Engl J Med* 1994;330:663–669.

Brescia MJ, Cimino JE, Appel K, Hurwich BJ. Chronic hemodialysis using venipuncture and a surgically created arteriovenous fistula. *N Engl J Med* 1966;17:1089–1092.

Brott TG, Hobson RW, Howard G, et al. Stenting versus endarterectomy for treatment of carotid artery stenosis. *N Engl J Med* 2010;363:11–23.

Chaikof EL, Brewster DC, Dalman RL, et al. The care of patients with an abdominal aortic aneurysm: the Society for Vascular Surgery practice guidelines. *J Vasc Surg* 2009;50: S2–S49.

Crawford ES, Coselli JS. Thoracoabdominal aneurysm surgery. *Semin Thorac Cardiovasc Surg* 1991;3:300–322.

Cronenwett JL, Johnston W, eds. *Rutherford's vascular surgery*, 7th ed. Philadelphia, PA: Elsevier Saunders, 2010.

Executive Committee for the Asymptomatic Carotid Atherosclerosis Study. Endarterectomy for asymptomatic carotid artery stenosis. *JAMA* 1995;273:1421–1428.

Moore WS, ed. *Vascular and endovascular surgery: a comprehensive review*, 7th ed. Philadelphia, PA: Elsevier Saunders, 2006.

North American Symptomatic Carotid Endarterectomy Trial Collaborators. Beneficial effect of carotid endarterectomy in symptomatic patients with high-grade carotid stenosis. *N Engl J Med* 1991;325:445–453.

United Kingdom Small Aneurysm Trial Participants. Long-term outcomes of immediate repair compared with surveillance of small abdominal aortic aneurysms. *N Engl J Med* 2002;346:1445–1452.

Venous and Lymphatic Disease

ANATOMY

The veins of the lower extremity are divided into the deep and superficial systems. The latter system consists of the great saphenous vein, the short (formerly the lesser) saphenous vein, and their tributaries. The great saphenous vein courses along the medial aspect of the leg from the medial malleolus to the groin and enters the deep system at the common femoral vein. Just prior to its entrance into the common femoral vein, the great saphenous vein receives five tributaries. The short saphenous vein courses up the posterior calf and enters the popliteal vein in the popliteal fossa. In some patients, it does not enter the popliteal but rather courses up the thigh to enter the saphenous vein. When this happens, the vein in the thigh is sometimes referred to as the vein of Giacomini. The deep system of veins consists of named venous trunks that coincide with the major arteries. It should be noted that below the knee, there are often two veins for every one artery. Connecting the deep and superficial systems are the perforator or communicating veins. These drain into the plexus of veins within the soleus and gastrocnemius muscles and together comprise the "muscle pump." Most of the perforators are clustered around the medial malleolus, with a few just above and below the knee.

The veins of the upper extremity include the radial, ulnar, brachial, axillary, subclavian and innominate deep veins, and the cephalic and basilic superficial veins. Most venous pathology (other than phlebitis) usually involves the veins of the lower extremity; hence, the majority of this chapter will deal with lower extremity conditions.

APPLIED VENOUS PHYSIOLOGY

Veins are richly supplied with valves. These bicuspid leaflets prevent blood from falling back down to the foot or hand in the erect position. The valves within the perforator veins also prevent blood from being squeezed out of the muscle pump into the superficial system when the muscle pump is activated during walking. In the normal subject, flow in the veins is toward the heart and is dependent on respiration, arterial inflow, position, and the activity of the muscle pump. Under resting conditions in the recumbent position, venous flow is phasic with respiration. In the lower extremity, flow is decreased during inspiration, since, although intrathoracic pressure becomes negative, intra-abdominal pressure becomes positive. With expiration, the temporary backup of blood that occurred during inspiration is released, and venous flow increases. During walking, when the muscle pump is active, blood is squeezed out of the muscle plexus of veins toward the heart, thus increasing flow in the deep system. Flow in the superficial system usually continues in an antegrade fashion. As the muscle pump relaxes within the walking cycle, blood is sucked into the muscle pump from the superficial system, thus refilling the deep plexus of veins. Provided that the perforator veins are competent, flow will be dominantly from the superficial system into the deep system and then to the heart.

Venous pressure at rest equals the weight of the column of blood from the point of estimation to the third interspace at the sternum. It should be remembered that venous valves prevent retrograde flow in the upright position but do not impede the effects of pressure. Thus, in the recumbent position, pressure at the ankle is approximately 10 mm Hg, whereas in the standing position, it equals 86 mm Hg. Furthermore, in the standing position, approximately 500 mL of blood will be accumulated in the veins of the leg. With exercise, the muscle pump lowers venous pressure in the dependent limb, reduces venous volume in the exercised area, and, as mentioned earlier, facilitates venous return to the heart.

With valvular destruction and chronic venous insufficiency, the hemodynamics of venous flow in the lower extremity is severely affected. Patients with primary varicose veins, in which only the valves of the saphenous system are incompetent, usually have minimal clinical manifestations, since functioning deep and perforator valves still allow for an efficient muscle pumping activity. If the deep and perforator valves are incompetent, efficacy of the muscle pump is greatly reduced, since during muscular activity blood will be directed not only toward the heart but also toward the superficial system. Venous pressure measurements obtained during walking will no longer show the significant reduction that occurs with muscular contractions. A state of ambulatory venous hypertension may thus result, and this may be aggravated if there is any proximal venous obstruction. This altered physiology results in diapedesis of red cells through the capillaries with destruction of hemoglobin and ultimate pigmentary changes in the skin. Edema and swelling may result, and, if it is complicated by lymphatic obstruction from fibrotic change of the edema fluid, capillary block and ultimately skin destruction may occur, resulting in chronic venous ulceration.

VARICOSE VEINS

Varicose veins may be primary or secondary. The majority of patients suffer from primary varicose veins, perhaps as a result of prolonged standing. Females are more commonly affected than males, with the varicosities usually manifesting during pregnancy. This is probably a result of hormonal changes rather than pressure effects, since the varicose veins usually begin to manifest in the first trimester, at which stage uterine growth has barely begun. An important congenital cause of varicose veins is the Klippel–Trenaunay syndrome, which manifests as varicose veins, cutaneous arteriovenous malformations, and, occasionally, gigantism of the involved extremities. Venograms of such patients may also demonstrate hypoplasia of the deep venous system. It is important to recognize these children, since venous interventions are generally contraindicated. A few patients may present with secondary varicose veins as a result of some other cause of arteriovenous fistulas, such as trauma. However, the majority of secondary varicose veins occur following valvular destruction from previous deep venous thrombophlebitis (DVT).

Clinical Manifestations

Most patients with varicose veins remain asymptomatic, their only concern being the cosmetic effects. However, some patients complain of an aching sensation that occurs after prolonged standing and which is relieved by rest. Occasionally, varicose veins may hemorrhage, especially when traumatized. First-aid treatment for such hemorrhage is elevation of the extremity with local pressure. A tourniquet should not be applied proximally, since this increases venous pressure and resultant bleeding. Superficial thrombophlebitis may also occur in a varicose vein (see later).

Treatment

Asymptomatic varicose veins require no therapy, but many patients will appropriately request treatment for cosmetic purposes. If symptoms are present, support stockings may decrease the sense of discomfort, but if it is persistent, or if recurrent episodes of superficial thrombophlebitis or hemorrhage have occurred, invasive treatment may be warranted. Treatment options have expanded considerably in the last decade. These include compression, compression sclerotherapy, stab avulsion phlebectomy, laser or radiofrequency ablation of the saphenous vein or perforators, and surgical stripping of the saphenous vein or any combination of the above. Controversy still exists as to which method achieves the best long-term results, but less invasive methods have gained in popularity.

Compression Sclerotherapy
Compression sclerotherapy involves the injection of an irritant substance into the vein while the vein wall is collapsed by elevation of the extremity. Compression is then maintained by wrapping the limb with a tight bandage or by using a surgical weight support stocking. The substance most commonly used for compression sclerotherapy is sodium tetradecyl sulfate with large veins requiring a 3% solution and smaller veins a reduced dosage. The results of compression sclerotherapy are variable. It appears to be most useful when the veins are localized to the below-knee area and when saphenous reflux is not present. Compression of veins in the thigh is often difficult, and the recurrence rate is higher. Complications include allergic reactions, toxic effects of an overdose of the sclerosant, thromboembolic phenomenon, ulceration of the skin from perivenous placement of the sclerosing agent, and recurrence. A method of mixing the

sclerosant with air or CO_2, so-called foam sclerotherapy, is increasingly being advocated. This technique may have a special role in the management of secondary groin varices following previous saphenous ablation or removal. It may also be beneficial for obliteration of perforators in patients with venous ulceration. However, there have been reports of amaurosis, migraine headaches, and, rarely, stroke especially in patients with a patent foramen ovale. More importantly, this technique is not currently FDA approved.

Phlebectomy

Outpatient excision of varicose vein clusters has increasingly replaced sclerotherapy. This technique can be done in the office under local or tumescent anesthesia. Small nicks are made with a no. 11 blade or equivalent instrument. Specially designed hooks are used to avulse the varicose vein cluster. The veins have no pain fibers, so as long as subcutaneous tissue is also not removed, the patient experiences no discomfort other than a pulling sensation which is well tolerated. Hemostasis is achieved by finger pressure and no sutures are required. The incisions can be closed with Steri-Strips. A surgical stocking can be used as the dressing and patients are instructed to maintain normal activity. The stocking can be removed after 2 days. Cosmetic results are excellent but recurrence is not infrequent. In patients with significant saphenous reflux, ablation or removal of the saphenous vein is often advised to decrease the incidence of recurrence.

Surgery

Many different variations of surgical removal of varicose veins have been described. In general, all involve disconnection of the greater saphenous vein from the common femoral (or the lesser saphenous vein from the popliteal) if these superficial veins are proven to be incompetent by clinical or noninvasive evaluation. The residual vein can be left in place (high ligation of the saphenous vein) or surgically stripped (stripping operation). However, all venous stripping operations have in common the removal of the greater saphenous or involved lesser saphenous vein using a stripping device that is passed from the distal vein at the knee or ankle to the groin and then removed, thus pulling out the surrounding vein. As described earlier, the remaining varicose tributaries are excised via separate local phlebectomy incisions. Specific complications of these operations include inadvertent stripping of the femoral artery or the deep femoral venous system,

injury to the saphenous nerve, ligation of the femoral vein, and pulmonary embolism (PE). Although high ligation can be performed under local anesthesia, stripping usually requires formal anesthesia or at least tumescent anesthesia performed in an operating room. Recovery is prolonged due to postoperative pain. High ligation alone is not infrequently followed by recurrent varicose veins, but even a full stripping may not prevent recurrence. Because of the morbidity of these procedures, radiofrequency or laser ablation is becoming the preferred therapy, although long-term data (i.e., >10 years) are still not available to ensure that these outpatient techniques offer superior protection from recurrence.

Saphenous Vein Ablation

Radiofrequency and laser devices have been developed to ablate the saphenous veins in situ without removal. Usually performed in an office or outpatient center, these procedures have rapidly supplanted stripping. The procedures are performed using tumescent anesthesia. This involves injection of approximately 200 mL of very dilute lidocaine into the perivenous space. This fluid not only provides anesthesia but also serves to compress the vein and cool the surrounding tissues. Ultrasound imaging is required to allow insertion of the fiber optic laser or radiofrequency catheter. Using ultrasound, the tumescence is delivered to the perisaphenous space. This fluid not only provides anesthesia but also serves to contract the vein more closely around the fiber or catheter and also acts as a heat sink to prevent inadvertent heat damage to surrounding tissue. Complications such as DVT, skin burns, and paresthesias are rare. Ultrasound proven ablation at 1 year is about 96% in most reported series. As with stripping procedures, residual varicose veins will require phlebectomy or sclerotherapy.

CHRONIC VENOUS INSUFFICIENCY

The clinical syndrome of chronic venous insufficiency can result from long-standing varicose veins but more often occurs from venous valvular dysfunction, most commonly caused by previous DVT. Patients complain of a sense of lower extremity discomfort that is worse in the late afternoon after standing and that is relieved by lying down. Examination of the legs may demonstrate varicose veins, pitting edema and swelling, brownish skin discoloration with thickening and scaling of the skin around the medial malleolus, or, ultimately, venous ulceration. These ulcers usually localize around the medial malleolus but may be more extensive and involve the entire leg and foot. They are commonly painless.

The diagnosis of chronic venous insufficiency can be supported by noninvasive techniques. They include use of the Doppler ultrasound flow detector to determine the direction of flow in the superficial and deep venous system. Retrograde flow of more than 0.5 seconds during a valsalva maneuver suggests valvular dysfunction. Photoplethysmography is increasingly being used to document chronic venous insufficiency. The photoplethysmograph measures skin capillary blood content. In normal controls, after five active dorsiflexions are performed in the sitting position, skin capillary blood content decreases as venous blood is pushed toward the heart. If valves are competent, these parameters will return to normal slowly, as arterial blood supply refills the extremity. The time taken for this to occur is called the venous recovery time (VRT). In patients with chronic venous insufficiency and valvular dysfunction, the VRT is shortened (<20 seconds). Primary and secondary chronic venous insufficiency can be defined by combining these tests with the use of a tourniquet placed below the knee. If such a tourniquet, which occludes the superficial veins, returns VRT to normal, it can be assumed that chronic venous insufficiency is caused by superficial venous dysfunction rather than deep. Failure of the VRT to improve with the use of a tourniquet suggests deep venous incompetence. Color duplex scanning has recently been proven to be a reliable method of demonstrating venous reflux, valve function, and location of perforators. Venograms are seldom necessary.

Management

Symptomatic improvement of patients with chronic venous insufficiency can usually be achieved using surgical support stockings, which offer a graduated pressure of 30 to 40 mm Hg to the extremity. Patients with advanced venous ulceration also require some method of delivering external compression. Standard therapy has usually consisted of an Unna's boot supplemented by an external elastic wrap or an Ace bandage. Newer techniques include use of special dressings supplemented by compression stockings, for example, Jobst UlcerCare. Once the ulcer is healed, stocking therapy should still be used to prevent recurrence. When these ulcers are recalcitrant to these conservative

forms of therapy, hospital admission with prolonged bed rest and possible split-thickness skin grafts may be required to achieve healing.

Surgical techniques for ulcer healing have been attempted. Direct venous valvular reconstructions by valve transposition (axillary or jugular venous valve) or valve repair (e.g., Kistner technique) have been described, but acceptable long-term results have rarely been reported. In the mid-20th century, Linton described subfascial ligation of perforators via a long medial incision. However, the morbidity of cutting through the fibrotic tissue associated with chronic stasis and ulceration was high, and so a less invasive technique using endoscopic techniques was devised (subfascial endoscopic ligation of perforator surgery or SEPS). However, although originally adopted with enthusiasm, difficulty in performing the SEPS procedures as well as early recurrent ulceration has resulted in a decline in the number of these procedures being performed. Direct ablation of perforators by radiofrequency, laser, or sclerotherapy now appears to be the more popular approach, but due to the novelty of these techniques, long-term data are not available.

THROMBOPHLEBITIS

The formation of blood clots within the venous system is called thrombophlebitis. This may occur in the superficial veins or deep veins.

Superficial Venous Thrombophlebitis

Superficial venous thrombophlebitis (SVT) usually occurs in patients who have varicose veins, although it may occur spontaneously in normal veins. If SVT is recurrent and associated with episodes of SVT in other unusual parts of the body, a diagnosis of migratory thrombophlebitis should be entertained and a workup instituted to attempt to detect some occult malignancy or hypercoagulable state. Rarely, SVT can be associated with a DVT. However, in general, SVT is a benign condition. Superficial phlebitis of the upper extremity veins is seldom spontaneous and is usually a result of venipuncture or intravenous catheters. It is increasingly seen these days in connection with peripherally inserted central catheter (PICC) lines.

Clinical Manifestations

SVT manifests with all the signs of local inflammation. These include redness, tenderness, local heat, pain, and swelling in the involved superficial vein. On occasion, SVT may be misdiagnosed as cellulitis; however, persistent fever is usually absent. The risk of PE is extremely low (<3%).

Management

Symptomatic relief is usually all that is required for such patients. This may be achieved by an anti-inflammatory analgesic such as indomethacin. Patients should be encouraged to continue ambulation, since bed rest may contribute to stasis and further aggravate the disease. Antibiotics are not required, since bacterial colonization of thrombus has not been demonstrated. The risk of PE increases if the phlebitis migrates up to the thigh especially if it comes close to the saphenofemoral junction. If this occurs, then ligation and division of the saphenous vein in the groin can be performed or the patient can be anticoagulated for a brief (1 month) period. Such a procedure can be done under local anesthesia. All patients with superficial thrombophlebitis should undergo some form of noninvasive testing to exclude an underlying, unrecognized DVT. Patients who have recurrent episodes of superficial thrombophlebitis occurring in varicose veins are candidates for phlebectomy and possibly saphenous ablation if incompetent.

Deep Venous Thrombophlebitis

DVT may occur spontaneously or as a result of some underlying inherited or acquired predisposing factor. The more common acquired risk factors include advanced age, hospitalization and immobilization, hormone replacement and oral contraceptive therapy, pregnancy and the recent postpartum state, prior venous thromboembolism (VTE), malignancy, major surgery, obesity, nephrotic syndrome, trauma, spinal cord injury, lengthy travel (generally >6 hours), varicose veins, antiphospholipid antibody syndrome, myeloproliferative disorders, and polycythemia. Heritable risk factors include factor V Leiden, prothrombin 20210A gene variant, antithrombin, protein C and S deficiency, and dysfibrinogenemias. In some patients, the etiology for the thrombophilia may have a heritable and acquired component. These include homocysteinemia; factors VII, VIII, IX, and XI elevation; hyperfibrinogenemia; and activated protein C resistance in the absence of factor V Leiden.

When multiple inherited and acquired risk factors are present in the same patient, a synergistic effect may occur, depending on the thrombophilia in question. For example, patients who are heterozygous for factor V Leiden are at only moderately increased risk for VTE (4- to 8-fold). However, when combined with the additional risk of oral contraceptive use, the risk for VTE increases approximately 35-fold, the same order of magnitude as someone who is homozygous for factor V Leiden.

Upper extremity deep vein phlebitis usually is associated with indwelling catheters such as PICC lines, ports, and dialysis catheters. However, spontaneous occlusion of the subclavian or axillary veins can be a result of thoracic outlet compression usually due to muscular compression or abnormal muscular bands (exertional axillosubclavian vein thrombosis or Paget–Schroetter syndrome).

Clinical Manifestations

The clinical diagnosis of DVT is extremely unreliable, and approximately 50% of patients may present without any major clinical findings. These findings include swelling, pain, local tenderness, and a fever spike. A palpable cord is seldom felt, and Homan's sign (pain in the calf with dorsiflexion of the foot) is present in only 25% of patients.

Because of the inaccuracy of the clinical diagnosis of DVT, further objective testing is required. However, since venograms themselves may induce phlebitis in 2% to 5% of patients, and since these procedures are painful, costly, and carry a small anaphylactic risk, noninvasive diagnostic techniques have been utilized. Duplex color ultrasound has supplanted older noninvasive techniques, and most physicians utilize these tests as the only diagnostic method foregoing venography. Accuracy rates for "named vein" phlebitis approaches 95% to 98%. A D-dimer blood test is often added to increase accuracy. This is especially helpful in delineating acute from chronic clot seen on duplex ultrasound. A negative D-dimer is very accurate in excluding DVT, but false positives are not infrequent especially postsurgery. The D-dimer is especially useful when duplex ultrasound is not available such as during the night hours. However, the most accurate method of diagnosing DVT includes use of D-dimer, ultrasound, and history and physical findings. The Wells' scoring system is especially helpful. However, venography may still be required in some patients (see Table 8.1).

Management

Patients with confirmed DVT require immediate anticoagulation. Since the anticoagulant effect of

TABLE 8.1	**Wells Criteria for Predicting Pretest Probability of Deep Vein Thrombosis. A Score of <1 is Low Probability, 1 or 2 is Moderate Probability, and >2 is High Probability**

Clinical Characteristic	Score
Active cancer (treatment ongoing or within previous 6 months or palliative)	1
Paralysis, paresis, or recent plaster immobilization of the lower extremities	1
Recently bedridden for more than 3 days or major surgery within 4 weeks	1
Localized tenderness along the distribution of the deep venous system	1
Entire leg swollen, calf swelling >3 cm larger than asymptomatic side (measured 10 cm below tibial tuberosity)	1
Pitting edema confined to the symptomatic leg	1
Collateral superficial veins (nonvaricose)	1
Previously documented DVT	1
Alternative diagnosis at least as likely as DVT	−2

Source: Wells PS, Anderson DR, Bormanis J, et al. Value of assessment of pretest probability of deep-vein thrombosis in clinical management. *Lancet* 1997;350:1795–1798.

warfarin takes about 3 to 5 days to become therapeutic, intravenous heparin, subcutaneous injections of heparin, or low-molecular-weight heparins will be required until therapeutic levels of warfarin have been achieved. Most upper extremity DVTs as well as infrainguinal DVTs can be managed as an outpatient with hospitalization being reserved for iliofemoral DVT or PE. Anticoagulant therapy with heparin should be started using a loading dose of 100 to 150 U/kg followed by continuous infusion of heparin at a dose of approximately 10 to 15 U/kg/hr. The anticoagulant effect of heparin should be monitored using the partial thromboplastin time (PTT) or activated clotting times. Adequate heparinization is achieved when these tests are prolonged to 1.5 times baseline. Once such levels are achieved, the test may be performed on a daily basis. Platelet counts should be performed every 2 to 3 days, since a few patients may manifest heparin-induced thrombocytopenia (HIT), whereby platelet consumption occurs with formation of platelet clots and increasing resistance to heparin's anticoagulant effect. Measurement of heparin antibodies may confirm the diagnosis of HIT. If the platelet count falls below 50,000, heparin therapy should be discontinued. Under such circumstances, direct thrombin inhibitors such as Hirudin or argatroban can be utilized. In general, patients with extensive DVT will require larger doses of heparin to achieve adequate anticoagulation. Low-molecular-weight heparins are increasingly replacing continuous infusion heparin due to ease of use, lower risk of HIT, and the absence of the need for PTT monitoring.

These drugs have weak antithrombin (factor IIa) activity but inactivate factor Xa and are given as a weight-adjusted dose. Routine laboratory monitoring is not necessary, but selective measurement of anti-Xa levels can be done in children or obese patients in whom high or low drug levels are anticipated.

Coumadin therapy is usually initiated at an oral dose of 5 mg of Coumadin daily. The goal of Coumadin therapy is the prolongation of the prothrombin time to 1.5 times baseline or an international normalized ratio (INR) of 2 to 3. Once this has occurred, heparin therapy can be discontinued. It is important that compression stockings be prescribed to decrease the sequelae of chronic venous insufficiency. The duration of chronic Coumadin therapy is controversial. Most physicians would agree with a 3-month course for a DVT that complicates a resolvable etiology such as recent orthopedic limb surgery. A spontaneous DVT without a predisposing event should be treated for at least 6 to 12 months. Patients who have recurrent DVT should probably be on Coumadin for life. Patients with antiphospholipid syndrome should also be considered for life-long anticoagulation. Patients with severe iliofemoral DVT and associated noncurable malignancy may require low-molecular-weight heparin long term instead of Coumadin.

Venous thrombectomy, although popular in Europe, is rarely performed in the United States. An indication may be to prevent limb loss in patients with incipient venous gangrene caused by massive iliofemoral venous thrombosis (phlegmasia alba and cerulea dolens). This rare complication is most often associated with DVT complicating metastatic malignancies. Tissue plasminogen activator, urokinase, and other lytic therapy have also been used with theoretical advantages of preservation of venous valve function in patients with iliofemoral thrombus. Definitive proof of benefit is, as yet, unavailable. However, lytic therapy associated with mechanical deformity and/or aspiration of clot using endovenous mechanical devices is gaining acceptance, especially if it can be performed within 14 days after the onset of thrombosis. A specific entity, May–Thurner syndrome, is a DVT associated with compression of the left iliac vein by the right iliac artery. This is often seen in women and responds well to clot lysis and endovenous stenting of the iliac vein.

Patients who have a contraindication to anticoagulation will require caval interruption using one of the many commercially available vena caval filters. These can be inserted with minimal morbidity via a femoral vein or jugular vein puncture using fluoroscopy or ultrasound for positioning in the vena cava below the renal veins. Prior to insertion, an inferior vena cavagram is recommended. Such a venogram will identify those patients with suprarenal clot, large vena cava, or double vena cava that would affect filter placement. Some newer filters can be removed up to 6 months after insertion if necessary.

Patients who develop spontaneous upper extremity DVT may benefit from lytic therapy, first rib resection, and possible stenting of the subclavian vein.

Prophylaxis

Various methods for the prevention of DVT in patients undergoing surgery have been described. These include full heparinization and coumadinization as well as minidose heparin, low-molecular-weight heparins, antithrombins, dextran, compression stockings, and intermittent sequential compression devices. Aspirin and antiplatelet drugs have also been utilized. Currently, the most popular methods of treatment involve combinations of minidose heparin (5,000 U subcutaneously [s.c.] b.i.d.) or s.c. low-molecular-weight heparins and/or lower extremity compression devices. Both methods have been shown to significantly decrease the incidence of DVT and PE. However, since some bleeding complications may still result from such prophylaxis, most surgeons reserve anticoagulation for high-risk patients, that is, orthopedic patients, especially those undergoing hip surgery, obese or elderly patients, and patients with a past history of thromboembolic disease. Intermittent pneumatic compression devices are widely utilized for DVT prophylaxis. Their efficacy is based on prevention of venous stasis as well as activation of fibrinolysis.

Pulmonary Embolism

Pulmonary embolism (PE) remains an important cause of postoperative mortality. The clinical spectrum may vary from completely subclinical to sudden death. Postoperative unexplained tachycardia is an extremely important pointer to the diagnosis of PE. Other manifestations include tachypnea, pleuritic chest pain, and hemoptysis. Arterial blood gases may demonstrate a respiratory alkalosis in the early stages, but with extensive pulmonary emboli, respiratory acidosis may develop. An electrocardiogram may show evidence of right heart strain with S waves in standard lead I and inverted T waves and Q waves in standard lead III. The chest x-ray may be completely normal or may show hypoperfused vascular markings. Ventilation-perfusion lung scans are often utilized for diagnosis, but a high false-positive rate makes them of limited value. Accordingly, spiral CT angiography has all, but abolished, the need for lung scans or conventional pulmonary angiography. The D-dimer may also be helpful.

Management of such patients involves general supportive care as well as heparin or low-molecular-weight heparin anticoagulation, followed by warfarin. Lytic therapy has also been used, but clinical evidence of improved mortality and morbidity has not been conclusively demonstrated. However, in patients who are clinically unstable because of the PE, lytic therapy may be lifesaving. If contraindicated, these critically ill patients may have to undergo pulmonary embolectomy.

Patients who have recurrent pulmonary emboli on adequate heparin therapy or those who have a contraindication to anticoagulation therapy will require a vena caval filter. With the recent development of filters that can be subsequently removed, temporary filters have sometimes been advised for high-risk patients such as multiple trauma victims or patients undergoing bariatric surgery.

LYMPHEDEMA

Lymphedema may be of primary or secondary origin. Primary lymphedema that occurs at birth is known as lymphedema congenital. When this occurs with a familial predisposition, the condition is referred to as Milroy's disease. Lymphedema that begins to occur during adolescence is much more common and is known as lymphedema praecox. The specific etiology of lymphedema praecox is not known but is related to hypo- and hyperplastic changes within the lymphatic system of the extremities. It does not carry familial tendencies.

Acquired lymphedema is the most common form of this condition and usually results from axillary or inguinal node dissection or persistent chronic venous insufficiency. Other rare causes include tuberculosis, actinomycosis, lymphogranuloma, Hodgkin's disease, and filariasis.

Pathophysiology

Lymphatic obstruction results in a failure of removal of capillary fluid transudation from the tissues. Since this fluid contains protein and fibroblasts, fibrous tissue builds up, thickening the skin and subcutaneous tissue and leading to further obliteration of lymphatic vessels. Thus, the natural history of lymphedema is continued progression. Symptoms occur because of the excess weight of the extremities. The lymphedematous limb is also predisposed to recurrent episodes of cellulitis, although this is less common in the praecox variety. Recurrent cellulitis further destroys lymphatics, thus aggravating the edema. Fungal superinfection of the thickened skin is not uncommon. Rarely, lymphangiosarcoma may develop in patients with long-standing untreated lymphedema (Stewart–Treves syndrome).

Diagnosis

The diagnosis of lymphedema is usually made on clinical grounds. Swelling often begins at the ankle and moves proximally. The edema is brawny and indurated. Often the edema is unilateral, but bilateral edema is not rare. The swelling is painless, and there is no evidence of inflammation. The temperature of the involved limb remains equal to that of the uninvolved extremities. Skin ulceration is almost never seen with lymphedema praecox. Lymphedema congenital is sometimes associated with other external abnormalities such as yellow fingernails, Turner syndrome, and Noonan syndrome. The "gold standard" for the diagnosis of lymphedema remains the lymphangiogram. This technique involves the injection of a vital dye into the web space between the digits of the infected extremities. This technique involves a cutdown and accordingly, the less invasive

technique of radionuclear lymphoscintigraphy using technetium-99m sulfur colloid has also been utilized. In most cases, however, clinical diagnosis will be sufficient.

Treatment

Since the clinical course of untreated lymphedema is unrelenting progression, attention should be given not only to local treatment but also to psychological support for the adolescent patient. In general, conservative measures suffice. These include use of a custom-fitted heavy-duty elastic support, modification of activity to permit intermittent periods of leg elevation, optimal foot hygiene, and prompt treatment of cellulitis, if this should occur. In addition, the use of high compression lymphedema pumps or massage therapy may be useful adjuncts in the management of these patients. Patients who suffer repeated attacks of cellulitis should be placed on antibiotic prophylaxis with penicillin 250 mg q.i.d. or erythromycin 250 mg q.i.d. for first week of every month. Fungal infections should be controlled, since these can lead to secondary bacterial involvement. Diuretics may also be prescribed intermittently to help decrease fluid accumulation. Surgical treatment seldom is required in the adolescent. However, later in life, if limb size becomes so extreme as to impinge on daily existence, surgical therapy may be warranted. The primary surgical techniques currently include one of two approaches: (a) debulking procedures, which involve removal of most of the subcutaneous tissue with a wound cover using the raised skin flaps or split-thickness skin grafts and (b) the creation of new lymphatics by pedicle flaps, omental transfer, or lymphatic venous anastomosis. These latter procedures are of dubious value and remain unproven.

QUESTIONS

Select one answer.

1. A 58-year-old male undergoes bariatric surgery. Two days later, he complains of pain in his right leg. On examination, it is not swollen but the calf is tender. The best screening test for detecting DVT of the lower extremities is
   a. D-dimer.
   b. Venous plethysmography.
   c. Phlebography.
   d. Venography.
   e. Venous duplex scan.

2. A 33-year-old female is upset by the appearance of her legs. On examination, she has extensive varicose veins but there is no discoloration or swelling. A venous duplex scan demonstrates reflux throughout a dilated saphenous vein. The deep veins are competent. Suitable therapy for improving the cosmetic nature of her legs would include
   a. Stab avulsion phlebectomy alone.
   b. Stab avulsion and laser or radiofrequency ablation of the saphenous vein.
   c. Compression stockings
   d. Foam sclerotherapy.
   e. SEPS procedure.

3. A 50-year-old woman suddenly develops painful swelling in her left leg. Duplex scan demonstrates occlusion of the left iliac and femoral veins. What statement is not true?
   a. A probable cause is compression of the iliac vein by the left iliac artery.
   b. She may harbor a hypercoagulable condition such as factor V Leiden.
   c. Treatment could include lytic therapy.
   d. A vena caval filter may be required.
   e. Treatment could include a venous stent.

4. A 55-year-old male requires bariatric surgery for obesity. He has a maternal family history of DVT and he has had a superficial phlebitis in his varicose veins twice before. Management should include all except

   a. Intermittent pneumatic compression during surgery.
   b. Possible low-molecular-weight prophylaxis perioperatively.
   c. Possible use of a removable vena caval filter prior to surgery.
   d. Preoperative blood tests to evaluate possible hypercoagulable tendency.
   e. Cancel surgery.

5. A 55-year-old male, heavy smoker who likes to lift weights develops a swollen left arm. Prior to this, he has noted tingling in his hand along the ulnar distribution. Management should include all except
   a. Lytic therapy to open the cephalic vein.
   b. Lytic therapy to open the axillary vein.
   c. Possible first rib resection.
   d. Possible placement of a venous stent.
   e. X-ray of his neck and chest.

SELECTED REFERENCES

Hobbs JT. Surgery and sclerotherapy in the treatment of varicose veins. *Arch Surg* 1974;109:793.

Rutherford R. *Vascular surgery*. 6th ed. Philadelphia, PA: Elsevier Saunders, 2005.

Strandness DE, Sumner DS. *Hemodynamics for surgeons*. New York, NY: Grune & Stratton, 1975:396–416.

Wells PS, Anderson DR, Bormanis J, et al. Value of assessment of pretest probability of deep-vein thrombosis in clinical management. *Lancet* 1997;350:1795–1798.

Wolfe JHN, Kinmonth JB. The prognosis of primary lymphedema of the lower limb. *Arch Surg* 1981;166:1157.

Diseases of the Breast

Breast cancer is the second most common cancer causing death among women in the United States (after carcinoma of the lung) and is the most common cause of death among women between 35 and 40 years of age. Epidemiologic variations are striking in different countries. The incidence of breast cancer in the United States continues to rise. Despite this increase in incidence, the mortality from breast cancer has recently begun to fall, possibly because of early detection and improvements in therapy.

PALPABLE BREAST MASSES

Although inspection precedes palpation during any physical examination, the most important initial presentation of breast cancer is a palpable mass in the breast detected by a patient or a physician. The etiology of breast masses is related to the age of the patient.

Fibroadenoma

From puberty until the late twenties, the most common cause of a discrete mass in the breast is a fibroadenoma. There may be a slight increase in size of the mass and some pain during the premenstrual period. Classically there is a well-defined mass with circumscribed edges that moves easily within the breast tissue (breast mouse). The natural history is often of fluctuation in size and eventual hyaline degeneration or calcification presenting as a stony hard mass in the postmenopausal period. Fibroadenomas can sometimes reach large dimensions in pubertal girls, pregnant women, and at menopause. These lesions have no malignant potential and are termed *giant fibroadenomas*. They are distinct from phyllodes

tumors. After age 25, it is not advisable to assume the diagnosis of fibroadenoma and a histologic diagnosis is necessary. Medullary carcinoma can mimic this picture absolutely with equally well-defined edges. Fibroadenomas should not be removed from the breast before the breasts are fully mature unless there is undue pain or unusual growth. Most surgeons wait until patients are in their twenties before removing these masses as the delay allows time for identification of patients with multicentric fibroadenomas, which can occur in up to 15% of patients. Most fibroadenomas can be removed under local anesthesia.

Phyllodes Tumors

Although the malignant variety of this tumor is the most common sarcoma of the breast, only 1 in 10 is malignant. Although these tumors resemble fibroadenoma on imaging studies, histologically the stroma is far more cellular. The peak incidence is in the fourth decade of life. The benign version of these tumors can be treated by local excision. There is a group of intermediate tumors referred to as "borderline" phyllodes tumors which should be excised with margins of at least 1 cm. The frankly malignant stromal sarcomas usually require a total mastectomy. Axillary lymph node dissection is rarely indicated.

Fibrocystic Disease

The most common cause of a breast mass in women particularly during their fourth and fifth decades is some variation of fibrocystic disease. Because of variable diagnostic criteria, it has been difficult to classify or examine the natural history of fibrocystic disease to determine its predisposition to malignancy. The clinical changes of fibrosis, epitheliosis, and cyst formation are so prevalent that the term disease may be a misnomer.

a. **The predominant single cyst** typically presents as a well-demarcated mass of recent origin occurring in women in their thirties and forties. The mass may vary in size becoming larger and more tenderer premenstrually. Fluctuation may not be appreciated because these lesions are frequently tense and situated in dense fibrous breast tissue. Ultrasonography can identify cysts but a simpler procedure for diagnosis is aspiration using a 22-gauge needle. Aspiration may be acceptable as the sole treatment for cysts if the following criteria are met:
   1. Total disappearance of the cyst.
   2. Absence of blood in the aspirate (blood may indicate an intracystic papilloma or carcinoma).
   3. Absence of recurrence of the cyst. (Recurrence of the cyst after 1 month indicates that the wall is still secreting and further aspiration attempts are unlikely to be successful.)

If any of these criteria are not met, the area of the cyst should be excised. Nonbloody fluid aspirated from a single cyst is usually not examined cytologically. However, recurrences may justify cytological studies.

b. **Lumpy breasts.** Breasts with diffuse masses associated with various manifestations of induration and multiple cyst formation represent the other extreme of fibrocystic changes. Detection of changes during examination is critical and may be aided by the following:
   1. Monthly breast self-examinations.

   2. Biannual examinations by the same physician (charting of the topography of the breast is often useful).

   3. Mammography. Mammograms at yearly intervals from age 40.

Although the malignant potential of this process is of little concern, the development of a carcinoma in a breast with these diffuse changes may be difficult to detect.

Fat Necrosis

Fat necrosis can occur at any age. It typically presents as a mass in a large fatty breast and may be associated with skin retraction, irregular edges, and even calcifications on mammography that mimic carcinoma. A history of trauma is present in only about half the cases and is not reliable for diagnosis.

Plasma Cell Mastitis

Plasma cell mastitis presents typically as a hard mass in the region of the areola during the perimenopausal period. Distended ducts are found with a marked round cell infiltrate. A chronic inflammatory response is caused by extrusion of duct contents into the surrounding interstitial tissue. Another manifestation of this condition is a chronic abscess developing in the subareolar area which can evolve after surgical drainage to form a persistent draining sinus in the area. Acute treatment of abscesses in this area requires incision and drainage and antibiotics. Repeated infections or persistent fistulae are often treated with excisional surgery involving the underlying duct or ducts.

Carcinoma of the Breast

The features of a breast mass suggestive of cancer include the following:

1. Site: Can be anywhere in breast but is most frequently found in the upper outer quadrant where there is the greatest mass of breast tissue.
2. Size: Size itself is of limited importance although a history of increase in size over several months is suggestive.
3. Shape: Irregular shape.
4. Consistency: A hard mass.
5. Surface: An irregular surface.
6. Edge: Poorly defined edges with extensions into the surrounding tissue.
7. Relations: Attachment to the skin or underlying fascia.

The above notwithstanding, the dictum still holds that any clinically definable solid mass detected in a woman older than 25 years demands histological verification.

FINDINGS ON INSPECTION

Polythelia

Multiple nipples are common findings in clinical practice. They can occur anywhere along the milk line (an ectodermal thickening in the 4.0-mm embryo from the midclavicle to the inguinal ligament). Most frequently they present inferior and medial to the nipple. This may be accompanied by polymastia (many breasts), which may become evident at puberty or during pregnancy. Amastia or athelia is frequently accompanied by underlying chest wall defects.

Breast Asymmetry and Nipple Inversion

These are frequently observed in otherwise normal breasts when they manifest for the first time at puberty. However, a recent change in a fully mature breast indicates a clear reason for further investigation.

Paget's Disease

Paget's disease presents as a red, thickened nipple with an eczematoid reaction. The surface can be scaly or moist. It is always associated with an underlying ductal carcinoma that is extending into the nipple areola surface. About half are associated with an underlying mass. If no detectable underlying mass is present, Paget's disease has an excellent prognosis when treated as a form of ductal carcinoma in situ (DCIS) with wide excision. Histologic diagnosis should be confirmed with a wedge or punch biopsy of the nipple-areola complex. The microscopic features of the lesion include Paget's cells in the epidermis, hypertrophy of the epidermis, and round cell infiltration. Paget's disease of the nipple accounts for 1% of breast cancer. Its importance stems from the fact that it is an early, curable cancer that can be detected on clinical examination.

Peau d'orange

Peau d'orange (skin of an orange) is a phenomenon caused by skin edema with apparent epithelial retraction. Hair follicles are anchored in the deep dermis, giving the appearance of an orange peel surface. The phenomenon may be seen in association with cellulitis or underlying abscess, but its notoriety rests in its association with breast cancer where dense infiltration of subdermal lymphatics causes skin edema and portends a poor prognosis. The appearance of skin edema in the dependent portion of the breast may be associated with extensive lymphatic metastatic involvement resulting in poor lymphatic flow.

Skin Dimpling

As an early sign of breast cancer, skin dimpling reflects the distorting effect of the desmoplastic reaction of breast cancer on Cooper's suspensory ligaments. These ligaments suspend the breast from the chest wall and extend from the pectoral fascia to the skin.

Malignant Ulceration

Malignant ulceration is a grave sign when found in association with breast cancer. Its prognosis is similar to that of metastatic disease.

ETIOLOGY OF BREAST CANCER

Family History and Genetics

Clinically the high-risk group includes women with first-degree relatives (mother, sister, daughter) particularly if the cancer appeared before menopause or was bilateral. In up to 10% of women with breast cancer there is an identifiable genetic marker.

Two genes have been fully sequenced: *BRCA1* on chromosome 17, also associated with ovarian carcinoma, and *BRCA2* on chromosome 13, also associated with ovarian and male breast and prostate cancer. Mutations in these two genes account for most known inherited breast cancer. Genetic testing of high-risk patients has become more available and is performed more frequently. The most effective management of patients with these genetic markers does involve ablative therapy of ovaries and breasts. Optimal timing of surgery and the efficacy of hormonal manipulation remain under investigation at this point. Penetrance for mutated genes is significant but may not be as high as originally thought (*BRCA1,* 55% to 85%; *BRCA2,* 37% to 85%). Quality of life issues are important in decision making.

Other Factors

A prolonged *menstrual history* particularly early menarche and late menopause is associated with a higher incidence of breast cancer. *Age of first full-term pregnancy* is also a significant factor. The younger the age at which a woman has had her first full-term pregnancy, the greater is the apparent protection against the development of breast cancer. *Previous exposure to radiation therapy* (e.g., mantle therapy for lymphoma) clearly predisposes to the development of breast cancer. *Mammographically dense breasts* are associated with an increased incidence of breast carcinoma, particularly in older women. This may represent an increased amount of susceptible fibroglandular tissue in these patients.

NIPPLE DISCHARGE

Discharge from multiple ducts bilaterally is most likely benign. If nipple discharge is persistent (galactorrhea) and not associated with recent pregnancy or breast feeding, it may be due to increased prolactin or thyrotropin levels. Medication history should be obtained since this is a common side effect of drugs.

Breast pathology, by contrast, is more commonly associated with spontaneous discharge from a single

duct. The discharge may be bloody or clear. The workup should include mammography and sonography. Cytology is usually not useful. If no breast pathology is revealed on imaging surgical excision of the offending duct is performed. The most common pathological finding is an intraductal papilloma. In situ and invasive cancers are found in less than 5% of duct excisions.

EARLY BREAST CANCER

Emphasis on early detection remains the most important method of reducing the mortality rate of this disease. The average doubling time of breast cancer on serial mammographic observations is estimated to be approximately 200 days.

Imaging

Mammography is the most effective means of screening for early breast cancer. For screening, the American Cancer Society recommends a yearly mammogram beginning at age 40. The radiation risks associated with x-ray mammography are minimal. Modern techniques allow in-depth dosage of 0.1 cGy for each of the two views conventionally used for mammography. On mammography early breast cancers are detected as groups of suspicious calcifications in about a third of mammographically detected cancers. Small densities with irregular speculated borders, with or without calcifications, are a typical finding. Architectural distortion and secondary signs of breast cancer such as an edema, thickening, and tethering of the skin may also be significant. Digital mammography has an advantage over analog mammography in screening women younger than 50 years of age.

Ultrasonography can distinguish cysts from solid masses. It has not been shown to be effective as a primary screening technique for breast cancer.

Magnetic resonance imaging (MRI) of the breast is particularly useful in young patients who are at high risk, such as patients with genetic markers for breast cancer (sensitivity in BRCA patients 85%). Breast MRI performed in women with known breast cancer is effective in detecting otherwise undiagnosed multicentric ipsilateral and contralateral lesions. In women who present with palpable axillary lymph nodes with adenocarcinoma and no clinical or mammographic evidence of breast cancer, MRI can reveal the primary tumor in up to 90% of patients.

Histologic Diagnosis

Needle core biopsies and surgical excisions are conventionally used for histological diagnosis of *palpable lesions*. Needle aspiration cytology cannot differentiate between invasive and in situ carcinoma and has not supplanted the histological three-dimensional requirement for pathological diagnosis.

Computer-assisted *stereotactically guided needle biopsies* of suspicious mammographic lesions have had an important impact on the diagnosis of early breast cancer. Adequate samples may be difficult to obtain in lesions close to the chest wall or close to the skin in the subareolar area. Calcifications may be extremely faint which can make this procedure technically difficult. The histological finding should be concordant with the imaging. If, for example, normal breast tissue is found on sampling a suspicious mammographic density, further wider sampling is necessary. Diagnosis of severe dysplasia or atypical ductal hyperplasia also necessitates wider sampling of the area.

Breast densities detectable with *ultrasound* can be sampled or localized using this imaging modality.

Surgical biopsy with needle localization can permit more extensive sampling of breast tissue. After radiographically placing a wire in the breast, the area to be removed can be stained with methylene blue. The wire can be used as a surgical guide to the area which is to be excised. In previously stereotactically biopsied breast a radiopaque clip can be left to facilitate later needle localization and excision.

DUCTAL CARCINOMA IN SITU

DCIS represents a spectrum of diseases which are a progression from atypical ductal hyperplasia to well-differentiated DCIS to the frankly neoplastic comedo carcinoma. Mammography and MRI have resulted in the increased diagnosis of this condition and these now account for one-third of mammographically detected carcinoma. Current management of lesions under 5 cm in diameter includes wide excision with clear histologic margins and radiation therapy to reduce the likelihood of recurrence. Selective management of lesions of less than 2.5 cm in diameter with only wide excision without irradiation has yielded acceptable results.

In widely dispersed or multicentric DCIS, mastectomy is the preferred approach. In patients undergoing mastectomy, a sentinel node biopsy is indicated because of the possible finding of undetected invasive

carcinoma in the histologic specimen. Hormone receptors (estrogen and progesterone) are obtained on a routine basis. Tamoxifen may be useful in reducing recurrences in receptor-positive cases. DCIS infrequently presents with a breast mass.

LOBULAR CARCINOMA IN SITU

Lobular carcinoma in situ does not present as a breast mass. It is most frequently found as an incidental finding in a biopsy specimen excised for another reason. It has a 90% incidence of multicentricity and 50% chance of bilaterality. Most patients with this condition never develop invasive carcinoma. When invasive carcinoma does occur, both breasts are equally at risk and most of the lesions are ductal in origin. Current management is nonoperative observation with lifelong surveillance. Use of tamoxifen reduces the probability of cancers developing. Bilateral mastectomy is uncommonly performed. The overall lifetime risk of developing invasive breast cancer is estimated to be 20%.

MARKERS

Hormone receptors (estrogen and progesterone) can be identified using histologic fixed sections. The presence of significant estrogen receptors (ERs) is associated with a 70% probability of a response to a change in the hormonal milieu. The figure is lower with brain, lung, and liver metastases. Negativity is associated with a 5% response. Hormone receptor-positive tumors are associated with a more prolonged time to metastatic recurrence, a higher response rate of metastases to hormonal manipulation and longer time from the appearance metastases until death. Overall, 70% of breast carcinomas are ER-positive. The figure is somewhat higher in postmenopausal women than in premenopausal women. The measurable receptors tend to be present at higher levels in older patients.

Her2/neu is a **human epidermal growth factor receptor** which is overexpressed in approximately 20% of invasive breast cancers. These tumors have been associated with a poor prognosis. However, the use of trastuzumab (Herceptin), an antibody against her2/neu, together with chemotherapy has significantly improved the outlook for these patients.

Triple negative tumors (ER, PR, and Her2/neu negative) are associated with the *BRCA1* gene mutation and are also found with increased incidence in the African American population without known genetic abnormalities. The histology is frequently referred to as basaloid. Triple negative tumors are associated with a poorer prognosis.

SURGICAL MANAGEMENT OF BREAST CANCER

Preoperative Evaluation

Preoperative evaluation of breast cancer is directed at determining within reasonable limits whether the carcinoma is regionally confined and amenable to cure through regional therapy. Clinical assessment remains an important modality in the preoperative evaluation. Those eligible for curative intent with regional therapy include those with Stage I and II tumors (i.e., tumors <5.0 cm without evidence of skin chest wall invasion and with or without ipsilateral mobile axillary lymph nodes). No signs of lymph nodes or other metastasis should be present beyond the surgically encompassable field. With tumors less than 2.0 cm in diameter with no palpable lymph nodes, the minimal preoperative evaluation should include a bilateral mammogram, bilateral MR image, and a computed tomographic scan of the chest and the abdomen. A history of joint pain or elevated alkaline phosphatase should be further investigated with a bone scan.

Breast Preserving Operations

Breast preserving operations have achieved results comparable to those seen with mastectomy for tumors less than 4 cm in diameter with or without palpable axillary lymph nodes. Although wide excision of the primary tumor is performed, the optimal margins of normal tissue are controversial. Acceptable results have been achieved with breast quadrant removal for tumors less than 2 cm; however, excisions with histologically free margins for tumors up to 4 cm have shown similar results.

Psychological and social issues may be relative contraindication to breast conservation. Risk of local recurrence is also important. Extensive intraductal carcinoma in the region of the primary invasive cancer is associated with an increased recurrence rate. Cosmetic factors may also be important (e.g., a large tumor in the small breast may result in a poor cosmetic outcome).

Imaging advances including digital mammography and MRI examinations may reveal previously undetected ipsilateral and contralateral lesions preoperatively and have resulted in a recent increase in the number of mastectomies. The effect on overall survival remains unclear.

When breast preserving operations are utilized, *radiation therapy* to the remaining ipsilateral breast tissue is given to a minimum of 5O Gy (conventionally in 200 cGy fractions). The use of higher-dose fractions with resulting shorter courses of therapy is currently under evaluation. The major effect of the radiation therapy is to destroy any remaining cancer cells and reduce the incidence of local recurrences in the affected breast and improve long-term survival. Partial breast irradiation is under investigation as a means of reducing recurrences close to the site of the original excision.

Axillary Lymph Nodes

Patients with palpable axillary lymph nodes are currently treated with full axillary lymph node dissection. Alternatively needle aspiration cytology can be used to determine pathological involvement. If positive, an axillary lymph node dissection is performed. If negative, a *sentinel node* can be sought. This is the first node to which the cancer will go via lymphatic spread. In patients with no palpable lymph nodes, the number of axillary lymph node dissections has been diminished by the utilization of the technique of sentinel lymph node biopsy. An injection of radioactive technetium 99 m sulfur colloid is made into the breast and a gamma probe is used to detect a radioactive lymph node in the axilla. A supravital dye (methylene blue or asulfidine) is used concurrently to define the node with blue staining. This allows for the detection and surgical removal of one or more sentinel nodes. These are frequently examined by frozen section at the time of surgery and in greater detail by permanent section with multiple sections and H and E staining. In addition, keratin antibodies can detect single epithelial cells in the lymph node. The absence of cancer cells in these sentinel nodes indicates a very low probability that the remaining lymph nodes in the axilla are involved with breast cancer. By contrast, if cancer cells are detected within the sentinel nodes, there is an increased likelihood that other lymph nodes are involved, and a full axillary lymph node dissection should be performed. Controversy exists in the interpretation of micrometastatic ($<$.2 mm) deposits detected by immunohistochemistry.

Radiation therapy following mastectomy has been demonstrated to decrease the incidence of local recurrence. Improvements in survival have been demonstrated in patients with four or more involved lymph nodes.

Extended surgical procedures (e.g., extended radical mastectomy or Urban's operation) include removal of portions of the sternum medial cartilages and internal mammary lymph nodes. These procedures are not regarded as standard therapy for operable cancer but may be useful for local disease control in selected cases.

ANATOMIC CONSIDERATIONS IN BREAST SURGERY

Lymphatics

The lymphatic drainage of the normal breast even in the medial aspect is predominantly toward the axilla. The medial intercostal lymph nodes are few in number (about four) and are predominately in the first, second, and third interspaces. By contrast the axillary lymph nodes are abundant. They are commonly regarded as distinct from the lower cervical lymph nodes but form a physiologic and anatomic continuum with these nodes. The deep breast tissue drains to the submammary plexus of lymphatics which lie superficial to the fascia overlying the pectoralis major. Hence removal of the fascia overlying the pectoralis major is required when performing a mastectomy.

Blood Supply

The *arterial* blood supply to the breast is dominated by the internal thoracic (internal mammary) artery. It also includes the lateral thoracic artery and the pectoral branches of the acromiothoracic artery. The *venous* anatomy generally follows that of the arteries. In addition, there is a communication of intercostal veins, which in turn communicate with the valveless vertebral system of veins, known as Batson's plexus. This route of spread is used to explain metastasis to the ribs and vertebra without pulmonary involvement.

Nerves

The *medial and lateral pectoral nerves* are so named because of their origin from the medial and lateral cords of the brachial plexus. The medial pectoral nerve enters the deep surface of the pectoralis minor muscle. After supplying a branch to this muscle, it then enters the pectoralis major. If the pectoralis minor muscle is

removed during an axillary lymph node dissection, partial denervation of the pectoralis major muscle results. However, removal of the pectoris may facilitate a more complete lymph node dissection. The lateral pectoral nerve penetrates the clavipectoral fascia (and hence is medial to the medial pectoral nerve) and enters the underside of the pectoralis major muscle.

The *thoracodorsal nerve* arises from the posterior cord of the brachial plexus, courses down the posterior axillary wall with the subscapular artery, and supplies the latissimus dorsi muscle. Injury to this nerve results in slight weakness of abduction and internal rotation.

The *long thoracic nerve (of Bell)* arises from the roots of the brachial plexus and innervates the serratus anterior muscle. Injury to this nerve produces a winged scapula and is often accompanied by severe shoulder pain.

The *intercostobrachial nerves* arise from the intercostal nerve and provide sensory innervation to the skin of the axilla and down the inner aspect of the upper arm. Injury will result in anesthesia of the affected area.

POSTOPERATIVE COMPLICATIONS

Seroma

Postoperative seroma may require repeated aspiration. It is best avoided by maintaining closed suction drainage until output falls to less than 50 mL/24 hr postmastectomy. Drainage should be avoided in breast preserving operations since inversion of the skin may affect the cosmetic outcome.

Infection

Signs of inflammation should be vigorously investigated and treated. Recurring episodes of infection can aggravate or precipitate lymphedema of the upper extremity.

Limitation of arm movement after lymph node dissection: Shoulder movement is not restricted postoperatively. Active exercise following axillary dissection should be avoided until the fifth postoperative day because of an increase risk of seroma and hematoma formation. At that point, a graduated exercise program may be useful.

Arm Edema

This may occur after axillary lymph node dissection and uncommonly after sentinel node biopsy. The prevention and aggressive treatment of infections and wounds of the ipsilateral upper extremity are paramount for the prevention of postoperative edema. Ongoing care of the skin and avoidance of intravenous lines is also important. Established lymphedema is treated with elevation, massage, compression garments, or mechanical pumps. Microsurgical procedures to reestablish lymphatic drainage are generally not useful.

Lymphangiosarcoma (Stewart-Treves Syndrome)

Lymphangiosarcoma may develop in the chronically edematous arm, frequently after radiation to the breast. On average it occurs nine or more years after mastectomy. It presents characteristically as a purple subcutaneous nodule and may grow rapidly. Lung metastases often appear. The 5-year survival is 30% but amputation can provide local palliation.

ADJUVANT THERAPY

Therapy designed to eliminate residual microscopic disease after locoregional therapy is known as adjuvant therapy. Adjuvant therapy should be considered in patients with characteristics associated with poor prognosis (e.g., undifferentiated histology, tumor size, and lymph node involvement). Recent advances include the assessment of molecular gene expressions involving groups of genes (signatures). These data are then used to define patient subgroups who will likely benefit from adjuvant therapy.

Chemotherapy

There is no uniform adjuvant chemotherapy protocol for all patients with clinically confined breast cancer. The most frequently used regimens include a combination of an anthracycline (e.g., doxorubicin), an alkylating agent (e.g., cyclophosphamide), and a taxane (e.g., paclitaxel).

Hormone Therapy

Indicated in estrogen and progesterone receptor-positive tumors. Tamoxifen is used in premenopausal patients. Aromatase inhibitors and tamoxifen are used in the postmenopausal patients.

Biological Agents

In human epidermal growth factor receptor (Her2/neu)-positive tumors the addition of trastuzumab (Herceptin) to adjuvant chemotherapy regimes has

been shown to improve survival. The optimal duration of treatment is not clearly defined.

LOCALLY ADVANCED CANCER

Patients with regionally confined but poor prognosis tumors are frequently treated with *neoadjuvant (preoperative) therapy*. These include patients with tumors larger than 5 cm or those with adhesions to the chest wall or with significant skin involvement. Histological diagnosis is essential before treatment is initiated. Treatment protocols similar to those used in the adjuvant setting are used as the initial therapy preceding surgery or radiotherapy. In addition to histology of the tumor, cytology may be used to stage axillary nodes. Further workup characteristically includes a computed tomographic scan of the chest, abdomen, and pelvis; bone scan; and possibly positron emission tomography (PET) scan.

Many of these tumors will respond to current chemotherapeutic regimens. On occasion, both clinical and pathological complete responses (no tumor found in subsequent mastectomy or other excisional therapy) are seen and are associated with an improved prognosis. Although it is difficult to define overall improvement in survival using neoadjuvant therapy, potential advantages include the ability to offer breast conservation and the prognostic information associated with complete responses.

PREGNANCY AND BREAST CANCER

Breast masses, particularly those discovered in pregnant women older than 25 years should prompt immediate evaluation. The mass should be aspirated and solid masses should undergo biopsy. Breast cancer during pregnancy often presents as advanced disease with an unfavorable prognosis. Localized carcinoma is usually treated by mastectomy. Radiotherapy is not given during pregnancy and adjuvant chemotherapy should be delayed until at least the second trimester. Occasionally termination of pregnancy may have to be considered in those patients with more advanced tumors where radiation and chemotherapy are urgently required for the welfare of the mother. In the absence of recurrent disease following successful treatment of breast cancer, avoidance or termination of pregnancy is not required.

CANCER OF THE MALE BREAST

Male breast cancer accounts for less than 1% of all breast cancers. Incidence may be increased in patients who have had previous radiotherapy and those who have had mumps or orchitis after age 20 years. There is an increased incidence in families with mutation of the *BRCA2* gene. Most tumors present with a firm mass under the nipple areolar complex. The prognosis is worse than that for women perhaps because of the close proximity of the chest wall, the greater age of the affected population, and the higher proportion of patients with lymph node involvement at the time of presentation. Treatment is wide mastectomy and sentinel node or axillary dissection. Most tumors are associated with elevated ER levels and adjuvant hormonal therapy may be considered. Ablative and additive hormonal manipulation has been shown to be useful for metastatic disease.

AXILLARY NODE ADENOCARCINOMA WITH NO APPARENT PRIMARY

Axillary node adenocarcinoma should be tested for estrogen and progesterone receptors as well as Her2/neu. A negative physical examination including thyroid, other lymph nodes, and regional melanomas should prompt further investigation. The primary is most likely to be in the breast and can be demonstrated on MRI in about 90% of cases. The prognosis seems better than in clinically detected breast cancers with an equivalent number of involved lymph nodes.

BREAST CANCER PROPHYLAXIS

The incidence of breast cancer can be diminished in high-risk populations. Both tamoxifen and raloxifene have been found to be effective in postmenopausal women.

DEVELOPMENTAL CONDITIONS

Nipple discharges at birth are a frequent result of removal of the infant from the high estrogen and progesterone maternal environment and an increase in prolactin production. It is usually a self-limiting disorder.

Precocious breast hypertrophy may be related to adrenal cortical and ovarian tumors. Boys can manifest a slight enlargement of breast tissue at puberty that subsides spontaneously with time. The initial breast development in pubertal girls is frequently asymmetric. Inadvertent removal of a breast "bud" can result in a severe cosmetic deformity.

BREAST ABSCESS

Breast abscess occurs most commonly during the first weeks of lactation. It is often caused by coagulase positive *Staphylococcus* and may be associated with suppuration and extensive destruction of breast tissue. These abscesses require aggressive early drainage to remove septated pockets and appropriate antibiotic therapy. In principle, an incision in the lower aspect of the abscess encourages dependant drainage. Streptococcal infections usually produce a cellulitis that can usually be controlled with antibiotics.

QUESTIONS

Select one answer.

1. A 31-year-old woman presents with a 2-cm mass in the upper outer quadrant of the right breast. It is well defined and has been present by history for 2 months. Your initial approach to this problem is to:
   a. Order a mammogram followed by a sonogram.
   b. Insert a needle to aspirate any fluid.
   c. Schedule an open biopsy.
   d. Reschedule an appointment in 6 weeks to reevaluate the problem clinically.

2. An 11-year-old girl is brought by her parents with a unilateral 1.5-cm mass underneath the areola on the right. Your approach to this problem should be:
   a. Observation only, as it is a "breast bud" which frequently develops asymmetrically.
   b. Excision, because with growth of the child the scar becomes less noticeable.
   c. Biopsy, as lymphomas occur in this age group.

3. The long thoracic nerve:
   a. Innervates the serratus anterior muscle.
   b. Courses down posterior to the axillary artery and vein because it arises from the roots of

the brachial plexus. Section of the nerve results in ipsilateral scapular prominence and shoulder pain.
   c. Both.
   d. Neither.

4. The incidence of breast carcinoma is lower:
   a. In the contralateral breasts of patients receiving tamoxifen.
   b. In young women.
   c. In women with no family history of breast carcinoma.
   d. All of the above.

5. Mammography:
   a. Is the most effective means of screening for breast carcinoma.
   b. Is more effective in detecting breast carcinomas in postmenopausal women.
   c. When normal, should not exclude biopsy of a palpable suspicious breast mass.
   d. All of the above.

6. Breast conservation surgery in breast carcinoma:
   a. Has resulted in major improvement in mortality and morbidity figures associated with this disease.
   b. Has resulted in durable survival data comparable to those for mastectomy for certain breast cancers.
   c. Should be recommended to all women suffering from breast carcinoma.
   d. Has resulted in a high incidence of serious radiation-related complications.
   e. Has resulted in diminution of the need for adjuvant chemotherapy and hormonal therapy.

7. In a patient with breast carcinoma, the clinical finding portending the worst prognosis is:
   a. Eczematous changes around the nipple areolar complex.
   b. Skin dimpling in the area of the tumor.
   c. The presence of a palpable 1-cm node in the axilla.
   d. Peau d'orange.

8. Statistically, the most powerful predictor of prognosis is:
   a. The presence of intramammary lymphatic involvement.

b. The grade of differentiation of the tumor.

c. The presence of marked intraductal carcinoma around the primary tumor.

d. The size of the primary tumor.

e. The number of axillary lymph nodes involved with metastatic tumor.

9. Ductal carcinoma in situ of the breast:

a. Is almost always bilateral.

b. Has become more frequently diagnosed as a result of mammography.

c. Cannot present as a palpable mass.

d. Is frequently associated with microscopic lymph node metastases.

10. A 33-year-old woman pregnant for the third time presents at 3 months with a 2-cm mass in the inner aspect of the left breast. A needle aspiration reveals no fluid. You would:

a. Arrange for a mammogram because multicentric lesions are common during pregnancy.

b. Consider termination of pregnancy because chemotherapy has been shown to be useful in node-negative premenopausal patients.

c. Expeditiously obtain a histologic diagnosis of the mass.

d. Wait until the third trimester because surgery is safer at that time.

SELECTED REFERENCES

Axelrod D, Smith J, Kornreich D, et al. Breast cancer in young women. *J Am Coll Surg* 2008;206(6):1193–1203.

Cameron JL. *Current surgical therapy: the breast: P641 ff. multiple authors.* Philadelphia, PA: Mosby Elsevier, 2008.

Cristofanilli M, ed. Inflammatory breast cancer. *Semin Oncol* 2008;35(1).

Foulkes, Smith IE, Reis-Filho JS. Triple-negative breast cancer. *N Engl J Med* 2010;363:1938–1948.

Levine MN, Ganz PA, Mamounas EP, eds. Breast reviews. *J Clin Oncol* 2008;26(5).

Newman L. Surgical issues and preoperative systemic therapy: *Cancer Treat Res* 2008;141:79–98.

Ronald Kaleya
Barbara Weinstein

Principles of Surgical Oncology

S urgery is the oldest effective therapy for cancer and it remains the most effective single modality in its treatment. Of the 1.5 million new cases of cancer diagnosed in 2008, surgeons were involved in the care of approximately 75% of cases. With the introduction of effective adjuvant and primary radiotherapy and/or chemotherapy as well as an acceptance of nonprogression as an acceptable oncologic end point, the older principles of surgical management of cancer and the cancer patient have been challenged. In the past, the surgeon attempted to extend the scope of resection to encompass all possible local and regional extension of cancer using increasingly radical and ablative procedures. Follow-up studies did not demonstrate improved survival or decreased local recurrence for the more radical and super-radical procedures when compared with conservative surgery in combination with other therapeutic modalities. Thus, multimodality therapy has become the standard of care for most cancers. Furthermore, combination therapy has reduced the scope of resection in some cases, permitting preservation of function and cosmesis. In some cases, neoadjuvant (preoperative) therapies have made unresectable or marginally resectable tumors amenable to surgical remediation. As a result of these trends in oncology, the general surgeon requires an intimate knowledge of the benefits and complications of these other therapies to provide optimal patient care.

The progress in chemotherapy, biologic agents, and radiation therapy (RT) has altered the timing, indications, and integration of surgical intervention for cancer. Nonetheless, the surgeon remains a central figure in cancer prevention, screening, diagnosis, treatment planning, management of complications of therapy, and palliative care.

TUMOR BIOLOGY, ONCOGENES, AND TUMOR SUPPRESSOR GENES

Most cancers arise from a single transformed cell. Most of these altered cells die spontaneously or fail to multiply. The average cell cycle is 3 to 5 days but may be as long as several months. It takes approximately 30 cellular doublings to form a clinically detectable 1 cm tumor containing 10^9 cells. The control of the cell cycle involves molecular pathways that either promote or restrict the normal cell cycle progression, or prevent normal apoptotic mechanisms. Growth factor oncogenes (e.g., platelet-derived growth factor, epidermal growth factor [EGF]) bind to receptors within the cell to promote growth and division. The growth factor receptor oncogenes lead to increased expression of cellular receptors, which in turn, increases cell proliferation (e.g., HER-2-neu an EGF receptor, c-KIT a platelet-derived growth factor receptor). The signal transduction oncogenes such as k-ras stimulate intermediary messengers of cell growth. Finally, the nuclear oncogenes can stimulate DNA transcription and cause cells to exit the G_1 cell cycle phase and enter the synthetic phase of cell division. Targeted therapies exploit these cell cycle control pathways to effect cancer control. Tumor suppressor genes prevent cell from leaving G_0 and G_1. Mutations in these genes cause dysinhibition and unregulated growth. Examples of tumor suppressor genes include p53 and the retinoblastoma (Rb) tumor suppressor genes.

CANCER SCREENING

Routine cancer screening has reduced the age-adjusted cancer-specific mortality especially in breast, cervical, and colorectal cancers. Large population screening,

TABLE 10.1	Relative Risk and Odds Ratio for Screening Populations		
	Disease+	**Disease−**	**Statistic**
Risk factor+	A	B	Risk of developing disease with risk factor (A/A+B)
Risk factor−	C	D	Risk of developing disease without risk factor (C/C+D)

Relative risk = risk of disease with risk factor/risk of disease without risk factor = (A/A+B)/(C/C+D).
Odds ratio A ≪ B and C ≪ D, therefore, A+B ~ B and C+D ~ D = (A/B)/(C/D) = AD/BC.

however, is usually ineffective with low-incidence cancers because of the low predictive values in the at-risk population. For a screening program to be effective, several criteria must be met. The population at-risk must be identified; the natural history of the disease can be altered favorably by earlier diagnosis and intervention; and the screening modalities must be accurate, available, and relatively inexpensive. The screening modalities include biochemical tests, physical examinations, molecular and genetic markers, as well as imaging and diagnostic tests. Outcome studies evaluating the efficacy of screening may be confounded by lead-time bias (diagnosis earlier without change in survival) and length-time bias. Length time bias describes differences in growth rates within identical histologic malignancies.

Screening at-risk populations is usually described by three statistics: relative risk, odds ratio, and lifetime risk. These parameters evaluate the contribution of each risk factor has on the development of a specific cancer. These parameters are described by a 2×2 contingency table (Table 10.1) Relative risk is a ratio of the fraction of patients with a risk factor and the disease to those without the risk factor with the same disease $[A/(A + B)]/[C/(C + D)]$. In most diseases, the number of patients without disease far outnumbers those with the disease $[(A \ll B)$ and $(C \ll D)]$. The relative risk can then be described in a simpler form called the odds ratio $[(A/B)/(C/D)$ or AD/BD]. These statistics do no define independence of the risk factors, therefore the relative risks and odds ratios are not additive.

Descriptive statistics for screening populations at risk for disease relate to diagnostic tests and are shown in Table 10.2. As seen in this figure, the prevalence of the disease in the population markedly affects the positive predictive value and the number

TABLE 10.2	Descriptive Statistics for Clinical Tests					
	50% Prevalence		**25% Prevalence**		**10% Prevalence**	
	Disease Present	**Disease Absent**	**Disease Present**	**Disease Absent**	**Disease Present**	**Disease Absent**
Test positive	40	5	20	7	8	9
Test negative	10	45	5	68	2	81
Sensitivity	80%		80%		80%	
Specificity	90%		90%		90%	
Prevalence	50%		25%		10%	
PPV	89%		79%		47%	
NPV	81%		93%		97%	

Sensitivity (true positive rate) = TP/TP + FN
Specificity (true negative rate) = TN/TN + FP
Prevalence (prior probability) = TN + FN/All
Positive predictive value = TP/TP + FP
Negative predictive value = TN/TN + FN
PPV, positive predictive value; NPV, negative predictive value.

TABLE 10.3	Screening Guidelines	
Test	**American Cancer Society Guidelines**	**USPSTF Guidelines**
Physical examination	>20	
Clinical breast examination	>20 q 3 years >40 yearly	Optional (not sufficient evidence to recommend)
Mammogram	Female >40 yearly	Every 1–2 years 50–69
Breast MRI	Female >40 with >20% LIFETIME RISK	Not discussed
Fecal occult blood test	Yearly >50	Yearly >50 years and <75 years
Fecal immunochemical test	Yearly >50	
Colonoscopy	At 50 and q 10 years Earlier if strong family history (1 first-degree relative <60 or 2 of any age)	At 50 and q 10 years to age 75

PSA and digital rectal examination	Discussion of screening at age >50 or
	  >45 in patients with first-degree
	  relative with prostate cancer
		Not recommended

Pap smear	3 years after onset of intercourse or
	  21, then q 1 year with Pap test
	  or q 2 year with liquid-based Pap test
		Q 3 years after onset of intercourse until 65
		  if consistently normal

MRI, magnetic resonance imaging; PSA, prostate-specific antigen.

needed to treat (screen). Because the efficacy of screening is greater when the prevalence of the disease is higher, screening is reserved for high-risk populations with highly sensitive and specific screening modalities. Patients having a genetic, familial, or biochemical predisposition to cancer are more suitable for screening programs. Table 10.3 lists the screening recommendations as published by the American Cancer Society and the United States Preventative Services Task Force (USPSTF) as of 2009.

Hereditary cancer syndromes comprise approximately 5% of breast, colon, and ovarian cancers. Broadly defined, hereditary cancer patients have two or more first-degree relatives with the same cancer, one of whom is younger than 50 years of age, earlier onset of the cancer in the index case, and multiple cancers in the same patient. These lineages exhibit excess numbers of cancers, synchronous and metachronous primaries, and earlier onset than the sporadic variety of the disease. Many of these cancers have been identified by a biologic or genetic marker (Table 10.4). Screening these populations may lead to earlier diagnosis and potentially increased survival. Commercial tests are available for *BRCA, MEN1, RET, APC, Rb1,* and *VHL.*

TUMOR MARKERS

Tumor markers (Table 10.5) are, in general, tumor antigens or products of tumor metabolism released into the general circulation. The markers are helpful in the diagnosis, monitoring, staging, localization, and treatment of several cancers. Tumor markers are not good screening tools because of the low sensitivity and specificity. Patients with known cancer can be monitored for recurrence.

BIOPSY TECHNIQUES

Frequently, the surgeon is called on to evaluate a clinically suspicious mass. A presumptive diagnosis is necessary prior to biopsy so the correct biopsy technique is used and the tissue is handled in an appropriate manner. There are four biopsy techniques: fine-needle aspiration biopsy (FNAB), core-needle biopsy, incisional biopsy, and excisional biopsy. Each technique has specific applications, benefits, and limitations.

Fine-Needle Aspiration Biopsy

Cells obtained by FNAB are aspirated through a 21-gauge needle, smeared on a glass slide, immediately

TABLE 10.4	**Cancer Family Syndromes**	
Gene	**Syndrome Name**	**Syndrome Characteristics**
BRCA1		Breast, ovarian, colon, prostate
BRCA2		Breast, ovarian, male breast, laryngeal, pancreatic
APC	Familial adenomatous polyposis	Colorectal adenomas and carcinoma, desmoids, duodenal, and gastric adenomas
MEN1	Multiple endocrine neoplasia type I	Islet pancreatic, parathyroid hyperplasia, pituitary adenomas
RET	Multiple endocrine neoplasia type II	Medullary carcinoma of thyroid, parathyroid hyperplasia, and pheochromocytoma
P16, CDK4	Familial melanoma	Melanoma, pancreatic adenocarcinoma
P53	Li-Fraumeni	Breast, sarcoma, pancreas
VHL	Von Hippel-Lindau	Pheochromocytoma, renal cell carcinoma
MSH2, MLH1, MSH6	Hereditary nonpolyposis colorectal carcinoma	Colon, gastric, endometrial
NF1	Neurofibromatosis type 1 (von Recklinghausen's disease)	Neurofibroma, neurofibrosarcoma, leukemia
NF2	Neurofibromatosis type 2	Acoustic neuroma, meningioma
Rb1	Familial retinoblastoma	Retinoblastoma, sarcoma, brain tumors, melanoma
PTEN	Cowden's disease	Breast, thyroid, endometrial

fixed with 95% alcohol, and stained with various stains. The specimens are examined for nuclear appearance, cellular cohesiveness, and mitotic activity. Cytologic evaluation requires a pathologist trained specifically in reading this type of specimen. Small needles retrieve too few cells, and large needles tend to aspirate cores of tissue unsuitable for cytologic examination. An adequate number of cells must be aspirated for an accurate evaluation. The FNAB is useful for evaluating a thyroid nodule; breast cancer; metastases to the liver, lung, or adrenal; and a suspected metastasis to a lymph node. The results of FNAB are often misleading in the diagnosis of suspected lymphomas, sarcomas, and intra-abdominal malignancies. In addition, a negative cytologic examination may be the result of sampling error rather than the absence of tumor. Many surgeons and pathologists suggest that definitive therapy for breast cancer can be carried out on the basis of cytology, but others urge caution with regard to using cytology as the definitive diagnostic test.

Core-Needle Biopsy

Core-needle biopsies obtain a small specimen that is suitable for paraffin embedding and routine histologic staining techniques. The core can be as large as a

TABLE 10.5	**Tumor Markers**	
Marker	**Tumor**	**Utility**
CEA	Colorectal, pancreas, breast, lung, gastric	P, M
AFP	Liver, germ cell	(S), D, P, M
HCG	Trophoblast, germ Cell	D, P, M
Calcitonin	Medullary thyroid cancer	D, M
PSA, PAP	Prostate cancer	P, M
Ca125	Ovarian	P, M
Ca19.9	Biliary/Pancreatic	P, M
Ca15.3, Ca27.29	Breast	M

S, screening; D, diagnosis; P, prognosis; M, monitoring.
CEA, carcinoembryonic antigen; AFP, alpha fetoprotein; HCG, human chorionic ganadotropin; PSA, prostate-specific antigen; PAP, prostatic acid phosphatase.

$2 \times 2 \times 10$ mm tissue fragment. This procedure can be carried out under local anesthesia. The only significant risk is the development of a hematoma and false-negative results. Because of better immunohistochemical straining techniques, core biopsy has supplanted FNA and open biopsy in the diagnosis of sarcomas, breast cancers, and lymphomas.

Incisional Biopsy

Incisional biopsies are useful for evaluating masses that have yielded equivocal results on core biopsy. The incision should be placed directly over the primary lesion; undermining is minimized, and the incision is planned in a manner that allows it to be included in the larger definitive resection. Drains and hematomas are avoided because they may increase the scope of a subsequent definitive surgical procedure.

Excisional Biopsy

Excisional biopsies are useful for small, superficial tumors. When possible, a rim of normal tissue is included in the specimen. Although there are no absolute upper limits of size for an excisional biopsy, in general, the excisional biopsy wound should be able to be closed primarily and be small enough to be included in a large definitive surgical field.

STAGING

The purpose of staging is to predict survival, standardize data collection permitting interinstitutional outcome comparisons, determine whether subsequent therapy is indicated, and evaluate the results of therapy. The TNM system as adopted by the American Joint Commission on Cancer is the most common staging system. The general rules governing the staging system are listed in Table 10.6.

There are several types of staging, including clinical, surgical, pathologic, and autopsy methods. After establishing a cancer diagnosis, the patient undergoes an appropriate extent-of-disease evaluation or clinical staging. This evaluation is based on the natural history of the particular cancer and the likely sites of metastatic and local spread. Surgical staging and pathologic staging predict survival better than clinical staging and are used to define populations eligible for adjuvant therapies.

TABLE 10.6	General Rules for American Joint Commission of Staging
Primary tumor (T)	
Tx	Primary cannot be evaluated
T0	Primary tumor occult
T1–3	Increasing size/local extent
Regional lymph nodes (N)	
Nx	RLN cannot be evaluated
N0	No RLN metastases
N1–3	Increasing RLN involvement
Distant metastases (M)	
Mx	Metastases cannot be evaluated
M0	Metastases absent
M1	Metastases present

RLN, regional lymph node.

PRINCIPLES OF SURGICAL ONCOLOGY

Local Surgical Therapy

The goal of cancer surgery is resection with a rim of normal tissue. Needless to say, the margins of resection must be pathologically free of tumor; however, the size of the margin is less well defined. Incomplete excision is useful only in cases where there are effective alternative therapies for the residual tumor, as in ovarian cancer. Incomplete resection is appropriate for palliation of symptoms (e.g., paraneoplastic syndromes, bleeding, or obstruction).

Lymphadenectomy

Regional lymph nodes are frequently the first site of metastases and are removed in the course of the primary therapy for most cancers. The presence of nodal disease may determine the need for adjuvant therapy in colorectal, breast, head and neck, and uterine cancers. The effect of regional lymphadenectomy on the survival outcomes of cancer remains speculative, whereas local disease control may be enhanced. Elective regional lymph node dissection has been replaced by sentinel node evaluation and selective node dissection in most malignancies.

Surgical Treatment of Locally Recurrent Disease

In general, locally recurrent disease should be treated similar to the primary cancer following an appropriate

extent-of-disease evaluation. A multidisciplinary team should evaluate the sequencing of surgery with the other therapeutic modalities.

Surgical Treatment of Metastatic Disease

Surgery for metastatic disease requires that the primary lesion can be controlled, all known metastatic deposits can be resected, and there is no other effective treatment for the disease. Workup prior to resection of a metastasis should be extensive and guided by the pattern of failure for the given disease (e.g., evaluation of the liver in cases of local recurrence of colon cancer). Evidence-based guidelines for preoperative imaging and testing have been published by the National Comprehensive Cancer Network (NCCN.org). If a metastasis is noted synchronously with the primary lesion, the procedure with the least likelihood of complete resection should be performed first to avoid unwarranted ablative surgery, as in the case of recurrent soft tissue sarcomas with lung metastases that would require an amputation as part of therapy. Should the lung metastases be widespread or unresectable, the utility of amputation is diminished.

Pulmonary Metastases

Among patients with a history of an extrathoracic cancer and a new lung nodule, 62% have a second primary, and 25% have a solitary metastasis. If the original cancer was a squamous cancer, most new nodules are new primaries. About half of the patients with a history of an extrathoracic adenocarcinoma have a solitary metastasis, whereas if the original cancer was melanoma or soft tissue sarcoma, almost all are metastatic lesions.

Workup should include chest computed tomographic scan, evaluation of other areas of common recurrence for the given primary, bronchoscopy if the lesion is central or large to exclude involvement of the mainstem bronchus, and thoracentesis for cytology when an effusion is present. FNAB is not necessary because resection must be carried out regardless of whether the cytology confirms the diagnosis. The patient should have adequate pulmonary reserve and an FEV1 greater than 1 liter.

The criteria for a pulmonary metastasectomy include the ability to control all disease with the resection, the absence of extrathoracic disease, and the expectation of adequate functional lung capacity following resection. The results of therapy are determined by the histology, the number of metastases, the interval between treatment of the primary and the recurrence (disease-free interval), and the completeness of resection.

Brain Metastases

Patients with brain metastases have a poor long-term survival. Indications for neurosurgical intervention include diagnostic uncertainty, a solitary metastasis, or placement of a drug delivery device. Predictors of improved long-term survival following resection of brain metastases include (1) a disease-free interval longer than 1 year following treatment of the primary, (2) better preoperative performance status, (3) relative radiosensitivity, (4) the extent of tumor resection (complete vs. partial), and (5) the extent of underlying cerebral dysfunction prior to surgery. Most metastatic brain tumors are treated with stereotactic RT.

Palliative Treatment of Cancer

Bleeding is a common complication of cancer and its therapy. It may result from the tumor itself, erosion into other structures, inflammation caused by chemotherapy or RT, or pancytopenia. The bleeding site should be aggressively localized preoperatively limiting the scope of surgery especially pancytopenic patients. Nonoperative measures including cauterization, laser ablation, and angiographic embolization, when applicable, are preferable to primary surgical intervention. Surgical intervention is indicated for continued bleeding despite nonoperative therapy.

Obstruction in the patient with a history of an intra-abdominal malignancy but no overt evidence of recurrence is caused by adhesions in the majority of cases. In contradistinction, patients with known peritoneal recurrence or malignant ascites are more likely to have malignant obstruction. In either case, initial management is decompression. Malignant obstruction rarely progresses to bowel necrosis and perforation. Preoperative evaluation should define an area of uninvolved distal bowel. Intestinal bypass is frequently required for malignant obstructions and is associated with 25% mortality. An additional 25% of patients never regain effective intestinal function. A gastrostomy is an option for those patients unable to undergo surgery or those in whom bypass is not possible.

Perforation is uncommon but more subtle in the immunocompromised host. It is treated similarly to nonmalignant perforations, although ostomies are used more liberally, and mortality is higher.

Inflammatory lesions are common following chemotherapy or RT. Because these inflammatory lesions can result in perforation of a hollow viscus or prolonged ileus, close observation is mandated. Typhlitis or neutropenic enterocolitis is common in leukemia patients treated with high-dose Ara-C. Neutropenic sepsis and ileus are treated with antibiotics and observation. Diarrhea is common following several of the chemotherapy regimens and can be treated symptomatically with antidiarrheal agents, a somatostatin analogue, and intravenous alimentation. These episodes are generally self-limited but can mimic ischemic or infectious colitis with an acute abdomen. Again, unless overt signs of an intra-abdominal catastrophe are present, nonoperative therapy is appropriate.

Principles of Medical Oncology

Normal cells have control points at each stage of the cell cycle. Malignant cells, either by loss of tumor suppressor genes or by overexpression of oncogenes, lose controlling pathways involved in cell division and proliferate unchecked. High growth fraction, the percentage of dividing cells, increases the cellular substrate requirements for nucleic acid and protein precursors needed by the rapidly proliferating cells. Chemotherapeutic agents exploit quantitative and qualitative differences between cancer and normal cells to achieve a selective effect. Enhanced uptake by the tumor cell, increased metabolic demand for substrates needed by the higher growth fraction, inadequate salvage pathways for needed metabolites, and the inability to repair sublethal damage are some of the differences used to increase tumoricidal activity while minimizing injury to normal cells.

Cells are generally insensitive to chemotherapy during the growth phase G_0 because most agents interfere with the production, translation, or transcription of nucleic acids. As a result, as more tumor cells go into this phase as a result of decreased blood supply and limitation of nutrients (Gompertzian kinetics), the entire tumor becomes more resistant to chemotherapy. In contrast, small, highly vascularized tumors tend to grow by exponential kinetics and are more sensitive to the actions of the cytotoxic agents. The principle of cytotoxic chemotherapy is to initiate therapy when the tumor burden is low, treat with the maximum tolerable dose (MTD), use multiple agents with non-overlapping toxicities, and escalate the dose when tolerated.

In contrast, the targeted therapies attempt to exploit molecular pathways specific to the tumor, such as overexpression of endothelial growth factor receptors or abnormal tyrosine kinase signaling pathways. These agents impede cellular growth only in those cells that express the specific targeted characteristics reducing toxicity.

General Characteristics of Chemotherapeutic and Targeted-Therapy Agents (Table 10.7)

Alkylating Agents

Alkylating agents cause interstrand cross-linking by binding to amino, sulfhydryl, carboxyl, and phosphate groups on DNA, RNA, and proteins, preventing transcription and translation and enzymatic activity. As a consequence of the broad activity, this class of drug is active throughout the cell cycle. Second malignancies, especially leukemia, are associated with these medications. The major treatment-associated toxicities include pancytopenia, hemorrhagic cystitis, and gastrointestinal complaints.

Platinum compounds, like the alkylating agents, bind to DNA, causing inter- and intrastrand cross-linkages, thereby disrupting DNA and RNA synthesis. Cisplatinum causes severe nephrotoxicity, and ototoxicity, and a nonreversible peripheral neuropathy. There is minimal myelosuppression, whereas bone marrow suppression is severe with carboplatinum. Oxaliplatinum has become a mainstay in the treatment of colon cancer. This group of drugs is less likely to cause leukemia than the alkylating agents.

Antimetabolites

The antimetabolites work at different steps in the production of nucleic acids. These agents tend to work best in rapidly dividing cells and are classified as cell cycle–dependent drugs. 5-Fluorouracil inhibits thymidylate synthetase, methotrexate inhibits dihydrofolate reductase, and Ara-C inhibits DNA polymerase. These agents inhibit enzyme systems because of their similarity to physiologic substrates. They can also be incorporated as false bases into the DNA or RNA, causing cellular dysfunction. The common adverse effects include mucositis and myelosuppression.

Antibiotics

The anthracycline antibiotics interfere with enzyme systems involved in DNA replication, disrupting translation and transcription. They are not cycle specific and are active in many solid tumors. They cause severe bone

TABLE 10.7	Chemotherapeutic and Targeted Therapy Drugs

Alkylating Agents

Alkyl sulfonates	Bisulfan	
Ethylenimines	Hexamethylmelamine	
	Thiotepa	
Nitrogen mustards	Chlorambucil	Cytoxan
	Cyclophosphamide	
	Ifosphamide	
	Melphalan	
	Mechlorethamine	
Nitrosoureas	Carmustine (BCNU)	
	Lomustine	
	Streptozocin	
Triazines	Dicarbazine (DTIC)	
	Temazolomide	
Platinum compounds	Carboplatin	
	Cisplatin	
	Oxaliplatin	
Antimetabolites	Capcitabine	Xeloda
	Cytarabine (Ara-C)	
	5-Fluorouracil	
	Gemcitabine	Gemzar
	6-Mercaptopurine (6-MP)	
	Methotrexate	
Antibiotics		
Anthracycline antibiotics	Daunorubicin	
	Doxorubicin	Adriamycin
	Epirubicin	
	Idarubicin	
	Mitoxantrone	
Other antibiotics	Actinomycin-D	
	Bleomycin	
	Mitomycin-C	
Mitotic Inhibitors		
Epothilones	Ixabepilone	
Taxanes	Docetaxel	Taxotere
	Paclitaxel	Taxol
Vinca Alkaloids	Vinblastine	Velban
	Vincristine	Oncovin
	Vinorelbine	
Topoisomerase Inhibitors		
Topoisomerase I	Irinotecan	CPT-11
	Topotecan	
Topoisomerase II	Etoposide	VP-16
	Tenoposide	
	Mitoxantrone	
Hormonal Agents		
Antiestrogens	Fulvestrant	Faslodex
	Tamoxifen	
	Toremifene	Fareston

(continued)

TABLE 10.7	Chemotherapeutic and Targeted Therapy Drugs (continued)	
Hormonal Agents (*continued*)		
Antiandrogens	Bicalutamide	Casodex
	Flutamide	Eulexin
	Nilutamide	Nilandron
Gonadotropin-releasing hormone antagonists	Leuprolide	Lupron
	Goserelin	Zoladex
Aromatase inhibitors	Anastrozole	Arimidex
	Exemestane	Aromasin
	Letrozole	Femara
Targeted Therapies		
vEGF binding	Bevacizumab	Avastin
EGF receptor antagonist	Cetuximab	Erbitux
HER-2/neu receptor antagonist	Trastuzumab	Herceptin
Tyrosine kinase inhibitors	Imatinib mesylate	Gleevec
	Gefitinib	Iressa
	Sorafenib	
	Sunitinib	Sutent

marrow suppression, alopecia, and mucositis. Cardiotoxicity following doxorubicin administration is pronounced at doses greater than 550 mg/m^2. Mitoxantrone acts similar to doxorubicin, with addition topoisomerase inhibition activity.

Topoisomerase Inhibitors

Topoisomerase I and II enzymes are involved in uncoiling the separate strands of DNA for translation and transcription. Therefore, the inhibitors of these enzymes decrease cellular turnover. They are associated with secondary malignancies, especially acute leukemia.

Mitotic Inhibitors

The mitotic inhibits prevent spindle formation or dissembly in metaphase, causing metaphase arrest. Cells caught in prolonged metaphase either die or fail to initiate subsequent divisions. This class of drug includes the taxanes, vinca alkaloids, and epothilones. The major toxicities include leukopenia, stomatitis, and neuropathy. Paralytic ileus is a consequence of vinca alkaloid therapy and should be treated expectantly.

Hormonal Agents

These medications alter the production or the endorgan activity of sex hormones. The reduction of hormone activity or concentration slows the growth of the sex hormone–responsive tumors. There are several classes of hormonal agents including the antiestrogens, antiandrogens, progestins, gonadotropin-releasing hormone analogues, and aromatase inhibitors (AIs). The antiestrogens and antiandrogens antagonize the effect of the natural sex hormones on the cellular and nuclear receptors. The gonadotropin-releasing hormone analogue antagonists cause a chemical castration, decreasing adrenal, ovarian, and testicular production of androgens and estrogens. In contrast, the AIs prevent peripheral aromatization of androgens to estrogen. The AIs may be more effective in the postmenopausal woman because the majority of estrogen is produced peripherally by this conversion.

Targeted Therapies

Targeted therapies are relatively new and help regulate cell division, angiogenesis, or programmed cell death (apoptosis). Bevacizamab is a monoclonal antibody that binds vascular endothelial growth factor (vEGF), making it unavailable to bind to the vEGF receptor. Cetuximab, a chimerized monoclonal antibody, binds to the vEGF receptor preventing binding of vEGF. Both of these drugs prevent cell growth by preventing the subsequent (downstream) growth pathways to be activated. Both these agents are approved for use in colorectal cancer. Similarly, the small molecule tyrosine kinase inhibitors antagonize the activity of downstream pathways and have been approved for use in gastrointestinal stromal tumors, renal cell carcinoma, and hepatocellular cancer. Trastuzumab binds to the HER-2/neu receptor found in breast cancer.

Biologic Response Modifiers

Biologic response modifiers alter the host's response to cancer. They are endogenous molecules used in pharmacologic dosages. Interferon enhances the antitumor activity of killer lymphocytes and macrophages. It enhances the expression of certain tumor antigens and alters enzyme systems involved with DNA synthesis. The major toxicities are flulike syndrome, leukopenia, and hepatic dysfunction. It is used for hairy cell leukemia and melanoma. There are currently no approved cancer vaccines or gene therapies for cancer.

Principles of Adjuvant Chemotherapy

Despite an adequate scope of resection, many cancers recur postoperatively suggesting the presence of microscopic residual disease. Adjuvant chemotherapy is an attempt to eradicate the residual disease to improve disease- and recurrence-free survival. Adjuvant chemotherapy requires effective agents against the specific cancer, and patients at risk for recurrence should be identified by prognostic factors and staging. This therapy is purported to be most effective in the immediate postoperative period when the tumor burden is low and the cellular growth kinetics are exponential. Patient-specific therapy, based on the molecular, genetic, and biochemical profile of the tumor, may be a better indication for adjuvant therapy and determinant of efficacy in individual patients. Commercial tests are available for breast and colon cancer recurrence risk stratification.

Treatment of Advanced Cancer

The use of chemotherapy in advanced disease is indicated if there are effective agents, the tumor is unresectable or the patient is nonoperable, the metastases are symptomatic, or the disease is progressing rapidly. Tumors poorly responsive to standard chemotherapy should be treated only in protocol settings.

Neoadjuvant (Preoperative) Chemotherapy

Neoadjuvant chemotherapy is an attempt reduce the scope of surgery, preserve function, decrease postoperative recurrence rates (as in rectal cancer), or to make a locally advanced tumor resectable. In a small number of studies, there may be a survival and/or disease-free survival advantage with preoperative therapy in breast, rectal, and gastric cancers.

RADIATION ONCOLOGY

Like surgery, RT generally affects the local recurrence rate with a limited impact on overall survival of the patient. Irradiation causes chromosomal breaks, directly or through free radicals generated from oxygen or water by the radiation. The irradiated cell appears normal until it attempts to divide. At the time of cell division the irradiated cell may die because of the aberration in the chromosomes, may produce nonviable progeny, may not be able to divide but may remain viable, may divide for several generations before dying, or may be unaffected. Cells are most sensitive to radiation during G_2 and metaphase. The effectiveness of RT may be enhanced by oxygen or radiosensitizers. Treatment planning can include the use of particles (superficial penetration) or high-energy photon (deep penetration). Furthermore, computerized guidance (intensity-modulated RT) allows precise targeting of the treatment region through multiple ports reducing injury to adjacent normal structures. The therapeutic index can be further enhanced by different fractionation or delivery methods, including hyperfractionation (multiple small doses), accelerated fractionation (multiple normal doses), accelerated fractionation (multiple normal doses), or interstitial therapy (brachyradiotherapy). The targeting, dose, and fractionation schemes are designed to enhance tumoricidal activity and minimize local tissue destruction.

In patients with head and neck cancer, nodal involvement in the neck is treated with adjuvant RT. The dose varies with the extent of nodal involvement, but usually 50 to 70 Gy is given. Toxicity in the head and neck area includes mucositis, pain, xerostomia, radiation caries, and osteoradionecrosis. Chest irradiation is frequently undertaken in the adjuvant setting following curative resection of lung cancers without proved benefit to the patient. Doses of 40 Gy to one lung or 20 Gy to both the lungs can cause severe radiation pneumonitis. The manifestations of radiation pneumonitis include cough, dyspnea, fever, and chest pain. It generally responds to steroid therapy.

Radiotherapy has been shown to reduce the local recurrence rates following resection of rectal carcinoma. In combination with chemotherapy, RT is the treatment of choice for squamous carcinoma of the anus, with cure rates that markedly exceed those of proctocolectomy for this disease. Severe radiation colitis is seen after 50 Gy and presents with symptoms of bleeding, tenesmus, and pain. Proctosigmoiditis is common during RT given for cancer of the uterus and uterine cervix. The effects of radiation are usually self-limited; however, steroid enemas and a low-residue diet may be helpful in the acute setting.

Radiation enteritis frequently occurs after only 40 Gy to the pelvis or abdomen. It causes severe nausea, vomiting, crampy abdominal pain, and

occasionally bleeding. Chronically, it may result in fistulas, obstruction, or malabsorption. The acute symptoms are treated with antispasmodics and antidiarrheal agents. The malabsorption can be severe and may require short- or long-term parenteral nutrition.

QUESTIONS

1. Which of the following cancer mass screening programs has been effective in reducing cancer specific mortality?
   a. Breast cancer.
   b. Colo-rectal cancer.
   c. Lung cancer.
   d. Cervical cancer.
   e. Thyroid cancer.

2. Which of the following tumor markers is effective as a screening tool for cancer?
   a. CEA
   b. AFP
   c. Ca125
   d. HCG
   e. Calcitonin.

3. Fine needle aspiration biopsies are *not* useful for which of the following entities?
   a. Thyroid nodules.
   b. Breast masses.
   c. Liver masses.
   d. Lymphadenopathy.
   e. Lung masses.

4. A patient presents with a 2 cm breast mass. Which of the following is the preferred method of diagnosis?
   a. FNAB
   b. Core biopsy.
   c. Excisional biopsy.
   d. Incisional biopsy.
   e. Excisional biopsy with normal margins.

5. A patient who had a colon adenocarcinoma resected 2 years prior now has a solitary pulmonary nodule in the periphery of the right lung. Which is the best next step in management?
   a. Bronchoscopy.
   b. Thoracentesis.
   c. Wedge resection.
   d. PET scan.
   e. FNA biopsy.

6. A patient being treated for ALL with ARA-C develops right lower quadrant pain with guarding and rebound. Which of the following should be the next steps in the management protocol?
   a. CT scan.
   b. Broad spectrum antibiotics.
   c. Bowel rest.
   d. Laparoscopic exploration.
   e. Appendectomy.

7. Which of the following is the treatment of choice for squamous carcinoma of the anus?
   a. Proctocolectomy.
   b. Radiotherapy alone.
   c. Local resection.
   d. Adjuvant chemotherapy.
   e. Radiotherapy with chemotherapy.

Match the following agents and their appropriate mechanisms of action:

8. Alkylating agents   a. vEGF binding

9. Vinca alkaloids   b. Interstitial cross-linkage

10. Tamoxifin   c. Binds to estrogen receptors

11. 5-Fluorouracil   d. Inhibits spindle formation

12. Bevacizomab   e. Inhibits thymidylate
    (Avastin)   synthesis

SELECTED REFERENCES

Devita VT, Hellman S, Rosenberg SA. *Cancer: Principles and Practice of Oncology*, 6th edition, Philadelphia, Lippincott William & Wilkins, 2001.

Tan MCB, Goedegebuure PS, Eberlein TJ in *Sabiston Textbook of Surgery*, Ch. 29, pp. 737–766, Philadelphia, Saunders-Elsevier, 2008.

Silberman H, Silberman AS. *Principles and Practice of Surgical Oncology: A Multidisciplinary Approach to Difficult Problems*. Philadelphia, Lippincott William & Wilkins, 2010.

Poston GJ, Beauchamp D, Ruers T. *Textbook of Surgical Oncology*. London, Informa UK Ltd 2007.

Bartlett DL, Thirunavukarasu P, Neal MD. *Surgical Oncology: Fundamentals, Evidence-based Approaches and New Technology*. New Delhi, Jaypee Brothers Medical Publishers 2010.

CHAPTER

11

Ronald N. Kaleya
Jacob Clendenon
Sagar Reddy

Melanoma, Sarcoma, and Lymphoma

MELANOMA

Melanoma is a malignant neoplasm of neural crest-derived melanocytes, Approximately 60,000 new cases and 8,100 deaths are anticipated in 2008 in the United States (1). It is now the fifth most common malignancy affecting males and the sixth in the US female population, accounting for 3% to 4% and approximately 1.5% of cancer deaths. The incidence of melanoma has increased to 650% over three decades, exceeding that of all other malignancies. Putting this increased risk into perspective, the lifetime risk for cutaneous malignant melanoma (CMM) was 1:1,500 for a person born in 1935 compared with 1:75 for a child born in 2000. As of 2004, there were 13.8 new cases of melanoma per 100,000 people in the United States. Coincident with the higher incidence, the virulence of the disease has decreased dramatically, with most patients presenting with thinner, localized, and therefore more curable lesions. The 5-year cancer-specific survival for patients with CMM was 32% in 1930 as compared with almost 90% in the late 1990s.

Demographics of Melanoma

Melanoma usually arises in the skin, but it also occurs in the anus, vulva, vagina, mucous membranes of the head and neck region, and uveal tract (Table 11.1). The trunk is the most common anatomic site for melanoma with the remainder equally distributed among the upper extremity, lower extremity, and head and neck region. There is a slight male predominance and the majority of melanoma is diagnosed in the Caucasian population (Table 11.2).

Pathogenesis

Many environmental, phenotypic, and genetic factors have been associated with increased risk for developing CMM (Table 11.3). Some of these risk factors have been causally related to the development of melanoma.

Environmental Risk Factors

Evidence supporting an actinic etiology (especially UVB radiation) of melanoma comes primarily from epidemiologic studies. The risk of melanoma is associated with the severity and number of blistering sunburns in childhood and adolescence. There is an increased rate of melanoma in people living closer to the equator within a single country. Migration studies have shown increased rates of melanoma for people who move from a low to high sun exposure region. In addition, melanoma incidence is higher within homogenous migrant ethnic populations with longer residence in the high sun exposure environment. CMM occurs more frequently in city dwellers and in office workers rather than outside laborers implicating severe intermittent sun exposure rather than total actinic exposure in the actinic etiology of melanoma.

Genetic Risk Factors

Several phenotypic characteristics are markers of increased melanoma risk. These include fair complexion, red or blonde hair color, and a tendency to burn or freckle rather than tan. Blue eye color is a weak independent risk factor. These risks may be surrogate markers for molecular and genetic differences in melanin production and response to ultraviolet radiation. Higher levels of melanin production, as seen in people with chronic sun exposure and dark-skinned individuals, reduce melanoma risk. Melanocytes, in response to UVB (280 to 320 nm), through differences in melanocortin-stimulating hormone receptor (MC1R) activity result in tanning or burning. Red headed and light skin people have polymorphisms in

TABLE 11.1	Anatomic Distribution of Melanoma
Skin	90%
Ocular	5%
Mucousal	1%
Unknown primary	4%
Anatomic site	
Trunk	32.4
Upper extremity	22.8
Head and neck	22.1
Lower extremity	20.5

TABLE 11.3	Risk Factors for Cutaneous Melanoma	
Risk Factor		**Relative Risk**
Pigmented lesions		
Familial DNS		148
Sporadic DNS		7–70
>20 Nevi		2–64
Congenital mole		17–21
White (vs. black)		12
Prior melanoma		5–9
First-degree relative		2–8
Immunosuppression		2–8
Excess sun exposure		3–5
Red hair		3
Sun sensitivity		2–3
Blue eyes		1.5

the MC1R, leading to their hair and eye phenotype as well as their burning response to UV radiation and thus presumably increased melanoma risk.

Personal or family history of melanoma places the patient at increased risk of developing CMM. Approximately 3% to 5% of patients with a past melanoma develop a second primary during their lifetime. First-degree relatives of a patient with melanoma have twice the risk of melanoma as the general population. Familial melanoma has been estimated to account for 8% to 12% of CMM. Patients with familial melanoma tend to have a higher incidence of atypical moles, earlier development of melanoma, and multiple primaries. Owing to an increased awareness, however, patients with familial melanomas tend to present at an earlier stage and may have a better overall survival. Chromosomal abnormalities have been found in familial atypical multiple mole melanoma syndrome (FAMMM) or atypical mole syndrome (AMS). In addition, a rare chromosomal defect, xeroderma pigmentosum, an autosomal recessive defect in DNA repair, is associated with a marked increase in melanoma incidence.

TABLE 11.2	Racial and Sex Distribution
Race	**%**
Caucasian	94.4
Hispanic	1.7
Black	0.7
Other	3.2
Sex	
Male	54.2
Female	45.8

Atypical Mole Syndrome (FAMMM, Dysplastic Nevi Syndrome)

Atypical mole syndrome (AMS) appears in both familial and sporadic settings. It is characterized by the presence of atypical (dysplastic) moles, which when multiple are considered potential precursors of melanoma as well as markers of increased melanoma risk.

The "typical mole" tends to be symmetric, is less than 6 mm, has uniform contour and color, and is sharply circumscribed. They are most commonly located in sun-exposed areas. In contrast, atypical moles are more likely to have indistinct borders, irregular contours, variegated colors (fried egg or target shaped), are larger (>6 mm), and can be located in sun-protected areas. Histologically, they tend to have a nested pattern of growth, nuclear atypia, indeterminate circumscription, and asymmetry. The National Institutes of Health has suggested that the term "atypical mole" be used with the clinical entity and the term "nevi with architectural disorder" for those that show histologic changes of atypia.

The classic triad of AMS includes the presence of more than 100 moles, one mole larger than 6 mm, and at least one with "atypical features." The syndrome has an autosomal dominant inheritance pattern with varying penetrance. The nevi that contain melanoma are frequently larger than 8 mm in diameter, develop after age 35, and occur in areas that are not exposed to the sun. The latency period for the development of CMM is unknown. The lifetime risk of melanoma has been stratified by the number of

TABLE 11.4	Lifetime Risk of Melanoma in Patients with Atypical Mole Syndrome		
Kindred Type	Descriptive Name	Characteristics	Risk
A	Sporadic	One relative has DN	27×
B	Familial	>Two relatives have DN	30–40×
C	Sporadic and melanoma	One relative has DN and melanoma	?
D1	Familial and melanoma	>Two relatives have DN and one has melanoma	?
D2	Familial and melanoma	>Two relatives have DN and melanoma	150×
D3	Familial and melanoma	Personal history of melanoma as well	500×

DN, dysplastic nevi syndrome (FAMMM syndrome).
Adapted from Kraemer KH, Greene MH, Tarone R, et al. Dysplastic nevi and cutaneous melanoma risk. *Lancet* 1983;2:1076.

relatives with the syndrome as shown in Table 11.4. AMS patients should undergo a thorough visual examination every 3 to 12 months, with all suspicious lesions evaluated by epiluminescence (surface) microscopy. The patient should perform self-examination with a full-length mirror and a hand-held mirror every 1 to 2 months. All moles should be charted and measured carefully. Photographs of specific moles should be obtained to document their stability. Any change in a mole on a patient with AMS should undergo biopsy to confirm its benign status.

Giant Congenital Nevi

Congenital nevi are present in 1% of neonates. Some of these nevi involve large portions of the body or portions of the face. By convention, small congenital nevi are those with a diameter less than 1.5 cm, intermediate moles are those between 1.5 and 2.0 cm, and giant congenital nevi are those that are larger than 20 cm in diameter or that encompass an orbit or a major portion of the face. The natural history of the giant nevi is unclear. Only 5% progress to melanoma. Excision eliminates the risk but may leave the child irreparably scarred. The small nevi do not pose an increased lifetime risk of melanoma.

Therapy for the intermediate and giant nevi should be individualized, considering the relatively small increase in risk and the potential disfigurement. Options for treatment include excision and grafting, excision after tissue expansion of the adjacent normal skin, curettage, dermabrasion, and ruby laser therapy. In most cases, treatment is withheld until the child is 6 months old for the giant nevi and until adolescence for the other nevi.

Pathology

Clark's microstaging system determines the level of the tumor by the depth of invasion into the layers of the skin (Table 11.5). This system tends to be subjective, requires multiple sections, and has significant interobserver variability. The Breslow microstaging system is less subjective and has become the standard (Table 11.6) for microstaging melanoma. The thickness of the tumor (reported in millimeters) is determined using an ocular micrometer. Every pathology report should include the elements listed in Table 11.7 because each may have prognostic significance beyond that included in the current American Joint Commission on Cancer (AJCC) staging system.

TABLE 11.5	Clark's Microstaging System for Melanoma
Level	Criteria
I	Confined to the epidermis; no invasion of the basement membrane
II	Into papillary dermis
III	Through papillary dermis, abutting reticular dermis
IV	Into reticular dermis
V	Into subcutaneous fat

TABLE 11.6	Breslow Microstaging System for Melanoma
Diameter (mm)	**Melanoma Designation**
0–1.00	Thin
1.01–2.00	Intermediate
2.01–4.00	
>4.00	Thick

Melanoma is divided into several distinct forms by its histologic characteristics, gross appearance, prognosis, and the duration of the respective radial and vertical growth phases. Nodular melanoma (NM) is considered monophasic because there is either a short or absent radial growth phase. The superficial spreading, acral lentiginous, and lentigo maligna melanomas (LMMs) are considered to be biphasic with a variable radial growth phase preceding the vertical growth phase.

Superficial Spreading Melanoma

Superficial spreading melanoma (SSM) is the most common type of melanoma, comprising approximately 70% of cases. It usually arises near or from a preexisting nevus. The peak incidence of SSM is during the fourth to fifth decade of life. Diagnosis is usually made after a preexisting lesion begins to bleed, becomes pruritic, or enlarges. Some series report a female predominance for SSM. It is, however, more prevalent on the legs of women and the trunks of men. The SSMs are typically flat and have irregular or notched borders with an average diameter of 2 cm at diagnosis. The invasive lesions tend to be larger than 2 cm, with loss of Langer's lines of the adjacent skin.

TABLE 11.7	Complete Pathology Assessment
Breslow Thickness	mm
Ulceration	Present/absent
Clark level	I–V
Lateral margins	Distance, mm
Deep margins	Distance, mm
Regression	Present/absent
Lymphovascular invasion	Present/absent
Vertical growth phase	Present/absent
Mitotic rate	Mitoses/10 HPF
Lymphocytic infiltrate	Present/absent/intensity

Although most are blue or black, the color is often variegated. White or gray areas are frequently seen within the lesions. Ulceration is uncommon, occurring in about 10% to 15% of cases at diagnosis. SSM has an intermediate prognosis.

Nodular Melanoma

Nodular melanoma (NM) accounts for 15% to 30% of cases. NM has a male predilection (2:1), has a peak incidence during the fifth to sixth decades, and does not arise from a preexisting nevus. NM has a significantly worse prognosis than SSM, in part, because it displays an earlier vertical growth phase. Similar to SSM, NM commonly affects the trunk in males and the lower extremity in females. The lesions are raised, symmetric, and generally darker than their SSM counterparts. Although only 5% of NMs are amelanotic, most primary amelanotic melanomas are of the nodular type. Approximately half of the NMs are ulcerated at the time of diagnosis.

Lentigo Maligna Melanoma

Lentigo maligna melanoma (LMM) accounts for only 4% to 10% of melanomas but up to 47% of melanomas of the head and neck. It occurs in areas of severe actinic skin damage and exhibits a prolonged radial growth phase and a delayed or absent vertical growth phase. The peak incidence is in the seventh to eighth decades of life and rarely if ever occurs before age 50 years. There is a slight female predominance that is attributed to the longer life expectancy of women. LMM commonly occurs on the temporal and malar regions of the face and the dorsal surface of the hands. At diagnosis, LMMs are larger than 3 cm and appear as a light brown stains on the skin. The margins of the lesions tend to be convoluted and lacey. LMM rarely recurs locally after excision and infrequently metastasizes. LMM has a good overall prognosis.

Acral Lentiginous Melanoma

Acral lentiginous melanoma (ALM) comprises 2% to 8% of melanomas in Caucasians and 35% to 60% of those found in the black population. The incidence of ALM peaks during the seventh decade of life. Most of these lesions are located on the soles of the feet and the palms of the hands. They exhibit an early vertical growth phase and therefore have a relative poor prognosis. ALMs are frequently larger than 3 cm at diagnosis. Though characteristically flat, nodularity may develop later in the course. The borders are irregular,

and the lesions are tan or brown. Most mucosal melanomas are of this subtype.

Subungual Melanoma

Subungual melanomas (SMs) are rare, accounting for only 2% to 3% of melanomas in the white population but a much higher percentage in the black population. Almost 75% are located on the great toe or thumb. They are often noted when the nail becomes detached from the underlying nail bed. Regional nodes are involved in more than 35% of cases at the time of diagnosis. SM occurs late in life and has a poor prognosis. Unlike the other types of melanoma, the prognosis is related to tumor thickness as well as (a) destruction of the nail bed; (b) location in the toe compared with other digits; (c) bony invasion; (d) lack of pigmentation; and (e) nodal involvement.

Differential Diagnosis

Several benign lesions can be mistakenly diagnosed as melanoma (Table 11.8). In general, acquired benign melanocytic nevi tend to be smaller than 5 mm in greatest diameter, symmetric, and uniformly pigmented. In contrast, melanoma tends to be larger than 8 mm and have variegated color and asymmetric

TABLE 11.8	**Differential Diagnosis**

Seborrheic keratosis: Waxy; unchanging; verrucous raised; and sharply delineated.
Junctional nevus: Usually <5 mm and rarely >10 mm; uniform pigmentation; preservation of Langer's line. Melanocytes at dermoepidermal junction. Rarely occurs after age 40 years.
Compound nevus: Palpable but similar to junctional nevus. May have excessive hair.
Dysplastic nevus: Nevus with architectural distortion and cytologic atypia; preserved epidermal rete architecture. Difficult to distinguish from melanoma in situ.
Halo nevus: Can undergo spontaneous regression. Differentiated from melanoma by symmetry and cytologic maturation.
Hemangioma: Bleeds more profusely than melanoma. Blanches with pressure.
Blue nevus: Less than 5 mm. Pigmented basal cell/ squamous cell carcinoma; long history; pearly nodules surrounding lesion.
Subungual hematoma: Can be drained by nail puncture. Moves with nail growth.

borders. More reliable indicators of melanoma are a change in size or color, the development of nodularity, ulceration, pruritus, and the discovery of a new pigmented lesion after age 40 years. The British have devised an ABCDE and seven-point checklist for diagnosing melanoma by nondermatologists (Table 11.9). The sensitivity and specificity of this system are 79% and 96%, respectively.

Prognostic Factors

Clinical and histologic features predict survival and age, sex, anatomic site, tumor thickness, ulceration, lymph node metastases (macroscopic vs. microscopic), and dissemination of disease.

Sex

The incidence of melanoma is about equal in men and women. The latter have thinner lesions that are more likely to be located on the extremity and less commonly ulcerated. Even when stratified by all pathologic risk factors, there is a survival advantage for women, site for site and stage for stage.

Age

Age at onset may be prognostically significant. Older patients present with thicker lesions. The median thickness of melanoma during the third decade is 1.1 mm compared with 2.8 mm for patients in the seventh decade of life. However, when stratified by thickness, survival is equivalent. Of interest, there is a correlation of younger age and increased incidence of sentinel node positivity even for thin lesions.

Anatomic Setting

The anatomic site of the primary lesion is an important prognostic variable. Extremity lesions, excluding those located on the hands and feet, have superior survival compared with head, neck, and trunk primaries, respectively. The purported poorer prognosis for lesions of the posterior back, arms, neck, and scalp (BANS area) has not been confirmed for clinical stage I melanoma. Only the scalp and neck lesions have a poorer prognosis. The BANS area lesions tend to behave more aggressively when the regional nodes are involved (clinical stage III).

Pregnancy

Approximately one-third of women who develop CMMs are in the childbearing age group. Women who are diagnosed with melanoma during pregnancy tend to have thicker lesions than age-matched controls;

TABLE 11.9	**Historical and Clinical Features of a Suspicious Skin Lesion and a Seven-Point Checklist for Diagnosis of Melanoma**

Historical features
    Change in color
    Change in size
    Bleeding
    Tenderness or pain
    Pruritus
    Family or personal history of melanoma
    Tendency to sunburn
    Prior sunburn frequency

Clinical features
    A: Asymmetry: Lesion is bisected visually, and the two halves are not identical
    B: Border irregularity: Border is not smooth or straight and is irregular or ragged
    C: Color variegation: More than one shade of pigment is present
    D: Diameter: It is >6 mm
    E: Elevation: Lesion is elevated above the skin surface
    Inflammation
    Crusting or bleeding
    Sensory change

Checklist
    Major criteria (2 points for each one present): Change in shape, size, or color
    Minor criteria (1 point for each one present): Inflammation, crusting or bleeding, sensory change, or diameter >6 mm
    If score is more than 3, biopsy is indicated

Adapted from Whited JD, Grichnik JM. The rational clinical examination. Does this patient have a mole or a melanoma? *JAMA* 1998;279(9):696–701.

however, there is no survival decrement stage for stage. Furthermore, pregnancy does not influence survival or recurrence rates in women previously treated for melanoma.

Staging

The AJCC revised the staging system to include most of these prognostic variables in 2002 (2,3) (Table 11.10). Both the clinical and pathologic staging systems have changed. The clinical staging system (Table 11.11) helps define the initial workup, whereas the pathologic staging system determines therapy and prognosis.

Surgical Treatment of Cutaneous Melanoma

Indications for Biopsy

Any pigmented lesion that enlarges, has variegated colors or irregular borders, changes color, develops nodularity, or becomes ulcerated should undergo biopsy. Pigmented lesions that are different from others on the same individual should be excised. Pigmented lesions that develop after age 40 years should be closely evaluated. In addition, any time there is doubt about the nature of a pigmented lesion, biopsy should be performed.

Options for Biopsy

Excisional biopsy is recommended for lesions less than 2 cm in diameter. The excision should include both underlying fat and 1 to 2 mm of adjacent normal skin to permit orientation by the pathologist. The defect can be closed primarily without the use of a skin flap or skin graft. An incisional biopsy is reserved for larger lesions. The clinically thickest part of the lesion should be the biopsy site. Punch biopsies are acceptable but should be at least 5 mm in diameter. In one study, the mean Breslow thickness was 0.66 mm for the incisional biopsy as compared with 1.07 mm at the time of complete excision. This discordance was therapeutically significant, changing the indication

TABLE 11.10	TMN Staging of Cutaneous Malignant Melanoma (AJCC 2002 Staging System for Cutaneous Melanoma) (2)		
Stage	**Criteria**	**Patients (%)**	**Survival (%)**
0	In situ melanoma (TisN0M0)		
IA	<1.00 mm without ulceration, or Clark level II/III (T1aN0M0)	47	>85 at 10 years
IB	<1.00 mm with ulceration, or Clark level IV/V (T1bN0M)		
	1.01–2.00 mm, or Clark level II/III (T2aM0N0)		
IIA	1.00–2 mm with ulceration, or level IV/V (T2bN0M0)	38	60 at 10 years
	2.01–4.00 mm without ulceration (T3aN0M0)		
IIB	2.01–4.00 mm with ulceration (T3bN0M0)		
	>4.00 mm without ulceration (T4aN0M0)		
IIC	>4.00 mm with ulceration (T4bN0M0)		
IIIA	Any thickness without ulceration 1–3 positive (micrometastases) (T1-4aN1-2aM0)	13	Median 3 years
IIIB	Any thickness with ulceration 1–3 positive (micrometastases) (T1-4bN1-2aM0)		
	Any thickness without ulceration 1–3 positive (macrometastases) (T1-4aN1-2bM0)		
	Any thickness with/without ulceration In-transit metastases/satellitosis without positive nodes (T1-4 a/bN2cM0)		
IIIC	Any thickness with ulceration 1–3 positive (macrometastases) (T1-4bN1-2bM0)		
	Any thickness with/without ulceration >3 positive nodes, In-transit metastases/ satellitosis with positive nodes, or matted nodes (T1-4 a/bN3M0)		
IV	Metastatic disease (TxNxM1 a/b/c)	2	Median 10 months
	M1 a—Distant skin, subcutaneous or nodes, LDH normal		
	M1b—lung metastases, normal LDH		
	M1c—other visceral metastases, normal LDH; Any metastases, elevated LDH		

LDH, lactate dehydrogenase.

for sentinel node biopsy (SNB) in 10% of patients undergoing an initial incisional biopsy.

Shave biopsies and electrodesiccation of pigmented lesions are mentioned only to condemn them. These techniques invalidate staging making therapeutic planning unreliable.

The prognosis for an SM is not only determined by thickness and ulceration but by nail bed destruction and bony invasion. After removing a piece of the nail, a portion of the lesion can be excised. Lesions involving the nail matrix should be excised horizontally and those of the nail bed longitudinally. Because all or some of the lesion can be attached to the nail plate, the nail itself should be submitted for pathologic evaluation. In cases where the tumor has grown through the nail, the exophytic component can be excised for diagnosis.

TABLE 11.11	Clinical Staging System for Melanoma

Stage	Criteria
I	Clinically node negative; <2.00 mm
II	Clinically node negative; >2.00
III	Metastases to regional nodes or in-transit metastases without nodal metastases
IV	Disseminated disease

Orientation of the Biopsy

Biopsies should be oriented in a fashion that does not compromise subsequent wide local excision and primary closure. Therefore, biopsy on the extremities is performed along the axis of the extremity, whereas those on the trunk are made in the direction of Langer's lines. Properly oriented biopsies reduce the need for skin grafts at the definitive surgical procedure.

Preoperative Assessment

The natural history of melanoma is unpredictable. The most common sites of metastasis are, in order of frequency, as follows: nodes and adjacent skin, lung, liver, brain, and bones. Most other visceral sites, such as the bowel, heart, eye, and bladder, are rare except in autopsy series. Therefore, once melanoma is diagnosed and prior to embarking on definitive therapy, the patient should undergo an extent-of-disease workup determined by the clinical stage of the disease (Table 11.11). Although many guidelines have been published, those outlined below are adapted from the NCCN 2009 (4) practice guidelines for melanoma.

Clinical Stage I and II (Clinically Node Negative) Disease

Although there is very low yield for a metastatic evaluations with clinical stage I and II patients, several authors suggest that a complete blood count, chest radiograph, lactate dehydrogenase, and liver function test be performed as baseline studies. Computed tomography (CT) and positron emission tomography (PET) imaging rarely change treatment planning in this group and are not recommended.

Occult Stage III (Clinical Stage I and II with Positive Sentinel Nodes)

The group of patients having no palpable inguinal adenopathy, satellitosis, in-transit metastases and clinically occult, pathology positive sentinel nodes do not benefit from more extensive radiologic evaluation.

Several studies evaluating CT, magnetic resonance imaging (MRI), and PET imaging suggest that these studies may be helpful in patients with macroscopic nodal disease, ulcerated and/or more than 4-mm-thick melanomas but not in cases of microscopic nodal disease (5,6).

Clinical Stage III Disease (Palpable Nodes, In-Transit Disease or Satellitosis)

More than 50% of clinical stage III patients will develop metastatic disease. The preoperative evaluation should include a fine-needle aspiration (FNA) biopsy of palpable nodes. Asymptomatic patients with laboratory abnormalities or palpable nodal disease (clinical stage III) may require a CT or MRI of the primary nodal drainage basin, the liver and lungs, but not the brain. There is controversy regarding the indications for CT/PET; however, it should be considered in all clinically node positive patients because of retrospective studies showing a change in therapy in 20% of clinical stage III patients (7). All patients should be examined for a second primary.

Margins of Resection

The controversy concerning optimal lateral margins of resection has been resolved with several prospective randomized trials (Table 11.12). The recommendations for margins (4) vary with Breslow thickness of the primary lesion. In situ melanoma is treated with 0.5 margins (not based on prospective trials). Invasive lesions less than 1 mm in depth (thin melanoma) can be treated with 1 cm margins without an appreciable increase in local recurrences; 2-cm margins are adequate for 1- to 4-mm melanomas. Melanomas thicker than 4 mm are treated with 2- to 3-cm margins, although these recommendations have not been supported by randomized trials. Most excisions can be closed primarily. Skin grafts are generally reserved for patients with large primaries or those with local satellitosis.

Melanomas located on the head, neck, and face (15% to 30% of CMM) pose a difficult oncologic and cosmetic problem. This site has a higher rate of nodal metastasis than other sites; recommendations for margins are the same as those for other cutaneous sites. In areas where 2 cm margins are unachievable or cosmetically unacceptable, skin grafts, Moh's microsurgery, or margins twice the largest diameter of the lesion can be considered. To date, there are no long-term studies supporting Moh's surgery for melanoma, and reduced margins are clearly a compromise of local recurrence and cosmesis.

TABLE 11.12	Trials of Excision Margins					
Study	Breslow Criteria (mm)	No. of Patients	Margin Comparison (cm)	Local Recurrence (%)	Survival (%)	Median Follow-Up (yr)
WHO (8)	0–1	612	1 vs. 3	1.6 vs. 0.6 (NS)	85 vs. 87	12
	1.2			4.2 vs. 1.5 (NS)		
Swedish Trial (9)	0.8–2	989	2 vs. 5	1.0 vs. 0.6 (NS)	NS	11
French Trial (10)	0–2	362	2 vs. 5	0.2 vs. 0.05 (NS)	NS	
Intergroup Trial (11)	1–4	468	2 vs. 4	1.7 vs. 0.8 (NS)	80 vs. 84	8
British Trial (12)	2–4	900	1 vs. 3	3.3 vs. 2.8	NS	5
	>4					

Head and neck mucosal melanomas are generally advanced at the time of initial therapy and tend to fail locally irrespective of the margins of resection. Similarly, anorectal melanoma and vaginal melanoma are associated with a dismal survival. With rectal melanoma, abdominoperineal resection seems to improve local control but not overall survival. Patients with localized and small rectal melanomas can be adequately treated with local excision.

SM in a digit other than the thumb is best treated with distal interphalangeal amputation. Melanoma involving the thumb can be treated with interphalangeal amputation. These recommendations are a reasonable compromise between the potential functional deficits and the possibility for cure.

Lesions involving the pinna can be treated with a wedge resection of the pinna, including the cartilage, with rotation of the remaining ear to achieve a reasonable cosmetic result. Melanoma on the sole must be treated in a fashion that maintains as much of the innervated weight-bearing surface as possible. Melanoma overlying the female breast should be treated similar to any other truncal lesion. Mastectomy is not indicated.

Depth of Resection

The controversy of whether to include the deep fascia during primary resection of a melanoma has been resolved. There is no difference in local recurrence rates, time to recurrence, or survival regardless of whether the fascia is resected.

Closure of the Defect

Local random flaps can be used to close the defect created during the initial treatment of CMM. Skin grafts can be used for large defects when needed. The use of skin grafts does not affect the outcome of the local therapy.

Treatment of Regional Nodes

Approximately 20% of patients with clinically uninvolved regional nodes have occult nodal micrometastases and 20% of patients with clinically palpable nodes are uninvolved when examined pathologically. The patients with thin melanomas (<1 mm) rarely have microscopic involvement of the regional nodes; those with thick lesions (>4 mm) frequently have microscopic nodal disease as well as systemic disease. Based on the assumption that micrometastases in regional lymph nodes, in part, give rise to disseminated disease, elective lymph node dissection (ELND) could theoretically delay or eliminate this progression. Although several retrospective studies have shown statistically significant improvements in disease-free and overall survival of patients who underwent ELND for intermediate thickness melanoma, three prospective trials failed to show a survival benefit for this procedure (13,14). In the Intergroup Melanoma Trial (14), patients with 1- to 4-mm melanomas were stratified by thickness, primary site, and ulceration and randomized to ELND versus observation. At 12 years, there was no significant benefit for elective node dissection. Thus, routine elective node dissection is no longer indicated for cutaneous melanoma.

Morton et al. (15) proposed that the absence of metastases, the first nodes draining a specific cutaneous area, is predictive of the remainder of nodes in that nodal basin. This concept was validated by performing SNB followed by a completion elective node dissection. The sentinel node is identified in more than 90% of cases, with a false negative rate of 3% to 4%. Late failure of the primary nodal basin following a negative sentinel node has been reported as high as

9%; however, much of this failure was due to inadequate pathologic examination of the sentinel node. Stratified by thickness, the risk of a positive sentinel node is 4%, 12%, 28%, and 44% for lesions with a Breslow thickness of less than 1.0, 1.01 to 2.0, 2.01 to 4.0, and more than 4 mm, respectively.

The Multicenter Selective Lymphadenectomy Trial (MSLT-1) (16,17), a study in which there was a 2:1 randomization of patients to SNB with completion node dissection for positive sentinel nodes or observation. After 5 years follow-up, the study confirmed that a negative sentinel node is predictive of improved survival. Seventy-two percent of patients undergoing completion node dissection for a positive sentinel node were alive at 5 years as compared with only 52% following therapeutic node dissection for patients recurring regionally in the observation group.

Lymphatic Mapping and Sentinel Node Biopsy: Method

Subdermal injection of technetium-99m–labeled sulfur colloid in four quadrants surrounding the primary lesion is performed followed by external lymphoscintigraphy. The scintigraphy identifies drainage to unexpected nodal basins and the presence of in-transit nodes. Prior to prepping and draping, a blue dye (isosulfan blue or methylene blue) is injected in similar fashion. Using an intraoperative gamma probe, the nodes draining this area are localized and exposed through a small incision. The marker dye highlights the "sentinel node," which undergoes frozen sections. Metastatic disease in the node is an indication for completion therapeutic node dissection. When no metastatic melanoma is found, the incision is closed expecting a 3% to 4% false-negative rate. Although there are proposals to limit the need for completion lymph node dissection (LND) to those with macroscopic nodal involvement (>0.2 mm), and despite the absence of any prospective study showing improved survival with completion node dissection, the standard of care as of 2008 for a positive sentinel node remains completion LND.

Indications for Sentinel Node Biopsy

The current recommendations for SNBx include all melanomas more than 1 mm, Breslow thickness melanoma less than 1 mm with ulceration, more than Clark level IV, mitotic rate more than 1/10 HPF. Even in thick lesion (>4 mm) where the risk of systemic failure is more than 50%, a negative sentinel node is a very strong prognostic factor for survival.

Sentinel Node Biopsy: Lymphoscintigraphy is Necessary

The extremities have fairly constant lymphatic drainage, but drainage from the trunk and head and neck regions can be ambiguous in as many as half of the cases. Multiple-node groups and unexpected drainage patterns can be found in these areas. SNB should therefore be directed by preoperative lymphoscintigraphy.

Morbidity of Node Dissection

The morbidity rate associated with LND is considerable, ranging from 25% to 81%. About 8% of patients develop lymphedema associated with functional deficits. Approximately one-fourth of patients develop lymphedema that does not impair function. Wound infection rates range from 4% to 45%. The average hospitalization is 8 days. In the Sunbelt Melanoma Trial, the morbidity of an SNB alone was 5% as compared with 23% for patients undergoing completion LND.

ELND for Head and Neck Melanoma

ELND for intermediate-thickness melanoma of the head and neck is area of controversy. The results from retrospective studies have and have not supported a survival advantage for ELND. However, in retrospective studies, there is a lower regional recurrence rates following neck dissection in node-positive patients as compared with observed patients. Based on these findings, elective neck dissections should be considered for the treatment of head and neck primary lesions. Most surgeons now use one of many modified neck dissection techniques that preserve the internal jugular vein, sternocleidomastoid muscle, and accessory nerve rather than using the classic radical neck dissection. SNB has not gained the same wide acceptance in the management of head and neck melanoma although in small studies, it seems to be as accurate as it is at other sites (18,19). As for other anatomic sites, SNB may be the best alternative to elective node dissection.

Extent of Node Dissection

The axillary dissection performed for upper extremity melanoma requires full dissection of levels I, II, and III. The groin dissections should initially include the inguinal (superficial) nodes. These nodes are examined by frozen section; and if involved, the iliac and obturator nodes are dissected. About 25% to 50% of patients with inguinal node involvement also have iliac node disease. Approximately 10% to 20% of patients with iliac node disease survive 5 years.

Treatment of Nodal Disease

Clinical Stage III Disease

Patients with clinically palpable lymphadenopathy should undergo therapeutic lymph node dissection (TLND) simultaneously with the treatment of their primary lesion if there is no evidence of systemic disease.

Stage III Disease with an Unknown Primary

Treatment of stage III disease without a known primary should be TLND. The survival is the same as for other patients with stage III disease. The areas that potentially drain (20) into the node basin should be examined with a UV (Wood's) lamp, and the mucous membranes, vagina and anus, are examined to uncover the occult cutaneous and mucosal primaries, respectively.

In-Transit Disease

In-transit disease is defined as subcutaneous or cutaneous metastases more than 2 cm from the primary lesion. There are several options for therapy, including isolated perfusion, tourniquet occlusion infusion, irradiation, intralesional therapy, cryotherapy, or systemic immunotherapy. Retrospective and anecdotal evidence shows isolated hyperthermic perfusion (IHP) to be effective in some cases.

Locally Recurrent Melanoma

Several series have reported 20% 5-year survival following resection of localized metastatic melanoma. Favorable prognostic factors for survival following resection of recurrent melanoma include regional versus distant recurrence; recurrence of an extremity versus a head, neck, or trunk primary; nodal versus nonnodal recurrence; and a disease-free interval of more than 1 year.

Adjuvant Therapy for High-Risk Melanoma

Patients with thick primary melanomas (>4 mm), in-transit disease, and regional nodal metastases relapse in more than 50% of cases. Interferon alpha-2b therapy was compared with observation alone and showed a significant increase in both disease-free and overall survival in the treatment arm. Disease-free survival increased from 26% to 37%, and the overall 5-year survival increased from 36% to 47%. Presently, routine adjuvant therapy is recommended consisting of 20 million U/m^2/day i.v. ×5 for 4 weeks followed by 10 million Units/m^2 three times a week for 11 months.

Advanced Disease

About one-third of patients with a single metastatic site can be rendered disease free by surgery. Isolated brain metastases should be resected to improve quality of life. There is no good chemotherapy for this disease. Immunotherapy, including interleukin-2 (IL-2)-LAK cell therapy and tumor necrosis factor, has only marginal, short-lived effects. Tumor vaccines, monoclonal antibodies, and other biologic response modifiers are still investigational treatments for advanced disease.

SOFT TISSUE SARCOMA

The soft tissue sarcomas (STSs) are a heterogeneous group of malignancies arising primarily from mesenchymal sites. There are at least 50 types of STS, each with different histologic and biologic characteristics. Although different STSs and malignant peripheral nerve sheath tumors (MPNSTs—not of mesenchymal origin) display different biologic properties, they have a similar natural history and management.

STSs can occur at any age. STS in pediatric patients is not discussed in this section. The median age for STS excluding pediatric and primary bone sarcomas is 49 years. Ninety percent of cases occur in Caucasians. The annual incidence of adult STS is approximately 8,000 cases. The lesions generally present as a painless mass that gradually enlarges. Symptoms are associated with encroachment of other organs (e.g., iliofemoral thrombosis with pelvic sarcomas). Because there are no distinguishing historical features of STS, the diagnosis is frequently delayed even under medical observation.

These tumors tend to invade locally. A pseudocapsule, composed of compressed tumor cells and normal tissue, is frequently present. The STSs disseminate almost exclusively by the hematogenous, rather than the lymphatic, route. Lymph node metastases are uncommon except in the synovial sarcomas, high-grade malignant fibrous histiocytomas, and epithelioid sarcomas. The lung is the most common site of metastasis for all STSs. Liver metastases are seen more frequently with the visceral and retroperitoneal sarcomas.

Pathology and Grading of Soft Tissue Sarcomas

The World Health Organization (21) classifies soft tissue tumors into four categories: benign, locally aggressive,

TABLE 11.13	WHO Classification of Soft Tissue Tumor (21)			
Class	**Potential for Local Recurrence**	**Potential for Metastatic Disease**	**Response to Reexcision**	**Treatment**
Benign	Rare, noninfiltrative	Very rare <1/50,000	Excellent	Local excision only
Locally aggressive	Common infiltrative pattern	Rare	Good	Wide local excision
Rarely metastasing	Common infiltrative pattern	<2%, not predictable by histology	Good	Wide local excision
Malignant	Common infiltrative	More common varies with grade/histology	Poor	Wide local excision, close follow-up for metastases

WHO, world health organization.

rarely metastasizing, and malignant. Sarcomas are classified by their cell of origin as rhabdomyosarcoma, leiomyosarcoma, synovial sarcoma, and liposarcoma (Table 11.13). The diagnosis of malignant fibrous histiocytoma (MFH), previously the most common subtype of sarcoma, is now a diagnosis of exclusion because of better immunohistochemical evaluation of cellular origin and has been largely reclassified as an undifferentiated pleomorphic sarcoma. The most common STSs are listed in (Table 11.14).

Histology and Immunohistochemical Analysis of a Soft Tissue Neoplasm

Immunohistochemistry is used to diagnose the cellular origin of an STS and to differentiate it from other tumors. The tissue is tested against a battery of immunohistochemical stains including vimentin, keratin, desmin, S-100, and others. Other methods are being used to stratify these tumors including gene expression profiling and cytogenetic studies.

TABLE 11.14	Common Soft Tissue Sarcomas by Location
Site	**Histology**
Extremity	LS; SS, MFH, FS, ES
Trunk	LS, LMS, MFH, desmoid
Retroperitoneum	LS, LMS
Head and neck	MFH, LS, FS, DFSP
Gastrointestinal	GIST
Genitourinary	LMS

LS, liposarcoma; SS, synovial sarcoma; MFH, malignant fibrous histiocytoma; FS, fibrosarcoma; ES, epithelioid sarcoma; LMS, leiomyosarcoma; DFSP, dermatofibrosarcoma protuberans; GIST, gastrointestinal stromal tumor.

Tumor Grade

Tumor grade in sarcomas is predictive of potential metastasis and mortality. Grading is subjective and there is a significant degree of interobserver discordance. It is based on the histology, cellularity, mitotic rate, necrosis, and cytologic heterogeneity of the neoplasm.

Specific Histologies
Liposarcoma

There are several subtypes of the liposarcomas, including the well-differentiated, myxoid, and pleomorphic varieties. These tumors commonly arise in the thigh, groin, shoulder, and popliteal spaces. The well-differentiated liposarcoma is rare, has a prominent pseudocapsule, and is associated with a 70% 5-year survival. The other, more common, poorly differentiated liposarcomas are associated with a 20% 5-year survival.

Malignant Fibrous Histiocytomas (Undifferentiated Pleomorphic Sarcoma)

The diagnosis of malignant fibrous histiocytoma (MFH) has decreased with the use of immunohistochemical and cytokeratin-staining techniques reclassifying a majority in other categories. It is now a diagnosis of exclusion. These tumors tend to occur in the deep soft tissues of the buttocks, thighs, arms, and neck and they infiltrate widely. They are more likely to have high-grade histology.

Leiomyosarcoma

Leiomyosarcomas can occur anywhere in the body but have a high incidence in the retroperitoneum and visceral sites. They have been reported to arise from

blood vessel smooth muscle. Although survival is associated with the grade, a small collected series looking only at this subtype showed that leiomyosarcomas in the extremities behave aggressively.

Dermatofibrosarcoma protuberans (malignant fibroblastic fibrous histiocytoma) is a low-grade fibrosarcoma of the trunk and head and neck region with a propensity for local recurrence. Metastases are rare, and wide excision is the most appropriate therapy for this tumor.

Desmoid tumors are classified as abdominal and extra-abdominal subtypes. The abdominal desmoids occur in women of childbearing age. They usually arise from the aponeurosis of the rectus abdominis muscle. Treatment is wide local excision. Estrogen receptors have been identified in some of these tumors, but the significance of this finding remains unclear. There is an association with scarring and some of the polyposis syndromes. In the latter cases, the tumors may become extensive and locally aggressive. These tumors may regress with the addition of some of the nonsteroidal anti-inflammatory drugs. This response is not predictable or well documented.

The extra-abdominal desmoids tend to occur in men in the thirties and forties. Although metastases are rare, they do occur. The locally aggressive nature of these lesions can cause significant morbidity and disability.

Diagnosis

Etiology

Most sarcomas arise without an identifiable cause. Trauma has been associated with the abdominal desmoid tumors (Table 11.15). Approximately 10% of patients with Von Recklinghausen's disease develop neurofibrosarcoma. Radiation therapy has been implicated in the development of sarcomas. In general, these radiation-induced sarcomas occur more than 10 years after therapy in poorly accessible areas of the head and neck; they respond poorly to therapy and have a rapidly progressive course. Chronic lymphedema following surgical lymphadenectomy or radiation therapy for breast cancer or melanoma is related to the development of lymphangiosarcoma of the affected extremity (Stewart-Treves syndrome). Several organic and inorganic chemicals are associated with hepatic angiosarcoma (Table 11.15). The androgenic anabolic steroids are notably included in this group.

TABLE 11.15 Etiology and Predisposing Factors for Soft Tissue Sarcomas

Trauma
Fracture site: fibrosarcoma
Burn: dermatofibrosarcoma protuberans
Foreign body: fibrosarcoma

Chemical
Alkylating agents
Vinyl chloride, Thorotrast, arsenic: hepatic angiosarcoma

Radiation
Both orthovoltage and megavoltage
Latency 2–25 years
MFH, extraskeletal osteosarcoma, fibrosarcoma

Lymphedema
Stewart-Treves syndrome (60% had radiation therapy)
Latency 8.6 years
Lymphangiosarcoma

Genetic
Von Recklinghausen's disease: neurofibrosarcoma
Gardner syndrome: desmoid fibrosarcoma of the mesentery
Li–Fraumeni cancer family syndrome
p53 Gene mutations: rhabdomyosarcoma
Synovial sarcoma: t(x:16)(p11.2; q11.2)

MFH, malignant fibrous histiocytoma.

Distribution of Soft Tissue Sarcomas in Adults

Sarcomas arise from mesodermally derived tissue and therefore occur where there is the greatest amount of muscle bulk. Half of the sarcomas occur on the extremities, one-fourth in the retroperitoneum, and one-fourth on the trunk and head and neck region.

Prognostic Factors

Several prognostic factors have been identified that predict survival and local recurrence, not all of which are independent of one another. Because some of the variables are dependent, there seems to be controversy as to which factors are the most important prognostic variables.

Survival

Histologic grade has the most prominent effect on survival, followed by the tumor size, depth, and site. The overall 5-year survival of high- versus low-grade sarcomas is 64% and 98%, respectively. Certain lesions always have high-grade histology and therefore

TABLE 11.16 **TMNG Staging of Soft Tissue Sarcomas and Survival**

Stage	Criteria	5-Year Survival (%)
IA (G1T1N0M0)	Grade 1, <5 cm	82
IB (G1T2N0M0)	Grade 1, >5 cm	
IIA (G2T1N0M0)	Grade 2, <5 cm	67
IIB (G2T2N0M0)	Grade 2, >5 cm	
IIIA (G3T1N0M0)	Grade 3, <5 cm	46
IIIB (G3T2N0M0)	Grade 3, >5 cm	
IIIC (GxT1–3N1M0)	Any grade or size, +nodes, no mets	
IVA (GxT3N0–1M0)	Bone or blood vessel invasion, no mets	10
IVB (GxTxNxM1)	Metastatic disease	

Mets, metastases.

have a poor prognosis. Included among them are the synovial sarcomas, clear cell sarcomas, MPNST, epithelioid sarcomas, and adult rhabdomyosarcomas. There is a linear relationship of size with risk of distant failure and survival. Patients with peripheral extremity sites tend to have a better survival than those with proximal extremity locations. Retroperitoneal lesions have a worse prognosis than the proximal extremity lesions. Some studies show better survival for young patients (<50), but this finding has not been reproduced in all of the large studies. Histology and necrosis are not independent variables for survival but, rather, a function of the tumor grade.

Local Recurrence

Grade, size, and depth of the primary do not affect the incidence of local recurrence. An inadequate margin of resection, however, does predict a higher frequency of local recurrence.

Staging

There are several staging systems for sarcomas. Because grade is such an important prognostic variable, it is the basis of the American Joint Commission on Cancer staging system (Table 11.16).

Treatment

Surgical Management
Indications for Biopsy

Any soft tissue mass that is enlarging or more than 5 cm in diameter and persists for more than 1 month should undergo biopsy. In addition, any new and enlarging mass in the adult should be considered for biopsy.

Options for Biopsy

The surgical management of a sarcoma is determined by the location, size, and grade of the tumor. Therefore, biopsy must be performed as the initial procedure. The pathologist requires a relatively large, fresh specimen to classify a sarcoma accurately. FNA biopsies are inadequate for initial evaluation of a suspected STS because it cannot reliably define the type of sarcoma or the grade. FNA is an excellent diagnostic test for recurrent or metastatic tumors. Core needle biopsies are acceptable if several cores of tissue are retrieved. An excisional biopsy is recommended for small tumors, whereas larger tumors should undergo an incisional biopsy. The biopsy incision is oriented along the axis of the extremity or in a manner that does not compromise a subsequent definitive operation. Improperly oriented biopsy incisions can limit the resection option or necessitate more extensive, debilitating surgery.

Preoperative Evaluation
Natural History of Sarcomas

The first site of metastatic spread for extremity and trunk STS is the lungs, whereas visceral and retroperitoneal sarcomas metastasize to the lungs and liver. The overall systemic failure rate of low-grade STS is 15% as compared with more than 40% for that of high-grade sarcomas. Preoperative extent of disease evaluation is therefore based on grade, histology, and size.

Low-Grade STS of the Extremities and Trunk

The current NCCN recommendations (22) for STS of extremities and trunk, even those less than 5 cm in diameter, include a chest CT scan and if possible a MRI or CT of the site of local disease. The chest CT is used for subsequent comparison and has a very low initial yield. A CT scan or MRI of the lesion allows better definition of the anatomic setting of the tumor and may help when planning the resection. MRI is considered the best test for extremity and head and neck sarcomas because bony artifacts are eliminated, multiple planes can be reconstructed, and the patient is not exposed to radiation.

High-Grade Sarcoma

Chest CT is mandatory for high-grade sarcomas because of the high incidence of lung metastases. Imaging of the primary is conducted in a similar fashion to the low-grade sarcomas. Positron emission imaging has a higher sensitivity and specificity in high-grade sarcomas and may be useful in this setting. At this time, the diagnosis of sarcoma is not an approved or reimbursable indication for a PET scan.

Retroperitoneal or Visceral Sarcomas

Abdominal CT scans are mandatory. Magnetic resonance angiography or CT angiography can be considered if there is suspicion of major vascular involvement.

Options for Therapy

Sarcomas should be treated by a team of physicians that includes a radiation oncologist, medical oncologist, and surgeon. The scope of the resection is determined by the anatomic setting of the tumor, its proximity to vital structures, its grade, the potential for cure, and the extent functional impairment that may result from ablative surgery. In addition, the patient must be willing to undergo the planned resection. In most cases, the combination of radiation therapy and surgery provides the best outcomes.

Margins of Resection

The resection should be planned to have as wide a margin as possible to prevent local recurrence. At a minimum, the margins of resection must be pathologically free of tumor. Involved surgical margins predict a higher rate of local recurrence but not lower survival. Patients who recur locally do have decreased overall survival. Adjuvant radiation therapy does not eliminate the higher risk of local recurrence in margin-positive resections. The tumor pseudocapsule should not be seen during the conduct of sarcoma surgery.

Limited margin resections (**LMRs**) are those where the margins are not pathologically involved, but the tumor is only one to two high-power microscope fields from the edge of the specimen. The LMR is not recommended due to the high rate of local recurrence. Limited margin resection (LMR) is considered adequate local therapy when combined with radiotherapy (RT) for all grade and stages of sarcomas.

Wide margin resections (**WMRs**) require a margin of at least 1 cm and this is the minimal acceptable margin if surgery is used as the sole modality. Usually, the recommended 1-cm margin cannot be achieved owing to anatomic constraints (i.e., bones, arteries, and nerves).

Muscle group resection is the prototype function sparing but oncologically sound procedure. It is applicable to the lower extremity exclusively. Because the proximal and distal portions of a muscle divided during a wide local resection perform no function, these procedures are no more disabling than the WMR. A problem arises when one of the margins of resection is close and RT is required. The RT must encompass the entire resection bed, necessitating larger radiation portals and higher overall doses with increased risk of radiation-induced complications. Muscle group resections and compartment resections provide no oncologic benefit over routine WMR.

Amputation causes significant functional impairment and has not been shown to provide a survival benefit. It does, however, limit local recurrence. Amputations should be avoided if a conservative limb-sparing option exists.

Alternative Therapy

Preoperative (neoadjuvant) radiation therapy in patients with extremity sarcomas has been advocated by some centers. Despite a higher incidence of local wound complications, survival and local control rates are comparable with that found with postoperative therapy. As the ability to precisely administer RT without substantial adjacent tissue damage improves, the role of preoperative radiation therapy will increase.

General Guidelines for Specific Sites

Sarcomas near or abutting neurovascular structures, bone, or joints or in the distal extremity are difficult to resect with adequate margins. For these lesions, amputation must be among the curative options. If the sarcoma abuts the pelvis, a hemipelvectomy should be considered. An internal hemipelvectomy preserves the leg for cosmetic and support purposes. Reconstruction of the pelvis with autoclaved autologous pelvic bone or preserved bone is also possible. Similarly, sarcomas near the shoulder or scapula may require intrascapulothoracic amputation (forequarter amputation) when no curative conservative option exists.

Although buttectomy alone has a 25% to 35% local recurrence rate for lesions of the gluteal region, more extensive resections have not been shown to improve local control and function. The sciatic nerve should be preserved if it is not involved.

Amputation is recommended for tumors involving the popliteal or antecubital fossae. Margins are limited by the nerves, arteries, and veins traversing these spaces and by the joint itself. An LMR with RT may be considered as an alternative. Locally recurrent disease following LMR and irradiation requires amputation.

Sarcomas of the trunk are difficult to treat because the margins of the abdominal and thoracic walls are thin, precluding adequate deep margins. The surgeon and the patient must be prepared to resect ribs and close the large defects with flaps and prosthetic materials. Adjuvant radiation has not been adequately evaluated for sarcoma in these sites.

Management of Positive Surgical Margins

Reexcision with curative intent for positive surgical margins in axial STS is successful in the majority of cases and translates into improved rates of local control. Radiation therapy can provide reasonable rates of local control in patients unable to undergo function or limb sparing re-resection for positive surgical margins due to anatomic constraints. Improved outcome for RT is associated with microscopic versus gross involvement of the margins, superficial location, and total radiation dose exceeding 64 Gy.

Adjuvant Radiation Therapy

Adjuvant radiation therapy reduces local recurrences but does not change the overall mortality associated with sarcoma of the extremity. For low-grade sarcomas with margins in excess of 1 cm, surgery is adequate. In small (<5 cm) low-grade tumors with margins less than 1 cm, adjuvant radiation should be considered. In contrast, larger low-grade sarcomas should receive adjuvant radiation therapy. All high-grade axial sarcoma patients, irrespective of the adequacy of the resection margins, are candidates for adjuvant radiation therapy. Radiation therapy can be administered externally or with the use of interstitial catheters (brachyradiotherapy).

Retroperitoneal Sarcoma

The mean diameter of a retroperitoneal sarcoma is about 20 cm at presentation. Leiomyosarcomas (25%), liposarcomas (21%), and fibrosarcomas (12%) are the most common types. These tumors should be resected through a transabdominal approach because 79% require resection of an adjacent structure or organ to achieve complete resection. Close or positive margins are the norm rather than the exception. The use of brachyradiation catheters or external beam RT has been advocated based on limited but compelling data. These patients should be followed by CT scans of the abdomen every 3 to 6 months. More than half of these tumors recur and require re-resection. The recurrences can appear more than 5 years after the initial therapy. Some have advocated either preoperative radiation or chemoradiation therapy in the unresectable or marginally resectable patients without convincing evidence of its efficacy.

Visceral Mesenchymal Neoplasms

The majority of visceral mesenchymal neoplasms are now called gastrointestinal (GI) stromal tumors (GISTs) because they are not derived from muscle precursors as was originally proposed. The remainders are leiomyomas, leiomyosarcomas, and schwanommas. Most GISTs (>95%) are positive for the CD117 antigen, a part of the transmembrane receptor tyrosine kinase. These tumors are postulated to derive from the interstitial cells of Cajal and are subtyped as spindle cell (70%), epithelioid (20%), and mixed (10%). They share histological but not immunohistochemical features of leiomyosarcomas, schwannoma, and MPNST. The difference between leiomyosarcoma and GIST is that the former stains for smooth muscle actin and desmin (muscle markers) but not for CD117.

The visceral mesenchymal neoplasms usually present with vague pain, bleeding, and a palpable abdominal mass. They are most common in the stomach but can arise anywhere in the GI tract. Preoperative evaluation includes CT scan of the abdomen looking for metastatic disease to the liver and endoscopic ultrasound with biopsy. Several approaches have been proposed including some radical procedures, but no survival advantage has been shown for the more radical procedures. Therefore, current surgical therapy is gross tumor resection with margins.

Prognosis is related to tumor size, mitotic rate, and location. Gastric neoplasms have a better survival than those found elsewhere in the genitourinary tract. Adjuvant imatinib mesylate (tyrosine kinase inhibitor) for completely resected GISTs is supported by a prospective trial that showed a significant reduction in recurrence at 14 months. Imatinib mesylate is also

used neoadjuvantly for unresectable disease and in the setting of metastatic disease.

Adjuvant Therapy

Forty percent of sarcoma patients die as a result of systemic, hematogenous metastases. Systemic adjuvant chemotherapy makes empiric sense in this situation. Several prospective and randomized trials have shown a small increase in the disease-free interval but no consistent survival benefit. Routine adjuvant chemotherapy off protocol is not advocated.

Treatment of Recurrent Disease

Eighty percent of recurrences are noted within 2 years of initial therapy. The routine follow-up for a patient with sarcoma includes chest CT every 3 months for 2 years then every 6 months for the next 2 years and annually thereafter. A physical examination of the primary site every 3 months and appropriate imaging studies of the surgical site if recurrence is suspected has been advocated.

About 15% of sarcomas fail locally. In the absence of distant metastases, local re-resection or amputation is indicated. Approximately 60% of patients undergoing complete re-resection of a locally recurrent sarcoma survive 5 years. This excellent survival may reflect the biologic behavior of the tumor rather than the efficacy of the reoperative surgery. The recurrence rate for retroperitoneal sarcomas is higher, and the long-term survival is lower.

The lung is the most common site of metastatic disease from STSs. In situations where pulmonary metastases are noted prior to treatment of the primary lesion, the patient must be carefully evaluated. If the primary lesion and the metastases appear resectable on preoperative studies, the patient is a candidate for staged surgery. The primary is resected first. In cases where lung metastases are noted on follow-up examination, they are resected if possible. Lung metastases are generally located peripherally, and resection does not sacrifice much lung parenchyma. Pulmonary functions (including FEV-1) should be obtained preoperatively to determine whether the patient can tolerate thoracotomy. Median survival for metastasectomy is 20 months, with 30% of patients surviving 5 years. The survival is not affected by the histology of the primary or the site of recurrence.

Advanced Disease

In general, treatment of advanced sarcomas is poor. The active agents include doxorubicin, dacarbazine (DTIC), ifosfamide, cyclophosphamide, actinomycin D, and cisplatin. At best, 20% of patients respond to chemotherapy. In the current trials, median survival increased from 4 months to 8 months.

LYMPHOMA

The surgeon's role in the treatment of nonintestinal lymphomas is limited to diagnosis, assessment of the extent of disease, evaluation of residual disease, and support during chemotherapy and radiation therapy.

Lymph Node Biopsies

Nodes are excised (not incised) if possible because the stromal architecture is important to the diagnosis. All nodes should be presented to the pathologist fresh without formalin fixation, allowing immunohistochemical analysis and immunophenotyping. In the future, the treatment of certain types of lymphomas will be based on the immunophenotype rather than the histologic class of the tumor.

Hodgkin's Disease

Historically, Hodgkin's disease was treated with irradiation, chemotherapy, or both. Patients with localized disease, stages IA or IIA, were candidates for RT alone and surgical staging was required. In the modern era, however, chemotherapy is the mainstay of treatment and staging laparotomy is no longer performed.

Non-Hodgkin's Lymphoma

Patients with non-Hodgkin's lymphoma present late stage III or IV disease. Occasionally, posttreatment laparotomy or laparoscopy is needed to differentiate residual disease from fibrosis.

Gastrointestinal Lymphomas

GI lymphomas represent 1% to 4% of all GI neoplasms. The GI tract is the most common extranodal site of lymphoma. Most are B cell lymphomas. About 55% occur in the stomach, 25% in the small intestine, and 20% in the colon. The incidence of gastric lymphoma peaks at the age of 62 years, whereas the other GI lymphomas occur at around age 50 years. These patients present with GI bleeding, obstruction, perforation (9% to 47%), abdominal pain, nausea, weight loss, and fatigue.

The therapy of gastric lymphoma has changed over the past 5 years (23). The majority are now classified as mucosa-associated lymphatic tissue (MALT) lymphomas of B-cell origin. *Helicobacter pylori* is a consistent etiologic agent. *H. pylori* produces an antigen leading to polyclonal B-cell proliferation. Most are low-grade MALT lymphomas and can be treated by eradication of *H. pylori*. High-grade MALT lymphomas and refractory low-grade gastric MALT lymphomas may need additional chemotherapy and/or radiation therapy. The survival is equivalent to surgery with gastric preservation. Surgery is reserved for treatment failures and perforation.

QUESTIONS

Select one answer.

1. Risk factors for the development of melanoma include all of the following *except*
   a. Fair hair.
   b. Light complexion.
   c. Green eyes.
   d. Multiple nevi.

2. The classic triad of the dysplastic nevi syndrome includes all of the following *except*
   a. Patient with more than 100 moles.
   b. One mole larger than 8 mm.
   c. Superficial spreading melanoma of one of the moles.
   d. One mole with atypical histologic features.

3. True statements with respect to melanoma include all of the following *except*
   a. Melanoma is increasing at a rapid rate.
   b. Most melanomas are more common in outdoor laborers than office workers.
   c. Melanoma has become less virulent.
   d. Melanoma is associated with xeroderma pigmentosum.

4. True statements with respect to superficial spreading melanoma include all of the following *except*
   a. SSM is the most common form of melanoma.
   b. Approximately half of the lesions are ulcerated at presentation.
   c. SSMs arise from or near a preexisting nevus.
   d. SSM has an immediate prognosis.

5. True statements with respect to NM include all of the following *except*
   a. NM is more common in females.
   b. Ulceration is common.
   c. Most amelanotic melanomas are of the nodular type.
   d. The lesions are raised and generally darker than the SSM counterparts.

6. True statements with respect to the prognosis of SMs include all of the following *except*
   a. Prognosis is related to destruction of the nail bed.
   b. Prognosis is related to the thickness of the tumor.
   c. Prognosis is related to bony invasion.
   d. Prognosis is related to the location of the lack of pigmentation.

7. Acceptable biopsy methods for a pigmented lesion include all of the following except
   a. Excisional biopsy.
   b. Punch biopsy.
   c. Shave biopsy.
   d. Incisional biopsy.

8. Optimal resection for melanomas of various sites include all of the following *except*
   a. SM of the thumb: interphalangeal amputation.
   b. SM of the third digit: distal interphalangeal amputation.
   c. Melanoma on the female breast: mastectomy.
   d. Melanoma of the thigh, 3 mm deep: wide local excision with 3-cm margins.

9. The following are true statements with respect to clinical stage II melanoma *except*
   a. If no primary is found, the patient should receive chemotherapy.
   b. Therapeutic node dissection is not indicated.
   c. Common sites of metastases include regional nodes, lung, liver, brain, and bones.
   d. About 20% of patients with positive regional nodes survive 5 years.

10. Adequate local therapy for an STS includes all of the following *except*
   a. Neoadjuvant radiation therapy followed by excision.
   b. Wide margin resection.

c. Limited margin resection.

d. Amputation.

11. True statements with respect to STSs include all of the following *except*

a. Lymphatic metastases are common and require lymphadenectomy when present.

b. Hematogenous spread is most common.

c. The pseudocapsule is made up of fibrous tissue and no tumor.

d. Lung metastases are the most common sites of initial failure.

12. Prognostic factors influencing survival include all of the following *except*

a. Size.

b. Grade.

c. Location.

d. Histology.

REFERENCES

1. Jemal A, Siegel R, Ward E, et al. Cancer statistics, 2008. *CA Cancer J Clin* 2008;58:71–96.

2. Balch CM, Buzaid AC, Soong SJ, et al. Final version of the American Joint Committee on Cancer staging system for cutaneous melanoma. *J Clin Oncol* 2001;19:3635–3648.

3. Balch CM, Cascinelli N. The new melanoma staging system. *Tumori* 2001;87:S64–S68.

4. NCCN Practice Guidelines in Oncology—Melanoma v. 2.2008. Available at: http://WWW.NCCN.org.

5. Aloia TA, Gershenwald JE, Andtbacka RH, et al. Utility of computed tomography and magnetic resonance imaging staging before completion lymphadenectomy in patients with sentinel lymph node-positive melanoma. *J Clin Oncol* 2006;24:2858–2865.

6. Miranda EP. Futility of positron emission tomography and other modalities in the initial radiographic screening of patients with melanoma. *Arch Surg* 2006;141:1050.

7. Choi EA, Gershenwald JE. Imaging studies in patients with melanoma. *Surg Oncol Clin N Am* 2007;16:403–430.

8. Cascinelli N. Margin of resection in the management of primary melanoma. *Semin Surg Oncol* 1998;14:272–275.

9. Cohn-Cedermark G, Rutqvist LE, Andersson R, et al. Long term results of a randomized study by the Swedish Melanoma Study Group on 2-cm versus 5-cm resection margins for patients with cutaneous melanoma with a tumor thickness of 0.8–2.0 mm. *Cancer* 2000;89: 1495–1501.

10. Khayat D, Rixe O, Martin G, et al. Surgical margins in cutaneous melanoma (2 cm versus 5 cm for lesions measuring less than 2.1-mm thick). *Cancer* 2003;97:1941–1946.

11. Balch CM, Soong S, Ross MI, et al. Long-term results of a multi-institutional randomized trial comparing prognostic factors and surgical results for intermediate thickness melanomas (1.0 to 4.0 mm). Intergroup Melanoma Surgical Trial. *Ann Surg Oncol* 2000;7:87–97.

12. Thomas JM, Newton-Bishop J, A'Hern R, et al. Excision margins in high-risk malignant melanoma. *N Engl J Med* 2004;350:757–766.

13. Cascinelli N, Morabito A, Santinami M, et al. Immediate or delayed dissection of regional nodes in patients with melanoma of the trunk: a randomised trial. WHO Melanoma Programme. *Lancet* 1998;351:793–796.

14. Balch CM, Soong SJ, Smith T, et al. Long-term results of a prospective surgical trial comparing 2 cm vs. 4 cm excision margins for 740 patients with 1–4 mm melanomas. *Ann Surg Oncol* 2001;8:101–108.

15. Morton DL, Scheri RP, Balch CM. Can completion lymph node dissection be avoided for a positive sentinel node in melanoma? *Ann Surg Oncol* 2007;14:2437–2439.

16. Morton DL, Thompson JF, Cochran AJ, et al. Sentinel-node biopsy or nodal observation in melanoma. *N Engl J Med* 2006;355:1307–1317.

17. Ross MI, Gershenwald JE. How should we view the results of the Multicenter Selective Lymphadenectomy Trial-1 (MSLT-1)? *Ann Surg Oncol* 2008;15:670–673.

18. Gomez-Rivera F, Santillan A, McMurphey AB, et al. Sentinel node biopsy in patients with cutaneous melanoma of the head and neck: recurrence and survival study. *Head Neck* 2008;30:1284–1294.

19. Tanis PJ, Nieweg OE, van den Brekel MW, et al. Dilemma of clinically node-negative head and neck melanoma: outcome of "watch and wait" policy, elective lymph node dissection, and sentinel node biopsy—a systematic review. *Head Neck* 2008;30:380–389.

20. Kirkwood JM, Tarhini AA, Moschos SJ, et al. Adjuvant therapy with high-dose interferon alpha 2b in patients with high-risk stage IIB/III melanoma. *Nat Clin Pract Oncol* 2008;5:2–3.

21. Fletcher CDM, Seigel R, Ward E, eds. *Pathology and genetics of tumours of soft tissue and bone.* Lyon, France: IARC, 2002.

22. National Comprehensive Cancer Network Clinical Guidelines in Cancer v.1.2008. 2008. Available at: http://WWW. NCCN.org.

23. Yoon SS, Coit DG, Portlock CS, et al. The diminishing role of surgery in the treatment of gastric lymphoma. *Ann Surg* 2004;240:28–37.

Gynecologic Disorders

BENIGN GYNECOLOGY

Knowledge of common gynecologic disorders is essential for the general surgeon. The purpose of this chapter is to review common gynecologic disorders that a general surgeon may encounter in daily practice.

ECTOPIC PREGNANCY

Although the majority of pregnancies are intrauterine, ectopic pregnancies are the leading cause of pregnancy-related deaths during the first trimester. With current laboratory tests and ultrasound imaging, the diagnosis and treatment can and should be made prior to rupture. Often patients will present with vague complaints and may be sent home with a misdiagnosis.

Definition

An ectopic pregnancy is a pregnancy that develops anywhere other than the endometrial lining of the uterine cavity. The most common site for ectopic pregnancy is the fallopian tube. Within the fallopian tube, the ampullary region is the most common site of implantation followed by the isthmic and fimbrial portions. Other ectopic sites include the ovary, cervix, hysterotomy (cesarean) scar, and peritoneal cavity.

Incidence

In the United States, it is estimated that 2 out of every 100 pregnancies are ectopic, and that these pregnancies account for 9% of all pregnancy-related deaths. The incidence of ectopic pregnancy has steadily increased in the United States since 1970 when the Centers for Disease Control and Prevention (CDC) first started collecting this information. At that time, the rate was 4.5 per 1,000 reported pregnancies.

This increase is thought to be secondary to two factors, an increased incidence of salpingitis and earlier detection of unruptured ectopics that may not have been detected and would have spontaneously resolved.

More than half of all ectopic pregnancies occur in women who have been pregnant three or more times, and only 10% to 15% occur in nulligravid women.

Etiology

The most important risk factor for ectopic pregnancy is prior pelvic inflammatory disease (PID), especially that caused by chlamydial infection. Other factors include prior ectopic gestation, prior tubal surgery, increasing age, cigarette smoking, diethylstilbestrol (DES) exposure, and a history of infertility. In about 40% of ectopic pregnancies, the cause cannot be determined and is thought to be a physiologic disorder that results in delay of passage of the embryo into the uterus so that the embryo is still in the tube when implantation occurs. Approximately one-third of pregnancies that occur in patients with tubal ligations are ectopic in nature. All contraceptive methods lower the overall risk of ectopic pregnancy by preventing ovulation or conception. However, in the rare case that a patient does conceive, ectopic pregnancy must be considered. Patients with copper and levonorgestrel containing intrauterine contraception have ectopic pregnancy rates, which are one-tenth that of those women not using contraception.

Symptoms

The symptoms that are classically associated with ectopic pregnancy include abdominal pain, amenorrhea, and vaginal bleeding (Table 12.1). These symptoms may be associated with several other processes

TABLE 12.1	Symptoms of Ectopic Pregnancy

Symptom	Prevalence (%)
Abdominal pain	95–100
Generalized	50
Unilateral	35
Shoulder	20
Back	5–10
Abnormal uterine bleeding	65–85
Amenorrhea	75–95
<2 weeks	45
<6 weeks	35
Syncope	10–18
Dizziness	20–35
Pregnancy symptoms	10–20
Nausea	15
Urge to defecate	5–15

Source: Reused with Permission from Beckmann CRB, Ling FW, Smith RP, et al. *Obstetrics and gynecology*. 5th ed. Philadelphia, PA: Lippincott Williams & Wilkins, 2006.

such as a threatened abortion, intrauterine pregnancy with coexistent appendicitis, ruptured hemorrhagic cyst, adnexal torsion, degenerating myomas, or endometriosis. However, given the potential catastrophic nature of a ruptured ectopic pregnancy, it is the responsibility of the physician evaluating these patients to rule out ectopic pregnancy.

Physical Exam

The most common findings on physical exam include adnexal tenderness, abdominal tenderness, and an adnexal mass (Table 12.2). Patients with a ruptured ectopic may present in shock, with rebound tenderness and peritoneal signs. However, symptoms are very variable even in patients with tubal rupture.

Diagnosis

History and physical exam together with ultrasound and laboratory tests are used to help make this clinical diagnosis.

Human chorionic gonadotropin (hCG) can be detected in serum and urine once implantation has occurred. Early in pregnancy, hCG rises in a curvilinear fashion up to day 41 of gestation and usually reaches a maximum level at approximately 10 weeks of gestation (~100,000 IU/L). The mean doubling time is 1.4 to 2.1 days, and in 85% of pregnancies, the level increases at least 66% every 48 hours. Initial assessment of the hCG level together with history, physical exam, and transvaginal ultrasound will help dictate further management.

In patients with an early gestation and minimal symptoms with an hCG level which is below the discriminatory zone (level of hCG when a normal intrauterine gestation would reliably be seen on ultrasound), repeat hCGs should be drawn to assess for an appropriate rise. Once the hCG has reached the discriminatory zone (hCG = ~2,000 IU/L), a repeat ultrasound should be done. In some patients, serum progesterone levels may also be helpful, as very low levels (<5 ng/mL) are consistent with nonviable pregnancies, whereas levels greater than 20 ng/mL are usually associated with normal intrauterine pregnancies. Transvaginal ultrasound is the most important component of the technical evaluation.

Ultrasound can detect an intrauterine gestational sac as early as 4 weeks + 2 days (1 to 2 mm), but it is dependent on the sensitivity of the ultrasound machine and the skill of the sonographer. By 5 weeks

TABLE 12.2	Physical Examination in Ectopic Pregnancy

Finding	Prevalence (%)
Abdominal tenderness	80–90
Peritoneal signs	
Ruptured ectopic pregnancy cases	50
Unruptured ectopic pregnancy cases	5
Adnexal tenderness	75–90
Unilateral	40–75
Bilateral	50–75
Cervical motion tenderness	50–75
Adnexal mass	30–50
Contralateral	20
Uterus	
Normal size	70
Enlarged	15–30
Orthostatic changes	10–15
Temperature >37°C	5–10
Vomiting	15

Source: Reused with Permission from Beckmann CRB, Ling FW, Smith RP, et al. *Obstetrics and gynecology*. 5th ed. Philadelphia, PA: Lippincott Williams & Wilkins, 2006.

of gestation, the sac is approximately 5 mm and should be detectable followed by a yolk sac, fetal pole, and cardiac activity in the subsequent days. When the hCG is above the discriminatory zone and these findings are absent, it is most consistent with a nonviable intrauterine pregnancy or an ectopic gestation. The presence of an adnexal mass or tubal ring sign in this setting is highly suggestive of an ectopic. The ultrasound also can assess for the presence of free fluid suggesting a ruptured ectopic pregnancy with hemoperitoneum and has replaced the use of culdocentesis. An algorithm for diagnosis and treatment of ectopic pregnancy is presented in Figure 12.1.

Treatment

Patients with a ruptured ectopic pregnancy should be managed expediently with a salpingectomy either via laparoscopy or laparotomy, depending on the patients' hemodynamic stability and the surgeon's capability to expeditiously stop the bleeding.

In all other patients, the decision is usually between medical management and laparoscopic surgery with salpingotomy or salpingectomy. Patients with a low hCG (<5,000 mIU) and small ectopic pregnancy size (<3.5 cm) may be excellent candidates for medical management with a single dose of methotrexate

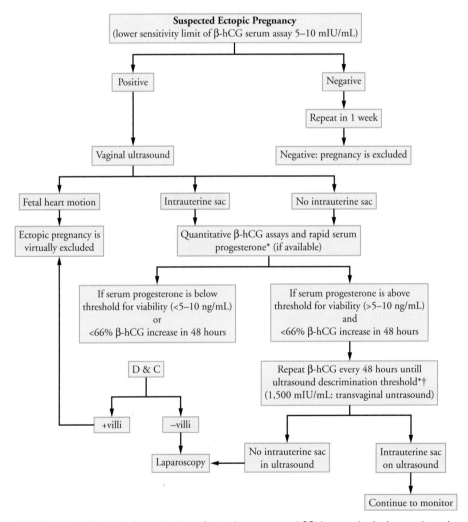

FIGURE 12.1. Algorithm for evaluation of ectopic pregnancy. hCG, human chorionic gonadotropin. (Reused with permission from Rock JA, Jones HW III. *TeLinde's operative gynecology.* 10th ed. Philadelphia, PA: Lippincott Williams & Wilkins, 2003.)

TABLE 12.3 Single-Dose Methotrexate Protocol for Ectopic Pregnancy Treatment

Day	Therapy
0	hCG, D&C, CBC,SGOT, BUN, creatinine, blood type + Rh
1	MTX, hCG[a]
4	hCG[b]
7	hCG

[a]In those patients not requiring D&C before MTX initiation (hCG <2,000 mIU/mL and no gestational sac on transvaginal ultrasound) days 0 and 1 are combined.
[b]With a 15% decline in hCG titer between days 4 and 7, follow weekly until hCG is <10 mIU/ml.
BUN, blood urea nitrogen; CBC, complete blood cell count; D&C, dilation and curettage; hCG, quantitative β-human chorionic gonadotropin; MTX, intramuscular methotrexate, 50 mg/m²; SGOT, serum glutamic oxaloacetic transaminase.
Source: Reused with Permission from Beckmann CRB, Ling FW, Smith RP, et al. *Obstetrics and gynecology*. 5th ed. Philadelphia, PA: Lippincott Williams & Wilkins, 2006.

(50 mg/m²) (Table 12.3). Successful resolution occurs in 92% of patients. Some patients may require a second injection, and follow-up is essential to assure complete resolution. Surgery is an excellent option for patients with more advanced ectopic pregnancies, ectopics with fetal cardiac activity, unreliable patients who will not return for follow-up post–medical treatment, or patients who have a contraindication to methotrexate.

PELVIC INFLAMMATORY DISEASE

PID is a nonspecific term that most often refers to inflammation caused by infection in the upper genital tract. This may include endometritis, salpingitis, oophoritis, myometritis, parametritis, or peritonitis. Sexually transmitted organisms, especially *Neisseria gonorrhoeae* and *Chlamydia trachomatis*, are implicated in many cases; however, microorganisms that compromise the vaginal flora, for example, anaerobic bacteria (including Bacteroides and gram-positive cocci), *Escherichia coli* and other gram-negative rods, *Actinomyces israelii*, and *Mycoplasma hominis* may be associated with some cases of PID. Acute PID is often difficult to diagnose because of the wide variation in signs and symptoms. However, early diagnosis is important, as delay in treatment can contribute to inflammatory sequelae in the upper reproductive tract. The differential diagnosis for PID includes acute appendicitis, urinary tract infections, pyelonephritis, diverticulitis, Crohn's disease, septic abortion, and viral gastroenteritis. Other noninfectious possibilities include ectopic pregnancy, adnexal torsion, ovarian neoplasia, endometriosis, and nephrolithiasis.

Diagnosis

The diagnosis of PID is usually based on clinical findings. According to CDC, treatment should be initiated in sexually active young women and other women at risk for sexually transmitted diseases if they are experiencing pelvic or lower abdominal pain, if no other cause for the illness other than PID can be identified, and if one or more of the following minimum criteria are present on pelvic examination: cervical motion tenderness (CMT) or uterine tenderness or adnexal tenderness. Other considerations, which may influence early initiation of empiric treatment, include evidence of lower genital tract inflammation or patients who have a high-risk profile. PID often occurs within the first 7 days of the menstrual cycle and in 85% of cases occurs postcoital.

Additional criteria may be used to enhance the specificity of the minimum criteria and support the diagnosis of PID include oral temperature 101°F (>38.3°C), abnormal cervical or vaginal mucopurulent discharge, presence of abundant numbers of white blood cell on saline microscopy of vaginal secretions, elevated erythrocyte sedimentation rate, elevated C-reactive protein, and laboratory documentation of cervical infection with *N. gonorrhoeae* or *C. trachomatis*.

Transvaginal ultrasound may be helpful to identify patients with pyosalpinges, tubo-ovarian complexes, or tubo-ovarian abscesses, as well as being helpful in evaluating for ectopic pregnancies. Other imaging modalities may aid in differentiating PID from acute appendicitis, nephrolithiasis, or diverticulitis. However, when the diagnosis is unclear based on clinical exam, laparoscopy is the gold standard to identify the etiology of the patients' pain. PID can be diagnosed by the appearance of indurated and edematous fallopian tubes with the presence of mucopurulent material, pyosalpinx, or tubo-ovarian abscess. Endometrial biopsy may be warranted in women undergoing laparoscopy who do not have visual evidence of salpingitis as some women with PID have endometritis alone. Although laparoscopy can be used to obtain a more accurate diagnosis, its use is not routinely employed when symptoms are mild and vague secondary to the associated risk and cost as well as the good success with empiric antibiotic regimens.

Treatment

Given the potential long-term sequelae of PID, health care providers should maintain a low threshold for the diagnosis and treatment of PID. Treatment regimens must provide empiric broad-spectrum coverage of likely pathogens. All regimens must be effective against *N. gonorrhoeae* and *C. trachomatis* and should have anaerobic coverage as well. Most patients can be treated on an outpatient basis. Hospitalization has been suggested if surgical emergencies (e.g., appendicitis) cannot be excluded; the patient is pregnant; the patient does not respond clinically to oral antimicrobial therapy; the patient is unable to follow or tolerate an outpatient oral regimen; the patient has severe illness, nausea and vomiting, and high fever; or the patient has a tubo-ovarian abscess. The most recent treatment recommendations from the CDC are outlined in Table 12.4. Patients undergoing

---

TABLE 12.4	**CDC Recommendations for Treatment of PID (April 2007)**

Recommended parenteral regimen A
  Cefotetan 2 g IV every 12 hours or
  Cefoxitin 2 g IV every 6 hours plus
  Doxycycline 100 mg orally or IV every 12 hours

Recommended parenteral regimen B
  Clindamycin 900 mg IV every 8 hours plus
  Gentamicin loading dose IV or IM (2 mg/kg of body
    weight), followed by maintenance dose (1.5 mg/kg)
    every 8 hours. Single daily dosing may be substituted.

Alternative parenteral regimens
  Ampicillin/sulbactam 3 g IV every 6 hours plus
  Doxycycline 100 mg orally or IV every 12 hours

Recommended oral regimen
  Ceftriaxone 250 mg IM in a single dose plus
  Doxycycline 100 mg orally twice a day for 14 days with
    or without
  Metronidazole 500 mg orally twice a day for 14 days or
  Cefoxitin 2 g IM in a single dose and Probenecid, 1 g
    orally administered concurrently in a single dose. Plus
  Doxycycline 100 mg orally twice a day for 14 days with
    or without
  Metronidazole 500 mg orally twice a day for 14 days or
  Other parenteral third-generation cephalosporin (e.g.,
    ceftizoxime or cefotaxime) plus
  Doxycycline 100 mg orally twice a day for 14 days with
    or without
  Metronidazole 500 mg orally twice a day for 14 days

CDC, Centers for Disease Control and Prevention; PID, pelvic inflammatory disease.

---

outpatient treatment should be reevaluated in 48 to 72 hours for signs of improvement (e.g., defervescence, reduction in abdominal tenderness, decreased CMT). Patients who do not improve require hospitalization, parenteral therapy, and additional diagnostic tests with possible surgical intervention such as diagnostic laparoscopy. HIV testing should be encouraged in all patients with acute PID, and repeat cultures for *N. gonorrhoeae* and *C. trachomatis* have been recommended by some specialists in patients known to have these pathogens. Male sex partners should be appropriately screened and empirically treated as well.

Tubo-Ovarian Abscess/Complex

A tubo-ovarian complex is a collection of pus within an anatomic space created by adherence of adjacent organs, involving the oviducts, ovaries, and sometimes the intestines. This process can evolve from a salpingitis and can usually be managed in a similar fashion to PID. When a tubo-ovarian complex is present, clindamycin or metronidazole may be added to the doxycycline for more effective anaerobic coverage.

Patients not responding to antibiotic therapy who desire future fertility may be good candidates for drainage under radiological guidance, colpotomy, or via laparoscopy. Patients with leaking or ruptured tubo-ovarian complexes may require extensive surgical treatment including hysterectomy and bilateral salpingo-oophorectomy. Patients being managed with medical therapy should be reimaged approximately 6 to 8 weeks after therapy to assure appropriate response to antibiotics. Patients with persistent masses may require surgical intervention.

Benign Adnexal Masses

A common finding during the work-up of a female patient that often concerns a surgeon is the incidental detection of an adnexal mass. Adnexal masses involving the ovary, tube, or the surrounding utero-ovarian ligaments must be thoroughly evaluated preoperatively to rule out malignancy. Table 12.5 outlines the benign ovarian tumors that may affect women.

Etiology

Functional ovarian cysts are extremely common in women in the reproductive years. Follicular cysts

TABLE 12.5 Benign Ovarian Tumors

Functional
Follicular
Corpus luteum
Theca lutein

Inflammatory
Tubo-ovarian abscess or complex

Neoplastic
Germ cell
Benign cystic teratoma
Other and mixed

Epithelial
Serous cystadenoma
Mucinous cystadenoma
Fibroma
Cystadenofibroma
Brenner tumor
Mixed tumor

Other
Endometrioma

Source: Reused with Permission from Berek JS. *Berek & Novak's gynecology.* 14th ed. Philadelphia, PA: Lippincott, Williams & Wilkins, 2007.

though usually small can reach up to 15 cm. These cysts grow in response to gonadotropins, are usually thin walled and simple in appearance on ultrasound, and will spontaneously resolve or rupture over a short period of time (<3 months).

Corpus luteum cysts, which produce progesterone postovulation, are usually small (4 cm) and asymptomatic. Neovascularization occurs 2 to 4 days after ovulation with blood from the theca zone filling the cyst cavity. Excessive bleeding within the cyst cavity can cause pain, and if the cyst ruptures, significant intraperitoneal bleeding can occur. The majority of corpus luteum cysts resorb. If the patient is hemodynamically stable with a negative hCG, these patients are managed with supportive care and observation, with a follow-up ultrasound in 4 to 6 weeks. These patients can present with an acute abdomen, and the differential must always include a ruptured ectopic pregnancy, appendicitis, ovarian torsion, ruptured endometrioma, or tubo-ovarian abscess. Women with a bleeding diathesis or on anticoagulants are more prone to develop hemorrhage from a ruptured corpus luteum cyst.

Theca lutein cysts are the least common functional cysts encountered and are commonly bilateral.

They are caused by excessive luteinization by hCG. Any condition that causes sustained hCG such as pregnancy, molar pregnancy, choriocarcinoma, and other hCG secreting tumors can initiate the process. On ultrasound, both ovaries are enlarged with multiple cysts ranging from 1 to 10 cm. Patients undergoing in vitro fertilization may develop these cysts, which may persist or enlarge in the event of conception.

Benign Neoplasms

Dermoid cysts (mature cystic teratomas) are the most common benign ovarian neoplasm. These cysts can be found at any age but is most common between 25 and 50 years of age. They are typically derived from all three germ cell layers and account for 90% of germ cell tumors of the ovary. They can range in size from a few millimeters to 25 cm and are often noted incidentally. The imaging often can be diagnostic revealing a complex ovarian mass with cystic and solid components with evidence of fat, bone, or teeth inside the cyst. One percent to 2% of dermoids can undergo malignant transformation. Occasionally, these masses can be the cause of an ovarian torsion or rupture, and as a rule, these masses should be removed. Benign teratomas occur bilaterally 10% to 15% of the time.

Serous cystadenomas are the next most common benign ovarian tumor accounting for 25% of neoplasms. These epithelial cysts occur most commonly in women in their 30s to 50s and can be bilateral in 15% of cases. On imaging, they can be large, are usually simple and unilocular. By comparison, mucinous cystadenomas are usually much larger on imaging and can be multiloculated containing a thick mucinous material. These cysts are usually unilateral and are typically seen in women in their 30s and 40s.

Solid neoplasms of the ovary include fibromas and Brenner tumors. Fibromas are the most common solid ovarian neoplasms, are derived from the fibrous stroma of the ovary, and account for 5% of benign ovarian neoplasms and 20% of all solid ovarian tumors. They are usually unilateral and can be associated with ascites and a right pleural effusion (Meigs' syndrome). Many fibromas are misdiagnosed as uterine fibroids. The size of these solid neoplasms can range from small nodules to extremely large masses weighing as much as 50 lbs. The larger the mass, the higher the incidence of ascites. These tumors have a low malignant potential. Brenner tumors (transitional cell tumors) are small fibroepithelial solid tumors of the ovary, which are commonly unilateral. These tumors are usually seen in women between 40 and 60 years of age and are often detected incidentally within mucinous cystadenomas and less commonly in serous cystadenomas and dermoids. They are rare and account for 2% of all ovarian tumors.

ADNEXAL TORSION

Ovarian torsion is one of the most common gynecologic surgical emergencies. Ovarian torsion refers to twisting of the ovary on its ligamentous and vascular supports, with resultant impedance in the blood supply to the ovary. Patients will often present with intermittent acute abdominal pain. The recognition of this condition is vital to salvaging ovarian function but can be very challenging as the symptoms are sometimes nonspecific. The differential diagnoses to consider includes ruptured corpus luteum, adnexal abscess, acute appendicitis, bowel obstruction, ectopic pregnancy, PID, degenerating fibroids, and endometriosis.

Ovarian cysts and neoplasms are associated with the overwhelming majority of cases of ovarian torsion. Torsion can occur at any time in a woman's life but occurs most frequently in women younger than 50 years. Normal ovaries have been described in 50% of children younger than 15 years with ovarian torsion. Ninety percent of neoplasms associated with torsion are benign. When ovarian torsion occurs, the lymphatic and venous outflow is compromised leading to marked ovarian enlargement, while the muscular arteries continue to perfuse the ovary. Ultimately, arterial flow can be occluded leading to ovarian ischemia with resultant necrosis, infarction, local hemorrhage, and peritonitis.

Patients with ovarian torsion may initially present with intermittent acute pain on one side. This pain may often be associated with nausea and vomiting which may confuse the diagnosis. On physical exam, a tender ovarian mass is identified in 70% of patients. A small percentage of patients will develop fever, which may be a marker of necrosis, especially in the setting of an elevated white blood cell count. Although the definitive diagnosis of ovarian torsion is made surgically, ruling out other potential causes can render a high index of suspicion. A pregnancy test can rule out an ectopic gestation, and computed tomography (CT) scan may be helpful in identifying appendicitis. The most useful test in identifying ovarian torsion is pelvic ultrasonography with Doppler velocimetry. In a patient with abdominal pain, an adnexal mass, and altered Doppler flow, the diagnosis is relatively easy. However, all these features are not consistently detected, and laparoscopy may be indicated to clarify the diagnosis. Swift operative evaluations in patients with lower abdominal pain, an ovarian cyst/mass, and diminished or absent blood flow may lead to preservation of ovarian function. Conservative management with laparoscopic ovarian detorsion is an effective management strategy if technically feasible. Even if the ovary initially appears dusky, detorsion should be attempted, as many of these ovaries will be viable with reperfusion. In the setting of severe vascular compromise or necrosis, unilateral salpingo-oophorectomy should be performed. In cases of childhood torsion with normal ovaries, or young women with only one ovary, oophoropexy, which involves tacking of the ovarian stroma to the pelvic sidewall with sutures, should be considered.

Fibroids

Introduction

Leiomyomas or fibroids are the most frequent pelvic tumor and are often noted incidentally in women undergoing exploratory surgery. These tumors are benign and have only 0.3% to 0.7% incidence of malignant degeneration. They are most commonly found in women in the fifth decade of life and can be found in 50% of black women.

Fibroids can vary in size from a few millimeters to filling the abdomen, and while they may be solitary, they are often multiple. Each myoma originates from a single muscle cell and is monoclonal. Myomas are often described by their location, which are submucous, intramural, or subserous (Fig. 12.2). Most fibroids are asymptomatic and only 20% of patients with fibroids will require surgical intervention. Symptomatic myomas are the primary indication for approximately 30% of all hysterectomies. Symptoms may include pressure, pain, dysmenorrhea, and abnormal uterine bleeding. Patients with fibroids that have a submucous component may present with heavy or irregular menstrual bleeding. Those with large intramural or subserous fibroids often have more pressure and bulk symptoms. Fibroids in general have a poor vascular supply and can often outgrow their blood supply leading to degeneration. The most common and mildest form of degeneration is hyaline degeneration. Patients who present with severe pain and peritoneal irritation may be undergoing acute muscular infarction or red degeneration of a myoma. Management is often supportive, but these tumors can become necrotic and infected requiring surgery.

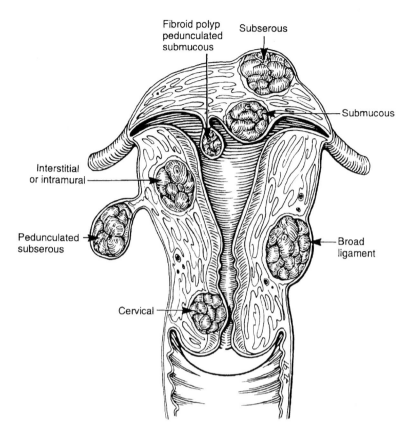

Fibroid polyp
pedunculated
submucous

Subserous

Submucous

Interstitial
or intramural

Pedunculated
subserous

Broad
ligament

Cervical

FIGURE 12.2. Common types of uterine fibroids. (Reused with permission from Beckmann CRB, Ling FW, Smith RP, et al. *Obstetrics and gynecology.* 5th ed. Philadelphia, PA: Lippincott Williams & Wilkins, 2006.)

Diagnosis

The diagnosis of fibroids can usually be made on physical exam by noting an enlarged, firm, irregular uterus. The differential diagnosis must include a pregnancy, adenomyosis, or an adnexal mass. Imaging with ultrasound is often helpful in identification and localization of myomas. Women with irregular bleeding should be evaluated for other causes, and in women older than 35 years, an endometrial biopsy should be performed to rule out endometrial cancer.

Treatment

Many options are available to manage patients with fibroids. In asymptomatic patients, observation is encouraged and no intervention is required. In postmenopausal women with rapid growth, there should be concern for leiomyosarcoma and surgery performed. Management of fibroids should be tailored to the patients' symptoms. Medical management with analgesics, oral contraceptives, Depo-Provera, and gonadotropin-releasing hormone (GnRH) agonists may all be effective in certain women. Patients who are more symptomatic or who fail medical management may benefit from other interventions.

Uterine artery embolization (UAE) has been shown to be effective in many patients and resolves bleeding problems in approximately 90% of patients treated, with up to a 50% decrease in fibroid volume. Patients with submucous myomas or large, pedunculated, subserous myomas may not be good candidates for this procedure. The infarction of a large pedunculated myoma can lead to an extensive intra-abdominal inflammatory process with potential bowel irritation or obstruction. Necrotic submucous myomas can become superinfected leading to sepsis. Approximately 15% of patients undergoing UAE will require further surgery secondary to failure or recurrence of fibroids.

Surgical options include laparoscopic, robotic-assisted laparoscopic, hysteroscopic, or open myomectomy as well as traditional hysterectomy.

Choice of procedure is dictated by the patient's symptoms and their desire for future fertility. Patients undergoing myomectomy must be aware of the risk of recurrence and that as many as one in four women will subsequently have a hysterectomy.

Two rare situations which may be encountered by the general surgeon are leiomyomatosis disseminata and Intravenous leiomyomatosis. Leiomyomatosis disseminata is a benign disease that mimics disseminated carcinoma and has small myomatous nodules over the surface of the pelvic and abdominal peritoneum. This condition is usually associated with a recent pregnancy. Intravenous leiomyomatosis is a rare condition where benign smooth muscle fibers invade and slowly grow into the venous channels of the pelvis. Although usually confined to the pelvis, rarely, the tumor has been reported in the vena cava and right heart.

Endometriosis

Introduction

Endometriosis is a condition whereby endometrial glands and stroma grow in an aberrant manner outside of the normal location within the uterine lining. Although benign, endometriosis can be a progressive, disabling disease with the potential of causing a multitude of symptoms ranging from mild dysmenorrhea to severe chronic pelvic pain and infertility. In some instances, endometriosis can behave like a malignancy by being locally invasive and infiltrative. The exact etiology of endometriosis is unknown; however, several theories have been proposed including retrograde menstruation, vascular/lymphatic dissemination, and coelomic metaplasia. Endometrial implants are usually located in the dependent areas of the pelvis. However, the location can be variable. Metastasis through vascular and lymphatic channels may explain the presence of endometrial tissue in these distant sites.

Epidemiology

Endometriosis is very common and predominantly affects women of reproductive age with a mean age of diagnosis between 25 and 30 years. It is estimated that approximately 5% to 15% of women are affected by this condition; however, the true incidence and prevalence are unknown. One-third of women are asymptomatic and it has been suggested that peritoneal implants are physiologic, and the finding does not necessarily confirm a disease process. For symptomatic patients, most estimates of the prevalence of endometriosis are 5% to 20% in women presenting with chronic pelvic pain and 20% to 40% of infertile women. Less commonly endometriosis can be seen in postmenopausal women, whereby exogenous estrogen stimulates endometrial implants, and in adolescents with obstructed outflow tracts and pelvic pain.

Clinical Diagnosis

Symptoms

The clinical manifestations of endometriosis are highly variable with one-third of women being asymptomatic.

The hallmark symptoms of endometriosis are cyclic pelvic pain and infertility. Dysmenorrhea usually begins 36 to 48 hours prior to the onset of menses and usually persists throughout menstruation and sometimes beyond this period. Endometriosis-associated pelvic pain can be diffused, unilateral, or bilateral and has been described as dull, achy, as well as a sensation of pelvic heaviness or fullness. Associated symptoms of nausea, diarrhea, and dyschezia may be present and pain may radiate to the back and thighs. Deep dyspareunia can occur, likely caused by disease in the posterior cul-de-sac, uterosacral ligaments, and rectovaginal septum. Although pain can be associated with menses, patients may also complain of intermenstrual pain.

As expected, extrapelvic endometriosis can present with a wide variety of symptoms reflective of the affected organs. Endometriosis has been reported in the gastrointestinal (GI) and urinary tracts, abdominal and episiotomy scars, breasts, extremities, lungs, pleural cavity, and peripheral nerves (Table 12.6).

| TABLE 12.6 | Sites of Endometriosis |

Site	Frequency (Percentage of Patients)
Most common	
Ovary (frequently bilateral)	60
Pelvic peritoneum over the uterus	
Anterior and posterior cul-de-sacs	
Uterosacral ligaments	
Fallopian tubes	
Pelvic lymph nodes	30
Infrequent	
Rectosigmoid	10–15
Other gastrointestinal tract sites	5
Vagina	
Rare	
Umbilicus	
Episiotomy or surgical scars	
Kidney	
Lungs	
Arms	
Legs	
Nasal mucosa	

Source: Reused with Permission from Beckmann CRB, Ling FW, Smith RP, et al. *Obstetrics and gynecology*. 5th ed. Philadelphia, PA: Lippincott Williams & Wilkins, 2006.

Signs

In addition to a detailed history, a thorough pelvic and rectal examination can provide valuable clues to the diagnosis of endometriosis. The external genitalia usually do not reveal any abnormalities. Speculum examination may demonstrate blue or red vaginal endometriotic lesions which are typically in the posterior fornix. Rectovaginal bimanual examination can reveal a uterus, which is often retroverted, with decreased mobility and a cervix which may be deviated. Uterosacral nodularities may be palpable with associated tenderness elicited. A palpable adnexal mass is suggestive of an endometrioma. Although useful and suggestive, the lack of these pelvic findings does not rule out endometriosis. In fact, compared with surgery, which is the gold standard for diagnosis of endometriosis, physical examination has poor sensitivity, specificity, and predictive value.

Imaging

Transvaginal ultrasonography is very helpful if an endometrioma, or "chocolate cyst," is present. The characteristic features of endometriomas on ultrasound are cystic masses with diffuse low-level internal echoes surrounded by an echogenic capsule. Internal septations or thickened nodular walls may be present. When these features are observed, transvaginal ultrasound has more than 90% sensitivity and almost 100% specificity. Unlike ultrasonography, magnetic resonance imaging (MRI) can detect peritoneal implants but this modality only identifies 30% to 40% of the endometriotic implants seen at the time of surgery. MRI can also be useful in the diagnosis of rectovaginal disease. The gold standard for the diagnosis of endometriosis is laparoscopy with histologic confirmation of excised endometriotic lesions. Classically, the implants have been described as "powder-burn" lesions which appear blue-black. However, they may appear vesicular, white, or red and "flame-like".

Differential Diagnosis

The differential diagnosis of a female patient with pelvic pain is extensive and includes many systems: gynecologic, urologic, gastrointestinal, musculoskeletal, neurologic, and psychiatric. Gynecologic causes in a nonpregnant patient include primary dysmenorrhea, endometriosis, chronic PID, leiomyomata with or without degeneration, adenomyosis, ruptured ovarian cysts, and ovarian torsion. A thorough review of systems can aid in the diagnosis of other nongynecologic causes of pelvic pain. Patients may also have irritable bowel syndrome, inflammatory bowel syndrome, diverticulosis, appendicitis, interstitial cystitis, urinary tract infections, nephrolithiasis, fibromyalgia, pelvic nerve entrapment, and lumbosacral disc disease. A detailed psychosocial history may reveal a history of sexual abuse and other psychiatric conditions.

Management

The treatment of patients with endometriosis must be individualized and should take into consideration the woman's age, desire for future fertility, severity of symptoms, and pelvic pathology. The treatment can be medical, surgical, or both.

Medical

The goal of medical management is to achieve a reduction or cessation of cyclic menstruation (amenorrhea), which in effect also suppresses activity within the endometriotic implants. This can be achieved through a variety of methods: Danazol, oral contraceptives, medroxyprogesterone, and GnRH agonists.

Surgical

The goal of surgery in the management of endometriosis is to restore normal anatomic relationships, remove visible disease, and delay or prevent future recurrences. Surgery can be definitive or conservative. Definitive treatment is reserved for patients who do not desire future fertility or who have advanced refractory disease. This involves a total abdominal hysterectomy, bilateral salpingo-oophorectomy, and removal of visible endometriosis.

For patients who desire future childbearing and who also have moderate-to-severe disease causing distortion of anatomy and adhesion formation, conservative surgical treatment is preferred. The goal of conservative surgery is to remove grossly visible endometriosis while trying to preserve ovarian function and restoring normal anatomy. The laparoscopic approach is preferred, as it is less likely to cause extensive scarring during the recovery period and the visualization is better with less tissue trauma. Peritoneal implants can be ablated using either monopolar or bipolar electrosurgery. Adhesions should be excised as opposed to simple adhesiolysis as the adhesions themselves may contain disease. The optimal management of endometriomas is controversial, but the rate of reoperation is lower after cystectomy than after drainage and ablation of the cyst wall. Patients with midline pain and dysmenorrhea may be candidates for presacral neurectomy and laparoscopic uterosacral nerve ablation. The former interrupts the sympathetic innervation to the uterus at the level of the superior hypogastric plexus, whereas the latter procedure ablates the midportion of the uterosacral ligaments. Patients with deeply infiltrative disease involving the bowel may require resection of a segment of bowel followed by anastomosis.

SURGERY IN PREGNANCY

Common Surgical Gastrointestinal Disorders Encountered During Pregnancy

Of all the pregnant women, 0.2% to 1% women require nonobstetric general surgery. The cardinal rule in these cases is that the mother always takes priority, as her well-being will usually benefit the fetus. Diagnosis and management of these disorders is usually the same with some specific challenges. Several anatomic and physiologic changes occur during pregnancy that must be taken into consideration and they include displacement of intraperitoneal organs by the gravid uterus, decreased venous return due to pressure exerted on vena cava, increased cardiac output and heart rate, physiologic anemia, leukocytosis, tachycardia, decreased gastric motility, increased gastric acidity, increased minute ventilation, and decreased functional residual capacity. Increased uterine size stretches the abdominal wall and compresses viscera which leads to decreased response to peritoneal irritation and altered or referred pain perception making localization more difficult. To complicate matters further, pregnancy symptoms can mimic GI disorders. Use of imaging is often a concern in the pregnant patient. Ultrasound is an excellent screening modality in pregnancy and safe. MRI can be used in complicated cases and CT scan when only absolutely necessary. The risk of fetal anomalies, growth restriction, or spontaneous abortion is not increased at exposure level of less than 5 rads and the average abdominal CT scan of 3.5 rads.

Appendicitis

Appendicitis affects 1 out of 1,500 to 2,000 pregnancies with equal frequencies in each trimester.

Perforated appendix is the number one cause for fetal loss in this condition. Right lower quadrant pain is the most reliable finding. However, in the fifth month, the appendix may shift above the right iliac crest and rotates medially. History and physical exam are the most reliable in making a diagnosis of appendicitis in pregnancy with a differential diagnosis that includes ovarian torsion, cysts, degenerating fibroids, pancreatitis, pyelonephritis, urolithiasis, and biliary tract disease. Ultrasound has a very high specificity if the appendix is seen (97%). Diagnostic laparoscopy is useful in equivocal cases, especially in early pregnancy, and has reduced the rate of false positive to 15%. In pregnant patients with a suspected appendicitis, preoperative considerations include maintenance of adequate hydration, availability of blood, avoidance of acidosis, deep venous thrombosis prophylaxis, and tocolytics used as required. Intraoperatively, patients should be positioned with slight left lateral displacement. Attention must be paid to protect the airway, as pregnant women are at increased risk of aspiration. The appropriate incision should be chosen to maximize exposure while trying to avoid excessive uterine manipulation. Fetal monitoring postoperatively is warranted dependant on the gestational age.

Biliary Tract Disease

Biliary tract disease is second most common GI disorder requiring surgery in pregnancy.

Biliary colic in pregnancy can be managed conservatively. One to 8 out of 1,000 pregnant women will suffer acute cholecystitis. Invasive procedures are well tolerated especially in second trimester. The presenting symptoms are the same as in nonpregnant patients as well as the typical lab findings of increased alkaline phosphatase and bilirubin levels. Jaundice, abnormal transaminases, or hyperamylasemia may be present in complicated biliary tract disease. The differential diagnosis includes appendicitis, pancreatitis, peptic ulcer disease, and hemolysis elevated liver enzymes and low platelet (HELLP) syndrome of pregnancy. The diagnosis is often made with the assistance of a right upper quadrant ultrasound. The management of these patients includes making the patients NPO (nil per os), antibiotics, analgesics, and hydration. If medical management fails or the patient has another repeat bout, second trimester cholecystectomy may be warranted and a laparoscopic approach is optimal.

Gynecologic Cancer

Gynecologic Malignancy

Every woman is at risk for developing a gynecologic cancer. It was estimated that in 2007 in the United States, there would be 78,000 new gynecologic cancers diagnosed and approximately 28,000 deaths. Screening can result in prevention and early detection especially in cervical cancer. Knowledge of family history and the availability of genetic testing for genes associated with cancer should also help further prevent or lead to more directed screening and hopefully earlier detection of gynecologic cancers. Awareness of physicians about the symptoms related to gynecologic malignancies may also lead to earlier detection and thus increase patients' survival.

Ovarian Cancer

Incidence, Morbidity, and Mortality
Ovarian cancer is the seventh most common cancer in women and the second most common female reproductive cancer, second only to uterine cancer. It is the most lethal of all gynecologic cancers causing more deaths than cervical and uterine cancer combined and ranks fifth in cancer deaths among women. The lifetime risk of developing ovarian cancer is approximately 1 in 70. In the United States, approximately 22,000 new cases are diagnosed annually, with about 15,250 deaths among US women. Survival in stage I is around 90%; however, only 20% of cases are diagnosed at stage I. Sixty-five percent to 70% of cases are advanced when diagnosed with a 5-year survival rate of 30% to 55%.

Risk Factors
The risk of epithelial ovarian cancer increases with age. The median age of diagnosis is 63 years old with 68.8% diagnosed after age 55 years. It is rare in women younger than 40 years. A familial history of breast or ovarian cancer is one of the most important risk factors. The Hereditary Ovarian Cancer Clinical Study Group found that patients who are BRCA1 carriers have a 60-fold increased risk and BRCA2 carriers have a 30-fold increased risk of developing ovarian cancer by the age of 60 years when compared with the general population. Patients with Lynch II syndrome or hereditary nonpolyposis colorectal cancer have a 13-fold greater risk of developing ovarian cancer than the general population.

Infertility and nulliparity also increase the lifetime risk of developing ovarian cancer. Aside from prophylactic oophorectomy, pregnancy and the use of oral contraceptives are the only factors that seem to decrease the risk of developing ovarian cancer.

Symptoms
In 2007, The Gynecologic Cancer Foundation came out with an ovarian cancer symptoms consensus statement. It stated that while historically ovarian cancer was called "A Silent Killer," studies reveal that the certain symptoms are much more likely to occur in women with ovarian cancer and include bloating, pelvic or abdominal pain, difficulty eating or feeling full quickly, and urinary symptoms such as urgency or frequency. Patients with persistent symptoms for more than several weeks should be evaluated for ovarian cancer. Several studies have shown that even early stage ovarian cancer can produce these symptoms.

Screening/Prevention
Currently, there are no effective screening tests available to help detect early ovarian cancer. Annual pelvic exams with attention to patients' complaints and maintaining a high index of suspicion are currently employed. In high-risk patients, transvaginal ultrasound and CA-125 blood tests on an annual or biannual schedule have been used, but the benefits have not been clearly proven. Screening of the general population using this algorhythm is costly and preliminary data from the Prostate, Lung, Colorectal, and Ovarian Cancer Screening Trial (PLCO) involving asymptomatic postmenopausal women showed a high rate of unnecessary surgeries and a low rate of ovarian cancer detection. However, most of the cancers detected by ultrasound were stage I/II as compared with CA-125, which detected cancers that were stage III/IV 90% of the time.

Diagnosis
Pelvic exam, including a rectal exam, even under anesthesia, have shown limited ability to identify adnexal masses, especially in patients with a body mass index of greater than 30. In premenopausal women, only 5% to 18% of adnexal masses picked up on physical exam will be malignant. In postmenopausal women, this number is much higher (30% to 60%) due to the higher prevalence of ovarian cancer in this age group. The differential diagnosis includes endometriomas, other benign neoplasms of the ovary, tubo-ovarian abscesses, and fibroids. A solid fixed mass especially if bilateral and in the presence of ascites should raise clinical suspicion. If an adnexal mass is detected, ultrasonography is essential to help assess the risk of malignancy. The size, consistency (solid, cystic, or mixed), laterality, presence of septations, nodularity, excrescences, and ascites should be assessed. Physical exam and ultrasound findings in conjunction with CA-125 help determine the likelihood of a mass being malignant and the need for consultation with a gynecologic oncologist (Fig. 12.3).

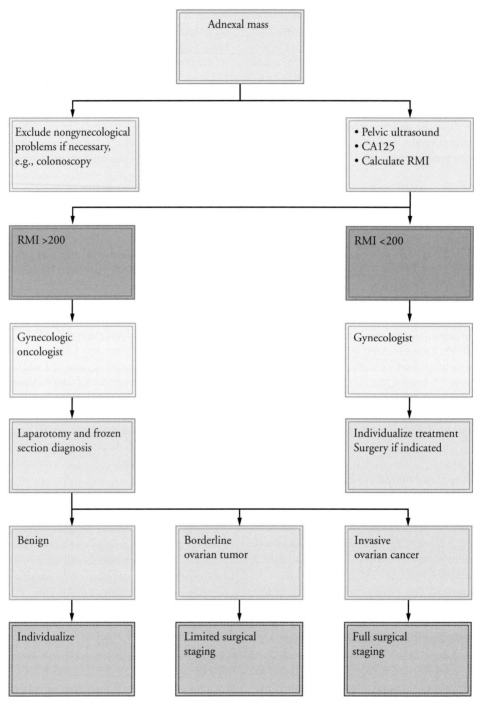

FIGURE 12.3. Preoperative evaluation of the patient with an adnexal mass. (Reused with permission from Berek JS, Hacker NF. *Berek & Hacker's gynecologic oncology.* 5th ed. Philadelphia, PA: Lippincott Williams & Wilkins, 2010.)

Postmenopausal women who have any one of the following should be referred to a gynecologic oncologist and they include ascites, a nodular fixed pelvic mass, evidence of abdominal or distant metastasis, elevated CA-125, and a family history of one or more first-degree relatives with ovarian or breast cancer. Premenopausal women similarly should be referred in the face of a suspicious pelvic mass. However, CA-125 is far less sensitive in premenopausal women and can be elevated in the face of many benign conditions. Therefore, a marked elevation (>200 U/mL) in CA-125 is used as a referral criteria in premenopausal women. The evaluation of women preoperatively should also include the exclusion of an extraovarian primary, which is metastatic to the ovary.

Differential Diagnosis

When the evaluation suggests the presence of ovarian cancer, the possible malignancies include primary epithelial ovarian carcinoma, which accounts for 90% of ovarian malignancies. Epithelial ovarian carcinomas can be subcategorized by type and include papillary serous histology, which accounts for 75% of epithelial ovarian cancers, mucinous cystadenocarcinoma (10%) endometrioid (10%) clear cell tumors, Brenner tumors, and undifferentiated carcinomas. Primary nonepithelial ovarian carcinomas include germ cell tumors (<5%), sex cord stromal, and small cell carcinoma. Malignant mixed mesodermal sarcomas of the ovary are rare but very aggressive in nature. Borderline or tumors of low malignant potential represent approximately 10% of malignant ovarian neoplasms. Metastatic disease to the ovary accounts for 6% to 9% of ovarian malignancies and may be the first clinical manifestation of a primary GI malignancy. Metastatic disease to the ovary coming from the GI tract is referred to as a Krukenberg tumor. These tumors, together with breast cancer, accounts for 50% to 90% of metastatic lesions to the ovary. Fallopian tube cancer can also be mistakenly attributed to the ovaries. Finally, primary peritoneal carcinoma also referred to as papillary carcinoma of the peritoneum is pathologically indistinguishable from papillary serous ovarian carcinoma but is characterized by normal ovaries, extraovarian involvement greater than ovarian involvement, a predominantly serous histology and surface involvement of less than 5 mm depth and width.

Staging

The International Federation of Gynecology and Obstetrics (FIGO) classification of ovarian cancer is presented in Table 12.7. Staging is based on extent of spread of tumor and histological evaluation of the tumor. Surgery remains the cornerstone for treatment of ovarian cancer. The role of surgery is to make a diagnosis, determine the extent of disease, and allow for debulking or cytoreduction. A staging procedure involves thorough inspection of the peritoneal cavity usually via a midline incision, although surgeons with advanced endoscopic skills have reported good success with laparoscopy. Cytological samples of free fluid should be obtained and if none is present, peritoneal washings should be done. Biopsy of suspicious areas should be done and subdiaphragmatic biopsies or scraping obtained. Total abdominal hysterectomy with bilateral salpingo-oophorectomy, pelvic and para-aortic lymph node sampling with removal of suspicious nodes, and omentectomy are required. Cytoreductive surgery or tumor debulking is indicted in most cases, as it is felt that adjunctive therapy is more effective when all tumor masses are reduced to less than 1 cm in size. Inspection of liver, spleen, and diaphragm with removal of all resectable lesions should be attempted if feasible.

Thorough staging is essential as subsequent treatment and prognosis will be determined by the pathologic or surgical stage of the disease. Upstaging is not infrequent based on final pathology. Incompletely staged women may require a second procedure to complete tumor resection or in some circumstances, chemotherapy can be initiated with subsequent surgical reassessment. Twenty-three percent to 33% of ovarian cancers are stage I at initial staging, 9% to 13% are stage II, 46% to 47% stage III, and 12% to 16% are stage IV. Because most ovarian cancer is advanced, adjunctive treatment using chemotherapy is usually necessary. First-line chemotherapy is with paclitaxel combined with a platinum compound intravenous or intraperitoneal. Recurrent disease may be treated with other agents which include doxorubicin, topotecan, gemcitabine, ifosfamide, hexamethylmelamine, etoposide, vinorelbine, and tamoxifen. Radiation therapy has only a limited role in managing ovarian cancer. Follow-up of these patients include physical exam, imaging with CT/ultrasound, and in epithelial tumors CA125. Figure 12.4 outlines a treatment scheme in patients with advanced-stage ovarian cancer.

Prognosis

The 5-year survival rate for stage I ovarian cancer is approximately 93%, for stage II 70%, for stage III 37%, and for stage IV 25%.

TABLE 12.7	FIGO Staging for Primary Carcinoma of the Ovary

Stage I	Growth limited to the ovaries
Stage IA	Growth limited to one ovary; no ascites containing malignant cells. No tumor on the external surface; capsule intact
Stage IB	Growth limited to both ovaries; no ascites containing malignant cells. No tumor on the external surfaces; capsules intact
Stage IC[a]	Tumor either stage IA or IB but with tumor on the surface of one or both ovaries; or with capsule ruptured; or with ascites present containing malignant cells or with positive peritoneal washings
Stage II	Growth involving one or both ovaries with pelvic extension
Stage IIA	Extension or metastases to the uterus or tubes
Stage IIB	Extension to other pelvic tissues
Stage IIC[a]	Tumor either stage IIA or IIB but with tumor on the surface of one or both ovaries; or with capsule(s) ruptured; or with ascites present containing malignant cells; or with positive peritoneal washings
Stage III	Tumor involving one or both ovaries with peritoneal implants outside the pelvis or positive retroperitoneal or inguinal nodes. Superficial liver metastasis equals stage III. Tumor is limited to the true pelvis but with histologically proven malignant extension to small bowel or omentum
Stage IIIA	Tumor grossly limited to the true pelvis with negative nodes but with histologically confirmed microscopic seeding of abdominal peritoneal surfaces
Stage IIIB	Tumor of one or both ovaries with histologically confirmed implants of abdominal peritoneal surfaces, none exceeding 2 cm in diameter. Nodes negative
Stage IIIC	Abdominal implants >2 cm in diameter or positive retroperitoneal or inguinal nodes
Stage IV	Growth involving one or both ovaries with distant metastasis. If pleural effusion is present, there must be positive cytologic test results to allot a case to stage IV. Parenchymal liver metastasis equals stage IV

These categories are based on findings at clinical examination or surgical exploration. The histologic characteristics are to be considered in the staging, as are results of cytologic testing as far as effusions are concerned. It is desirable that a biopsy be performed on suspect areas outside the pelvis.

[a]To evaluate the impact on prognosis of the different criteria for allotting cases to stage IC or IIC, it would be of value to know if rupture of the capsule was (a) spontaneous or (b) caused by the surgeon, and if the source of malignant cells detected was (a) peritoneal washings or (b) ascites. FIGO Annual Report, Vol 26, *Int J Gynecol Obstet* 2006;105:3–4.

Source: Reused with Permission from Berek JS, Hacker NF. *Berek & Hacker's gynecologic oncology*. 5th ed. Philadelphia, PA: Lippincott Williams & Wilkins, 2010.

SPECIAL CONSIDERATIONS FOR THE GENERAL SURGEON

Breast Cancer Patients and Prophylactic Oophorectomy

Most epithelial ovarian cancers are sporadic, with familial or hereditary patterns accounting for 5% to 10% of all malignancies. The BRCA1 and BRCA2 genes are associated with genetic predisposition to both breast and ovarian cancer. Women with breast cancer who carry these mutations are at a greatly increased risk of ovarian cancer as well as a second breast cancer. The lifetime risk of ovarian cancer is 54% for women with BRCA1 mutation and 23% for those with a BRCA2 mutation, and for the two groups together, there is an 82% lifetime risk of breast cancer. The value of prophylactic oophorectomy in these patients has been documented, with a reduction of BRCA-related gynecologic cancer by 96%. There is a 4% risk of developing primary peritoneal cancer. The additional benefit of prophylactic oophorectomy is a subsequent decrease in breast cancer by 50% to 80%. Furthermore, quality-adjusted survival estimate analysis has shown an expected increase in life expectancy of 3 to 5 years in patients with BRCA1 or BRCA2 mutations who have a prophylactic oophorectomy. This should be performed once childbearing is completed, and until that point, use of oral contraceptives should be considered.

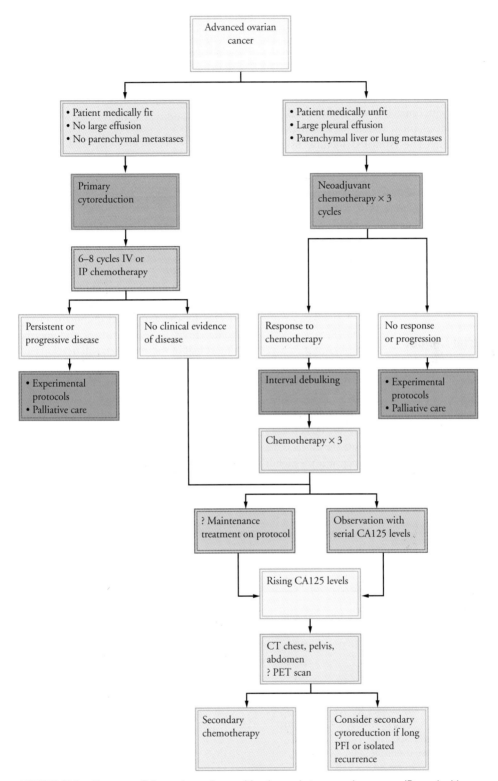

FIGURE 12.4. Treatment Scheme for patients with advanced stage ovarian cancer. (Reused with permission from Berek JS, Hacker NF. *Berek & Hacker's gynecologic oncology.* 5th ed. Philadelphia, PA: Lippincott Williams & Wilkins, 2010.)

Lynch II Syndrome (Hereditary Nonpolyposis Colorectal Cancer Syndrome)

HNPCC syndrome includes multiple adenocarcinomas including colorectal, ovarian, endometrial, and breast cancers. Patients with Lynch II syndrome have a 13-fold greater risk of developing ovarian cancer than the general population. The estimated lifetime risk for endometrial cancer is 40% to 60%. The mean age at diagnosis is 50 years old. Patients with this syndrome should begin endometrial surveillance with endometrial sampling every year beginning at 30 to 35 years of age as well as transvaginal ultrasound to evaluate the ovaries. Hysterectomy/oophorectomy should be discussed after completion of child bearing. Oophorectomy should be considered during exploratory laparotomy or laparoscopy for colorectal cancer or breast cancer in these patients.

Endometrial Cancer

Introduction

According to the American Cancer Society, cancer of the uterine corpus is the fourth leading cause of new malignancies in women, after breast, lung, and colon and rectal cancer. It is estimated that there were 40,100 new cases and 7,470 deaths in 2007. Although uterine cancer is the most common gynecologic malignancy, it is the eighth leading cause, or 3%, of all cancer deaths in women.

Malignant changes within the uterus can arise in the endometrial lining, the muscle, the stroma, or a combination of epithelial and stromal cells. These changes give rise to endometrial adenocarcinomas, leiomyosarcomas, stromal sarcomas, and carcinosarcomas, respectively.

Endometrial adenocarcinomas are further divided into type I and type II derivatives:

- *Type I*—Most common form of carcinoma of the endometrium. Associated with conditions of unopposed estrogen excess. Good prognosis.
- *Type II*—Accounts for approximately 10% of endometrial cancers. Includes papillary serous and clear cell adenocarcinomas. Women tend to be older and growth of tumor is rapid and aggressive.

Epidemiology

Most cases of endometrial carcinoma are sporadic; however, some cases are hereditary. Women in families affected by the autosomal dominant HNPCC syndrome are at increased risk of endometrial cancer. Almost half of these women will develop endometrial cancer, which is the most common extracolonic malignancy. The majority of affected women are postmenopausal, but approximately 25% of cases occur in the premenopausal population. The increasing incidence has been attributed to the aging population and to environmental factors that are associated with excessive and unopposed endogenous and exogenous estrogen exposure. The risk factors and their associated

TABLE 12.8	Comparison between Type I and Type II Endometrial Cancers	
	Type I	**Type II**
Clinical features		
Risk factors	Unopposed estrogen	Age
Race	White > black	White = black
Differentiation	Well differentiated	Poorly differentiated
Histology	Endometrioid	Nonendometrioid
Stage	I/II	III/IV
Prognosis	Favorable	Not favorable
Molecular features		
Ploidy	Diploid	Aneuploid
K-ras overexpression	Yes	Yes
HER2/neu overexpression	No	Yes
P53 overexpression	No	Yes
PTEN mutations	Yes	NO
Microsatellite instability	Yes	NO

Source: Reused with Permission from Barakat RR, Markman M, Randall ME. *Principles and practice of gynecologic oncology.* 5th ed. Philadelphia, PA: Lippincott Williams & Wilkins, 2009.

relative risk are listed in Table 12.8. Tamoxifen, a selective estrogen receptor modulator, has antiestrogenic effects on breast tissue but has stimulatory effects on the endometrium. Its use is associated with a 6.4- to 7.5-fold increased risk of endometrial cancer which should be weighed against the benefit of its use in patients with a history of breast cancer.

Clinical Diagnosis
Symptoms
Unlike ovarian cancer, which is often diagnosed at a later stage, almost three-fourths of patients with endometrial cancer are diagnosed with stage I disease. Patients typically have abnormal bleeding: postmenopausal bleeding or menometrorrhagia in premenopausal women.

Diagnosis
Diagnosis is usually made by an office endometrial biopsy. If unable to obtain tissue, a diagnostic hysteroscopy and dilation and curettage is helpful and allows directed biopsies. An endometrial echo of less than 5 mm on transvaginal ultrasound in postmenopausal women with bleeding has a 99% negative predictive value for malignancy. However, persistent vaginal bleeding and a thickened endometrial lining warrant further evaluation.

Screening
There is no screening test for endometrial cancer. Careful examination of the known risk factors would conclude that reduction or elimination of the modifiable risk factors is key to prevention. This would include weight reduction, control of blood pressure and blood sugar, and avoidance of unopposed estrogen exposure, both endogenous and exogenous. Abnormal uterine bleeding should also be evaluated promptly.

Management
Staging
In 1988, FIGO changed the staging criteria of endometrial cancer from a clinical to a surgical staging system. Adequate staging requires a total abdominal hysterectomy, bilateral salpingo-oophorectomy, pelvic washings, and, at a minimum, removal of suspicious pelvis and para-aortic lymph nodes. However, complete pelvic lymphadenectomy and resection of enlarged para-aortic nodes is recommended for high-risk patients (e.g., grade 3, deep myometrial invasion, cervical extension, serous, or clear cell histology). An omentectomy should also be performed for patients with serous or clear cell adenocarcinomas. The staging system for uterine cancer is listed in Table 12.9.

Although, surgery is considered the main treatment for endometrial cancer, radiation therapy can be used in patients who are either poor surgical candidates or who have advanced disease. For stage I disease, however, the results are inferior for primary radiation; one

---

TABLE 12.9   FIGO Surgical Staging of Endometrial Carcinoma (1988)

Stage	Description
IB G123	Invasion to less than one-half of the myometrium
IC G123	Invasion to more than one-half of the myometrium
IIA G123	Endocervical glandular involvement only
IIB G123	Cervical stromal invasion
IIIA G123	Tumor invading serosa, adnexa, or both and/or positive peritoneal cytology
IIIB G123	Vaginal metastases
IIIC G123	Metastases to pelvic and/or periaortic lymph nodes
IVA G123	Tumor invades bladder, bowel mucosa, or both
IVB	Distant metastases, including intra-abdominal and/or inguinal lymph node

Rules related to staging
1. Because corpus cancer is now surgically staged, procedures previously used for differentiation of stages are no longer applicable (e.g., the findings of dilation and curettage to differentiate between stage I and stage II). It is appreciated that a small number of patients with corpus cancer may be treated primarily with radiation therapy. If that is the case, the clinical staging adopted by FIGO in 1971 would still apply, but use of that staging system would be noted.
2. Ideally, the width of the myometrium is measured along with the width of tumor invasion.

Source: Reused with Permission from Beckmann CRB, Ling FW, Smith RP, et al. *Obstetrics and gynecology.* 5th ed. Philadelphia, PA: Lippincott Williams & Wilkins, 2006.

study showed an 87% 5-year survival rate for surgically treated patients compared with 69% for the pelvic radiation group. The decision to proceed with adjuvant postoperative therapy should be based on prognostic factors identified from surgical staging.

Patients are considered to be at low risk for recurrence if they have

• Grade 1 or 2 histology *and*
• Stage IA or IB

The intermediate-risk group have

• Stage IC *and* grade 1 or 2 histology *or*
• Stage IA *or* IB and grade 3 histology

Patients at high risk for recurrence include those with

• Stage IC, grade 3
• Stage II or greater, regardless of tumor grade
• Papillary serous or clear cell histology
• Lymphovascular invasion (LVI) or lower uterine segment tumor involvement

Adjuvant radiation does not reduce overall survival in patients with low-risk stage I disease although it may decrease pelvic recurrence rates. In women with a high risk of recurrence or persistent disease, adjuvant therapy is recommended. The management of the intermediate-risk group is more controversial. Patients within this group have been further substratified into high risk and low risk based on identifiable risk factors: older than 70 years, invasion of tumor into outer third of myometrium, and presence of LVI. In a post hoc analysis done in a study by the Gynecology Oncology Group, patients in the "high-risk" intermediate group were shown to have a reduction in local recurrence at 2 years with adjuvant radiation. Women with carcinosarcoma, papillary serous, and clear cell adenocarcinomas are treated with chemotherapy as well as radiation therapy for all stages but stage IV, which is treated only with chemotherapy.

Prognosis
The survival rates for patients with endometrial adenocarcinoma are 86%, 66%, 44%, and 16% for stages I through IV, respectively. The overall survival rate is 72.7%.

Cervical Cancer

Incidence
In the United States, cervical cancer has seen a marked decline secondary to advances in our knowledge related to the causative agent and recognition of its premalignant precursors. It was estimated that in 2007, there would be approximately 11,150 new cases of invasive cervical cancer diagnosed and approximately 3,670 deaths. Most new cases occur in patients who have not had regular Pap smear screening. Cervical cancer usually affects women between the ages of 30 and 55. The majority of cervical cancers are squamous cell (85% to 90%) with 10% to 15% being adenocarcinomas.

Symptoms
Many cases of cervical cancer are asymptomatic. The presenting symptoms for cervical cancer may include postcoital bleeding, excessive discharge, and abnormal bleeding between periods.

Risk Factors
Infection with high-risk human papilloma virus (HPV) is associated with almost all cases of cervical cancer.

HPV infection is extremely common in young, sexually active women and only a small percentage will develop cervical disease. Smoking, HIV infection, and young age at first intercourse are also risk factors for development of cervical cancer. Failure to be screened with annual Pap smears prevents early diagnosis of premalignant conditions which when appropriately managed can avoid future development of cervical cancer.

Screening
Over past 50 years, deaths from cervical cancer have been reduced by 74% through the routine use of screening Pap smears. The Pap is able to detect precancerous changes long before malignancy develops. The addition of HPV surveillance has further added to our ability to determine whether an abnormal Pap smear requires further investigation as well as allowing for less frequent screening if cervical cytology and HPV testing are both negative. Testing for high-risk strains of HPV is appropriate for women older than 30 years or reflexively in response to an atypical Pap smear. HPV type 16 (60%) and 18 (20%) are the most common types associated with cervical cancer.

Prevention
The approval of an HPV vaccine in June 2006 should be a significant factor in further decreasing the incidence of cervical cancer. Gardasil was FDA approved for girls/women ages 9 to 26 years old. Large clinical trials have shown effectiveness in preventing precancerous lesions of the cervix.

TABLE 12.10	Clinical Stages of Carcinoma of the Crevix Uteri

Stage	Characteristics
I	Carcinoma is strictly confined to cervix (extension to corpus should be disregarded)
IA	Preclinical carcinoma
IA1	Minimal microscopically evident stromal invasion
IA2	Microscopic lesions no more than 5 mm deep measured from base of epithelium surface of glandular from which it originates; horizontal spread not to exceed 7 mm
IB	All other cases of state I: Occult cancer should be marked "occ"
II	Carcinoma extends beyond cervix but has not extended to pelvic wall; involves vagina but not as far as lower third
IIA	No obvious parametrial involvement
IIB	Obvious parametrial involvement
III	Carcinoma has extended to pelvic wall; on rectal examination, there is no cancer-free space between tumor and pelvic wall; tumor involves lower third of vagina; all cases with hydronephrosis or nonfunctioning kidney should be included, unless they are known to have another cause
IIIA	No extension to pelvic wall, but involvement of lower third of vagina
IIIB	Extension to pelvic wall, hydronephrosis, or nonfunctioning kidney caused by tumor
IV	Carcinoma has extended beyond true pelvis or has clinically involved mucosa of bladder or rectum
IVA	Spread of growth to adjacent pelvic organs
IVB	Spread to distant organs

Source: International Federation of Gynecology and obstetrics (FIGO) Staging Classification, revised 1985.
Source: Reused with Permission from Beckmann CRB, Ling FW, Smith RP, et al. *Obstetrics and gynecology.* 5th ed. Philadelphia, PA: Lippincott Williams & Wilkins, 2006.

Probably, the most effective means of prevention will be early vaccination prior to the onset of sexual activity, coupled with appropriate screening with Pap and HPV.

Staging and Treatment

Cervical Cancer is clinically staged (Table 12.10) because most patients are treated only with radiation therapy. Clinical staging is often inaccurate and when patients are surgically explored, upstaging often occurs secondary to metastases to the pelvic and para-aortic lymph nodes. Surgery has a role only in local-ized disease *or* in salvage after central, localized recur-rence following radiation. Microinvasive carcinoma of the cervix can effectively be treated with total hys-terectomy, with a 5-year survival of almost 100%. Stage Ib cervical cancer can be treated with either a radical hysterectomy with pelvic lymph node dissec-tion or radiation therapy. Surgery is often chosen for treating stage Ib and early stage IIa cervical cancers par-ticularly for smaller tumors and younger patients to

attempt to salvage the ovaries. Radiation therapy with brachytherapy and teletherapy are often used with approximately 85 Gy delivered to point A and 50 to 65 Gy to point B. Combination of chemotherapy, cis-platin, a radiation sensitizer, with radiation is often used to optimize results.

Complications of radiation are dose related and tend to occur even 1 year or more after therapy and include nausea and diarrhea, radiation inflammation of the bladder and bowel with potential scarring, ulceration, bleeding, and fistulization. Approximately one-third of patients will develop tumor recurrence with the majority located in the pelvis.

Prognosis

The prognosis of cervical cancer is related to the tumor stage and lesion size, depth of invasion, and spread to lymph nodes. The 5-year survival rates for patients with cervical cancer is 95% for stage 1a, 80% for stage 1b, 64% for stage II, 38% for stage III, and 14% for stage IV.

Vulvar Cancer

Introduction

The vulva collectively refers to the external female genitalia and includes the labia majora, mons pubis, labia minora, clitoris, vestibule of the vagina, Bartholin's and Skene's glands, and the vaginal orifice. Cancer of the vulva accounts for approximately 4% of gynecologic malignancies and 0.6% of all cancers in women. In the United States, it was estimated that 3,460 women would be diagnosed with vulvar cancer and approximately 870 women would die of this disease in 2008.

Squamous cell carcinoma is the predominant histological type, representing about 90% of all vulvar cancer cases. Melanomas are the most common non-squamous cell malignancy of the vulva, accounting for 4% to 5% of cases. The remainder is composed of other cell types such as Bartholin's glands adenocarcinomas, basal cell carcinoma, and sarcomas. Paget's disease of the vulva is an intraepithelial adenocarcinoma, which accounts for less than 1% of all vulvar malignancies. This rare condition may have an underlying invasive adenocarcinoma and is often associated with a synchronous malignancy in other organs (e.g., breast, bladder, rectum, cervix).

Epidemiology

Vulvar cancer is typically a disease of postmenopausal, older women with half of all cases diagnosed between ages 60 and 79 years. However, one series reported that 15% of cases occurred in women younger than 40 years. Vulvar carcinoma in situ is usually seen in the 40- to 55-year age group and premalignant changes, vulvar intraepithelial neoplasia, are being seen in increasing frequency amongst even younger women. This is likely related to infection with the HPV, which is associated with vulvar carcinoma.

In addition to HPV, other risk factors include granulomatous disease of the vulva, diabetes, hypertension, smoking, and obesity. In addition, a prior history of cervical or vaginal carcinoma is a risk factor for developing a malignancy of the vulva.

Clinical Diagnosis

Symptoms

Patients often have a long history of vulvar pruritus but some may be asymptomatic. Women may complain of irritative symptoms, such as vulvar pain, burning and discomfort with urination, or they may present with a lump or an ulcer.

Diagnosis

The appearances of the lesions are variable. They classically appear white, but lesions may be red or pigmented. Patients may also present with an ulcerated vulvar lesion. Grossly obvious lesions should be biopsied. Application of 3% acetic acid prior to colposcopy of the vulvar with sampling of whitish areas can help to identify dysplastic or malignant areas. An office punch biopsy can be utilized to obtain tissue, making sure to include some surrounding skin and underlying stroma. The differential diagnosis of vulvar lesions includes herpes simplex, lichen sclerosis, seborrheic keratoses, and other dermatoses.

Staging

The staging system for vulvar cancer is surgical and was modified in 1994 by FIGO. Table 12.11 lists the staging system.

Management

In treating vulvar carcinoma, the goal is to perform the most conservative surgery, which is also curative, to decrease disfigurement and psychosexual morbidity. For lesions that are localized, radical local excision is as effective as radical vulvectomy in preventing recurrences. For advanced disease, primary surgical excision is preferable if it is possible to resect the lesion, with negative margins, without causing urinary and fecal incontinence. If surgery would result in diversion of urine or bowel contents, primary radiation therapy may be desirable. An algorithm for the management of locally advanced vulvar cancer is outlined in Figure 12.5. If the patient is not an operative candidate, radiation can be used as the primary modality for treatment. This approach can have severe sequelae including radiation dermatitis, fibrosis, and ulceration.

Prognosis

The overall survival rate at 5 years for vulvar cancer stages I through IV are 71.4%, 61.3%, 43.8%, and 8.3%.

Vaginal Cancer

Introduction

Vaginal cancer is less common than malignancies of the cervix and vulva and account for approximately 2% to 3% of gynecologic malignancies. It was estimated that, in 2008, there would be 2,210 new cases of and 760 deaths from vaginal cancer in the United States.

TABLE 12.11	Staging for Carcinoma of the Vulva

FIGO surgical staging

Stage 0	
Tis	Carcinoma in situ; intraepithelial carcinoma
Stage I	
T1 N0 M0	Tumor confined to the vulva and/or perineum; <2 cm in greatest dimension; nodes are not palpable
Stage II	
T2 N0 M0	Tumor confined to the vulva and/or perineum; >2 cm in greatest dimension; nodes are not palpable
Stage III	
T3 N0 M0	Tumor of any size with:
T3 N1 M0	1. Adjacent spread to the lower urethra and/or the vagina, or the anus, and/or
T1 N1 M0	2. Unilateral regional lymph node metastasis
T2 N1 M0	
Stage IVA	
T1 N2 M0	Tumor invades any of the following: upper urethra, bladder mucosa, rectal mucosa, pelvic, and/or bilateral regional node metastasis
T2 N2 M0	
T3 N2 M0	
T4 any N M0	
Stage IVB	
Any T	Any distant metastasis, including pelvic lymph nodes
Any N, M1	

TNM clinical staging (rules for staging are similar to those for carcinoma of the cervix)

T	Primary tumor
Tis	Preinvasive carcinoma (carcinoma in situ)
T1	Tumor confined to the vulva and/or perineum; <2 cm in greatest dimension
T2	Tumor confined to the vulue and/or perineum; >2 cm in greatest dimension
T3	Tumor of any size with adjacent spread to the urethra and/or vagina and/or to the anus
T4	Tumor of any size infiltrating the bladder mucosa and/or the rectal mucosa, including the upper part of the urethral mucosa and/or fixed to the bone
N	Regional lymph nodes
N0	No lymph node metastasis
N1	Unilateral regional lymph node metastasis
N2	Bilateral regional lymph node metastasis
M	Distant metastasis
M0	No clinical metastasis
M1	Distant metastasis (including pelvic lymph node metastasis)

FIGO, Federation of Gynecology and Obstetrics; TNM, tumor, node, metastasis.
Source: Reused with Permission from Beckmann CRB, Ling FW, Smith RP, et al. *Obstetrics and gynecology*. 5th ed. Philadelphia, PA: Lippincott Williams & Wilkins, 2006.

Epidemiology

Squamous cell carcinoma accounts for 80% to 90% of all cases of primary vaginal cancers and is a disease of older women. Rarer kinds of vaginal cancer include DES-associated clear-cell adenocarcinoma, melanoma, and mesenchymal tumors. Of the mesenchymal tumors, embryonal rhabdomyosarcoma has a variant, sarcoma botryoides, which is the most common malignant vaginal tumor in the pediatric population. Leiomyosarcoma is the most common sarcoma in adults.

Risk factors for vaginal cancer include the HPV, age (≥60 years), smoking, and a history of cervical and vulvar cancer. Intrauterine DES (a medication that was

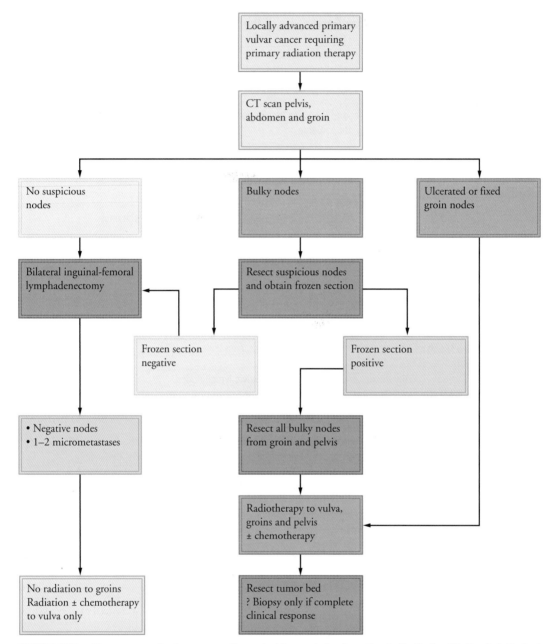

FIGURE 12.5. Management of vulvar cancer. (Reused with permission from Berek JS, Hacker NF. *Berek & Hacker's gynecologic oncology.* 5th ed. Philadelphia, PA: Lippincott Williams & Wilkins, 2010.)

last used more than three decades ago to prevent miscarriage) exposure is a risk factor for the clear-cell type.

Clinical Diagnosis
Symptoms

Precursor lesions and early stage primary vaginal cancers may be asymptomatic, but more advanced lesions can cause abnormal vaginal bleeding, pelvic pain, and urinary or bowel dysfunction.

Diagnosis

Advanced disease can be detected on pelvic examination. Tumors are usually located in the upper, posterior wall of the vagina. Abnormal cytology through

TABLE 12.12	Clinical Staging of Vaginal Carcinoma

Stage	Description
0	Carcinoma in situ
I	Carcinoma limited to the vaginal mucosa
II	Carcinoma involving the subvaginal tissue but not extending onto the pelvic wall.
III	Carcinoma extending onto the pelvic wall
IV	Carcinoma extending into the mucosa of the bladder or rectum or distant metastases

Source: Reused with Permission from Beckmann CRB, Ling FW, Smith RP, et al. *Obstetrics and gynecology*. 5th ed. Philadelphia, PA: Lippincott Williams & Wilkins, 2006.

the use of Pap smears can detect precursor lesions, vaginal epithelial neoplasia, and early stage disease. Directed biopsies during colposcopy can localize dysplastic areas and provide tissue for diagnosis.

Staging

Primary vaginal malignancies are clinically staged. FIGO staging system is listed in Table 12.12. To determine the extent of disease, it is important to perform a thorough pelvic and rectal examination, usually under anesthesia, cystoscopy, proctoscopy, intravenous pyelogram, and chest x-ray. Pelvic CT can also be used to evaluate inguinal and pelvic lymph node involvement and spread of local disease.

Management

Given the rarity of this malignancy, patients should be managed by specialists in the field of gynecologic oncology. Treatment should be individualized and will depend upon disease stage and site of vaginal involvement. The goal is to preserve a functional vagina for most women. Given the close proximity of the bladder and rectum, surgery can be very difficult and thus has limited utility in most cases. Radiation therapy, therefore, is the treatment modality of choice.

However, surgery can be considered in the following situations:

- *Stage I disease involving upper posterior vagina:* Radical hysterectomy, upper vaginectomy (at least 1-cm margin), and pelvic lymphadenectomy in patients with the uterus in situ. If the uterus was previously removed, radical upper vaginectomy and pelvic lymphadenectomy can be performed

- Ovarian transposition in young women prior to radiation therapy
- Primary pelvic exenteration for patients with stage IVA disease
- Pelvic exenteration for central recurrence after primary radiation therapy

Prognosis

A study of 193 patients from the MD Anderson Cancer Center in Houston reported 5-year survival rates of 85% for 50 patients with stage I disease, 78% for 97 patients with stage II, and 58% for 46 patients with stages III to IVA.

QUESTIONS

1. The diagnosis of ectopic pregnancy can usually be made with serial β-hCGs and transvaginal ultrasound.
2. The earliest sign of an intrauterine pregnancy on ultrasound is a gestational sac and can generally be seen by the time of the first missed menses.
3. The incidence of ectopic pregnancy has been decreasing over the past 30 years.
4. Medical management of an ectopic pregnancy is successful in approximately 90% of patients treated.
5. The diagnosis of pelvic inflammatory disease requires pelvic pain, cervical motion tenderness, and a fever.
6. Definitive diagnosis of ovarian torsion requires absence of flow on Doppler velocimetry.
7. The most common benign ovarian neoplasm is a dermoid cyst.
8. Three percent to 7% of fibroids will undergo malignant degeneration.
9. The proper positioning of the pregnant patient undergoing a surgical procedure is with slight left lateral displacement.
10. The hallmark symptoms of endometriosis are cyclic pelvic pain and infertility.
11. Ovarian cancer is the most common gynecologic malignancy.
12. Ovarian cancer is usually diagnosed at stage I or II.
13. Ovarian cancer is a silent killer and no symptoms are reliably associated with this disease.
14. Patients who are BRCA1 carriers have a 60-fold increased risk of developing ovarian cancer by age 60 when compared with the general population.

15. A benefit of prophylactic oophorectomy in BRCA-positive patients is a subsequent decrease in breast cancer by 50%.

16. The most common presenting symptom of endometrial cancer is postmenopausal bleeding.

17. Only 50% of patients with cervical cancer will test positive for HPV infection.

18. Vaccination with Gardasil in patients aged 9 to 26 years is recommended to help prevent HPV infection and the development of cervical cancer.

19. Melanomas are the most common nonsquamous cell malignancy of the vulva, accounting for 4% to 5% of cases.

SELECTED REFERENCES

American Cancer Society. *Cancer facts & figures, 2008.* Available at: www.cancer.org/downloads/STT/2008CAFFfinalsecured.pdf.

Barakat RR, Markman M, Randall ME. *Principles and practice of gynecologic oncology.* 5th ed. Philadelphia, PA: Lippincott Williams & Wilkins, 2009.

Beckmann CRB, Ling FW, Smith RP, et al. *Obstetrics and gynecology.* 5th ed. Philadelphia, PA: Lippincott Williams & Wilkins, 2006.

Berek JS. *Berek & Novak's gynecology.* 14th ed. Philadelphia, PA: Lippincott, Williams & Wilkins, 2007.

Berek JS, Hacker NF. *Berek & Hacker's gynecologic oncology.* 5th ed. Philadelphia, PA: Lippincott Williams & Wilkins, 2010.

Boyle KJ, Torrealday S. Benign gynecologic conditions [review]. *Surg Clin North Am* 2008;88(2):245–264, v.

Denny L, Hacker NF, Gori J, et al. FIGO committee on gynecologic oncology. Staging classifications and clinical practice guidelines for gynaecologic cancers. *Internat J Gynecol Obstet* 2000;70:207–312.

Diagnosis and treatment of cervical carcinomas. ACOG Practice Bulletin No. 35. American College of Obstetricians and Gynecologists. *Obstet Gynecol* 2002;99:855–867.

Elective and risk–reducing salpingo-oophorectomy. ACOG Practice Bulletin No. 89. American College of Obstetricians and Gynecologists. *Obstet Gynecol* 2008;111:231–241.

Lindor NM, Petersen GM, Hadley DW, et al. Recommendations for the care of individuals with an inherited predisposition to Lynch syndrome: a systematic review. *JAMA* 2006;296(12):1507–217.

Management of adnexal masses. ACOG practice bulletin no. 83. American College of Obstetricians and Gynecologists. *Obstet Gynecol* 2007;110:201–214.

McWilliams GD, Hill MJ, Dietrich CS III. Gynecologic emergencies [review]. *Surg Clin North Am* 2008;88(2):265–283, vi.

Medical management of ectopic pregnancy. ACOG practice bulletin no. 94. American College of Obstetricians and Gynecologists. *Obstet Gynecol* 2008;111:1479–1485.

Parangi S, Levine D, Henry A, et al. Surgical gastrointestinal disorders during pregnancy [review]. *Am J Surg* 2007;193(2):223–232.

Peipert JF, Ness RB, Blume J, et al. Clinical predictors of endometritis in women with symptoms and signs of pelvic inflammatory disease. *Am J Obstet Gynecol* 2001;184:856–864.

Rock JA, Jones HW III. *TeLinde's operative gynecology.* 10th ed. Philadelphia, PA: Lippincott Williams & Wilkins, 2003.

Speroff L, Fritz MA. *Clinical gynecologic endocrinology and infertility.* 7th ed. Philadelphia, PA: Lippincott Williams & Wilkins. 2005.

Stenchever MA, Droegemueller WD, Herbst AL, et al. *Comprehensive gynecology.* 4th ed. St. Louis, MO: Mosby, Inc., 2001.

The role of the generalist obstetrician–gynecologist in the early detection of ovarian cancer. ACOG committee opinion no. 280. American College of Obstetricians and Gynecologists. *Obstet Gynecol* 2002;100:1413–1416.

2007 State of the State of Gynecologic Cancers. *Fifth annual report of the women of America.* Available at: http://www.thegcf.org/whatsnew/Ovarian_Cancer_Symptoms_Consensus_Statement.pdf.

Updated recommended treatment regimens for gonococcal infections and associated conditions—United States, April 2007. Available at: http://www.cdc.gov/STD/treatment/2006/updated-regimens.htm.

Pediatric Surgery

The aim of this chapter is to acquaint the general surgeon with some of the key points regarding major problems in general pediatric surgery. For more detailed information, the interested reader can refer to one of several excellent textbooks of pediatric surgery.

CARE OF THE PEDIATRIC PATIENT

Monitoring

All infants and children who undergo general anesthesia need the following monitors.

1. Precordial or esophageal stethoscope
2. Blood pressure cuff, manual or automated (Dynamap, Infrasonde)
3. Electrocardiogram
4. Temperature probe
5. Pulse oximeter

Additional monitoring aids may be necessary in selected cases. These include an arterial line, central venous catheter, and urinary catheter. In rare situations (open heart surgery), a pulmonary artery catheter is useful.

Temperature

Infants' relatively large body surface area in proportion to their weight in combination with little subcutaneous fat render them highly susceptible to rapid loss of heat. This problem is magnified if the child is exposed to a usually cold operating room and undergoes surgery during which body cavities are opened. These manipulations result in heat loss through radiation, evaporation, and convection. To compensate for the heat loss, infants increase their metabolic rate, but a small baby or seriously ill child may not have the energy stores to increase its caloric output to maintain normothermia. The resulting hypothermia can cause respiratory and myocardial depression.

Therefore, all children who undergo surgery with anesthesia should have a temperature probe inserted and the core temperature monitored. Appropriate places to monitor are the rectum or the esophagus. Skin temperature should be monitored as well. Every effort should be made to reduce heat loss, including keeping the extremities and the head covered whenever possible. The operating room should be warmed, and the immediate area surrounding the patient can be heated with infrared heating lights, especially during induction of anesthesia and when lines and monitors are being placed. The child is placed on an appropriately controlled heating mattress; all anesthetic gases are heated, as are all intravenous fluids and blood products. Older children need to have their temperature monitored as well to alert the anesthesiologist to the onset of malignant hyperthermia.

Fluids

Infants have a resting metabolic rate approximately three times that of an adult, or about 100 kcal/kg/day. Their fluid needs therefore are correspondingly about three times that of the adult (Table 13.1).

In addition to the above, all ongoing losses such as nasogastric, ileostomy output, and severe diarrhea should be measured and replaced by the appropriate electrolyte-containing fluid. Adequacy of fluid replacement can be monitored by following urine output and specific gravity. Normal urine output in a child is approximately 0.5 to 1.0 mL/kg/hr. Newborns have immature renal tubules that are not able to concentrate the glomerular filtrate as thoroughly as those of older infants. Urine-specific gravity more than 1.015 therefore indicates that the kidney is

TABLE 13.1	Maintenance Fluid Needs in Infants
Weight (kg)	**Fluid Needs (mL/kg/day)**
1–10	100
11–20	50 (+1,000 mL)
21+	20 (+1,500 mL)

concentrating urine maximally and that fluid replacement should be increased. In addition to water needs, the infant has electrolyte and glucose requirements. Sodium and potassium maintenance is 2 to 3 mEq/kg/day. Neonatal glucose levels are lower than those of the older child, hypoglycemia being defined for this age group as a serum glucose of less than 30 mg/dL. The infant is dependent on the glycolysis of existing glycogen homeostasis. Stress such as surgery, sepsis, or trauma can rapidly deplete these stores, resulting in hypoglycemia with subsequent seizures and brain damage. Therefore, all infants should have blood glucose levels monitored. All intravenous solutions given to them should contain glucose. Premature or small-for-gestation-age (SGA) infants may require a continuous 10% glucose solution to maintain normoglycemia.

Calories

The surgeon caring for the infant or child is often faced with treating a patient whose gastrointestinal (GI) tract is unable to accept enough calories to maintain normal growth and development. Prolonged inadequate nutrition in the infant may have severe consequences. The immune system, already not well developed even in the normal, healthy young infant, is compromised further, and sepsis is more likely to occur with devastating results. Wound healing is impaired, which can lead to anastomotic leaks, disruption, and wound dehiscence. In addition, prolonged malnutrition may have adverse long-term effects on the brain, which is undergoing rapid development during the early months of life. Intravenous alimentation for a period exceeding 1 week should be started in any child in whom adequate enteral nutrition cannot be given. One can use either the peripheral or central route and infuse approximately 100 cal/kg/day. If the central route is to be used, a cuffed catheter is inserted percutaneously or via cutdown, so the tip of the catheter lies at the junction of the superior vena cava and right atrium. When intravenous alimentation is initiated, periodic determinations of serum glucose, electrolytes, calcium, and liver function are needed. Although most children do quite well on intravenous alimentation, even for prolonged periods, some problems do occur with this technique, the most common of which is liver dysfunction. Cessation of the alimentation usually reverses the complications if they are diagnosed early. There is some evidence that fish oil emulsions containing high levels of omega-3 fatty acids may prevent this complication.

SURGICALLY CORRECTABLE CAUSES OF RESPIRATORY DISTRESS

Choanal Atresia

Atresia of the nares is a rare anomaly occurring in approximately 1:60,000 live births. If not recognized promptly, choanal atresia may result in severe respiratory distress in the newborn. This condition results from a bony obstruction of the posterior nares behind the palate at the level of the sphenoid bone. Because the newborn is an obligatory nose-breather, the obstruction effectively blocks the upper airway. Diagnosis is based on the inability to pass a feeding tube through the nose into the pharynx. Further information can be obtained by instillation of a water-soluble contrast agent into the nose with the patient lying supine.

Initial treatment is aimed at providing a secure airway for neonates until they can breathe spontaneously through the mouth. In most cases, this can be accomplished by inserting an oral plastic airway, which is taped securely in place. In the interim, feeds are accomplished through a small feeding tube placed through the mouth. After several weeks most infants learn to breathe by mouth, and the airway can be removed and normal feeds started.

Definitive surgery for choanal atresias is usually postponed until the child is about 1 year old. Two approaches are used, each having its proponents: the transnasal and the transpalatal. The results in either case are usually highly satisfactory. Most children undergoing surgery to correct this condition lead a normal life without further problems. Newer modalities to repair choanal atresia including endoscopic procedures through either the nasal or retropalatal approach using lasers of microdebriders have been used with some success in even neonates and young infants.

Congenital Diaphragmatic Hernia

Congenital diaphragmatic hernia is one of the most common conditions causing respiratory distress in the newborn that is amenable to surgical correction. In most series, the reported incidence is approximately 1:4,000 live births. In the usual case, a hernia of variable size at the posterolateral foramen of Bochdalek, most commonly on the left, results in protrusion of the abdominal contents into the chest, thereby compressing the ipsilateral lung and causing a shift of the mediastinum to the right. Studies have shown that both the ipsilateral and contralateral lungs are affected, with a diminution in the number of alveoli. The pulmonary arterial vasculature is deficient as well, because its development parallels that of the airways. In addition, the pulmonary arteries have hypertrophic muscles in their media, making them highly sensitive to hypoxia, hypercarbia, and acidosis.

Although most infants with diaphragmatic hernia present shortly after birth and quickly experience severe respiratory distress needing ventilatory assistance, others become symptomatic only during the next 24 hours. A few infants who suffer from diaphragmatic hernia are just mildly symptomatic with occasional grunting and tachypnea, and the diagnosis may not be made for several weeks after birth. Many fetuses with diaphragmatic hernia are being diagnosed by means of ultrasonography. These babies are then delivered in a major medical center where expert neonatology and pediatric surgical services can expedite treatment. In utero repair of the hernia is feasible and has been done in more than 20 patients at one medical center; this technique is appropriate in selected fetuses with a large hernia or when the liver is herniated. In those cases, the lungs will become severely hypoplastic if the hernia is not repaired early. Another approach in treating large diaphragmatic hernias in fetuses is to occlude the fetal trachea with a balloon. This results in increased lung growth, improves lung compliance, and helps reduce the abdominal contents from the chest. The balloon is then removed when the fetus is close to term.

On physical examination, the infant with a congenital diaphragmatic hernia usually has a scaphoid abdomen. Auscultation reveals a heart that is displaced to the right and absent bowel sounds on the left. Peristaltic sounds are heard occasionally on the affected side. A chest radiograph reveals a left hemithorax filled with air-filled loops of bowel and a shift of the mediastinum to the right with compression of the right lung. Occasionally, cystic adenomatoid malformation mimics a diaphragmatic hernia; if any doubt exists, an upper GI series with barium can clarify the diagnosis. Once the hernia is diagnosed, a nasogastric tube in inserted and placed on suction to prevent gaseous distension of the bowel, which would further compromise the lung. If the infant is in respiratory distress, he or she should be intubated and placed on a respirator. Ventilation by mask in contraindicated.

An arterial catheter is inserted to determine the acid–base balance and the PO_2. Every effort is made to combat hypoxia and hypercarbia, as these conditions are potent stimuli for pulmonary vasoconstriction. It may necessitate placing the child on either a conventional or high-frequency respirator and starting inotropic support. If these modalities prove unsuccessful, there are several other options available, including the use of vasodilators, the most potent of which is tolazoline (Priscoline), or starting the infant on inhaled nitric oxide. The latter has been remarkably successful in reducing pulmonary hypertension and reversing persistent fetal circulation. Should these measures fail, the child is placed on extracorporeal membrane oxygenation (ECMO), a complex, labor-intensive technique available only in major medical centers. In most cases, venoarterial ECMO is used via the internal jugular vein and common carotid artery. ECMO reverses the acid–base and oxygen problems without subjecting the baby to severe barotrauma and allows the severe pulmonary vasoconstriction to reverse. Some centers operate on the infants while they are on ECMO. The more conservative approach is to wean the infant off ECMO and then operate. Almost all surgeons now believe that, in all cases, the baby should be stabilized for at least 48 hours after birth to allow for stabilization of the pulmonary vasculature before undertaking surgery. There is no need or place for emergency middle-of-the-night surgery in these babies.

Most surgeons use a transverse abdominal incision. The abdominal contents are removed from the chest, and any sac present is excised. The diaphragmatic defect is closed with interrupted nonabsorbable sutures. A chest tube may be left in the pleural space and connected to a water-seal apparatus; suction should not be used. No attempt is made to hyperinflate the hypoplastic lung. Some surgeons insert a chest tube in the contralateral pleural space prophylactically, as many infants are subject to pneumothoraces during the postoperative period when high ventilatory settings may be necessary. The viscera are inspected for atresias or other obstructions (e.g., Ladd's bands). If found, they are repaired. The abdominal contents are then returned to the peritoneal cavity, and the abdominal wall is closed in layers. Occasionally, this presents a difficult challenge, as the peritoneal cavity is often markedly underdeveloped because the bulk of the viscera were in the chest during fetal development. In such a case, a temporary Silastic chimney closure may be needed (see "Omphalocele and Gastroschisis," later). For most cases, however, layered closure of the abdominal wall is possible.

Removal of the abdominal contents from the chest and closure of the diaphragm results in marked improvement of the respiratory condition in most children. Some have a transient improvement in their condition, the so-called honeymoon period, and then begin to deteriorate. In most of these cases, the lung volume is adequate for survival, but a progressive right-to-left shunt due to pulmonary vasoconstriction is occurring. If therapy with vasodilators and conventional ventilators fails, infants are started on inhaled nitric oxide; should that fail, they are placed on ECMO.

Survival of infants with congenital diaphragmatic hernia who are symptomatic during the first 12 hours of life has improved somewhat with the advent of ECMO. Some centers are reporting an almost 80%

survival rate, but some of these children have severely compromised lung function and may well need lung transplantation as they get older. Infants who need ECMO have about a 50% survival rate. Reduced-size transplants using lobes have been performed in a number of centers with encouraging results. Another new technology being evaluated and undergoing clinical trials is perfluorocarbon ventilation. These new agents produce little toxicity and have been shown to reduce lung pathology and improve gas exchange. They may have an important role to play in the treatment of congenital diaphragmatic hernia (1).

Tracheoesophageal Fistula

Anomalies that occur during development of the trachea and esophagus are common causes of respiratory problems in neonates. The types most commonly found are atresias of the esophagus, often associated with a fistula between the esophagus and the trachea. Several anatomic variants are extant (Fig. 13.1).

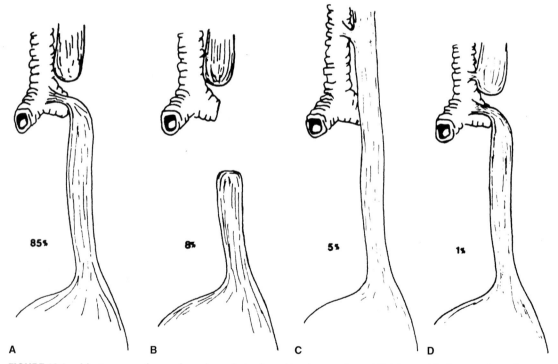

85%   **8%**   **5%**   **1%**

A   **B**   **C**   **D**

FIGURE 13.1.   Most common forms of esophageal atresia and tracheoesophageal fistulas and their percentage of occurrence. **A:** Proximal esophageal atresia with a fistula between the distal esophagus and the trachea, present in 85% of all cases. **B:** Isolated esophageal atresia without a fistula, present in 8% of all cases. **C:** H-type tracheoesophageal fistula without esophageal atresia, found in 5% of cases. **D:** Esophageal atresia with fistulas between the upper and lower esophageal pouches; occurs in 1% of all cases.

Signs and Symptoms

There may be a history of maternal polyhydramnios. Ultrasonography during the third trimester of pregnancy may reveal a dilated upper esophagus in the fetus, making the diagnosis highly likely. The infant usually presents in the newborn nursery as a "mucousy" baby needing frequent oral suction; a choking or cyanotic spell may occur when the baby is first fed. An attempt to place a nasogastric tube is unsuccessful because the tube meets resistance in the midthorax. Physical examination of the baby may reveal an SGA neonate. The abdomen may be scaphoid if an isolated atresia is present or distended if there is a large fistula between the esophagus and trachea. About 10% of these infants have an imperforate anus. Other conditions found in association with tracheoesophageal fistula are congenital heart disease, Down syndrome, and renal anomalies.

The diagnosis can be confirmed by radiography with a radiopaque nasogastric tube left in place as far as it will advance. The catheter typically stops at the level of the fifth interspace. The proximal esophagus may be seen as a slightly dilated air-filled pouch. If a fistula is present between the trachea and the esophagus, air is present in the stomach and bowel. Isolated atresia without fistula is seen as a gasless abdomen. Additional findings that may be noted on radiographs are vertebral anomalies, a pulmonary infiltrate, or an abnormally shaped heart shadow. If the clinical picture is still unclear, 0.5 mL of liquid barium can be instilled in the nasogastric tube, the radiograph obtained, and the barium quickly aspirated back. Under no circumstances should water-soluble contrast be used. In the most common form of esophageal atresia, the blind upper esophageal pouch is clearly delineated. In rare situations, a fistula is found between the upper esophagus and the trachea. Babies with an H-type fistula present later in life (several months old) with recurrent pneumonia.

Treatment

Once the diagnosis has been established, the child is moved to an intensive care unit with the head elevated. The pharynx and proximal pouch are kept empty of secretions by placing a Replogle tube in the upper pouch and maintaining it on continuous suction. Administration of broad-spectrum antibiotics is begun. If there are no contraindications, definitive surgery is performed.

An extrapleural approach is used through a right thoracotomy. The tracheoesophageal fistula is divided, and an end-to-end esophagoesophagostomy is performed. Many surgeons add a feeding gastrostomy during the same operation to enable early postoperative enteral feeding, bypassing the anastomosis. Definitive surgery is deferred if the child's condition does not permit such a major procedure (i.e., prematurity, pneumonia, or severe congenital heart disease). In such cases, a feeding gastrostomy can be performed even under local anesthesia if necessary to prevent aspiration of highly acidic gastric contents into the trachea until the fistula can be closed. The fistula is closed at a later time through a thoracotomy. The child can then be fed and his or her condition stabilized until esophageal continuity can be established.

In some instances, especially in cases of pure esophageal atresia, the long gap between the upper and lower esophageal pouches makes primary repair difficult. Additional length on the upper pouch can be obtained by performing one or more circular myotomies on the upper pouch. Other options include extracorporeal traction with a repair done approximately 10 days to 2 weeks later, once the two ends of the esophagus have come together. If the distance cannot be bridged, one can perform a cervical esophagostomy (spit fistula) as a first stage repair and then a gastric, jejunal, or colon interposition when the child reaches the age of about 1 year.

Complications following repair of esophageal atresia are relatively common: leaks, strictures, disruptions, and recurrent fistula. They usually result from performing the anastomosis under tension. Most small leaks seal spontaneously. Strictures are usually managed by repeated dilatations. Recurring strictures may indicate that the baby has significant gastroesophageal reflux, a condition that occurs in up to 30% of these infants. Gastroesophageal reflux is often difficult to treat by medical means only and may require an antireflux operation (Nissen fundoplication). In otherwise normal full-term infants, the survival rate with tracheoesophageal fistula and esophageal atresia is 80%. The long-term prognosis for these children is excellent. The keys to good results are early recognition of the condition and intensive care during the perioperative period.

GASTROINTESTINAL TRACT OBSTRUCTION

Infantile Hypertrophic Pyloric Stenosis

Pyloric stenosis is a common condition, with an incidence of about 1:900 live births in the white population and 1:2,000 live births in the black population. Its etiology is unknown. It is not a congenital lesion and is rare during the first week of life. Male infants with pyloric stenosis outnumber female infants, 4:1, and the firstborn boy is the most common infant stricken. Some hereditary factors have been noted; infants of mothers who have had pyloric stenosis as infants are more likely to develop the condition. The pathophysiology is unknown. When examined histologically, the pyloric muscle is hypertrophic and edematous. Some believe that the triggering mechanism is an allergic response to milk curd proteins hitting a spastic pylorus.

Other theories include a redundant pyloric mucosa and decreased levels of nitric oxide synthase.

Signs and Symptoms

These otherwise healthy infants usually present at about 4 to 6 weeks of age with increasingly frequent vomiting of undigested formula shortly after feeds. The vomiting intensifies over the course of several days to several weeks, becoming more projectile and causing the infant to lose weight. Careful examination of the conjunctiva may show evidence of mild jaundice. Peristaltic waves may be seen crossing the upper abdomen. The careful examiner can feel an olive-shaped mass in the upper abdomen in about 85% of all cases. Finding this mass is pathognomonic of pyloric stenosis and constitutes sufficient evidence to warrant surgery. In infants where careful examination has failed to reveal the pyloric tumor, a barium swallow is done carefully with the physician looking for the characteristic elongated, markedly narrowed pyloric channel. Ultrasonography has proved accurate for delineating the dimensions of the thickness and length of the pylorus and is useful in infants in whom the olive is not felt on physical examination. Infants with prolonged vomiting have a hypokalemic, hypochloremic, metabolic alkalosis; a certain percentage of infants are jaundiced with elevated indirect bilirubin. The latter is probably caused by a deficiency in hepatic glucuronyl transferase.

Treatment

After fluid and electrolyte deficits have been appropriately corrected, a pyloromyotomy is performed using the Ramstedt technique. The traditional approach has been through a right upper quadrant verse incision. Newer techniques used are: a curved supraumbilical incision leaving a virtually unnoticeable scar and laparoscopic pyloromyotomy. Any of these techniques work well and result in a low morbidity and essentially no mortality. Fluids are slowly resumed about 12 hours after surgery and are gradually increased in strength

and volume. Most infants can be discharged 2 to 3 days after surgery. Some vomiting during the postoperative period is common, but it settles down once the stomach regains normal tone. Complications, which are rare, include perforation of the mucosa, usually at the duodenal end of the pyloric tumor, and incomplete pyloromyotomy resulting in persistent postoperative vomiting. The prognosis for children with pyloric stenosis is extremely good, and they should lead normal lives.

Duodenal Obstruction

Obstruction of the duodenum occurs once in about 5,000 live births. The obstruction can be total, which is termed an atresia, or the lumen may be patent but markedly constricted, resulting in a stenosis. Most of the obstructions occur at the second portion of the duodenum, usually distal to the ampulla of Vater. A duodenal obstruction occasionally seen is annular pancreas, in which the duodenum is circumferentially surrounded by pancreatic tissue. An intrinsic atresia or stenosis is common with this condition.

Signs and Symptoms

In some cases, the diagnosis is suspected antepartum if the mother is noted to have polyhydramnios. The condition can be confirmed by means of ultrasonography. The neonate usually presents during the first day of life with vomiting, most often bilious, as the usual obstruction is distal to the ampulla. There is usually little abdominal distension because the distal bowel is completely collapsed. The neonate may have normal stools even if the duodenum is atretic.

Physical examination is usually not helpful. One should check for the stigmata of Down syndrome, as about one-third of all neonates with duodenal obstruction are found to have this chromosomal abnormality. Other anomalies found occasionally are esophageal atresia and imperforate anus.

The diagnosis is simple to establish. Plain films of the abdomen reveal the classic "double bubble" sign (i.e., gas-filled distended stomach and proximal duodenum). There is no reason to use a contrast agent unless the plain films are inconclusive, as occurs in some cases of duodenal stenosis.

If surgery is delayed (for evaluation of a murmur, possible Down syndrome), a contrast x-ray study is performed to eliminate the possibility that the baby does not have a midgut volvulus, a life-threatening condition that can present as a double bubble much like duodenal atresia.

Treatment

The child is positioned with the head elevated and the stomach is decompressed using an appropriately sized nasogastric tube. Dehydration is corrected with intravenous fluids. Supplemental fluids may be needed to compensate for ongoing nasogastric losses. Because the stomach can be effectively decompressed with a nasogastric tube, there is no reason to perform emergency surgery. If one strongly suspects a chromosomal abnormality, the infant can be maintained on this regimen until chromosomal studies are carried out and the parents are informed of the diagnosis with certainty.

Operation is performed as soon as the child's condition is stable and the appropriate facilities are ready. Two operations are commonly used: duodenoduodenostomy and duodenojejunostomy. They are both side-to-side anastomoses that bring together the proximal dilated duodenum and the small intestine beyond the obstruction. One should not dissect the duodenum excessively, because inadvertent damage to the common duct may result. If possible, one should avoid performing a gastrojejunostomy in a newborn because it carries with it the well-known risk of future ulcer development. Many pediatric surgeons add a Stamm-type gastrostomy to the operation to help keep the stomach empty during the first few days until the anastomosis is patent and the child is able to tolerate oral feeds. A formula containing small curds such as Nutramigen may help speed oral feeding. Some vomiting may occur for up to 2 weeks postoperatively, but it should settle down as the stomach regains normal tone and edema resolves. If there are no other serious anomalies, the prognosis is excellent, and the infant should lead a normal life.

Intestinal Atresia

Atresias of the jejunum and ileum occur commonly. Relative to the length of the ileum, atresias are much more common there than in the jejunum. Their pathogenesis has been worked out quite well by Louw and Bernard, who showed that subjecting fetal puppies to intrauterine selective mesenteric arterial ligation results in atresia of that segment of the bowel supplied by the corresponding arterial branch. It is believed that a large percentage of intestinal atresias result from intrauterine vascular accidents to the mesenteric vasculature. Several types of atresia are found, ranging from an atretic segment that may involve just the mucosa, with an intact seromuscular coat, to a more common type where there is loss of continuity of an entire segment of bowel, often with an associated gap in the intervening mesentery. A rarer type is a proximal atresia with a markedly shortened bowel and mesentery, the so-called apple-peel atresia, with a precarious arterial blood supply arising from distal branches of the superior mesenteric artery.

Signs and Symptoms

The signs and symptoms depend to a great extent on the site of the atresia. Many of the mothers have not had polyhydramnios, which is only found in about one-fourth of cases. Bilious vomiting is common, occurring in about 85% of all cases of jejunal atresia. The more distal the atresia, the more pronounced is the abdominal distension. Infants with more proximal atresia vomit earlier than those with more distal atresia and may pass normal meconium. Physical examination usually shows a distended abdomen. Otherwise the examination may be completely normal. Other anomalies are relatively uncommon.

Plain films of the abdomen show distended gas- and fluid-filled loops of small bowel with air–fluid levels on the upright view. In the newborn, it is difficult to differentiate between small and large bowel on plain films. Therefore, to be sure that the loops seen on plain films are those of small bowel, one should perform a barium enema. The enema shows a small, unused colon (microcolon), confirming the presence of small bowel obstruction.

Treatment

Once the diagnosis has been established, a nasogastric tube is passed and connected to suction; fluid and electrolyte losses are corrected. When the infant's condition has stabilized, surgery is performed expeditiously. It is important to remember than it is virtually impossible to decompress the distal small bowel adequately with a nasogastric tube. Therefore, any unnecessary delay in surgical decompression may result in necrosis of the intestine.

At surgery, the entire intestinal tract is explored to make sure that no other atresias or stenoses are present. The bulbous dilated end of the atretic bowel is resected, and an end to end or end to side in anastomosis is performed; any mesenteric defect found is closed. Before completing the anastomosis, the surgeon inserts a catheter into the distal bowel and injects saline to be sure that there is no distal atresia.

Once the postoperative ileus is resolved, feeds are begun slowly. If a major section of bowel is missing, or if the ileocecal valve has been sacrificed, a short-gut syndrome may be encountered, in which case it may take several weeks to several months for the residual intestine to adapt. Parenteral nutrition or, in less extreme cases, predigested formulas such as Alimentum may be necessary.

Malrotation

During embryonic life, the intestinal tract elongates rapidly and undergoes a complex rotational process that, among other things, accounts for the small bowel mesentery being diagonally based, running from the ligament of Treitz in the left upper quadrant to the cecum in the right lower quadrant. This broad base allows the small intestine enough motility for normal peristalsis while preventing it from twisting to the point where it compromises its blood supply. Abnormalities in this rotational process are not uncommon and may lead to several entities, by far the most common of which is midgut volvulus. In this condition, the entire midgut from the duodenum to the midtransverse colon is suspended from a narrow pedicle, rendering it unstable and subject to twisting. During the course of normal peristalsis, the intestine rotates on its pedicle, thereby compromising its blood supply. If the condition is not recognized quickly, the bowel infarcts, leaving the baby totally dependent on parenteral nutrition unless he or she is given a bowel transplant.

Signs and Symptoms

The most common symptom is bilious vomiting in a previously well infant. Most of these infants are about 1 month old or younger, but children (or for that matter even adults) of any age can be affected. Because the obstruction occurs in the third portion of the duodenum, abdominal distension need not be present. Guaiac-positive nasogastric aspirates or stools may or may not be present. Some infants quickly go into shock if gangrenous bowel is present.

If one suspects midgut volvulus (i.e., bilious vomiting by an infant), the diagnosis must be confirmed or ruled out expeditiously because bowel viability is at stake. A plain abdominal radiograph is not usually helpful, especially at an early stage. The most direct approach to the diagnosis of this condition is by an upper GI series. Barium flows into the proximal duodenum, and the flow is cut off in a bird's beak shape at the twist of the midgut. Even if there is no obstruction to flow (i.e., a midgut volvulus), if the duodenum does not have its characteristic C shape with a ligament of Treitz in the left upper quadrant, the baby has

intestinal malrotation. The infant should be prepared for immediate surgery. An upper GI series is much more definitive than a barium enema, since the latter examination only defines the position of the cecum away from its normal location in the right lower quadrant, suggesting malrotation and possible volvulus.

Treatment

An upper transverse abdominal incision is used. The first thing one usually sees is small bowel with the transverse colon lying posteriorly. The entire bowel is delivered into the incision and the volvulus derotated, usually in a counterclockwise direction. Several turns may be necessary to obtain complete derotation. Only obviously necrotic bowel is resected; marginally viable bowel is left in situ unless it is only a small segment. In all cases where marginally viable bowel is left in place, a second-look operation is planned for 24 hours later. One next divides all peritoneal bands running across the duodenum to the right parietal peritoneum, the so-called Ladd bands. All kinks in the duodenum must be straightened. In some cases, there is an intrinsic stenosis of the duodenum, and it should be dealt with in the usual manner. The pedicle of the small bowel mesentery is splayed out so the duodenum lies in a straight, vertical line to the right of the vertebral column and the ascending colon on the left. Every effort is made to make the root of the mesentery as wide as possible to prevent recurrence of the volvulus.

Because the procedure results in the cecum coming to rest in the left abdomen, an appendectomy is performed. Most surgeons do not fixate the bowel to itself or to the abdominal wall, pointing out that such procedures are not necessary, as recurrence of volvulus is rare. Others disagree and advocate that the distal small bowel be sutured to the left colon, thereby ensuring that the root of the mesentery remains broad based.

Once the postoperative ileus has resolved, the infant is begun on progressive feeds. Unless a large percentage of the small bowel has been removed, the prognosis should be excellent. Fortunately, as mentioned earlier, recurrence of this condition is rare.

Meconium Ileus

Meconium ileus is an entity in which the neonate's meconium becomes inspissated in the ileum, causing an obturator-type obstruction. The cause for this condition usually is pancreatic insufficiency secondary to mucoviscidosis or cystic fibrosis. Two forms of the disease are recognized: simple meconium ileus, occurring in about two-thirds of patients, and complicated meconium ileus, occurring in the remaining one-third. Infants with simple meconium ileus show signs of intestinal obstruction during the first 2 days of life: abdominal distension, bilious vomiting, and absence of meconium stools. Rubbery, dilated loops of bowel are often seen and palpated. The anus may appear stenotic, and examination may reveal a tight rectum with only a small amount of sticky meconium present. Plain abdominal radiographs show dilated loops of bowel without air–fluid levels because the inspissated meconium is too viscous to layer out. Instead, a ground-glass appearance may be noted, representing gas and meconium in the ileum.

Complicated meconium ileus represents the complications of the disease: volvulus, atresias, perforations, peritonitis, and pseudocysts. These infants are much sicker, presenting with symptoms shortly after birth. Abdominal distension is marked, and the abdominal wall is often edematous and erythematous. A mass is found occasionally. Abdominal radiographs may show free air, a large mass, calcifications, or a large, formless intestinal loop representing a gangrenous loop of small bowel.

Diagnosis

Treatments for simple and complicated meconium ileus differ greatly, so it is of utmost importance to diagnose the infant's condition as quickly as possible. If the infant's condition suggests simple meconium ileus, a barium enema is performed. The colon appears small (microcolon), as little or no meconium has passed into it during fetal life. Some pellets of inspissated mucus may be seen. Refluxing the barium through the ileocecal valve reveals inspissated meconium in the ileum, confirming the diagnosis. The enema helps differentiate meconium ileus from the other entities that present in similar fashion, such as Hirschsprung disease, ileal or jejunal atresia, meconium plug syndrome, and hypoplastic left colon syndrome.

Treatment

Simple Meconium Ileus

Helen Noblett, an Australian pediatric surgeon, introduced a method for nonoperative decompression of the small intestine by means of a hyperosmotic radiopaque enema. This technique has dramatically decreased the mortality of this condition.

The infant is started on intravenous fluids until good urine output is obtained and parenteral antibiotics are begun. The stomach is decompressed with a nasogastric tube. The agent used, meglumine diatrizoate (Gastrografin), is extremely hypertonic, having an osmolarity of 1,900 mOsm/L. When given as an enema, the sudden increase in intraluminal osmolarity draws water into the intestine at the expense of the intravascular volume. It is therefore of critical importance to carefully monitor the infant's vital signs, hematocrit, serum electrolytes, and osmolarity during and after the enema. The influx of fluid within the small intestine loosens inspissated meconium and thereby relieves the obstruction.

The enema is usually followed by passage of liquid meconium and gas over several hours. Abdominal distension should decrease as the obstruction is relieved. If no relief is obtained, a second enema may be performed. The risk of perforation increases with repeated enemas, and so they should be done only by experienced pediatric radiologists. If, despite a technically successful enema, the obstruction is not relieved, the intestines must be decompressed surgically.

If the Gastrografin enema has been successful, infants are started on acetylcysteine (Mucomyst) via nasogastric tube, and once they are able to tolerate a diet, they are placed on pancreatic enzyme supplementation and on formulas containing medium-chain triglycerides such as Portagen. A sweat test is performed to the infant to confirm the diagnosis. Because the condition is hereditary, being passed on by an autosomal recessive gene, the parents are given genetic counseling because the chances of a subsequent child having cystic fibrosis are 1:4.

Complicated Meconium Ileus

Children with complicated meconium ileus are often critically ill, being septic, hypovolemic and acidotic, and in shock. The intense abdominal distension may interfere with diaphragmatic movement and may cause respiratory embarrassment. Several hours of intensive care is needed to stabilize these infants, restore the circulating blood volume, and combat the acidosis. Broad-spectrum antibiotics are begun, and a nasogastric tube is inserted. If need be, these children are intubated and placed on a respirator. They are then taken to the operating room, and the abdomen is explored. Sites of obstruction, perforation, or necrosis are identified, and all obviously nonviable bowel is removed.

Atresias, sometimes multiple, may be found and should be repaired in end-to-end fashion. If an obstruction of the ileum is present, an enterotomy is performed over the most dilated loop and the contained meconium evacuated. A 4% solution of acetylcysteine is flushed into the obstructed bowel to help free the highly tenacious meconium from the mucosa. This procedure may have to be repeated until the obstruction is relieved. There are several options for the management of the opened bowel. Most surgeons favor bringing out the bowel as an enterotomy until bowel function returns to normal. Equally good results are obtained by a double-barreled ileostomy or by an end-to-side enterostomy of the Bishop-Koop or Santulli types. Once GI function has recovered, the infant is started on pancreatic enzymes given by mouth to enhance absorption. Medium-chain triglyceride-containing formulas are more easily tolerated by these infants and are the preferred choice. GI tract continuity should be restored only after the infant is making steady weight gain and has a well-adjusted caloric intake.

These children have a lifelong tendency to manifest GI problems, including meconium ileus equivalent, intussusception, and rectal prolapse as well as cirrhosis and portal hypertension. Although the prognosis of these children is guarded in view of the systemic nature of the underlying disease and its serious consequences, aggressive medical and surgical management has made marked advances in prolonging their lives so that middle-age adults with cystic fibrosis are now alive.

INTUSSUSCEPTION

Unlike most of the other conditions discussed earlier, intussusception rarely affect infants during the first month of life; this age group accounts for only 0.3% of all cases. The peak incidence in several large series was at 7 to 8 months of life, with the incidence dropping off rapidly after 1 year of age. Intussusception is the invagination of a portion of intestine into itself. The portion by far most commonly affected is the ileum, which is intussuscepted into the ascending colon. On occasion, the intussusception extends all the way to the rectum.

Signs and Symptoms

The classic case involves a child who is usually well, perhaps having had a viral-like condition 1 or 2 weeks prior, and is awakened from sleep with sudden severe abdominal pain causing him or her to cry and draw up the legs. The bout may last a few minutes and then stop. These attacks are almost always accompanied by vomiting, and most infants pass normal stools either during or shortly after the attack. Following the attack, the infant becomes well, taking feeds until another attack begins. These attacks then occur at more frequent intervals, with the stools becoming mixed with blood, so-called current jelly stools. If the attacks are allowed to continue, the infant becomes lethargic and dehydrated, and abdominal girth begins to increase.

On examination early in the course of the condition, the child may look well and have a soft, nontender abdomen without evidence of peritonitis. A mass can be palpated in more than 85% of cases. The mass is usually in the right side of the abdomen, although on occasion, it is present on the left side as well. It is usually sausage shaped. In cases of very long intussusception, a rectal mass can be palpated. There are reports of intussusception being mistaken for rectal prolapse. It is important to emphasize that early in the course of intussusception, the child has a soft, nontender abdomen. An acute abdomen manifests in cases where intestinal necrosis has already occurred. Low-grade fever is not uncommon and is most often found in the young infant.

Laboratory examinations are not helpful early in the course of the condition. A plain abdominal radiograph sometimes suggests a mass in the right lower quadrant. Other suggestive findings on radiography are absence of gas in the transverse colon, absence of stool in the left colon, and signs of small bowel obstruction. The mainstay of diagnosis is the history; if the history is suggestive of the condition, one should go ahead with further diagnostic maneuvers regardless of what the radiograph shows.

The child is started on intravenous fluids, and if there are signs of small bowel obstruction, a nasogastric tube is inserted to decompress the stomach. Appropriate blood samples are obtained, including one for typing and one to hold. The pediatric surgeon is notified, who then contacts the operating room so that no unnecessary delay is encountered should the child need emergency surgery.

Diagnosis and Treatment

Since it was introduced in the United States by Ravitch in 1947, the barium enema has been the main diagnostic and usual therapeutic modality for children with uncomplicated intussusception (i.e., in whom there is no obvious peritonitis). More and more pediatric centers are now using other modalities for diagnosis and treatment. A more modern approach for suspected intussusception is abdominal ultrasonography, looking for the characteristic doughnut sign. A positive ultrasound scan is then followed by hydrostatic reduction using an air enema performed under fluoroscopic control using pressures of 80 to 110 mm Hg. The air enema is less expensive than the traditional barium enema and is associated with fewer complications should perforation occur. This technique has become the standard and has replaced the barium enema. If barium is used then, the guidelines set forth by Ravitch and McCune in their classic study on the subject (2) should be closely followed to avoid bowel perforation. The enema can or bag should be raised no more than 3.5 feet above the child's abdomen, and the abdomen is not manipulated in any way whatsoever. The enema is stopped if there is no advance of the column of barium after 10 minutes. One must be sure that there is reflux of barium into the distal ileum before being confident that the intussusception has been completely reduced. In most reported series, the intussusception was reduced about 75% of the time by hydrostatic means alone. Once the reduction is accomplished, the child is kept in the hospital overnight, as a small percentage of cases tend to recur during the first 12 hours following reduction.

Infants for whom hydrostatic reduction is unsuccessful are taken to the operating room for operative reduction. A right transverse abdominal incision is made, and the intussusception is identified. The bowel just distal to the intussusception is compressed, driving the intussuscepted bowel proximally. The proximal bowel should not be pulled on because it invariably leads to a tear and spillage of intestinal contents. Failure of reduction often indicates the presence of gangrene, usually at the lead point, in which case a limited resection and primary anastomosis is performed with care to minimize spillage. Most surgeons recommend performing an appendectomy at the time of operative reduction.

The older the child, the more likely it is that an anatomic lead point will be found. Among the conditions causing intussusception are Meckel diverticulum, intestinal lymphoma, cystic fibrosis, polyps, and intramural bleeds as found in Henoch-Schönlein purpura. Older children (those older than 4 years) should have a workup for these conditions even if the barium enema was successful. The mortality for intussusception should be minimal. Prompt diagnosis of the condition enables most of these children to undergo successful hydrostatic reduction, obviating the need for surgery.

HIRSCHSPRUNG DISEASE

Hirschsprung disease is a congenital megacolon caused by the absence of ganglia within the mesenteric and submucosal plexi of the distal large bowel. The zone of aganglionosis is just proximal to the dentate line and extends for a variable distance proximally. Most cases involve the rectosigmoid only. Total colonic aganglionosis, however, is by no means rare, representing about 15% of the cases. Aganglionosis extending up to the jejunum, and even more proximally, has been reported. Most of the involved infants are full term and otherwise healthy. The most common associated anomaly is Down syndrome. Some evidence suggests that a hereditary factor is involved. The incidence reported is approximately 1:10,000 live births, depending on the series studied. The usual rectosigmoid Hirschsprung disease is three to five times more common in male infants than in female infants.

Signs and Symptoms

The most common presenting symptom is an abnormality in the passage of meconium, usually delayed passage. Ninety percent of healthy full-term infants pass their first meconium within the first 24 hours of life. More than 95% have passed meconium by day 2. Some infants with Hirschsprung disease pass a small, hard piece of meconium and then nothing else, except following rectal stimulation.

Other signs and symptoms seen are those of intestinal obstruction (i.e., vomiting, often bile-stained, and abdominal distension). Rectal examination in the typical case of Hirschsprung disease may be helpful in making the diagnosis. Typically, the distal rectum is narrow and empty, and the proximal rectum or rectosigmoid is dilated and stool-filled. Upon withdrawal of the examining finger, an explosive evacuation of stool and gas takes place, often resulting in decompression of the distended abdomen.

A plain abdominal radiograph shows distended air- and fluid-filled loops of bowel. In the neonate, it is impossible to distinguish between large and small bowel on plain films. Because unrelieved large bowel obstruction can be quickly followed by enterocolitis, which is associated with significant morbidity and mortality, it is of utmost importance to make the diagnosis expeditiously. The first examination usually performed is a barium enema. Again, the barium enema should be the infant's first enema. It is totally inappropriate to perform saline enemas in the neonate without having first done a carefully performed barium enema. A plain catheter is introduced into the rectum just above the internal sphincter, and barium is injected slowly by means of a syringe under the guidance of image intensification and fluoroscopy. In older infants, one should see a dilated proximal colon that tapers down to a cone-shaped transitional zone representing the beginning of the aganglionosis. The distal aganglionic bowel is narrow and does not contract. One frequently sees an area of saw-toothing and spasticity in the bowel just proximal to the transitional zone. This may be seen even in the neonate. In normal infants, the barium is usually evacuated within 24 hours. Barium retained beyond this period is suggestive of Hirschsprung disease.

In the neonate, where the barium enema may not be diagnostic of Hirschsprung disease, a rectal biopsy is done. (One may dispense with this procedure in the older child with a classic history, examination, and barium enema.) The biopsy may be done at the bedside using a suction apparatus. Because there is normally a narrow zone of aganglionosis just proximal to the dentate line, the biopsy is performed at least 1.5 cm above the dentate line. This type of biopsy is deep enough only to obtain submucosa. The fresh specimen is stained for cholinesterase activity. A positive biopsy demonstrates increased uptake of the stain in the hypertrophic nerve fibers present, confirming the diagnosis of Hirschsprung disease. If the pathologist is unable to make the diagnosis, a full-thickness biopsy of the rectal wall is performed under general anesthesia. In the older infant (older than 2 weeks), Hirschsprung disease can be diagnosed using anorectal manometry. In the normal individual, distension of the proximal rectum results in relaxation of the internal sphincter. This reflex is mediated by the intramural ganglia. In Hirschsprung disease, no such relaxation occurs. The test is not accurate in infants younger than 12 days and therefore cannot be relied on to make the diagnosis.

Treatment

Some pediatric surgeons favor performing a decompressing colostomy when Hirschsprung disease is diagnosed. It can be either a transverse colostomy or

a sigmoid colostomy just above the area of aganglionosis. A piece of colonic wall is sent to the pathologist at the time of colostomy to be sure that ganglia are present. At this time, one may perform multiple seromuscular biopsies to determine the level of aganglionosis (the so-called leveling colostomy), thereby helping and guiding the surgeon for the next stage. Between ages 6 months and 1 year, an elective pull-through operation can be performed. The most widely used procedure today is the endorectal pull-through operation as modified by Cilley et al. (3). The procedure involves resecting the aganglionic bowel segment, performing a rectal mucosectomy to just above the dentate line, bringing normally innervated intestine through the seromuscular cuff created, and performing an end-to-end anastomosis 1.5 cm above the dentate line. The procedure gives a highly satisfactory result with minimal morbidity.

If hirschsprung disease (HD) is diagnosed in a timely fashion in the newborn before the colon has become distended, most surgeons will perform a one stage pull-through operation before the infant is discharged. This will eliminate the need for colostomy and decrease the risk of enterocolitis. The pull-through can be performed using the open or laparoscopic approach depending on the surgeon's degree of expertise in performing advanced laparoscopy.

This traditional approach, which requires three separate operations, has been modified by many pediatric surgeons in recent years to eliminate the need for multiple operations. A number of centers are now advocating performing a primary pull-through operation without colostomy in otherwise healthy neonates who are stable and can be decompressed with enemas prior to surgery (4). A number of surgeons have reported performing the pull-through procedure using laparoscopic techniques, obviating the need for an extensive laparotomy (5). If the aganglionosis is limited to the rectosigmoid, another option is to perform a transanal pull-through without any abdominal component.

IMPERFORATE ANUS

Even though one would think that infants with imperforate anus would be diagnosed immediately after birth, there are numerous instances of the diagnosis being delayed for 1 to 2 days. The incidence of imperforate anus is about 1:5,000 births. There are several manifestations of the condition, and the operative correction of the condition depends on the type found.

Types of Imperforate Anus

Anal Stenosis

Anal stenosis is similar in female and male infants. The rectum has descended in normal position, but the anal canal is stenotic. The diagnosis is easy, and treatment is straightforward. A simple anoplasty is performed during the neonatal period, and the results are generally good. As with all other deformities of the anus and rectum, there may be associated anomalies within the urologic, cardiac, or skeletal system. A screening workup is therefore done before these children are discharged, including radiographs of the sacrum and ultrasonography of the kidneys and heart.

Membranous Imperforate Anus

In membranous imperforate anus, the embryonic membrane covering the anus has not disappeared. On examination, the anal dimple appears normal, but the lumen of the anus is covered by a thin membrane. Often meconium is seen bulging underneath the membrane. Treatment is straightforward and involves incising the membrane. This condition is similar in female and male infants. The usual screening workup is done before discharge.

Rectal Agenesis

The next two types of imperforate anus are low (infralevator) rectal agenesis and high (supralevator) rectal agenesis. The anatomy of these two conditions is different in male and female infants, so each sex is discussed separately.

Low Imperforate Anus

Male Infants. Examination of the perineum reveals no orifice. An anal dimple may be seen, or, in some cases, heaped-up tissue at the site of the normal anus. Stimulation of the area may result in the normal anal wink reflex. The external genitalia are usually normal. With these low lesions, there is usually no communication between the rectum and the urinary system, so the examination of the urine is normal, not showing the presence of meconium (Fig. 13.2).

Female Infants. The term "low imperforate anus" in these children is a misnomer. The rectum does have an opening, but it is ectopic, usually anterior at the fourchette. Careful examination of the vulvar area

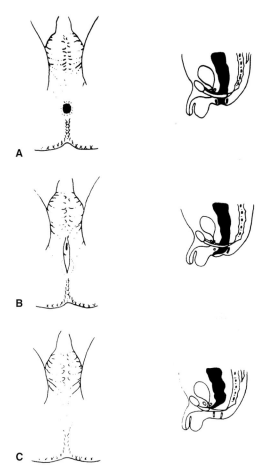

FIGURE 13.2.   Most common forms of imperforate anus in male infants. **A:** Normal anatomy. **B:** Low imperforate anus with rectoperineal fistula. **C:** High imperforate anus with rectourethral fistula.

reveals a small orifice in the posterior wall of the vulva. The opening can be catheterized with a small feeding tube and meconium expressed (Fig. 13.3).

High Imperforate Anus

Male Infants. The external appearance of the infant is similar to that of the infant with low imperforate anus. There is usually a fistula between the rectal pouch and urinary system, however, most often at the urethral–bladder neck junction. A careful urinalysis shows meconium in the urine. On occasion, meconium is seen at the tip of the penis, confirming the presence of a fistula.

Female Infants. The fistulous opening of the rectum is high in the vagina. Vaginoscopy can be performed

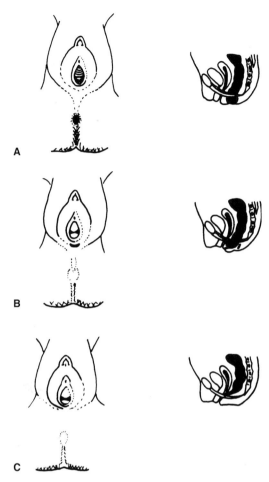

FIGURE 13.3. Most common forms of imperforate anus in female infants. **A:** Normal anatomy. **B:** Low imperforate anus with rectoperineal fistula. **C:** High imperforate anus with rectovaginal fistula.

using an otoscope or cystoscope and the rectal orifice found and cannulated. Rarely, one encounters a rectocloacal fistula or the so-called one-hole perineum where only one orifice is present in the perineum. This common cloacal channel may extend for several centimeters as one tract before it branches, giving off the urethra, vagina, and rectum.

Diagnosis

The most important part of the workup for an imperforate anus in the neonate is determination of the level of the end of the rectum and whether a fistula to the urinary or genital system is present. Anomalies in

which the rectum has descended below the level of the levator sling can be managed by a perineal anoplasty without colostomy. The high (supralevator) conditions are best managed by a diverting colostomy. Definitive correction is deferred until the child is older, weighing about 8 to 10 kg.

If the baby has passed meconium in the urine, the diagnosis is a high imperforate anus. No other diagnostic studies are necessary. Either a transverse or sigmoid colostomy is performed. Because a fistulous tract between the rectum and urinary system exists, it is important to irrigate the distal bowel at the time of colostomy to decrease the chance of persistent urinary sepsis.

If there is no meconium in the urine, one must differentiate between a low lesion and a high lesion. The most widely accepted method is the Rice-Wangensteen radiographic technique. This examination is done after the baby is at least 6 hours old, and the swallowed gas has had a chance to reach the rectum. A radiopaque marker is placed on the perineum where the anus should be, and the baby is turned upside down in a lateral position with the hips flexed. This position allows the gas in the rectum to rise as high as possible. A line is drawn between the posterior portion of the pubis and the lowest portion of the sacrum, the so-called pubococcygeal (PC) line. If air is seen to pass beyond this line on the radiograph, the infant has a low (infralevator) lesion, which can be treated by an anoplasty without a colostomy.

If air is not seen beyond the PC line, the infant is presumed to have a high lesion, and a colostomy is performed. This examination is not foolproof, however; gas may not pass all the way to the end of the rectum, especially in young neonates. Thus, one may perform an unnecessary colostomy in an infant for a low lesion. If air does seem to extend past the PC line, however, one can be confident that the bowel has traversed the levator sling. To be absolutely sure before proceeding with an anoplasty, some surgeons advise performing a perineal tap with a large-bore needle to gauge the thickness of the intervening tissue before finding meconium. Unless one is absolutely confident that the child has a low lesion, it is better to perform a colostomy than to risk damaging the delicate pelvic musculature, which would result in lifelong incontinence.

Treatment

Definitive surgery is postponed until the baby is thriving and weighs about 8 to 10 kg. A variety of surgical techniques exist. The important point of any procedure is to identify the levator sling of the puborectalis muscle and pass the bowel through it before bringing it down to the perineum.

The operative technique used at present by most pediatric surgeons is posterior sagittal anorectoplasty. A midline presacral incision is made down to the external sphincter. The voluntary muscle complex is identified and divided in the midline. The blind end of the rectum is identified, the fistula to the urinary tract is ligated and divided, and the rectum is tapered and brought down through the muscle and sutured to the perineum. Once the anal anastomosis has healed well and is of adequate caliber, the colostomy is closed. Complications of surgery for high imperforate anus are not uncommon. The most common is an everted anus with rectal mucosa protruding beyond the skin, causing a wet anus that becomes chronically irritated and finally ulcerates. The second, even more serious, complication is incontinence. Many children with high imperforate anus have delayed continence of stool and flatus. Sometimes, continence is achieved only when the children reach puberty. The reasons for this delay are not known. Even sophisticated testing cannot pinpoint the specific problem. Occasionally, the cause for the incontinence is that the bowel has not been brought through the levator sling. In such cases, a second pull-through is done, again being careful to identify the levator complex.

The low or ectopic imperforate anus in the female infant can be treated during the neonatal period by a simple cutback procedure. The anal opening close to the fourchette is brought farther posteriorly by incising the perineal skin. The rectal mucosa is then sutured to the skin with interrupted absorbable sutures. As the child gets older, the anal opening tends to separate from the vulva, giving an acceptable cosmetic result.

The overall results of surgery for children with imperforate anus are good. Most have a good result with no soiling. About 12% in a large series from the Children's Hospital of Pittsburgh were considered to have a poor result after long-term follow-up.

NECROTIZING ENTEROCOLITIS

Necrotizing enterocolitis (NEC) has become one of the most common abdominal emergencies for the newborn and is the most common abdominal surgical emergency in the premature infant. The condition occurs almost exclusively in newborns who are stressed or premature. Its causes are multifactorial and include decreased blood flow to the mesenteric vessels, increased bacterial proliferation in the gut, and the presence of incompletely digested feeds in the bowel. The small and large intestines become edematous and ischemic and can undergo liquefaction necrosis and perforate. Early in the course of the disease, the infant's signs are vague and nonspecific: lethargy, temperature instability, apneic or bradycardic spells, ileus, and then occult blood and mucus in the stools. As the disease progresses, there may be increased abdominal distension, erythema, and edema of the abdominal wall. Radiographs may show distended loops of bowel, pneumatosis intestinalis, and portal venous gas. If perforation has occurred, there is free air.

When the diagnosis is established, the infant is resuscitated, the stomach is decompressed with a nasogastric tube, and broad-spectrum systemic antibiotics covering GI tract flora are given. Serial abdominal radiographs are obtained every 6 to 8 hours to look for evidence of perforation. If perforation has occurred, laparotomy is performed; the obviously gangrenous bowel is resected, and the ends of viable bowel are exteriorized. Any marginally affected bowel is left in situ to prevent a short-gut syndrome later on.

Very small infants, especially those weighing a 1,000 g or less, may benefit from undergoing a less stressful procedure. There are a number of studies showing that perforations in this high-risk group can be often treated by primary peritoneal drainage alone sometimes accompanied by subsequent rescue laparotomy in those cases where there is evidence of continued metabolic instability.

With aggressive medical care, NEC can be treated by medical means alone in 50% of cases. The mortality and morbidity from NEC are still high but have improved, as critical care of the premature infants has become more effective in salvaging this at-risk population. NEC is one of the major causes of short-gut syndrome as discussed earlier.

ABDOMINAL WALL DEFECTS

Omphalocele and Gastroschisis

There are several defects of the abdominal wall at or near the umbilicus. A fair amount of confusion exits as to the exact terminology and embryology of these defects.

Omphalocele is a defect in the development of the abdominal parietes at the umbilical cord. Most investigators believe that this condition is explained by failure of the normally herniated abdominal viscera to return to the embryonic celom during the third week of development. Clinically, one finds a newborn with a large percentage of the small and large intestines present within a sac at the umbilicus. The umbilical cord emerges at the apex of the sac. The extent of the defect is variable. Large defects are not uncommon, and the liver may be found within the sac. The sac may be intact or may have ruptured during pregnancy or delivery.

Gastroschisis is a defect in the development of the abdominal parietes lateral to the umbilical cord. The cord is usually normal, and the defect is to its right. There is never a peritoneal sac. Unlike omphalocele, in gastroschisis the only extruded organs are the large and small intestines.

Associated anomalies are much more common with omphalocele than with gastroschisis. They include trisomy 21, trisomy D, cardiac defects, diaphragmatic hernias, and bladder exstrophies. In addition, all neonates with omphalocele have nonrotation of the midgut. The anomalies one sees with gastroschisis are related to the defect itself. They are usually areas of atresias or stenosis of the bowel, probably resulting from compression of the bowel between the abdominal wall and the extruded viscera.

Diagnosis of these conditions is obvious. The most important points in the management of the babies are keeping them normothermic and well hydrated. The exposed viscera should be covered with warm saline pads, over which a plastic sheeting is placed to prevent evaporative water loss. A nasogastric tube is inserted to prevent the intestines from filling up with swallowed gas. Antibiotics are started, and a rapid review of systems is begun. Newborns with omphalocele are especially prone to develop hypoglycemia. Intravenous infusions with 10% dextrose are administered.

The small defects are easily corrected with layered closure of the abdominal wound. Closure of the large defects is accomplished by most surgeons using the technique pioneered by Schuster (6). Dacron-reinforced Silastic sheeting is sutured to the fascial ring circumferentially, creating a pouch for the viscera. This pouch is covered with antiseptic solutions such as povidone–iodine (Betadine), and meticulous attention is paid to sterile technique. All attendants who handle the infant wear masks, gloves, and gowns.

Over the next 10 to 14 days, starting at day 2, the viscera are progressively reduced out of the pouch and returned to the peritoneal cavity, which gradually expands. This is done in the intensive care unit under sterile conditions. The infant is then brought back to the operating room for removal of the pouch and closure of the abdominal wall.

Other techniques used are the creation of large skin flaps bilaterally and placing the viscera in the large ventral hernia created, closing only the skin. When the child is older, usually at the age of 2 years, a secondary operation is done to close the abdominal wall defect. For cases of an intact omphalocele, Gross devised a technique of painting the intact sac with 2% aqueous mercurochrome solution. A solid eschar is formed followed by slow epithelialization of the sac.

Most surgeons use the Silastic pouch technique even though there are potentially serious complications: separation of the pouch from the fascia, sepsis, and intestinal gangrene from pressure on the bowel against the Silastic pouch at the fascial ring. Infants with gastroschisis or omphalocele often have a prolonged ileus and intestinal dysmotility. It may take weeks to months until they are able to tolerate oral intake, during which time intravenous alimentation is necessary.

The prognosis for these conditions has improved dramatically with the advent of total parenteral nutrition and with the introduction of the Silastic pouch techniques. Most of the infants who die do so as a result of the cardiac defect or chromosomal abnormality.

Inguinal Hernia

Inguinal hernias during infancy result from failure of the processus vaginalis, which is normally open in the fetus, to close. The open processus allows small intestine or other abdominal viscera to protrude, incarcerate, and strangulate. The incidence of inguinal hernia during infancy is high, and hernia surgery is by far the most common general surgical procedure performed on infants. Three times as many boys as girls are affected; right inguinal hernias are more common than left.

The diagnosis of inguinal hernia in infants is straightforward. The mother or pediatrician notices a groin bulge, especially when the infant cries or strains. If the patent processus is complete and extends to the scrotum, the infant has an inguinal-scrotal hernia.

The complications of hernias are frequent and serious, and they vary inversely with the age of the infant: the younger the infant, the more likely are complications. The most frequent is incarceration of intestine leading to strangulation and necrosis. Pressure of the incarcerated intestine on the delicate spermatic vessels running through the inguinal canal can also lead to ischemic necrosis of the testicle. Therefore, all inguinal hernias should be repaired surgically when discovered. No minimum age or weight is used to determine suitability for surgery. In the case of the premature infant, most surgeons operate when the infant is ready for discharge from the nursery.

Infants older than 50 weeks postconception can be operated on a same-day-surgery basis. They are admitted in the morning to a separate unit; a physical examination, blood count, and urinalysis are performed; and if they are normal, the infant is taken to the operating room; most can be discharged the afternoon of surgery.

Infants who were born prematurely have a tendency to develop postanesthesia apneic spells and should be observed at least 12 hours postoperatively; some surgeons advocate hospitalizing this group of patients overnight following a general anesthetic. This problem can be avoided by performing the hernia repair under spinal anesthesia, a technique that is becoming more widespread. Children with medical problems (e.g., upper respiratory tract infections or anemia) should have their surgery deferred until the condition is resolved.

As mentioned earlier, *incarceration* of the inguinal hernia is not an infrequent problem. The infant presents with a tense, somewhat tender inguinal bulge that may extend to the scrotum. Frequently, the abdomen is distended, and the infant may have vomited before the parents sought medical attention. Unless there is evidence of peritonitis, one may attempt reduction of the hernia. The older infant is sedated and kept in bed with the legs and pelvis elevated. The simple combination of sedation and the effects of gravity are often enough to reduce the incarcerated viscus. Should these measures fail, taxis on the hernia can reduce it in most cases. The infant is then admitted, and the edema is allowed to subside for about 12 to 24 hours before repair is undertaken. If attempts at reduction are unsuccessful, immediate surgery is needed. This can be an extremely difficult operation because of the edema and friability of the tissues. Extreme care is needed not to injure the vas deferens and the spermatic vessels.

Controversy exists even today as to the advisability of operating on the contralateral side. The younger the child, the greater the likelihood of finding a contralateral hernia that has gone unnoticed. As the infant gets older, a hernia, if present, would have been obvious, so a contralateral exploration on an older child tends to be less rewarding. The incidence of metachronous hernias in childhood is about 10%. Therefore, many surgeons will not perform a routine contralateral exploration except for those high-risk groups. These include premature infants, infants who have high intra-abdominal pressure due to presence of a V-P shunt, children with ascites, or children who have a strong family history of inguinal hernias.

Complications of hernia surgery include injury to the vessels or to the vas deferens. Recurrence is rare, about 1%, and results from incomplete removal of the sac infection or from a ligature that is too distal. In experienced hands, these complications should be minimal.

Hydroceles are common during infancy. In most cases, the fluid is slowly resorbed over the first several months after birth, so that by the time an infant is 1 year old, the hydrocele is completely resorbed. An additional number of hydroceles resolve over the second year of life. Hence, hydroceles need not be operated on during the first year. Some surgeons operate on them when they have persisted beyond the first year, but others wait until the child's second birthday. In all cases, the hydrocele should be explored through an inguinal incision, because the most common cause of a persistent hydrocele in the child is a small patent processus vaginalis that allows peritoneal fluid to trickle down into the scrotum while the child is up and about.

Umbilical Hernia

Umbilical hernias are common during infancy but, unlike inguinal hernias, are usually asymptomatic: the likelihood of intestinal obstruction or strangulation is extremely low. Most of these hernias close progressively as the child gets older. With few exceptions, umbilical hernias need not be repaired until the child reaches school age. The parents should be discouraged from taping over the protuberant hernia, as it can cause skin irritation.

BILIARY ATRESIA

There are several causes of persistent hyperbilirubinemia in the infant. Among them are liver dysfunction secondary to an infection such as toxoplasmosis, rubella, or cytomegalovirus; metabolic causes; and anatomic causes (i.e., biliary atresia). Advances in the surgical management of the child with biliary atresia have lent a great deal of urgency to the importance of an early diagnosis. Unfortunately, no single or combination of examinations enables the clinician to make the diagnosis with any degree of certainty, so there is still a place for exploratory laparotomy in the child with persistently elevated direct bilirubin levels.

Signs and Symptoms

The infant with biliary atresia is usually full term, with no other congenital anomalies. The jaundice may be mild at first and masked by the physiologic jaundice most neonates have. The early stools may be normal meconium and may contain bile pigment. The infant is usually discharged and is brought to the pediatrician with jaundice after several weeks at home.

On examination, the infant appears well. The liver and spleen are usually of normal size. Rectal examination shows acholic, clay-colored stools. The urine is dark. A variety of laboratory examinations have been used to differentiate jaundice on the basis of biliary atresia from that due to other nonsurgical conditions. They include radiologic techniques such as the rose bengal nuclear medicine scan and the hydroxy iminodiacetic acid (HIDA) scan. These two tests show no excretion of the radioisotope by the liver into the bowel. Unfortunately, they are not specific for atresia, as severe neonatal hepatitis with cholestasis but a normally patent biliary tree gives the same results. Among the more promising serum tests is an enzyme test for lipoprotein-X, which is severely elevated in biliary atresia and mildly elevated in nonsurgical conditions. Unfortunately, there is a fair amount of overlap between values obtained in those with biliary atresia and those with severe hepatitis.

Several centers have reported accurate diagnosis using real-time ultrasonography. An experienced ultrasonographer should be able to identify the gallbladder and common duct and their dimensions in a normal infant. The common duct in biliary atresia is atretic, enabling the ultrasonographer to make the diagnosis. More experience must be obtained before we can rely on this test for the diagnosis. In the interim, the most accurate test is the operative cholangiogram at laparotomy.

Treatment

It is the author's belief that all infants with persistent direct hyperbilirubinemia with acholic stools require a laparotomy. If the laparotomy confirms the diagnosis, hepaticoportoenterostomy is performed. Because the results of this operation are markedly poor after the age of 12 weeks, the laparotomy must be done before the child is 2 months old. At laparotomy, the gallbladder, if present, is cannulated; a cholangiogram is obtained and the biliary tree anatomy delineated. The atretic common duct is identified and dissected proximally as high as the bifurcation of the portal vein. A Roux-en-Y loop of jejunum is brought up to the transected portal tract and is there anastomosed.

The results of the operation depend in part on the histology of the bile ductules at the level of the anastomosis. Patients who have bile ductules larger than 150 μm at the time of the portoenterostomy have a good prognosis, generally obtaining good bile flow and no cirrhosis. Those patients in whom the bile ductules are less than 50 μm or in whom no epithelial-lined ductules are found have a poor prognosis, with poor bile flow, recurrent bouts of cholangitis, and ultimately progressive cirrhosis. The younger the patient, the greater are the chances that favorable histology will be found.

The prognosis following surgery for biliary atresia remains guarded. About half the children have sustained bile drainage after portoenterostomy. In most series, though, half of these patients have progressive biliary cirrhosis leading to portal hypertension and ultimately liver failure. These children should be referred to a center specializing in pediatric transplantation. Liver transplantation has proved successful, with 76% of children alive and well at 5 years with no signs of rejection.

QUESTIONS

Select one answer.

1. A newborn infant begins having bilious vomiting on day 2 of life. Which of the following investigations is most likely to give the proper diagnosis?
   a. Sonogram.
   b. HIDA scan.
   c. Upper GI series.
   d. Barium enema.
   e. CT scan.

2. Which of the following is likely to be found in a 6-week-old with a 4-day history of nonbilious projectile vomiting?
   a. Cl = 110.
   b. pH = 7.30.

c. $HCO_3 = 30$.

d. $K = 4.8$.

e. $PO_2 = 70$.

3. A full-term infant fails to pass meconium at 48 hours of age. Which is the most likely diagnosis?
   a. Duodenal atresia.
   b. Jejunal atresia.
   c. Hirschsprung disease.
   d. Esophageal atresia.
   e. Colonic atresia.

4. Which of the following anomalies is the most common?
   a. Proximal esophageal atresia with a tracheoesophageal fistula to the distal pouch.
   b. H-type tracheoesophageal fistula.
   c. Isolated esophageal atresia without a fistula.
   d. Esophageal atresia with tracheoesophageal fistulas to the proximal and distal pouches.
   e. Esophageal atresia with a tracheoesophageal fistula to the upper pouch.

5. Which of the following is not true of babies who have duodenal atresia?
   a. About 30% have Down syndrome.
   b. Most of the atresias are distal to the ampulla of Vater.
   c. There is a strong likelihood that other atresias will be found.
   d. The correct operation to repair the anomaly is duodenoduodenostomy.
   e. The mother may have had polyhydramnios.

6. Which of the following techniques should be used to reduce an incarcerated inguinal hernia in a 6-month-old infant?
   a. Sedation.
   b. Traction.
   c. Elevation.
   d. Ice packs.
   e. All of the above.

7. A 2-year-old girl has an umbilical hernia. Which of the following is the recommended plan of treatment?
   a. Surgery within the next few months.
   b. Surgery at the age of 5 years.
   c. Strapping the umbilical defect.

d. Surgery only if the hernia becomes incarcerated.

e. Surgery at the age of 12 years.

8. An 1,800-g premature infant presents with abdominal distension, lethargy, and stools positive or occult blood. Which of the following investigations needs to be done?
   a. Radiography of kidneys and upper bladder.
   b. CT scan.
   c. Sonogram.
   d. HIDA scan.
   e. Barium enema.

9. A 2,000-g infant with necrotizing enterocolitis is found to have portal venous gas. Which of the following procedures is in order?
   a. Continued medical therapy.
   b. Abdominal paracentesis.
   c. HIDA scan.
   d. Immediate surgery.
   e. Adding Cipro to the antibiotic regimen.

10. A 2-week-old infant is found to have a hydrocele. Which is the best course of treatment?
    a. Surgery at the age of 6 months.
    b. Surgery at the age of 2 years.
    c. Aspiration of the hydrocele.
    d. Transscrotal hydrocelectomy at the age of 2 years.
    e. None of the above.

REFERENCES

1. Clark RH, Hardin WD Jr, Hirschl RB, et al. Current surgical management of congenital diaphragmatic hernia: a report from the congenital diaphragmatic hernia study group. *J Pediatr Surg* 1998;33:1004.
2. Ravitch MM, McCune RM Jr. Reduction of intussusception by hydrostatic pressure, an experimental study. *Bull Johns Hopkins Hosp* 1948;82:550.
3. Cilley R, Statter M, Hirschl R, et al. Definitive treatment of Hirschsprung's disease in the newborn with a one-stage procedure. *Surgery* 1994;115:551–556.
4. Langer JC, Fitzgerald PG, Winthrop AL, et al. One-stage versus two-stage Soave pull-through for Hirschsprung's disease in the first year of life. *J Pediatr Surg* 1996;31:33.
5. Georgeson KE, Feunfer MM, Hardin WD. Primary laparoscopic pull-through for Hirschsprung's disease in infants and children. *J Pediatr Surg* 1995;30:1017.
6. Schuster SR. A new method for the staged repair of large omphaloceles. *Surg Gynecol Obstet* 1967;125:837.

SELECTED REFERENCES

Boley SJ, Lafer DJ, Kleinhaus S, et al. Endorectal pull-through procedure for Hirschsprung's disease with an anastomosis. *J Pediatr Surg* 1968;3:258.

Breaux CW Jr, Rouse TM, Cain WS, et al. Improvement in survival of patients with congenital diaphragmatic hernia utilizing a strategy of delayed repair after medical and/or extracorporeal membrane oxygenation stabilization. *J Pediatr Surg* 1991;26:333.

Campbell BT, McLean K, Barnhart DC, et al. A comparison of laparoscopic and open pyloromyotomy at a teaching hospital. *J Pediatr Surg* 2002;37:1068.

Grosfeld JL, O'Neill JA, Coran AG, et al., *Pediatric surgery*. 6th ed. Philadelphia, PA: Mosby Elsevier, 2006.

Kleinhaus S, Weinberg G, Gregor MB. Necrotizing enterocolitis in infancy. *Surg Clin North Am* 1992;72:261.

Louw JH, Barnard CN. Congential intestinal atresia: observations on its origin. *Lancet* 1955;2:1065–1067.

Pena A. *Surgical management of anorectal malformations.* New York: Springer-Verlag, 1990.

Vacanti JP, Shamberger RE, Eraklis A, et al. The therapy of biliary atresia combining the Kasai portoenterostomy with liver transplantation: a single center experience. *J Pediatr Surg* 1990;25:149.

CHAPTER 14

Ronald J. Simon
Melvin Stone

Trauma

T rauma is not something that happens to the other person or in "that" part of town. It is something that touches each of us directly, as a victim or family of a victim, or indirectly, as the one responsible for the care of an injured person. The statistics remain staggering. According to the statistics from the Centers for Disease Control and Prevention (CDC) in 2005, death relating to trauma was the fifth most common cause of death at all ages. Its incidence was more than twice that of acquired immunodeficiency syndrome (AIDS)-related deaths. Trauma is the number one cause of death in the 0- to 44-year age group. Although statistics from the Federal Bureau of Investigation (FBI) show a 3% reduction in violent crimes, 1.8 million violent crimes were still reported. One of every five people in major metropolitan areas is subjected to a violent crime. The frequency with which accidents and violence occur in our society necessitates a complete knowledge of the management of patients who have been traumatized.

This chapter highlights the management of patients after sustaining injury. It starts with the ABCs of resuscitation and evaluation and then moves to the management of injuries in specific body regions. It must be remembered that this chapter serves as an overview. More complete descriptions of management issues can be found in books referenced at the end of the chapter.

PRIMARY SURVEY

It is good to know that a few things you learned as a resident still hold true today. Specifically, I am referring to the ABCs of the primary survey of the trauma patient. Airway and breathing—assessing the adequacy of the airway and the effectiveness of one's breathing—are the initial priorities after the arrival of a trauma patient. Do not be lulled into a false sense of security by the presence of an endotracheal tube placed in the field. It is amazing, considering the conditions under which these tubes are placed, that so many are done correctly. But, there is a real percentage that is not so always assess the placement of these tubes. The second benefit of assessing the airway is that it allows you to do a quick mini-neurologic examination. If a patient does not follow commands, the airway may need to be secured. A general rule of thumb is that patients with a Glasgow Coma Scale (GCS) of less than 8 should have airway control.

If control of the airway is necessary, endotracheal intubation is the method of choice. Nasotracheal intubation of a spontaneously breathing patient is no longer considered the treatment of choice. In-line immobilization of the neck is required if there is the possibility of a spinal injury. Most people now agree that intubation using a two-person technique for in-line immobilization is adequate protection for the cervical spine. If intubation cannot be performed because of massive facial injuries or other factors, a surgical airway via a cricothyrotomy tube is recommended. One of the more difficult decisions we have to make is when to abandon attempts to obtain a standard airway and perform a surgical one. I allow three attempts; if they are unsuccessful, I opt for a surgical airway.

Once the airway has been controlled and breathing established, one's attention turns to the adequacy of circulation and establishing intravenous access. Although pulse and blood pressure are the most accessible measures, they are not the best for determining the adequacy of circulation. (A discussion on "shock and resuscitation" follows this section.) After most injuries, intravenous access should be established regardless of whether you believe the circulation to be adequate.

Their location depends on the mechanism and location of the injury. After a penetrating injury, the lines are placed between the injury and the heart. The lines should never be placed distal to the injury. It is recommended that two intravenous lines be inserted. Intravenous lines should be short and large, with 14- to 16-gauge angiocaths being optimal for peripheral lines. Triple-lumen central venous pressure (CVP) lines are inadequate, as their length and small lumen size make them unsuitable for rapid-volume infusions.

Venous cutdowns have joined nasotracheal intubations in the book of "Things we did in the past but don't do anymore." If peripheral access is unobtainable, central access using a 7 French Swan introducer via a subclavian, internal jugular, or femoral approach is the method of choice.

The next phase of the ABCs of the primary survey is assessment of "D"isability, which in essence is a mini-neurologic examination. It involves assessment of mental status by calculating the GCS, checking the papillary light response, and checking motor function in all four extremities.

The final phase is "E"xposure or a quick full body examination. Make sure that the patient is fully exposed and that areas such as the axillae and groin creases have been checked for injuries. This is especially true for a patient who has sustained penetrating injury. One should be careful that an electrocardiogram (ECG) lead does not inadvertently cover a wound or obscure the physical exam.

After this initial phase or primary survey, which should take only a few minutes, radiographs are obtained. X-rays should be used judiciously and should not delay patient resuscitation. These films can be taken in the resuscitation area with a portable x-ray unit. After penetrating injury, the need for radiographs depends on the nature and location of the injury. The evaluation of a patient after blunt injury is less focused, as it is designed to evaluate for occult multisystem injury. The initial survey usually consists of three films: chest, pelvis, and lateral cervical spine. I always insist on a chest radiograph first because the most immediately life-threatening injuries would be in the chest (i.e., pneumothorax or hemothorax).

Blunt trauma patients may safely forgo any radiographic evaluation of the C-spine if they have none of the Nexus criteria on physical exam. The Nexus criteria are (a) midline cervical tenderness, (b) altered level of consciousness, (c) evidence of intoxication, (d) neurologic deficit, and (e) presence of painful dis-

tracting injury. During the Nexus study, 99.8% of cervical spine injuries were identified using these criteria. If patients failed to meet the Nexus criteria, they will need full radiographic evaluation for the cervical spine. Three x-rays views are required to evaluate the cervical spine: anteroposterior (AP), lateral, and odontoid. Computed tomography (CT) scan may used in lieu of plain x-rays to evaluate the cervical spine. Recent data strongly suggest that CT scan for the evaluation of the spine has greater sensitivity and specificity than plain films. In addition, it may facilitate the evaluation of the patient who will also require a head CT. For the patient with neurologic deficits, magnetic resonance imaging (MRI) is recommended to rule out any soft tissue lesions such as ligamentous or spinal cord injury which cannot be detected with plain films or CT. It should be stressed that CT or MRI are only appropriate for the hemodynamically stable patient.

The *Focused Abdominal Sonography for Trauma* (FAST) has been developed to help evaluate the injured patient. The FAST exam can be quickly done at the bedside as adjunct to the primary survey. Using ultrasound, it evaluates the pericardial sac and the abdomen for fluid. The FAST exam will be discussed in further detail in later sections of this chapter.

SHOCK AND RESUSCITATION

Blood pressure and pulse are poor indicators of the shock state. It is not that a hypotensive patient is not in shock, he is. It is that the normotensive patient can fool you. Shock is defined as a state in which oxygen delivery is inadequate to meet demand. When less than 25% of blood is lost, the blood pressure is maintained by systemic vasoconstriction, and blood is shunted away from nonvital organs such as the gut. A prolonged reduction in gut blood flow has been implicated in the development of multiple system organ failure. Thus, despite a normal blood pressure, there can be isolated organ ischemia that if not treated may result in an adverse outcome.

If blood pressure and pulse are poor indicators for shock, what is better? The most available indicator is base excess, which has been shown in numerous studies to be a good indicator for the presence of shock. What appears to be most helpful is not the numeric value itself but the trend of the numbers and the speed with which these numbers normalize. The presence of a base deficit by itself suggests the recent presence of anaerobic metabolism. If the base deficit increases with time despite resuscitation, it suggests that anaerobic metabolism is still occurring and there is either ongoing bleeding or the efforts at resuscitation have been inadequate to restore perfusion. A good rule of thumb is that the base deficit should be resolved or at least reduced by half within 24 hours.

The lactate level is another measure for predicting the level of shock and the adequacy of resuscitation. It usually takes some time to see the test results, though, which may limit its usefulness. As with base deficit, the direction and rate at which the values move provide important information about the status of the patient and the resuscitation.

In the early to mid-nineties, there was a great deal of attention given to fluid management during resuscitation in the prehospital phase and in the emergency department (ED). The major controversy involved how much fluid to give a hypotensive patient after a penetrating truncal injury. Several studies had shown in both animals and humans that giving volume when bleeding is uncontrolled resulted in increased blood loss and higher morbidity and mortality. Many believe that patients with penetrating truncal injury should not spend time in the ED being resuscitated. The place for this patient is in the operating room (OR) with rapid control of bleeding. With this in mind, aggressive fluid management aimed at restoring a "normal" blood pressure should not delay definite bleeding control. Indeed, a balanced and careful approach of "permissive hypotension" whereby a less than normal blood pressure (systolic blood pressure [SBP] 80 to 90 mm Hg) is acceptable until bleeding can be controlled. A target of SBP 80 to 90 mm Hg or mean arterial pressure (MAP) of 60 to 65 mm Hg may achieve the ultimate goal of organ perfusion yet limit increased hemorrhage. In the patient with a suspected central nervous system injury (traumatic brain injury or spinal cord injury), a slightly higher target of SBP 90 mm Hg to avoid outright hypotension is appropriate. Similarly, in a patient who sustained a significant blunt injury, a rapid and diligent search for, and control of, bleeding is essential for optimal patient outcome.

The next issue is *what* to give. This problem is much simpler. If a patient is hypotensive, the fluid of choice is blood. Otherwise, crystalloid (0.9% normal saline or lactated Ringer's solution) can be used as the initial resuscitation fluid. What is commonly overlooked during the resuscitation is that all fluids, blood, or crystalloid, should ideally be warmed to 41°C. Another point learned from the recent military experiences is that the previously taught ratio of 4 units of packed cells to 1 unit of fresh frozen plasma allows for the development of coagulopathy and the over resuscitation with crystalloid. More emphasis on a 1:1 or 2:1 ratio of blood to plasma seems to be leading toward better outcomes (less adult respiratory distress syndrome, less compartment syndromes).

MANAGEMENT OF SPECIFIC INJURIES

Head Injury

Head injuries are the major cause of death in trauma patients. The diagnosis is usually straightforward. Any patient admitted after a traumatic event with altered mental status undergoes head CT scan. Do not make the mistake made by hundreds of inexperienced physicians: assuming that altered mental status is secondary to drugs or alcohol only to find out several hours later when a pupil blows that this intoxicated patient also has a large subdural hematoma that has caused herniation. My teaching is that a patient is never drunk until he has a negative head CT scan. Whether to obtain a head CT scan on every patient with a transient loss of consciousness (LOC) but who has a GCS of 15 on arrival in the ED is controversial. Some argue that if the head scan is negative and there are no other injuries, the patient can be discharged. Others prefer to admit the patient overnight for observation without a CT scan. Any change in mental status indicates the need for CT scan. Of course, the middle ground also exists, where all people with a brief LOC undergo head CT scanning and are admitted for observation. Neither of these protocols is right. The one you follow must depend on the reliability of the patient population and whether admitted patients are observed or simply "housed" in the hospital.

The indications for surgical repair vary with the neurosurgeon. There is no disagreement that a subdural or epidural hematoma that is causing a mass effect with midline shift should be decompressed, but a 1-cm subdural hematoma in a neurologically intact patient is now simply observed by many. Whether to débride a gunshot wound (GSW) of the head is unclear. Most neurosurgeons believe that the débriding process removes more viable tissue than it saves and so do not débride these wounds.

Medical management of intracranial hypertension has changed. The American Association of

Neurological Surgery has come out with new guidelines for management of the head-injured patient. Hyperventilation is no longer done unless the patient is herniating or has refractory intracranial hypertension that has not responded to other methods of control. If hyperventilation is to be used, the PCO_2 is kept between 30 and 35 mm Hg. This change has come about because of changing attitudes toward the benefits of maintaining cerebral blood flow versus the potentially adverse effects of reduced blood flow during hyperventilation-induced vasoconstriction.

Few words raise my blood pressure more than hearing a neurosurgeon say "keep them dry." That thinking again is based on the misconception that low pressure is good even at the sacrifice of flow. Head-injured patients must be kept **euvolemic** to optimize blood flow to ischemic areas of the brain. Euvolemia, though, does not mean hypoosmotic. Serum osmolality should be kept around 300 to 310 mmol/dL, which can be achieved with mannitol or furosemide (Lasix). Neither should be given to a hypovolemic patient, as it may cause hypotension, which along with hypoxemia are the nemesis of head-injured patients.

Class II and III data have demonstrated hypertonic saline's ability to reduce intracranial pressure (ICP). It has been used as a continuous infusion to elevate the serum sodium into the 150 to 160 range. The elevated sodium is thought to stabilize ICP. Hypertonic saline has also been use as a bolus in an attempt to rapidly lower ICP.

Neck Injuries

Referencing the "zones" of the neck are required when discussing penetrating neck injuries. The neck is traditionally divided into three different zones that provide a guideline for managing the injury. As demonstrated in Figure 14.1, the zones are defined as the following: zone 1, manubrium to cricoid cartilage; zone 2, cricoid cartilage to the angle of the mandible; zone 3, angle of the mandible to the base of the skull. In a patient who is hemodynamically stable, selective management is the norm in dealing with injuries in zone 1 and zone 3 because examination and operative exposure of these zones are difficult. Selective management involves some combination of CT scan, angiogram, endoscopy, and dynamic swallowing exams to better define the type and location of an injury. For example, a vascular injury in zone 1 may require a median sternotomy for proximal control of

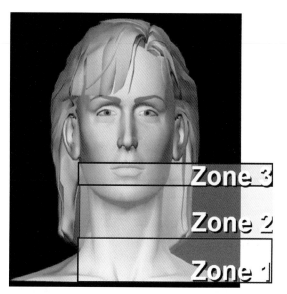

FIGURE 14.1.   Zones of the neck.

the right subclavian or either common carotid, while if the left subclavian is injured, proximal control is best obtained via a left posterior lateral thoracotomy. In zone 3, vascular exposure may require disarticulation of the mandible, or for more distal injuries, angiography and embolization may be the only therapeutic option.

Because zone 2 offers a relatively easy operative approach, there had been a classic controversy since the Korean War on the merits of mandatory exploration versus selective management. Due to mounting evidence in the 1990s that supports selective management over mandatory exploration, the current standard supports taking only patients that display "hard" signs suggestive of aerodigestive or vascular injury immediately to the OR. Hard signs include hemodynamic instability or active bleeding, enlarging or pulsatile hematoma, airway compromise, and extensive subcutaneous air.

Those patients without "hard" signs or who have "soft" signs that include dysphagia, voice changes, and hemoptysis may be candidates for selective management. For most centers, the standard initial diagnostic test for those patients undergoing a selective approach is helical CT. CT scan has the distinct advantage of being a "one-stop" diagnostic shop for the hemodynamically stable patient who would otherwise require panendoscopy and the angio suite. Level II evidence supports CT angiography as acceptable test for vascular injury. CT scan also offers information on missile trajectory through soft tissue to decide whether further testing or intervention is needed. Lastly, CT provides important diagnostic information on spine fractures or spinal cord injury. Of note, selective management using physical exam and CT can miss the occasional esophageal injury. If the diagnosis is missed for 12 hours, mortality is 5% to 25% and increases with time. Any suspicion for esophageal injury requires an esophagoscopy (rigid or flexible) or active contrast swallow depending on the expertise and resources that are available and the patient's ability to perform the exam. Instilling Gastrografin passively through a nasogastric tube pulled up into the esophagus prior to performing a CT will lead to missed injuries. Patients unable to actively swallow should undergo endoscopy.

It should also be mentioned that there is increasing acceptance for the use of intravascular stents for the treatment of nonbleeding vascular injuries (pseudoaneurysms, intimal flaps) in all zones of the neck, especially zone 1.

Thoracic Injuries

Rib fractures remain a common injury for the traumatologist. Management of a patient with multiple rib fractures remains a challenge specifically in regard to pain control. This is especially important in the elderly who are more likely to develop pneumonia and have a higher mortality following multiple rib fractures. It is better to prevent the pulmonary complications associated with rib fractures because once atelectasis has developed, it is difficult to reverse. Most awake patients will benefit from a patient-controlled analgesia (PCA) regimen using morphine or fentanyl. These patients are then transitioned to oral opiates with or without a nonsteroidal anti-inflammatory drug to further reduce pain and inflammation. For those patients where PCA is not adequate, the standard of care is the use of an epidural catheter. Epidural analgesia provides the best long-lasting pain relief, and has been shown to have the best improvement of pulmonary mechanics following chest trauma especially when injuries are bilateral. Rib block, although effective for one or two isolated fractures, is not helpful when there are multiple fractures. The pain relief obtained from it is short lived and for prolonged control would involve two to three blocks per day. This is beyond the time capabilities of most surgeons and would be tolerated by only the most masochistic patient.

Ribs broken in two places create a flail segment. The problem with this flail segment is that it moves in a paradoxical fashion relative to the rest of the rib cage. That is, during inspiration it moves inward and during expiration it moves outward. This abnormal movement increases the work of breathing. If the flail segment is large, the work of breathing may be so increased as to require that the patient be intubated. Adequate pain relief is probably the best way to avoid unnecessary intubation. It was once believed that the paradoxical motion resulted in hypoxemia but has been shown not to be true. If hypoxemia is present, it appears to be related to the pulmonary contusion underlying the flail segment.

The remaining myth in the management of patients with rib fractures and pulmonary contusions is how to manage the fluid status. In the past, it was thought that patients with a pulmonary contusion should be kept dry. This is not true. It is correct that hypervolemia should be avoided in the presence of pulmonary contusion. Maintaining a euvolemic state allows adequate organ perfusion while limiting third space fluid accumulation in the injured segment.

Blunt Cardiac Injury

Blunt cardiac injury (BCI) represents a wide spectrum that can range from a mild cardiac injury manifested only by ECG changes to the less common cardiac chamber rupture. (Cardiac chamber rupture will be discussed in the next section.) Mild BCI was previously called "cardiac or myocardial contusion," and this generated much confusion in the literature and made it difficult to accurately defined/diagnosed this group of patients. In 1998, an ad hoc committee of the Eastern Association for the Surgery of Trauma (EAST) proposed using the term BCI and it gave recommendations on the diagnosis and management of this group of patients. Based on an extensive literature review by this committee, the following conclusions were reached: all patients in whom the diagnosis is suspected should have an ECG on admission. If the ECG is normal, no further diagnostic maneuvers are needed, as the diagnosis is ruled out. If the ECG is abnormal (arrhythmia, ST changes, ischemia, heart block, and unexplained sinus tachycardia), the patient should be admitted for 24 to 48 hours for observation with continuous cardiac monitoring. If a patient is unstable, echocardiography appears to be the best test to detect the wall motion abnormalities associated with more severe BCI. Creatine phosphokinase values are not helpful for predicting complications.

Cardiac Chamber Rupture

Cardiac rupture is rarely diagnosed in the ED, as most of these patients die in the field. Ventricular ruptures are uniformly fatal, though rupture of the atria has been successfully repaired. The key to salvage is early recognition. If an unstable patient arrives, and a source in the abdomen, pelvis, and chest has been ruled out, this diagnosis must be considered. Evaluation for Becks' triad (elevated CVP, muffled heart sounds, and hypotension) should be done, but the diagnostic tests of choice is the pericardial view of the FAST exam. (At centers where readily available, transthoracic or transesophageal echocardiogram can substitute or confirm the FAST exam.) If the patient is stable, then a subxiphoid pericardial window can confirm or clarify the results of sonography. Some patients may present in cardiopulmonary arrest and an ED thoracotomy via an anterolateral approach may be used as a last ditch effort to salvage the patient.

Thoracic Great Vessel Injury

Although blunt rupture of the aorta and other great vessels in the thorax are not uncommon, it is uncommon to see them in the ED. About 80% to 90% of patients with a great vessel injury die before reaching the hospital. The most important factor in making this diagnosis is a high index of suspicion based on the mechanism of injury and some key clinical findings. Table 14.1 lists some of these high risk factors. Once one's awareness has been raised, the most commonly used screening test is the chest radiograph. Common findings great vessel injuries are listed in Table 14.2. It must be remembered that a negative chest radiograph does not rule out the diagnosis. As many as one-third

TABLE 14.2	Some Chest Radiographic Findings Associated with Traumatic Rupture of the Aorta

Superior mediastinal widening
Loss of definition of the aortic knob
Obliteration of the outline of descending aorta
Deviation of esophagus to the right at T4 more than
    1.0–2.0 cm
Obliteration of the aortopulmonary window
Tracheal deviation to the right
    apical cap
Depression of left main stem bronchus more than
    40 degrees
Widened paravertebral stripe
Fracture of first or second ribs
Fractured sternum, especially in younger individuals
Thickened and/or deviated paratracheal stripe

of patients with rupture may have an initially normal chest radiograph.

The role of CT scanning in the diagnosis of great vessel injury has been controversial, and aortography has traditionally been the gold standard for the diagnosis of great vessel injury. However, new advances in CT technology have increased its accuracy. Its use as the definitive diagnostic study is increasing at many centers where aortography was previously the standard diagnostic test after chest radiograph. Many still believe that CT is most useful as a screening tool. When used in this fashion, the scan is evaluated for the presence of a mediastinal hematoma which is usually associated with a blunt aortic rupture. In addition, it may pick up other aortic wall or intraluminal findings suggestive of aortic injury. If there are findings on CT that are suggestive of aortic injury, a formal aortograph is then done to ascertain the extent of the injury and provide a road map for operative repair. If the CT has no suspicious findings and there is a low suspicion for injury, the patient can be observed.

Where available, some centers may use transesophageal echocardiography in addition to the above-mentioned modalities. Its use is highly dependent on the availability of an interested echocardiologist, but it may play an important role in certain clinical situations. We have used transesophageal echocardiography in the OR in patients who had to be taken rapidly to the OR for bleeding control and required prolonged OR procedures. In this scenario, echocardiography can be performed in a semiemergent setting. If it is

TABLE 14.1	Clinical Features Suggesting Possible Traumatic Rupture of the Aorta

High-speed deceleration injury
Multiple rib fractures
Fractured first or second rib
Fractured sternum
Hoarseness or voice change without laryngeal injury
Hypertension, especially in the upper extremities
Superior vena cava syndrome
Systolic murmur, especially interscapular
Pulse deficits

negative, definitive operative procedures can be performed. If it is positive, some thoracic surgeons still require an aortogram, whereas others are willing to operate based on the echocardiographic results. Without this procedure, temporizing procedures may need to be done so that a timely angiogram can be obtained.

The most common site for injury of the aorta is at the aortic isthmus, which is the area between the left subclavian artery and the ligamentum arteriosum. The second most common site is in the ascending aorta. Once the location has been determined, if and how to repair the problem becomes important. There are two methods for open repair the aorta: one uses cardiopulmonary bypass while the other is clamp and sew. The major concern with the latter procedure is the development of paraplegia during cross clamping. What is apparent from the literature is that the incidence of paraplegia is related to expertise and not how the procedure is done. If the repair can be performed with 30 minutes or less clamp time, the incidence of paraplegia rivals that using bypass. Therefore, the recommendation is that unless there is expertise in the rapid repair of such injuries, some type of bypass should be utilized. Endovascular stenting is emerging as a first-line treatment in a subset of patients with blunt aortic rupture. Although there are yet only small series reported, the low mortality (0% to 12%) as compared with the operative repair (0% to 55%) and the almost 0% rate of paraplegia make this technique attractive. The patients with injury in the proximal descending aorta are most suitable for endovascular stenting. Limited large data series and lack of available appropriate size stents remain an issue.

There is a role for nonoperative management and/or purposeful delay of operation in blunt aortic injury. It should be considered in patients in whom the risks of surgery are high: (a) severe head injury; (b) risk factors for infection such as, burns, sepsis, and heavily contaminated wounds; (c) severe multisystem trauma with hemodynamic instability and/or poor physiologic reserve. There is evidence that delayed or nonrepair of injuries *in high-risk patients* has a better outcome than attempting repair.

If there is going to be a delay in treatment, medical management is important. The cornerstone of such management is the reduction of shear forces on the aorta, which is achieved by tight control of blood pressure using β-blockers. Vasodilators such as nitroglycerine and nitroprusside should be avoided as they do not reduce shear forces. SBP should be maintained below 120 mm Hg. Preventing gagging due to naso-gastric tube manipulation or suctioning with its resultant transient rise in blood pressure is also important.

The order of management of associated injuries is important. For example, in an unstable patient with a widened mediastinum and a grossly positive FAST or diagnostic peritoneal lavage (DPL), the decision should be to go to the OR first for control of intra-abdominal hemorrhage and worry about the possible aortic injury once the patient has been stabilized.

Penetrating Injuries to the Chest

According to careful reviews in the literature, resuscitative or emergency room thoracotomy is a procedure that provides little benefit to the patient and incurs high risk to providers and high cost to the system. Careful analyses have shown the subgroups of patients who may benefit from this procedure. Overall survival varies from 0% to 20%. The highest survival rates are in patients who arrive *in extremis* after a penetrating cardiac injury. In this scenario, control of the injury can be rapidly and directly achieved. Therefore, resuscitative thoracotomy is not indicated for the patient with blunt trauma and who arrives to the ED in cardiac arrest. No matter what the mechanism, patients with no signs of life in the field have no chance of survival, and thoracotomy should not be performed. The groups of patients who appear best served by this procedure are those with penetrating injury to the chest or extremities who have signs of life either during transport or after ED arrival. These patients fare significantly better than those with penetrating injury to the abdomen because rapid control of bleeding is possible in the chest or the extremities. Although one may restore vital signs in patients with severe intra-abdominal injuries, these patients just rebleed once blood pressure has been restored and die before or soon after definitive control of the bleeding is established.

The great majority of penetrating trauma to the chest, approximately 85%, can be managed with tube thoracostomy alone. Classic indications for OR thoracotomy or thoracoscopy in the patient **not** *in extremis* are (a) chest tube output more than 1,500 mL after insertion; (b) chest tube output of 200 to 300 mL/hr for 3 hours; (c) chest radiograph with significant retained hemothorax after chest tube insertion; and (d) large air leak with hypoxemia. Whether to perform a left or right thoracotomy or a median sternotomy is determined by the location of the injury and the expected organ injured. It should be remembered that for proximal and mid tracheal and esophageal

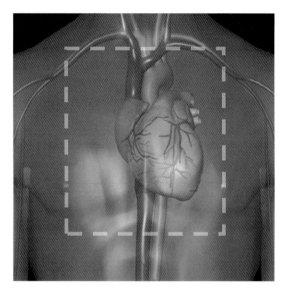

FIGURE 14.2. Cardiac zone of risk.

injuries, a right posterolateral thoracotomy is the preferred incision while the distal segments are better exposed via a left posterolateral thoracotomy.

Figure 14.2 demonstrates another area of concern in patients who are stable after sustaining penetrating thoracic injuries. The outlined box represents an area where the risk of cardiac injury is the highest. Reports of unsuspected injuries, as high as 23%, have been reported in patients sustaining penetration in this area (especially after stab wounds [SWs]). Although the pericardial window has been the mainstay in the diagnosis of these injuries, many centers are resorting to using the pericardial view of the FAST exam in these patients as a means of noninvasive, rapid evaluation to determine if there is a pericardial effusion. Our experience has been that the ED staff, surgery residents, and trauma attendings are quite proficient at the FAST exam. It is the rare occasion that the cardiologist is called in to verify the FAST exam with a formal echocardiogram. When there is the additional concern of a mediastinal injury, some centers evaluate both the heart and the mediastinum using thoracoscopy.

Transmediastinal GSWs often present a dilemma. These patients usually present in one of two ways: (a) *in extremis* after sustaining an injury to the heart, pulmonary hilum, or great vessel or (b) in stable condition with minimal evidence of life-threatening injury. Concern involves four basic structures: heart, great vessels, tracheobronchial tree, and esophagus. GSWs to the heart and great vessels are rarely occult, unlike

SWs to these organs, and will usually present with obvious signs or a patient in extremis. Angiography in these patients is usually not possible and injuries are discovered in the OR. In the stable patient, however, there may be occult mediastinal injuries. Although the pericardial window or echocardiogram were the traditional tools to rule out an occult injury to the heart, the FAST exam complemented by CT have emerged as the procedures of choice after the initial CXR in the stable patient with a transmediastinal GSW. The great advantage of CT is that it provides a roadmap of the possible trajectory of the missile; subsequently, the traumatologist can determined what other diagnostics, if any, are necessary. For example, CT can be used to help determine if further diagnostic tests are required to evaluate the esophagus with a transmediastinal GSWs with a posterior trajectory.

Esophageal injuries are notoriously subtle on initial presentation and often fatal when they present in a delayed fashion. Mortality rates for esophageal injuries if repaired within 12 hours vary from 5% to 25% depending on associated injuries. If repair is delayed 12 to 24 hours, the mortality doubles, and it triples if repair is delayed more than 24 hours. A CT scan showing findings suggestive of a trajectory in the posterior mediastinum, such as subcutaneous air, would prompt the traumatologist to obtain an esophagoscopy or an esophagogram to rule out injury.

The approach to operative repair depends on the location of the injury. If the wound is in the proximal or midesophagus, operative repair should be via a right posterolateral thoracotomy. Injuries to the distal third of the esophagus are best approached via a left posterolateral thoracotomy. It is best to repair the esophagus in two layers and to buttress the repair. In the upper esophagus, this can be achieved with either a wrap of pleura or intercostal muscle. In the lower esophagus, a gastric fundal wrap may be used.

Blunt Abdominal Trauma

Thorough evaluation of the abdomen after blunt injury remains a critical part of the evaluation of the trauma victim. Missed intra-abdominal injury remains the most common cause of *preventable* trauma deaths. The methods used to determine the presence of an injury depends on patient stability and available resources. Although DPL was once the "gold standard," in the evaluation of the abdomen, it has been replaced in most scenarios by ultrasound and CT scan. Although ultrasound has been the gold standard

<table>
<tr><td>

TABLE 14.3 **Criteria for Evaluating the Abdomen**

</td></tr>
</table>

Unexplained hypotension
Equivocal or unreliable examination
Inability to observe patient (need for surgery for associated injury)
Multiple lower rib fractures
Pelvic fracture

<table>
<tr><td>

TABLE 14.4 **Strengths and Weaknesses of CT Scan**

</td></tr>
</table>

Strengths
  Noninvasive
  Good for retroperitoneal injuries
  Organ specific
  Provides grading of solid organ injury
Weaknesses
  Never scan unstable patient
  Misses bowel injuries
  Expensive
  Time consuming
  Need cooperative patient
  Weight limitations

in Europe for years, it is now being used routinely in the United States as a quick and easy way to detect the presence of free fluid in the abdomen.

The general criteria for evaluating the abdomen are listed in Table 14.3. These criteria simply suggest that evaluation is necessary; they do not define the type of evaluation needed that is determined by the clinical condition of the patient. Basically, the evaluation of a patient with BAT is determined by the patient's stability. If the patient is unstable, then the priority is to find out whether the patient is bleeding and if so, where. Most centers have replaced the use of DPL with ultrasound, which we previously referred to as FAST (more on that in a moment). If the FAST shows free fluid in the abdomen, then it is presumed that intra-abdominal hemorrhage is the etiology for the instability and the patient should be taken to the OR for exploration. If ultrasound is not available then a DPL is still an acceptable option with a grossly positive DPL being the indication to go to the OR. If the patient is stable, then FAST can be used as a screening tool to determine whether or not to get a CT scan. A negative FAST would indicate that observation without CT scanning is adequate. A positive FAST in this circumstance does NOT mean a trip to the theatre (operating theatre); in this circumstance, it indicates a need for CT scanning to better evaluate the abdomen in an attempt to better define the source of the fluid. More on this in the sections on management of blunt trauma to the liver, spleen and pancreas. Table 14.4 reviews the pros and cons of CT scanning.

The role of ultrasound by surgeons has changed many aspects of the early management of patients with BAT. Although the Europeans have been using ultrasound in the evaluation of trauma patients for many years, its use in the United States took off in the early 1990s. The method by which ultrasound was used by trauma surgeons became known as Focused Abdominal Sonography for Trauma, or FAST. Since its introduction, FAST has been shown to highly accurate in detecting fluid in the abdomen when in excess of 400 cm^3. Its ability to detect fluid below that level is more user dependant. As the majority of injuries with less fluid rarely require either surgical or radiologic intervention, the lack of sensitivity at these levels does not take away from its usefulness. As stated earlier, the strength of FAST is as a screening tool. The procedure for doing it requires evaluation of four areas of the abdomen, the right and left upper quadrants, a cardiac view, and a suprapubic view. The presence of fluid in one of these quadrants is sufficient to considerate it a positive test. Adequate training is critical for proper performance and interpretation of this modality and it is important that this occurs before one begins utilizing this technology. Table 14.5 lists the strengths and weaknesses of ultrasound.

<table>
<tr><td>

TABLE 14.5 **Strengths and Weaknesses of Ultrasonography**

</td></tr>
</table>

Strengths
  Noninvasive
  Rapid
  Inexpensive
  Repeatable
  Sensitive for the presence of fluid
  Can evaluate heart
Weaknesses
  User dependent
  Misses bowel injuries
  Need cooperative patient
  Weight limitations
  Nonspecific

TABLE 14.6 Strengths and Weaknesses of DPL

Strengths
  Rapid
  Easy to teach
  Highly sensitive to the presence of injury
  May detect bowel injury
  Inexpensive

Weaknesses
  Invasive
  Iatrogenic complications
  Misses retroperitoneal organ injuries
  High rate of unnecessary laparotomy
  Nonspecific
  Difficult to do in obese or uncooperative patients

DPL, diagnostic peritoneal lavage.

DPL could be used for all of the criteria outlined in Table 14.3. The only absolute contraindication for DPL is when there is an obvious need for laparotomy. Relative contraindications include third-trimester pregnancy and multiple previous abdominal operations. Table 14.6 lists the strengths and weakness of DPL. The criteria for evaluating the results of DPL are listed in Table 14.7.

TABLE 14.7 Criteria for Interpretation of Lavage Results After Blunt Abdominal Trauma

Positive findings
  Aspiration of 5 mL blood
  Lavage fluid comes out Foley catheter or chest tube
  RBC >100,000/mm^3
  WBC >500/mm^3
  Amylase >175 U/mL
  Presence of bile, bacteria, and/or particulate matter

Indeterminate findings
  Aspiration of <5 mL of blood
  RBC 50,000–100,000/mm^3
  WBC 100–500 mm^3
  Amylase 75–175 U/mL

Negative findings
  No blood aspirated
  RBC <50,000/mm^3
  WBC <100/mm^3
  Amylase <75 U/mL

Management of Blunt Solid Organ Injury

Although nonoperative management of blunt *splenic* injury was initiated in children, it rapidly became the standard for management in the adult. The major criteria for nonoperative management in adults are that the patient be hemodynamically stable and that there is no concern for hollow-viscus injury. If the injury extends into the hilum on CT (grade 4 or 5) or there is a blush of contrast in the injured area, noninvasive management cannot be effective and an angiographic approach should be pursued. Although some surgeons operate if the CT shows evidence of bleeding, most will first attempt angiographic embolization of the source of bleeding. Proponents of early surgery for splenic injury have demonstrated a high splenic salvage rate when operation is done early rather than when conservative management has failed. In an unstable patient, operative management is the treatment of choice.

Nonoperative management of *hepatic* injuries uses basically the same criteria as for the spleen. Injuries near the porta hepatis carry a higher failure rate than more peripheral injuries. Active bleeding demonstrated by hemodynamic instability or a blush on CT should be treated with angiographic embolization or laparotomy. Severe liver injuries remain a surgical challenge. We believe in the adage: "if it ain't bleeding, don't touch it." Stirring up bleeding in the depths of the liver can have disastrous consequences. Less severe injuries can often be controlled with direct pressure and patience. On occasion, liver sutures and an omental pack may be effective. With severe injuries, vascular control using the Pringle maneuver (clamping the porta hepatis) may be necessary, followed by thorough packing of the injury and angiography. If packing does not control the bleeding, the finger fracture technique can be used to reach the site of bleeding. Lateral injuries can be treated with resectional débridement. It is important to drain most injuries of moderate and greater degree because bile leaks are common after these injuries and may not be evident immediately.

Blunt and penetrating injuries to the *pancreas* are handled in a similar fashion. The key concept is conservative operative management. In general, there is no role for nonoperative management. The location of the injury and the presence or absence of a ductal injury usually determines the treatment. Proximal and distal injuries that do not involve the duct can usually be managed by drainage alone. If there is involvement of the distal duct, distal resection is the treatment of choice. Splenic salvage is recommended only in the stable patient with isolated injury. Proximal injuries that involve the pancreatic duct are more complex to manage. Distal pancreatectomy is inappropriate for injuries to the right of the superior mesenteric vessels, as it would produce a state of pancreatic insufficiency. How the proximal pancreas is handled is determined by the status of the duodenum. If the duodenum is badly injured, pancreaticoduodenectomy is indicated, which is rarely performed. Many would argue that a full pancreatico-duodenectomy should not be performed at the initial operation. Bleeding and any intestinal spillage should be controlled at the first operation and the patient stabilized and resuscitated. The definitive operation can then be performed during the initial 24 to 48 hours after injury. If the duodenum is not injured but the proximal duct is, then the proximal duct is ligated and a distal pancreatic enteric anastomosis is performed. If ductal injury is unclear or the patient is too unstable for pancreatic enteric anastomosis, wide drainage is a reasonable option. If the duct is intact, even significant proximal injuries may be able to be adequately managed by drainage alone. One could consider placement of a stent in the pancreatic duct in these cases. It is important to drain all pancreatic injuries. There is support in the literature for the use of somatostatin after pancreatic injury to reduce the incidence of fistula formation.

Penetrating Abdominal Trauma

Management of penetrating abdominal injuries depends on numerous factors, including the mechanism of injury, the location of the injury, and the clinical status of the patient. GSWs are different from SWs. The mortality due to GSWs (5% to 15%) is significantly higher than that due to SWs (1% to 2%). The incidence of intra-abdominal injury is also higher with GSWs (92% to 98% vs. 15% to 25%). Most GSWs that penetrate the abdomen require surgery because of the high incidence of injury. Such is not the case for SWs, where the abdomen is regionalized to determine optimum management.

SWs to the **anterior** abdomen create no intra-abdominal injury in 20% to 40% of cases. If all patients with injury to this area were explored, an unacceptably high negative laparotomy rate would occur. If one limits exploration to those with hypotension, evisceration, or peritonitis, the negative laparotomy rate is reduced to 15%. How best to evaluate those who do not meet those criteria is controversial. DPL is not helpful for SWs to the anterior abdomen because DPL may be negative in the presence of injuries to the bowel and diaphragm or positive in patients with small liver and spleen injuries that have stopped bleeding. Laparoscopy can be performed but requires general anesthesia, and running the small bowel can be time consuming. We believe in careful observation. In a series by Ivatury et al., hemodynamically stable patients with benign abdomens were followed by serial examinations. They found that 75% did not need laparotomy, and the negative laparotomy rate was 3%. There did not appear to be any morbidity or mortality associated with observation.

The management of SWs to the flank and back are different. These injuries are special because of the risks associated with retroperitoneal colon injuries. There are proponents for doing triple-contrast CTs, DPL, and laparoscopy. I believe that CT and laparoscopy can be useful in specific patient groups. For SWs to the flank that are between the anterior and midaxillary line, CT scanning with oral and rectal contrast has become the diagnostic test of choice. It is useful for evaluating peritoneal penetration and colon injuries. Any hematoma or air seen near the colon mandates exploration.

For SWs to the back, the preferred method of evaluation is the CT scan. There is a belief that the optimal way to perform this scan is with oral, rectal, and intravenous contrast. This preference may be met with resistance from radiologists, and the scans are performed with intravenous and oral contrast alone. If it is performed in this manner, it is critical that enough contrast is given and time is allowed to obtain adequate filling of the colon. Any air or hematoma seen around the colon dictates the need for laparotomy or laparoscopy.

Penetrating injury to the area of the thoracoabdomen has its own scheme of management. Studies have shown a 20% to 30% incidence of occult diaphragm injury after penetrating injury to this region. The morbidity and mortality of diaphragmatic hernia from a missed injury has led some to advocate mandatory laparotomy for all patients with injury to this area. If followed, a 75% negative laparotomy rate would result, making this kind of approach less than optimal. Some believe that DPL is a good option here. This choice is again less than perfect as positive lavage can occur from small injuries to the liver and spleen, and there have been many reports of a false-negative DPL in the presence of a diaphragmatic injury. This area must also be subdivided by injuries to the right and left. I believe that the optimal method for evaluating penetrating injury to the left thoracoabdominal area is laparoscopy. It is minimally invasive and highly sensitive for detecting diaphragmatic injuries. Injuries to the right thoracoabdominal area are probably not an issue, as the liver seals the diaphragmatic hole, and the risk of herniation is low.

Management of Colon Injuries

Repair of a penetrating injury to the colon, like most other injuries discussed so far, is determined by patient stability and the extent of the bowel injury and contamination. Injuries to the right and transverse colon should be primarily repaired under most circumstances. Primary repair or resection plus anastomosis are acceptable procedures. If a left colon or sigmoid injury is present, a primary repair can be performed if the patient is stable, there is minimal contamination, and there are no major associated injuries (pancreatic injury is probably the worst). Although primary repair is the preferred method for reconstruction, if one is unsure colostomy is the safest choice.

Rectal injuries are managed by diversion. A sigmoid loop colostomy is the best option as is can be reversed without going back into the abdomen. Although in the past, distal washout and presacral drainage has been recommended, neither one of these procedures has been shown to be of any benefit in civilian injuries and should no longer be performed.

DAMAGE CONTROL: OPERATIVE STRATEGY IN THE UNSTABLE PATIENT

It is important to know when injuries should *not* be definitively repaired but should be temporized and the final treatment delayed. This is the concept of "damage control." The basic philosophy follows three points: (a) the OR is a bad place for resuscitation; (b) resuscitation takes precedence over definitive repair; and (c) cold, acidotic, coagulopathic patients do not do well in the OR. When a hypotensive, acidotic patient is in the OR, the operative strategy would be to control hemorrhage and intestinal contamination and then move the patient to the ICU for resuscitation. Bowel repairs

should be limited to simple repairs or stapling of injured segments to stop spillage. Intestinal continuity need not be restored at this time. The abdomen should be closed rapidly once these repairs are achieved. Temporary closure is accomplished with an intravenous bag (Bogota bag), a prosthetic patch (e.g., Gortex or Vicryl), or a VAC abdominal dressing.

The underlying theory is that these patients remain in a state of shock with progressive acidosis and organ injury. If this cycle continues, even if the patient eventually makes it off the table, there is a significantly increased risk of developing multiple organ failure. Using the principles of damage control, resuscitation is accomplished in the ICU under a more controlled setting and at a more rapid pace. Once the patient has been resuscitated, definitive repairs can be performed in the OR under optimal circumstances. This method of treatment has been shown to salvage severely injured patients with a significant reduction in morbidity and mortality.

PELVIC FRACTURES

No chapter on trauma management would be complete without a discussion on the management of pelvic fractures. This injury often complicates our ability to manage a multiply injured patient. The usual issue is whether an unstable patient with a pelvic fracture is bleeding from vessel injury in the pelvis or an associated intra-abdominal injury, which occurs in about 5% to 10% of patients with these fractures.

The key management principle is rapid evaluation of the abdomen. Options for evaluation include DPL, FAST, and CT (stable patients only) depending on patient stability. When DPL is performed in the presence of a pelvic fracture, a supraumbilical tap using the open technique should be used to avoid entering the pelvic hematoma, which would result in a false-positive tap. In an unstable patient, if the FAST or DPL shows evidence of blood, it can be presumed that the instability is from an intra-abdominal source and the patient taken to the OR for exploration. If the DPL or FAST is negative, it can be presumed that the bleeding is from the pelvis.

The optimal method for control depends on the type of pelvic fracture. The four major classifications are open book, lateral compression, vertical shear, and a combination of these types. With an open book fracture pattern, there is an increase in pelvic volume.

The bleeding vessels with this type of injury are usually veins from the sacral plexus. The best way to control this bleeding is by reducing the pelvic volume. This can be done by either placing an external fixator on the pelvic rim to reduce the pelvic volume or by wrapping the pelvis with a sheet or a commercially available product. This reduction in volume often increases the pressure on the pelvic veins enough to stop the bleeding. If either one of these methods does not control the bleeding, it is presumed that the bleeding is from an arterial source and an angiogram is obtained with the hope of visualizing and embolizing the source of bleeding.

If one of the other fracture patterns is present, the pelvic volume is not increased and external fixation is not a viable alternative. With these fractures, bleeding from small arteries such as the pudendal or obturator artery is more common. Unstable patients with these injuries should have their abdomens rapidly evaluated by DPL or ultrasonography and, if negative, be taken emergently for angiography for evaluation and potential treatment. A pelvic wrap can be placed in these fractures also but are less likely to be efficacious.

CONCLUSIONS

This chapter reviews basic management principles for the trauma patient. The most important reminders are a high level of suspicion and attention to detail. Current data suggest that arresting hemorrhage and resuscitation should take priority over definitive therapies.

QUESTIONS

Select one answer.

1. A 25-year-old man arrives after sustaining a GSW to the right lower quadrant. He is explored and found to have laceration to the right colon encompassing 75% of the circumference. He is hemodynamically stable, and there is minimal local contamination. The correct procedure would be to
   a. Perform an ascending loop colostomy.
   b. Resect the injury and bring up an end-colostomy and mucous fistula.
   c. Exteriorize the repair and drop it back in after 5 to 7 days if intact.
   d. Perform a primary repair.
   e. Perform a resection and anastomosis.

2. A complete cervical spine evaluation after a motor vehicle accident should include
   a. Careful clinical examination.
   b. Lateral radiograph including the top of T1.
   c. Anteroposterior view.
   d. Odontoid view.
   e. All of the above.

3. The first priority during evaluation of a multiply injured patient who is hypotensive is to
   a. Establish intravenous access.
   b. Obtain blood for crossmatch.
   c. Perform a mini-neurologic examination.
   d. Assess the airway.
   e. Search for occult bleeding.

4. A 36-year-old woman arrives with stable vital signs after sustaining a SW to the neck just lateral to and above the cricoid cartilage. There is a slowly expanding hematoma lateral to the wound. The next step in management would be
   a. Observation.
   b. Angiography to better define bleeding source.
   c. Neck exploration
   d. Esophagography and observation.
   e. CT scan.

5. A 34-year-old man arrives at the ED hypotensive after being involved in a motorcycle accident. He has an angulated right femur, facial trauma, and a tender abdomen. Initial films revealed an unremarkable chest radiograph, normal lateral cervical spine, and an open-book pelvic fracture. Despite 2 L of crystalloid, he remains hypotensive. The next step in management is
   a. Exploratory laparotomy.
   b. CT scan of the abdomen.
   c. FAST or DPL.
   d. Angiography.
   e. None of the above.

6. The preferred fluid for a patient who arrives at the ED hypotensive after sustaining a GSW to the chest is
   a. Normal saline 0.9%.
   b. Ringer's lactate solution.
   c. 5% Albumin.
   d. Blood.
   e. 5% Hetastarch.

7. The most important determinant for the need for aortography in a patient at risk for blunt aortic injury is
   a. Clinical suspicion.
   b. First rib fracture.
   c. Morphology of aortic knob.
   d. Sternal fracture.
   e. Myocardial contusion.

8. A 52-year-old woman is involved in a high-speed motor vehicle crash. She is initially hypotensive but normalizes with volume. A CT scan of the abdomen is performed and shows free fluid around the spleen and a 2 cm hyperdense area in the lower pole of the spleen. The most appropriate management of this finding would be
   a. Splenectomy.
   b. Angiographic embolization.
   c. Admit and observe in ICU setting.
   d. Repeat CT scan in 24 hours.
   e. Factor VII.

9. A 68-year-old man is involved in a high-speed motor vehicle accident. He is unconscious and hypotensive with systolic pressure of 80 mm Hg on arrival at the ED with a distended abdomen. Initial radiographs reveal a minimally displaced pelvic fracture and normal cervical spine; the chest radiograph shows a widened mediastinum, loss of aortic contour, and deviated nasogastric tube. Despite blood transfusion, he remains hypotensive. FAST shows free fluid in the subhepatic and pelvic areas. The next step in management is
   a. Head CT scan.
   b. Pelvic angiogram.
   c. Aortogram.
   d. Emergency thoracotomy.
   e. Exploratory laparotomy.

10. A 48-year-old man is stabbed in the right upper quadrant. He arrives in the ED hypotensive and with abdominal tenderness. He is taken emergently to the OR for laparotomy. At exploration, he is found to have a 5-cm laceration to the dome of the liver that is no longer bleeding. No other injuries are found. The next step in managing this injury would be
    a. Pringle maneuver.
    b. Pringle maneuver and finger fracture exploration of the injury.
    c. Exploration of the injury.
    d. Drain injury and close the abdomen.
    e. Close the abdomen and get an angiogram.

SELECTED REFERENCES

Bickell WH, Wall MJ, Pepe PE, et al. Immediate versus delayed fluid resuscitation for hypotensive patients with penetrating torso injuries. *N Engl J Med* 1994;331:1105.

Eastern Association for the Surgery of Trauma. Trauma practice guidelines. Available at: http://www.east.org/Portal/Default.aspx?tabid = 57. Accessed February, 2011.

Feliciano DV, Mattox KM, Moore EE, eds. Trauma. 6th ed. New York, NY: McGraw Hill, 2008.

Hirschberg A, Mattox K. *Top knife: art and craft in trauma surgery*. Castle Hill Barnes, UK: Tfm Publishing, 2005.

Hoffman JR, Mower WR, Wolfson AB, et al. Validity of a set of clinical criteria to rule out injury to the cervical spine in patients with blunt trauma. National Emergency X-Radiology Utilization Study Group. *N Engl J Med* 2000;343: 94.

Ivatury RR, Cayten CG, eds. *The textbook of penetrating trauma*. Baltimore, MD: Williams & Wilkins, 1996.

Statistics on violence in America. National Center for Health Statistics and FBI Web pages. Available at: http://www.cdc.gov/nchswww/nchshome.htm and http://www.fbi.gov/publish.htm. Accessed February, 2011.

Wilson RF, Walt AJ, eds. *The management of trauma: pitfalls and practice*. Baltimore, MD: Williams & Wilkins, 1996.

CHAPTER 15

Stuart Greenstein   Amy Lu

Daniel Glicklich   Richard S. Schechner

Jane Yang   Vivian A. Tellis

Transplantation

In the past two decades, there have been remarkable advances in solid organ transplantation due to improvements in surgical technique, organ preservation, and the general management of patients. Transplantation of the kidney, heart, and liver has become as safe and effective as to be the standard of treatment for many conditions. Intestinal transplants have become more common with almost 200 performed in 2007, and almost 500 pancreas transplants and 1500 lung transplants were performed that same year.

In fact, there have been more than 430,000 transplants performed to date, with over 28,000 performed in 2007 alone. However, the availability of organs for transplantation lags far behind the need. The number of potential donors in the population has been estimated at 50 per million, even after exclusion of those with contraindications. An increasing number of living donors have been used, but approximately 100,000 people remain on an organ waiting list. As a result, the criteria for both living and cadaveric donors have been extended, and investigation in the use of partial organ donations, xenografts, and even cloning has increased.

In this chapter, we provide a broad overview of various clinical aspects of transplantation, referring most often to kidney transplantation, as kidneys are by far the most commonly transplanted organ. The similarities and differences to transplantation of the heart, lung, liver, pancreas, and small bowel are discussed. We provide an overview of the immunologic basis for the immune response and the related topics of rejection and immunosuppression. The indications, contraindications, and results of the transplantation of various organs, the complications of surgery and of immunosuppression, and the role of various regulatory agencies are also addressed.

INDICATIONS AND CONTRAINDICATIONS FOR TRANSPLANTATION

The potential solid organ transplant recipient must have irreversible progressive and severe damage to a vital organ system. For example, a glomerular filtration rate of less than 10 cc/min is considered end-stage renal disease (ESRD). At this degree of renal impairment, a patient may have few uremic symptoms. In fact patients who receive a renal transplant before the need for dialysis have better allograft survival than those who get transplanted after two or more years on dialysis. In contrast, patients with end-stage heart, lung, liver, and small bowel disease are usually quite ill at the time of transplantation. The presence of advanced cardiac or vascular disease concomitantly with ESRD may cause patients to be ruled out as transplant candidates. Other contraindications to transplantation include aggressive malignancy, uncontrolled infection, severe dementia, uncontrolled mental illness, noncompliance with medical regimen, self-destructive, and antisocial behavior. Finally, lack of adequate social support and no insurance may preclude transplantation.

Another important factor to consider is the existence of other safe alternatives to transplantation, from corrective cardiac surgery or partial liver resection to the administration of exogenous insulin for uncomplicated diabetes. It is important to consider whether the risks of the immunosuppression that will follow the transplantation are justified, especially if another treatment can be safely applied. Ultimately, the transplantation of any organ should result in a significant improvement in the quality of life, as well as in life expectancy in the recipient.

TABLE 15.1	Most Common Etiologies of Renal Failure Requiring Renal Transplantation

Diabetes mellitus types I and II
Hypertension
Glomerulonephritis
Polycystic kidney disease
Urologic disease

INDICATIONS FOR RENAL TRANSPLANTATION

Although patients with ESRD can be maintained on dialysis, life expectancy has been shown to be improved after transplantation. The most common etiologies of ESRD for which transplantation is performed are diabetes mellitus and hypertension (Table 15.1). Although many of the 500,000 patients with ESRD are potential candidates, a great number are ruled out because of severe coexisting multiorgan disease or other conditions. Most renal transplant recipients are on maintenance dialysis at the time of transplantation. Transplantation can be carried out before dialysis becomes necessary ("preemptive" transplantation), particularly if a suitable living donor is available. The median age of both donors and recipients is rising, and age is no longer a major determining factor. Transplants are being performed on infants as well as septuagenarians. Transplantation in children must be aggressively pursued, as physical and emotional growth becomes stunted on dialysis.

PREPARATION FOR TRANSPLANTATION

Patients with ESRD have an increased likelihood of significant cardiovascular and peripheral vascular disease. Many patients should undergo exercise stress testing, formal cardiologic evaluation, and tests for vascular disease. All potential renal transplant recipients are tested for HIV 1 and 2, hepatitis B and C, Epstein–Barr virus (EBV), cytomegalovirus (CMV), and syphilis. Patients who are HIV-positive may be transplant candidates if the following pertains: there is no detectable viral load on antiretroviral therapy, there is clear compliance with medical therapy, CD4 counts are greater than 200/mm^3 and there are no opportunistic infections or malignancy.

Patients from endemic areas may need screening for intestinal parasites, especially strongyloides, malaria, Chagas' disease, histoplasmosis, and coccidiomycosis. All patients should have skin testing for tuberculosis. Patients with symptoms suggestive of gastrointestinal or urologic disease may need specific investigation. The patient's own kidneys are usually left alone; nephrectomy is reserved for indications such as severe ureteropelvic reflux, massive calculus disease, or infection, which if left untreated may pose a problem after transplantation. All patients should undergo age- and gender-appropriate cancer-screening tests.

Immunologic Testing and Preparation

The term "tissue typing" is loosely applied to a series of tests that may have a bearing on the choice of donor and on the patient's chances of receiving and retaining an organ.

Red Blood Cell Agglutinin Testing

Organ distribution follows rules similar to those for blood transfusion: type O kidneys may be transplanted into all recipients, but type O recipients can receive only type O kidneys, whereas AB-type recipients can receive kidneys of all blood types. In practice, kidneys are generally allocated to the type-specific recipient. With the scarcity of organs, it is particularly inappropriate to transplant type O kidneys into recipients who can receive organs of other types.

Histocompatibility Testing

The cells of every organism carry proteins known as major histocompatibility (MHC) antigens, important for allograft immune reactivity. The greater the differences between individuals, the greater the chance the recipient will reject the tissues or organs from the donor. However, other mechanisms also participate in the destructive process since grafts between perfectly matched pairs can be rejected, whereas those between disparate pairs may survive. In humans, MHC antigens are encoded by a set of genes located on chromosome 6 and designated human leukocyte antigens (HLAs). The antigens are distributed at several loci (A, B, C for class I; DR, DP, DQ for class II). The greatest clinical importance is focused on matching at the A, B, and DR loci. There are more than 120 antigenic specificities. Not all antigens can be clearly identified, as cross-reactions do occur. Each person inherits a "set" of antigens (one A, B, and DR) known as a "haplotype" from each parent. For most individuals, it is possible to identify all six antigens at the A, B, and DR loci. These haplotypes, identified by HLA serotyping, are used to determine the degree of similarity between prospective donors and recipients. This simplifies the process of identification of possible donors within a family, as only four possible permutations exist for the two "halves" of each parent. When a patient has several siblings, there is a 25% chance that one of them is identical at all loci (six-antigen match), a 25% chance of a total mismatch, and a 50% chance of being haploidentical (half-matched). Obviously, matches between parents and offspring can only be haploidentical (except in small populations in which inbreeding has resulted in a limited gene pool).

Matching has important connotations. Six-antigen matches continue to have the best long-term results and require the least amount of immunosuppression. Graft survival is excellent for six- and five-antigen matched cadaver kidneys; with lesser degrees of matching, the data are conflicting. Currently, if a medically suitable six-antigen matched recipient is identified for a kidney anywhere in the United States, it is mandatory for the kidney to be offered to the recipient. For all other kidneys, a computer-assisted allocation is made based on HLA matching, time waiting, and degree of sensitization.

It must be stressed that typing of HLA antigens does not give any indication of compatibility. It is important to determine whether a potential recipient has soluble antibodies against a potential recipient.

Cytotoxic Crossmatch

In a direct test of compatibility, the serum of a potential recipient is incubated with the lymphocytes of potential donors. Care must be taken to exclude autoantibodies (some patients have immunoglobulin M [IgM] antibodies that react universally and have no bearing on transplantation) and to confirm that the reaction occurs at room temperature. Lysis of the donor cells (a "positive crossmatch") signifies the presence of a circulating antibody that is destructive to the donor. Therefore, the crossmatch is essential before any renal transplant is performed, living or cadaver. Transplantation despite a true positive crossmatch usually leads to the aggressive, immediate loss of the graft (hyperacute rejection). With liver transplantation (LTX), a positive crossmatch does not seem to be of importance, possibly because destructive antibodies

are phagocytosed within the Kupffer cells of the liver itself. Due to time constraints, crossmatching generally has not been utilized for heart transplantation, although it does not seem to have major significance. However, since catastrophic hyperacute cardiac rejections have been reported in sensitized recipients and with retransplantation of the heart, crossmatching is selectively practiced. Recently, intensive plasmapheresis has been employed in selective patients to remove the antibody and carry out transplantation despite an antibody.

Antibody Testing

Antibody status is most commonly assessed using a panel of lymphocyte donors, representing the most commonly occurring HLA antigens. The sera of potential recipients are tested against this panel to determine the percentage of panel donor cells that are lysed by the recipient serum. This percent panel-reactive antibody (% PRA) provides a measure of the reactivity of the patient; a patient with a high PRA (sensitized patient) has difficulty obtaining a compatible kidney and may be at high risk for graft loss. Causes of such sensitization include previous transplants, blood transfusions, and pregnancy. The test is carried out when a patient is first placed on the waiting list and at intervals thereafter.

Specific anti-HLA antibodies can be identified by using a panel of polymer beads coated with purified HLA antigens using ELISA techniques. This recently introduced and very sensitive assay can be used to detect clinically important donor-specific anti-HLA antibody (DSA) before and after transplantation.

Blood Transfusion

Before cyclosporine immunosuppression, patients who had received blood transfusions were noted to have improved graft survival. After cyclosporine was introduced, this "transfusion effect" was no longer apparent; the deliberate use of blood transfusion as an immunosuppressive technique has all but disappeared. This is also true of "donor-specific transfusion" in which a live donor's blood was given to the recipient over several weeks before transplantation.

Other Investigations

Additional tests are carried out as necessary. Patients suspected of having circulating antibodies may be tested for antivascular endothelial antibodies or antiglomerular basement antibodies. Patients with a history of recurrent thrombotic events should be tested for hypercoagulable disorders.

Choice of Donor

A kidney may be obtained from a cadaveric donor or from a living donor (related or unrelated). Several factors must be taken into account to make a reasonable and prudent choice. First, kidneys can function well from a living or a cadaveric donor, as long as the donor is free of renal disease, hypertension, and systemic disease. However, the survival of kidneys transplanted from living donors is superior to that from other sources. This difference is best appreciated in terms of "half-life": the mean time that elapses for 50% of a cohort of transplanted kidneys to cease functioning. For patients receiving deceased donor renal transplants, the half-life is 11.6 years. For a one haplotype living related donor (LRD) transplant recipient, the half-life is 14 years and for a two-haplotype matched living related kidney recipient, the half-life is 24 years. Kidneys from living unrelated donors (LURDs) have results comparable to one haplotype LRDs. Spouses comprise most LURDs although there is a yearly increase of living altruistic donors. For the recipient, the long-term benefits of live donor kidneys include less immunosuppression and a reduced risk of rejection and loss of the kidney. Additional advantages of LRDs/LURDs are minimal waiting time and immediate diuresis (and consequently avoidance of dialysis and a shorter hospital stay). The disadvantage is that a healthy person (donor) must undergo a major operation without tangible benefit. The operative mortality risk for the donor is 3:10,000. There is also a small (<1%) risk of complications, such as infection or bleeding. A live donor has a normal life span, as can be noted from the fact that life insurance companies do not increase the premium payments of kidney donors.

Live Donors

The willing donor who is crossmatch compatible must undergo extensive preoperative evaluation, including a history and physical examination, chest radiography, ECG, and routine blood tests. The donor should be in excellent health and a grade I anesthetic risk. There must be no systemic disease that threatens the donor or the kidney. Requirements include normal creatinine clearance or radionuclide GFR, 24-hour urine protein

excretion, urinalysis, and urine culture. The crossmatch is repeated, and if it still shows compatibility, the final step before the transplant is a test to determine the anatomy of both kidneys and the number of arteries on each side; this is usually done with spiral computed tomography (CT).

The *operative technique* for live donor nephrectomy is an operation unlike any other in surgery. A healthy person undergoes the risk of a major operation for no direct benefit. Maximum care in handling tissues must be exercised, both for the sake of the donor and for the kidney functions immediately upon reimplantation in the recipient.

Currently, approximately 90% of donor nephrectomies in the United States are performed laparoscopically, mostly through a transperitoneal approach, while some use a retroperitoneal approach. Laparoscopic donor nephrectomy causes less pain and allows the patient to have a shorter hospital stay.

Open Donor Nephrectomy

After induction of anesthesia, the patient is placed in the lateral position over a kidney rest with a central venous line and Foley catheter in place to monitor fluid balance. A flank incision is made and carried through the bed of the twelfth rib. The peritoneum is retracted medially and Gerota's fascia opened. The ureter is dissected as far distally as possible. The renal artery and vein are dissected to their connections to the great vessels. For the left kidney, the adrenal and gonadal veins are divided between ligatures. If the right kidney is being removed, the mobilization must go right up to the vena cava. During dissection, urine output is carefully monitored, and fluids and diuretics are administered as necessary to ensure a brisk diuresis.

When donor and recipient teams are ready, the ureter is divided. In some centers, heparin is given before vascular clamps are placed across the renal artery and vein (on the right, the venous clamp is placed on the vena cava). The vessels are divided with the maximum possible length compatible with safety. The kidney is removed from the field, flushed with cold electrolyte solution, and taken to the recipient operating room. The stumps of donor vessels are secured. If heparin was given, it is reversed with protamine. Hemostasis is carefully ensured and the wound is closed.

Laparoscopic Donor Nephrectomy

The patient is placed in a lateral decubitus position, with the side of the kidney being removed superior, with the flanks hyperflexed. For a left nephrectomy, a veress needle is inserted into the left subcostal area and the abdomen insufflated. Three ports are used, with their placements varying by institution. The approach used at our institution is to place a 12-mm port in the umbilical region, one in the left lateral border of the rectus, just inferior to the first port, and then a 5-mm port in the epigastrium, approximately 2 inches inferior to the xiphoid. A 30° scope is used for visualization.

After the colon is reflected medially and either the spleen (for a left nephrectomy) or liver (for a right nephrectomy) is mobilized, the tissues surrounding the kidney are freed. The ureter is mobilized, the renal artery and vein dissected, being careful to ensure they are freed from their attachments to any surrounding tissue. The ureter, renal arteries, and veins are stapled and divided and the kidney removed via a vertical infraumbilical incision or a Pfannensteil incision. The kidney is removed from the field, placed in frozen saline slush, and the renal artery flushed with heparin.

Cadaver Donors

Organ Recovery and Distribution Network

Because most of the costs of renal transplantation are paid through Medicare coverage, the U.S. government has asserted its interest in and authority over the acquisition and distribution of organs. The Health Care Financing Administration (HCFA) awarded the contract to the United Network for Organ Sharing (UNOS), which has responsibility for all organ recovery and distribution. The 50 states are divided into 11 geographic regions. Representatives of each region, including donor and recipient advocates, surgeons, medical specialists, ethicists, and representatives of health organizations form the national policy-making board.

Within each region are one or more organ procurement organizations (OPOs), which are responsible for organ recovery in their geographic areas; distribution of organs occurs first on a regional and then on a national basis, according to definitive criteria, which differ with the organs concerned. The complexities of donor identification, declaration of death and donor maintenance, and organ distribution have given rise to a group of professionals, the transplant coordinators, with expertise in the field. In most cases, the hospital personnel who recognize that a patient may be a potential donor need only to call their regional OPA,

and much of the subsequent responsibility (as detailed below) is then assumed by them.

Organ Donor Identification

Organ donation should be considered whenever death is imminent in an individual free of transmissible disease, such as sepsis and malignancy. It should be possible to sustain perfusion of the vital organs until the final determination is made. In practical terms, the cause of death is usually a sudden intracranial event, such as trauma or a cerebrovascular accident. There is no absolute age requirement; organs from 80-year-old donors have been successfully transplanted. Although one organ may be known to be diseased, others may be salvageable (e.g., the kidneys from an alcoholic with cirrhosis). Any organ that is to be used must have acceptable function and be unaffected by disease or trauma. A kidney donor must generally be free of renal disease, hypertension, or systemic diseases known to affect kidneys. Different criteria apply for donation of other organs (Table 15.2). For example, in addition to absence of disease affecting the organs, heart, liver, and lung transplants must be matched in size to the prospective recipient. Finally, consent of the next of kin is required in the United States before organs are removed. In some European countries, organ removal is permitted so long as the family does not raise an objection. Because of the extreme shortage of organs, in the last few years, transplant programs have explored ways of increasing the number of potential donors through the use of expanded criteria donors (ECDs) and the use of organs from donors after cardiac death (DCD). The use of these organs has an increased relative risk of failure compared to standard criteria donors. However, when used in selected patient populations, they have been found to show good results. Furthermore, many programs are now using kidneys from donors who are hepatitis C positive in recipients who are hepatitis C positive. This "expanded" use of organs has allowed for continued growth in the number of deceased donors over the last few years.

Declaration of Death

In the United States, cadaver donors are determined to be dead by cerebral criteria ("brain death"), but circulation and ventilation are artificially maintained until organ removal. The advantage of pronouncement by cerebral criteria is that the operative procedure is carried out under controlled circumstances, and retrieved organs are therefore in better condition.

TABLE 15.2	Criteria for Exclusion of Organ Donors[a]			
Criterion	**Kidney**	**Heart**	**Liver**	**Pancreas**
Age (years)	>70	>60	>80	>50
Malignancy	+	+	+	+
Sepsis	+	+	+	+
Intravenous drug abuse	+/−	+/−	+/−	+/−
+Hepatitis B or C, HIV	+/−	+	+	+
Prolonged hypotension	+	+	+	+
DIC	+	+	+	+
Donor size incompatible	−	+	+	−
Abnormal ECG	−	+	−	−
Abnormal BUN, creatinine	+/−	−	−	−
Abnormal LFT	−	+/−	+	−

BUN, blood urea nitrogen; HIV, human immunodeficiency virus; DIC, disseminated intravascular coagulopathy; ECG, electrocardiogram; LFT, liver function tests.

[a]The crisis in organ availability prompts continued re-evaluation of criteria. For example, kidneys from older donors or those with known hypertension or diabetes may not be ruled out. A biopsy is often done and based on the degree of glomerular senescence or arteriolar disease, a decision may be made to use the kidney for an older recipient. Some have advocated using two suboptimal kidneys in a single recipient to provide adequate renal mass.

Without such criteria, donors are taken to the operating room, artificial support is discontinued, and organs are harvested after cessation of heartbeat. Under these circumstances, the chance of retrieving viable organs is reduced dramatically.

Cerebral criteria for death are as follows. (a) The cause of brain damage must be known. (b) There must be no brain-generated response to any neural stimulus (Table 15.3). These findings must occur under circumstances of normothermia and in the absence of drugs that may depress brain function, such as alcohol and barbiturates. When these clinical criteria are met, they can be confirmed by the finding of an isoelectric electroencephalogram (EEG) or a radionuclide scan or cerebral arteriogram that demonstrates an absence of cerebral blood flow. There is a clear distinction made between death and coma. However hopeless the prognosis for recovery of cerebral function, the diagnosis of death cannot be made unless all criteria are rigidly observed.

Maintenance of the Potential Donor

Once a potential donor has been identified, considerable time may elapse before death can be diagnosed with certainty and consent obtained. During this time, care and maintenance of the donor is critical. Most donors by this time are dehydrated, so massive fluid infusion is required. There may have been blood loss, which must be replaced, and the administration of colloid, together with diuretics, may be indicated. The choice of intravenous fluid is dictated by the circumstances; initially, isotonic solutions such as normal saline or lactated Ringer's solution may be required. If diabetes insipidus has set in, sodium is avoided and dilute glucose solutions are used; if the volume of dilute urine is too great to be effectively replaced, the administration of pitressin may be necessary. Recently, the use of thyroid replacement hormones has become widespread because of their effect on blood pressure maintenance. Prostaglandins may also play a role, when heart and or lung retrieval is to occur. The need to maintain good diuresis to preserve kidney function must be balanced against the possibility of fluid overload, which may compromise the heart or liver. The use of vasopressors also requires discretion. In all patients, meticulous asepsis must be

TABLE 15.3	Criteria for Absence of Brain Function

No pupillary response to light
No corneal reflex
No eye movement with doll's eyes or caloric testing
No motor response to supraorbital pain
No cough reflex
Apnea

observed in the care of catheters, endotracheal tubes, and so on. Blood chemistries should be obtained to monitor the function of liver, kidneys, and pancreas; cultures of blood and of other sites should be obtained to determine the presence of infection. Finally, serologic tests for hepatitis B and C, CMV, and HIV should be obtained.

Retrieval of Organs

As with any other surgical operation, cadaver donor nephrectomy must be conducted with maximum care, minimum blood loss, and preservation of all vital structures. This is even more important (and more difficult) when multiple organs are retrieved, which is increasingly the norm.

An incision is made from the sternal notch to the pubis. The chest and abdomen are opened simultaneously. A thoracic team isolates the great vessels and passes vessel tapes around them in preparation for removal. Simultaneously, an abdominal team dissects and isolates the blood supply to the liver: the isolation of hepatic artery or arteries and portal vein must be done without compromise to other viscera, such as the pancreas and kidneys. The distal aorta is encircled and supraceliac dissection is done for placement of a clamp. When all preliminary dissection has been completed, the patient is heparinized, the distal aorta is cannulated, the aorta is cross-clamped above the celiac axis, and preservation solution is flushed into the distal aorta, cooling all abdominal organs. Venting the vena cava above the diaphragm provides outflow. The thoracic team simultaneously cools and removes the heart. The abdominal organs are removed sequentially, with the blood vessels to each being carefully preserved. Once the needed organs are removed and packaged, the spleen and a large number of lymph nodes are also removed to provide a source of lymphocytes for HLA typing and crossmatching.

When only the kidneys are to be retrieved, the abdomen is opened through a full midline incision, which may be converted to a cruciate incision. The right colon is mobilized and, together with the small intestine, retracted above and to the donor's left. The aorta and vena cava are visualized and traced up to the renal arteries and veins. The superior mesenteric artery is identified, ligated, and divided. Dissection is continued cephalad on the aorta to allow room for a clamp or a tie proximal to the renal arteries. Both kidneys are mobilized, so they are attached only by the renal vessels to the aorta and vena cava. Care is taken to preserve the ureters throughout their length

and to leave a sheath of adventitial tissue attached to them. The ureters are divided close to the bladder. The donor is given 20,000 units of heparin and the distal aorta is cannulated. The aorta and vena cava are ligated and divided distally and then mobilized cephalad by dividing pairs of lumbar vessels between clips until both kidneys are now completely free and attached only by the proximal aorta and vena cava. At this point, a clamp is placed across the proximal aorta and cold preservation solution is flushed through the aortic cannula. The vena cava, which is also clamped proximally, is opened distally to provide outflow. In this fashion, both kidneys may rapidly be flushed free of blood and cooled. Once cooling is accomplished, the aorta and vena cava are transected proximally, the kidneys are removed, immersed in cold solution, and then separated and packaged in sterile insulated containers immersed in ice for transportation.

Preservation

Preservation of solid organs is based on the premise that deep hypothermia reduces metabolic requirements. The initial step is for all solid organs to be flushed *in situ* using iced preservation solution (via cannulation of the distal aorta in the donor, as already discussed). Reduction of the core temperature to 0°C causes cellular metabolism to slow by a factor of 12 to 13 and the requirements for ATP and oxygen to be reduced markedly. However, the anaerobic state leads to acidosis and paralysis of the Na–K pump, which increases interstitial edema and causes cell swelling and ultimately cell death.

The ideal preservation solution minimizes cell swelling, prevents intracellular acidosis, and restricts interstitial expansion during the perfusion period. It also prevents injury from oxygen-derived free radicals and provides a substrate for the generation of high-energy phosphate compounds during the reperfusion period. The University of Wisconsin (UW) lactobionate solution comes closest to achieving these goals. It contains impermeable osmotic agents (potassium lactobionate and raffinose) that minimize cell swelling and exert an effective oncotic pressure to reduce interstitial swelling, a hydrogen ion buffer (phosphate), and precursors for ATP production (adenosine). It also contains glutathione and allopurinol to counteract oxygen-free radical injury. Preservation time using UW solution has been extended up to 72 hours for the kidney and pancreas and up to 30 hours for the liver. Therefore, UW solution has largely supplanted Collins solution for solid organ preservation.

The University of Wisconsin preservation solution has the following ingredients:

Component	Action
Potassium lactobionate	Osmotic agent
Raffinose	Osmotic agent
Phosphate	Buffer
Adenosine	Precursor to ATP production
Glutathione	Free radical scavenger
Allopurinol	Free radical scavenger

As an alternative to cold storage, kidneys may also be preserved by pulsatile perfusion. After being flushed and cooled, the kidneys are connected via a cannula in the aorta or renal artery to the pulsatile perfusion apparatus. A plasma solution or modified UW solution is perfused through the cannula; it emerges through the renal vein and is collected in a chamber in which flow can be measured. After filtration and aeration, it is recirculated. The temperature is maintained at 4°C. In addition to providing a longer preservation time, this method permits measurement of pressure and flows and can thus provide a means of assessing viability. Preservation for more than 72 hours is regularly achieved. These extended preservation times allow a kidney to be sent anywhere in the world. It should be cautioned, however, that in prospective randomized clinical trials comparing perfusion and static storage in matched-donor pairs little significant difference has been shown between the two methods up to 24 hours. Therefore, from an immunologic, economic, and functional point of view, for routine preservation, static storage is the norm, while pulsatile preservation is increasing for the use of ECD and DCD donor organs.

SURGICAL TECHNIQUES FOR RENAL TRANSPLANTATION

The standard approach for transplantation of the kidney is through an extraperitoneal incision in the iliac fossa. The peritoneum is retracted medially and the iliac vessels are exposed. The renal vein is usually anastomosed end to side into the external iliac vein. The renal artery may be similarly anastomosed to the external iliac artery or anastomosed end-to-end to the divided hypogastric artery. The vascular clamps

are then released. When good flow to the kidney is confirmed, the ureter is attached to the bladder using an antireflux implantation. Modification of the technique may be required because of the presence of vascular disease, urologic abnormalities, or gross disparity in size, such as an adult kidney in an infant. In the latter case, the vascular anastomoses are done to the aorta and the vena cava through a standard midline incision. Care must be taken that hemostasis is absolute. If possible, division of large lymphatics is avoided; if unavoidable, these lymphatics must be ligated to prevent the occurrence of a lymphocele. Frequent, liberal irrigation of the wound is carried out with antiseptic solution. If surgical drains are used, they should be of the closed suction variety.

Of equal importance to surgical technique is management of the recipient before and during the operation. Most patients should be dialyzed within the 24 to 48 hours preceding the operation to ensure optimum body chemistry. Perioperative prophylactic antibiotics are given. Some immunosuppressives are more effective if started preoperatively. Caution should be exercised in the use of anesthetic agents that are predominantly excreted by the kidney, with special reference to muscle relaxants: a patient with acute tubular necrosis may otherwise have respiratory paralysis for an extended period. Attention must also be given to adequate fluid management. Despite renal failure, recipients may be fluid-depleted as a result of preoperative dialysis, intraoperative blood and insensible loss, and perhaps a large urine volume from the newly transplanted kidney. Inadequate administration of fluid may result in renal shutdown. We routinely monitor the central venous pressure as a guide to fluid and diuretic therapy. It is customary to administer diuretics after the vascular clamps are released in the recipient. Mannitol and furosemide are usually given singly or in combination. Finally, those who have not received any immunosuppressive agents prior to the procedure should receive them during the operation.

TRANSPLANTATION IMMUNOLOGY

The long-term success of transplantation depends on the prevention of graft rejection while simultaneously preserving the ability of the recipient to respond to other foreign antigens. For the most part, the immune process is mediated through the actions of lymphocytes. Totipotent cells of the bone marrow differentiate into precursors of the various cellular elements of the blood. Lymphocytes undergo maturation in the thymus (T cells) or in other various areas, such as bone marrow, spleen, and Peyer's patches (B cells). B cells are large and short-lived, whereas T lymphocytes are small and long-lived.

The multiple roles of T cells may be classified according to function: cytotoxic cells (T_C) whose principal function is to effect destruction, helper cells (T_H), which aid in the differentiation of other lymphocytes, and suppressor cells (T_S) which curb cytotoxic functions and thus permit tolerance. The T_S cells act as a balance to the T_C cells. T lymphocytes are better classified by specific cell surface antigens, known as cluster of differentiation (CD) receptors. Many CD antigens exist, but CD4 and CD8 are probably the best known. They generally, but not absolutely, correspond to the functional description of the T cells. Generally, T_H cells are $CD4^+$ and react with class II molecules (e.g., HLA DR), whereas T_C cells are usually $CD8^+$ and react with class I molecules, HLA A and B. All T cells also carry the cell antigen recognition complex, $CD3^+$.

The T cells diffuse through body tissues, entering the bloodstream from the thymus. They enter the lymph nodes through venules and afferent lymphatic channels. Lymphocytes leave the nodes via efferent lymphatics, which merge with other channels, to enter the bloodstream via the thoracic duct. Because lymph flowing into the nodes also contains antigens and dendritic cells, the stage is set for the first encounter in the immune response. Foreign antigen can directly stimulate small numbers of T_H, T_C, and B cells to perform their respective functions, but rejection appears to depend mostly on the effects of lymphokines (Fig. 15.1).

Normally quiescent, T cells require two separate signals to become activated. A foreign antigen is ingested by an antigen-presenting cell (APC), usually a macrophage or dendritic cell, which processes it in a way that permits recognition by the clone of T_H cells that possess the CD3 complex specific for that antigen. With the double signals from the APC and the antigen, interleukin (IL)-1 is secreted, stimulating the clone of T_H cells to proliferate and release IL-2. This is a critical point in the process. IL-2 is essential for the further differentiation and proliferation of antigen-stimulated T_C cells. It also acts as a stimulus for the further proliferation of T_H cells, both escalating and perpetuating the process. IL-2 stimulates interferon (IFN), which mobilizes macrophages

and causes many cells to increase their expression of MHC antigens on the surface, thereby increasing their vulnerability. Finally, IL-2 is necessary for the stimulation of resting B cells to proliferate and differentiate into plasma cells, which produce antibodies. Inhibition of IL-2 may therefore play a significant role in the abrogation of the immune response. In addition to the processes described, some T_H cells remain as memory cells to respond to that same antigen in the future. T_S cells are also stimulated to proliferate and act as a balance to the cytotoxic cells.

The CD4+ T lymphocytes have been subdivided into two groups: T_H1, which stimulate a cell-mediated response, and T_H2, which stimulate a humoral response. T_H1 cells produce IFNγ, which stimulates the endothelial cells and the APCs, and that they secrete IL-2, which stimulates the activation of T cells. The T_H2 cells produce IL-4 and IL-10, both of which inhibit differentiation of the T_H1 cell line, as well as IL-5, which stimulates B cell growth, eosinophilia, and immunoglobulin secretion. Studies suggest that an immune response predominated by T_H1 cells may be more acutely damaging, while T_H2 cells are more predominant in chronic rejection. Further research is investigating the actions of all of the specific cytokines involved.

Cell adhesion molecules (Table 15.4) are now recognized as integral in the acute rejection process. The activation of T cells and endothelial cells causes upregulation and expression of various cell adhesion molecules. These cell adhesion molecules are part of the integrin family and are important not only in the migration of T cells but also in promoting activation of the lymphocytes. CD28 is one of this family of molecules that binds with one of the B7 family of proteins that resides on APCs, stimulates the production of high levels of cytokines and chemokines, as well as promotes T cell proliferation. CTLA-4, similar in structure to CD28, instead inhibits the early steps of T cell activation and thus the immune response.

If unchecked, the immune process continues until the antigen is destroyed by two mechanisms: cellular rejection, through the agency of lymphokines (e.g., tumor necrosis factor); and humoral rejection, caused by soluble antibodies released through the activation of B cells. Numerous lymphokines (including interleukins) have been identified. Understanding these processes has allowed us the building blocks to arm ourselves against both the prevention and the treatment of rejection.

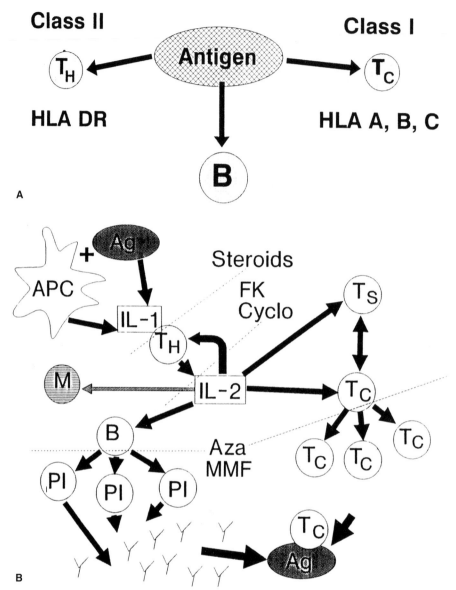

FIGURE 15.1. **A:** Immune response: antigen-activated cells. Class I molecules of the antigen (usually HLA A, B, C) stimulate CD8+ cytotoxic cells (T_C); class II (HLA DR) stimulate CD4+ helper cells (T_H). B cells are also stimulated directly. **B:** Immune response: lymphokine-activated cells. Action of immunosuppressive agents. Antigen (Ag) and antigen-presenting cells (APC) send separate signals, which cause IL 1 to be secreted by the helper (T_H) cell. T_H secretes IL 2, which (i) stimulates further proliferation of T_H; (ii) stimulates B cells to differentiate into plasma cells (PI), which secret antibody; (iii) stimulate cytotoxic (T_C) cells to proliferate; (iv) causes T_S cells to proliferate while maintaining a balance with T_C cells; and (v) causes some T_H cells to become memory cells (M) to react to future stimuli. Dotted lines show action of drugs: corticosteroids act by blocking production of IL-1, cyclosporine (*Cyclo*) and tacrolimus (FK) by blocking IL-2, and Azathioprine (*AzA*) and mycophenolate mofetil (MMF) by inhibiting cell proliferation.

TABLE 15.4	Common Cell Adhesion Molecules
T Cells	**Antigen-presenting Cells**
LFA-1 (CD 11 a/18)	ICAM-1 (CD 54), ICAM-2
CD 28	B7-1 (CD 80), B7-2 (CD 86)
CTLA4	B7-2 (CD 86), B7-1 (CD 80)
VLA-4 (CD 49 d/29)	VCAM-1 (CD 106)

PREVENTING REJECTION

Except between identical twins, transplantation without immunosuppression is uniformly unsuccessful. The earlier approaches—massive steroid doses, total body irradiation, and thoracic duct drainage—have largely given way to more selective immunosuppression, in smaller doses.

Until 1984, two drugs (prednisone and azathioprine) formed the cornerstone of immunosuppressive therapy; since then cyclosporine has become the mainstay. In addition, polyclonal and monoclonal antibodies, although mainly used to treat rejection, are also used as part of induction protocols. Calcineurin inhibitors (Cyclosporine or Tacrolimus) are the drugs of choice; they are usually given with low-dose steroids, often in combination with a third drug (Table 15.5).

1. *Corticosteroids.* These agents block the activation of IL-1 and thus indirectly IL-2. They also have an anti-inflammatory effect, which may help minimize the rejection injury (IL-1 was previously called endogenous pyrogen). Most centers now use a low-dosage schedule (e.g., total daily dose of 25 mg/d achieved within the first month), which has resulted in a significant decline in complications while kidney and patient survival has improved. The dose is tapered until a low maintenance level is achieved. In children and selected adults, minimization or total withdrawal of steroids may be possible.

2. *Cyclosporine.* Cyclosporine (CsA), a fat-soluble extract of fungal origin, has revolutionized transplantation since the first reports of its clinical use in 1978. It blocks secretion of IL-2, the essential stimulus to the further proliferation and differentiation of T cells. Cyclosporine has been found to work only on resting T cells, not activated ones. CsA binds to its intracellular binding protein, cyclophilin. Cyclophilin is an example of a class of intracellular receptors found in T cells known as immunophilins. Two such proteins have been described: cyclophilin and FK binding protein (FKBP) (see below). This CsA–cyclophilin complex, in turn, inhibits calcineurin. Calcineurin is an enzyme involved in the activation of genes responsible for the immune response by a mechanism that has not yet been elucidated. By inhibiting calcineurin, CsA blocks secretion of IL-2. It must be administered intravenously or orally in an oil-based solution or in capsules.

It was initially hoped that CsA alone would be effective, but rejection usually ensues unless a second agent is given. In the United States, CsA is used with small doses of corticosteroids. Unfortunately, CsA is nephrotoxic and its use in renal transplantation can cause clinical dilemmas. With deceased donor kidneys,

TABLE 15.5	Immunosuppressive Agents	
Agent	**Action**	**Toxicity**
Corticosteroids	Blocks IL-1	Physical appearance, hyperglycemia, avascular necrosis of bone
Cyclosporine A	Blocks IL-2	Hepatotoxicity, nephrotoxicity, hirsutism, gingival hyperplasia, hypertension
Azathioprine	Blocks cell proliferation	Bone marrow suppression, hepatotoxicity
Antilymphocyte globulin (ALG)	Lymphocytolytic	Thrombocytopenia, leukopenia, fever, serum sickness
OKT3	Blocks T cell effector function	High fever, chills, GI symptoms, pulmonary edema
Tacrolimus (FK506)	Blocks IL-2	Tremors, headache, nephrotoxicity, glucose intolerance, hyperkalemia
Mycophenolate mofetil	Blocks cell proliferation	Nausea, vomiting, diarrhea
Sirolimus	Blocks IL-2 action	Inhibits wound healing, hyperlipidemia, thrombocytopenia.

early graft dysfunction often occurs; and to avoid toxicity, it is common not to use CsA until good renal function has been established. During this period of uncertainty, the use of antilymphocyte globulin (ALG or ATG) or the IL-2 blocking monoclonal antibodies, such as basiliximab or daclizumab, offers high degree of protection against rejection until the kidney has recovered sufficient function for CsA to be started. Later in the course, an elevated serum creatinine level may pose a problem: It may be due to CsA toxicity, which would require reduction of CsA dosage; or it may be secondary to acute rejection, which would mandate augmented immunosuppression. When the clinical circumstances are unclear, measurement of blood levels of CsA may be helpful; needle biopsy of the kidney can also be useful by establishing the presence or absence of rejection.

3. *Tacrolimus (FK 506).* Tacrolimus is a macrolide antibiotic derived from a fungal source. Although structurally dissimilar to CsA, its mechanism of action is similar. Essentially, both work by blocking IL-2 expression and production. Like CsA, Tacrolimus works by binding to its cytoplasmic receptor, FKBP. In a mechanism similar to that described for CsA–cyclophilin, FK–FKBP inhibits the T cell's calcineurin, which in turn renders the T cell unable to produce IL-2. Tacrolimus is approximately 500 times more potent than CsA.

Originally used to rescue patients suffering from steroid- or OKT3-resistant rejection, Tacrolimus has become one of the basic immunosuppressive agents used for kidney and liver allograft recipients. Several prospective, randomized clinical trials have demonstrated that the efficacies of CsA and FK506 as initial therapy after renal allograft transplantation are similar. These studies have shown that (a) the nephrotoxicities of the two agents were similar; (b) there was decreased hypertension, cholesterol, gingival hyperplasia, and change in physical appearance; but (c) there was increased neurotoxicity (e.g., headaches, paresthesias) and pancreatic beta-cell toxicities (insulin requiring diabetes mellitus) with Tacrolimus.

Tacrolimus is rarely given as an initial intravenous dose but usually is switched within 24 hours to an oral formulation. Tacrolimus and CsA are not given together, as their mechanisms of action are similar, and when used in combination they may have an increased nephrotoxic effect. Like CsA, Tacrolimus is metabolized in the liver. The therapeutic window for

this agent is narrow so it is important to monitor the 12-hour trough blood levels in patients on Tacrolimus.

Cyclosporine and Tacrolimus and Sirolimus (see below) are metabolized through the cytochrome P-450 enzyme system of the liver, as are many commonly used therapeutic agents. Thus the use of erythromycin or ketoconazole may result in augmentation of the effect of CsA and FK and possibly toxicity, whereas rifampin and diphenylhydantoin may cause a reduction of the CsA and FK level and precipitate rejection. One must always be alert to the possibility of drug interactions in patients on these agents.

4. *Azathioprine.* Azathioprine (AZA), one of the earliest agents, continues to play a role in transplantation. A derivative of 6-mercaptopurine, it is an antimetabolite that acts more peripherally in the immune process by blocking DNA synthesis and by inhibiting cell division. The action is nonspecific and affects all dividing cells. Bone marrow suppression is a common complication, and the white blood cell (WBC) count must be monitored carefully.

The clinical difficulties often encountered with the use of CsA have led many centers to adopt a "triple therapy" protocol, wherein all three agents (prednisone, AZA, CsA) are used in relatively small doses, thereby minimizing the toxic effects, and the immunosuppressive effects are additive. Because each works at a different point in the process, it is an appealing approach. It also offers some protection if one of the agents must be discontinued.

5. *Mycophenolate mofetil.* A modified ester of mycophenolic acid (a fermentation product of several *Penicillium* species), mycophenolate mofetil (MMF), is effective when taken orally. Essentially, MMF blocks *de novo* purine synthesis. Unlike most cells, lymphocytes (T and B) rely on this pathway more than the salvage pathway for purine synthesis, and so MMF prevents T and B cell proliferation. MMF also appears to decrease smooth muscle proliferation within blood vessels. Its mechanism of action is similar to that of azathioprine in that both agents are antiproliferative medications. Currently, MMF is being used at many centers as part of the primary immunosuppressive regimen. It has also been used in patients with chronic rejection and for acute rejection that is refractory to standard therapy. Azathioprine and MMF are not used together because they are both antiproliferative agents. There are several known adverse effects of MMF, the most prominent being gastrointestinal

effects (diarrhea, nausea, vomiting) and dose-responsive leukopenia and thrombocytopenia.

6. *Antilymphocyte globulin/thymoglobulin.* Antilymphocyte globulin (ALG) or antithymocyte globulin (ATG) is an antiserum to human lymphocytes, created in animals (rabbits, horses, goats). The globulin fraction is extracted from the serum of the animal and contains a potent polyclonal antilymphocyte antibody that acts by destroying or masking T cell antigens; it may also promote the development of suppressor cells. It is relatively nonselective and has effects on other cellular elements of the blood. Administered in dilute intravenous solution into a central vein, it has three principal uses: induction therapy, initial prophylaxis during a period of graft dysfunction, and treatment for established acute rejection.

7. *Muromonab CD3 (OKT3).* Among the first of a new generation of products, OKT3 is a hybridoma product. It is engineered by fusion of a strain of immortal mouse myeloma cells with cells from a mouse immunized against human lymphocytes. Cells selected for their specific activity against the CD3 antigen recognition complex are then propagated. The resultant monoclonal antibody is specific, consistent, and predictable. It is not subject to biologic variability like the polyclonal ALG and does not affect the other cellular elements of blood. One of the disadvantages is the fact that antibodies develop against the mouse antibody (anti-idiotype antibodies), which renders the product ineffective after some time. Other adverse effects are the initial physiologic reactions to the first few doses of OKT3, including fever, diarrhea, and sometimes bronchospasm, pulmonary edema, and meningeal irritation. Thus, patients must be adequately prepared by diuresis or dialysis to remove excess fluid and by premedication to mitigate the severity of the initial response. OKT3 is most useful for the treatment of acute rejection, but it is occasionally used for initial prophylaxis or induction.

8. *Anti-IL-2 monoclonal antibodies.* With the development of monoclonal technology came the development of specific antibodies that interfere with IL-2 and thus interfere with the upregulation of the T cytotoxic cell. Unlike Thymoglobulin, these drugs either in the form of basiliximab or in the form of daclizumab can be administered peripherally and do not have the same toxic effects. They do not cause a cytokine release syndrome and are relatively benign with regards to side effects. They are used for induction therapy.

9. *Sirolimus (rapamycin).* Rapamycin is another macrolide antibiotic derived from a fungal source found in Rappanui (Easter Islands). This agent is structurally similar to Tacrolimus, but its mechanism of action is different. Unlike Cyclosporine or Tacrolimus, rapamycin does not block IL-2 expression and production; rather, it blocks cytokine-mediated signal transduction (e.g., IL-2 and IL-2 receptors), thereby preventing cell proliferation. Because the mechanism of action is different from that of the calcineurin inhibitors and because rapamycin and the calcineurin inhibitors appear to block cell proliferation at different steps, there is much work focusing on using these two agents in combination. It is thought that the calcineurin inhibitors and rapamycin may work synergistically and that the dose requirements of the two agents can be reduced without compromising adequate immunosuppression. Rapamycin has been looked upon as a nephron-sparing drug allowing for either CNI minimization or withdrawal.

Other Approaches

In addition to chemical agents, experimental efforts are being directed toward biologic methods to induce tolerance. Administration of donor bone marrow simultaneously with the organ and selective irradiation of the recipient prior to transplantation are two such approaches. New, highly specific monoclonal antibodies are being designed to disable the mechanisms specific to the graft while leaving all other mechanisms intact. Because recognition of a foreign antigen requires two signals, blocking one of them is a potential avenue to creating tolerance. CTLA4Ig is a synthetic agent that competes for the CD-28 binding site on the lymphocyte. Because it has great avidity for the ligand, it has been successfully used experimentally to create tolerance. Clinical trials in humans are under way.

REJECTION

Classification

Total abolition of the immune response is impractical and undesirable, so rejection occurs despite prophylactic drug regimens. It is frequently simplified into "humoral" and "cellular" types, but there is considerable overlap.

Pure humoral (*hyperacute*) rejection occurs when a kidney is transplanted into a patient who has circulating antibodies to donor antigens. These antibodies

TABLE 15.6	Criteria for Categorizing Rejection	
Type	**Mechanism**	**Pathology**
Hyperacute	Circulating antibodies	Endothelial swelling, platelet thrombi, glomerular and arteriolar thrombosis, fibrinoid necrosis
Acute	Cell-mediated	Edema, lymphocytic infiltration, hemorrhage
Chronic	? Antibody-mediated	Endothelial thickening, fibrosis, vascular occlusion

attack the vascular endothelium of the graft, resulting in endothelial damage, platelet aggregation, and rapid vascular occlusion of the graft (Table 15.6).

More common is the *acute rejection* "crisis." This process requires recognition of a foreign antigen by host lymphocytes, the creation of effector cells, and finally the destruction or attempted destruction of the graft. Although acute rejection is more common during the first few months after transplantation, it can occur at any time. Histologic examination of acute rejection reveals massive infiltration of the interstitium, tubules (tubulitis), glomeruli (glomerulitis), and vascular endothelium (arteritis) with lymphocytes and monocytes, together with edema and some protein deposition within Bowman's space (Fig. 15.2). It should be noted that severe, transmural arteritis involving the whole arterial wall (endothelium, medial smooth muscles, media) involves not only lymphocytes and mononuclear cells, but also polymorphonuclear leukocytes. To standardize how pathologists and transplant physicians around the world define rejection and attempt to elucidate the most effective immunosuppressive regimen for patients suffering from acute rejection, the Banff classification was developed. Renal biopsies are graded in ascending order depending on the severity of the acute rejection (Table 15.7).

Finally, *chronic rejection* (chronic allograft dysfunction [CAD]) is a process that takes place over weeks, months, or years. It consists of a gradual restriction of the blood supply, starting with subendothelial thickening and fibrosis, and results in the eventual loss of the kidney (Fig. 15.3). In the age of such potent immunosuppression regimens, chronic rejection has become a dominant cause of graft loss.

Diagnosis and Treatment

Hyperacute rejection, usually apparent in the operating room, presents as a rapid vascular occlusion that occurs despite an apparently patent anastomosis. The manifestations may be delayed by some hours, in which case it presents as a rapid loss of function of the graft. Investigations such as radionuclide scanning, duplex sonography, and arteriography demonstrate the loss of blood supply. There is no treatment except the immediate removal of the graft. The key is in prevention and can be usually, but not always, prevented by a reliable crossmatch.

Chronic rejection also has no treatment and is a diagnosis of exclusion. Care must be exercised that a treatable lesion is not missed. When a patient who has apparently had good function for a period of time demonstrates gradual deterioration of renal function, the cause must be investigated. In the absence of any other explanation, such as renal artery stenosis or ureteral stenosis, the diagnosis of chronic rejection may be assumed and can be confirmed by biopsy. Because there is no treatment, immunosuppression is continued until such time that the patient once again requires dialysis or can receive a new transplant.

An acute rejection crisis is usually an easily recognizable syndrome, a combination of an acute inflammatory response and acute renal failure. The patient may have fever, tenderness over the graft site, and leukocytosis, as well as oliguria, hypertension, proteinuria, and an elevated serum creatinine level. The clinical syndrome may be mild, such as a minimal rise in creatinine or a minor elevation in temperature with no other clinical symptomatology, and the diagnosis is sometimes difficult to establish. It is important that other causes of some of these findings are not missed. A urinary leak may cause localized pain and tenderness, fever, leukocytosis, and oliguria. A viral infection, such as CMV, can similarly present with fever and creatinine elevation. Loading the patients with steroids in these other situations would clearly be disastrous.

A renal biopsy is standard procedure to confirm the diagnosis of acute rejection and to assess the severity

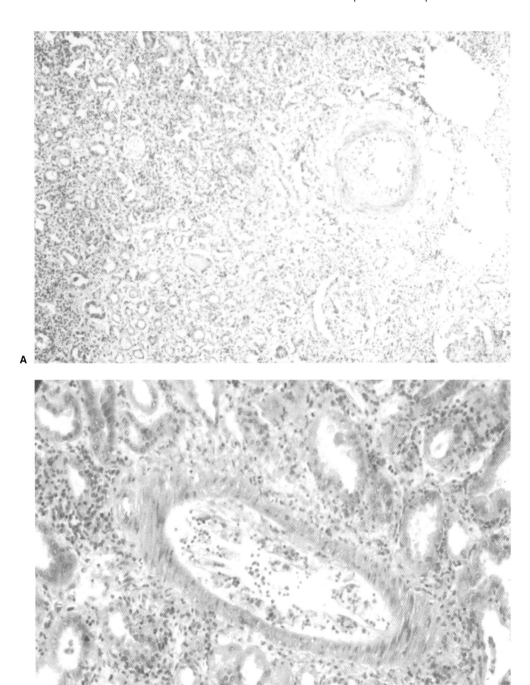

FIGURE 15.2.   Acute rejection: histologic appearance, under low power **(A)** and high power **(B)** light microscopy, of a core-needle biopsy specimen of kidney. Note edema and diffuse infiltration with mononuclear lymphocytes; vasculitis is manifested by infiltration and endothelial swelling and proliferation. Glomeruli show swelling, but the architecture is preserved. (H&E)

TABLE 15.7	Banff Diagnostic Categories for Renal Allograft Biopsies	
Category	**Definition**	**Pathology**
Normal	No abnormalities	No glomerular abnormalities; no cellular infiltration; no tubulitis; no vascular abnormalities
Antibody Mediated rejection (ABMR)		Documentation of circulating antidonor antibody and C4 d, allograft pathology
	Type I	ATN- like minimal inflammation
	Type II	Capillary and or glomerular inflammation and/or thromboses
	Type III	Arterial
Chronic active antibody-mediated rejection (CABMR)		C4 d+, circulating antidonor antibodies; evidence of chronic injury, such as glomerular double contours, peritubular capillary basement membrane multilayering, interstitial fibrosis/tubular atrophy, fibrous arterial intimal thickening
Borderline changes	Suggestive of rejection (nondiagnostic)	No intimal arteritis present, mild or moderate focal cellular infiltrate; mild tubulitis and/or mild glomerulitis
Acute T cell mediated rejection (TCMR)	Grade IA	Significant interstitial infiltrate (>25% of parenchyma affected) and foci of moderate tubulitis
	Grade IB	Significant interstitial infiltrate (>25% of parenchyma affected) and foci of *severe* tubulitis
	Grade IIA	Mild to moderate intimal arteritis
	Grade IIB	Severe arteritis comprising >25% of the luminal area
	Grade III	Transmural arteritis and/or fibrinoid changes and necrosis of medial smooth muscle cells with lymphocytic infiltrate
Chronic active T-cell-mediated rejection		Intimal fibrosis with mononuclear cell infiltrate, formation of neo-intima (chronic allograft arteriopathy)
Interstitial fibrosis and tubular atrophy		No evidence of any specific etiology, includes vascular and glomerular sclerosis; graded by tubulointerstitial features

of the rejection (Table 15.7). If immunostaining shows the presence of C4 d in a peritubular capillary distribution, antibody or humoral mediated rejection is likely and specific treatment with plasmapheresis and intravenous immune globulin is indicated. In this setting, peripheral blood testing for donor-specific anti-HLA antibody is important. The titer of the antibody can be used to guide therapy. Renal sonography with Doppler studies to assess the vascular resistivity index and rule out obstruction is usually done. Radionuclide scanning is helpful to assess renal perfusion.

Acute rejection can usually be reversed with treatment. First-line therapy is usually intravenous high-dose methylprednisolone. Secondary therapy may include thymoglobulin or high-dose Tacrolimus. Plasmapheresis with intravenous immune globulin or Rituximab, a monoclonal antibody therapy directed at CD20, an important B cell surface protein, might be indicated if biopsy reveals that the patient is undergoing an antibody-mediated rejection.

COMPLICATIONS OF TRANSPLANTATION

Complications of transplantation may be considered in three broad categories: complications due to the immunosuppressed state, those engendered by the surgical operation, and those due to the medications used.

Complications of the Immunosuppressed State

General impairment of host defenses occurs at extremes of age, in the presence of certain malignancies, after chemotherapy for malignancy, in patients with immune deficiency syndromes, and in patient's

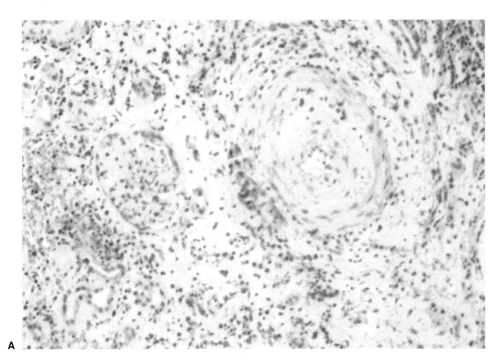

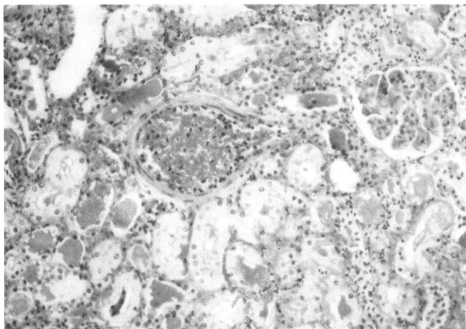

FIGURE 15.3. Chronic rejection: histologic appearance of core-needle biopsy specimen of kidney under low power **(A)** and high power **(B)** light microscopy. Note in **(A)** the extensive fibrosis, almost total obliteration of the vascular lumen by proliferative endarteritis, areas of tubular atrophy, and patchy lymphocytic infiltrate. (H&E)

immunosuppressed after transplantation. One consequence of immunosuppression is increased susceptibility to infection from all sources, including bacterial, viral, fungal, rickettsial, protozoan, and parasitic. Vigilance is therefore required during the management of these patients. Aggressive evaluation is carried out for minor temperature elevations and vague syndromes such as malaise and joint pains cannot be ignored.

Most infections, if diagnosed early, can be treated effectively with the appropriate agent. If infection is life threatening (e.g., meningitis or severe viral pneumonia), immunosuppression is terminated to allow host defenses to recover. This may result in loss of the kidney, which is preferable to the death of the patient. For less-severe infections, high doses of immunosuppressive drugs are usually reduced; if doses are already low, they are usually continued unless it is apparent that the therapeutic agent is not effectively reversing the infectious process. Whenever possible the specific agent for the bacteria, viruses, or parasites involved is administered. Infections after transplantation generally fall into predictable, and thereby sometimes preventable, patterns.

First Transplant Month

During the early postoperative period, infections that include those in any surgical patient (e.g., pneumonia, urinary tract infection, line sepsis). Special care must be exercised to prevent their occurrence and to treat any event rapidly and aggressively. Infection during this period may also result from donor causes inadvertently transmitted with the transplanted organ. As mentioned previously, careful screening of donors is critical.

Reactivation of latent herpes simplex virus (HSV) can also begin during the early postoperative period. Viruses of this category can be controlled, though not eradicated, with the use of acyclovir.

One to Six Months

Opportunistic infections are most likely to manifest during the first 1 to 6 months. Cytomegalovirus (CMV) is a common viral infection, the clinical presentation of which ranges from a mild nonspecific febrile illness to lethal multiorgan failure. Milder forms may require no intervention or a modest reduction of immunosuppressive agents. Serious forms require aggressive management, including drawing a blood gas to detect hypoxia that may be seen even before chest radiographs become abnormal and pathologic diagnosis, by aspirate, bronchoscopy, or open lung biopsy, to confirm the disease. The risk of CMV infection is greatest in those recipients treated with thymoglobulin for induction therapy and those patients who received a CMV positive organ (D+) and they were CMV seronegative (R−).

Treatment then consists of cessation of immunosuppression except for stress doses of steroids and the administration of hyperimmune serum and antiviral agents such as ganciclovir or foscarnet. Other viral infections (e.g., HSV, herpes zoster, and EBV) are also likely to occur during this period. Acyclovir is useful for managing some of these problems. Recently, BK virus has been found to be a cause of renal transplant dysfunction. Treatment of this viral infection consists of reduction in the immunosuppressive medications.

Pneumocystis pneumoniae is also often seen within the first 6 months and requires aggressive diagnostic measures when the diagnosis is suspected. Treatment is with sulfamethoxazole and trimethoprim (Bactrim) or pentamidine. Both have also been used as effective prophylaxis.

After 6 Months

Patients with stable graft function on low-dose immunosuppression usually have similar infections to other people in the community. Patients who have received high-dose therapy or repeated rejection treatment continue to be at risk for opportunistic infection.

There is also an increased risk of malignancy in all immunosuppressed patients. This is particularly true of skin malignancies, such as squamous cell and basal cell carcinomas and malignancies of the lymphoid system. The former are most notable in regions of excessive sunshine, such as southern California and Australia. Patients should be carefully monitored for new skin lesions, which must be aggressively removed as they appear.

With posttransplant lymphoproliferative disorder (PTLD), the general incidence of lymphoma ranges from 1% in kidney recipients to 4.5% in heart–lung recipients. Lymphomas constitute 22% of all cancers in transplant recipients, compared with 5% in the general population. PTLD occurs predominantly in extranodal sites, with a particularly high incidence of involvement of the central nervous system, which is rare in the general population. Rather than being associated with a particular drug, PTLD appears to be a consequence of heavy immunosuppression. Thus patients with prolonged or repeated courses of thymoglobulin or OKT3, especially if these agents are combined with others, are at greater risk.

Oncogenic viruses such as EBV or human herpesvirus-8 may play a role, especially in children. In addition to reducing immunosuppressive treatment, the use of antiviral agents, such as acyclovir, may help reduce the incidence. Once PTLD has occurred, 30% of the cases regress with withdrawal of immunosuppression. Many patients do require systemic chemotherapy treatment.

Complications of the Surgical Operation

After surgery, hematomas, seromas, infections, and disruptions can occur as with any wound. The patient is predisposed to these complications by virtue of poor nutrition, edema, hypoproteinemia, platelet dysfunction, and anemia; the effects of steroids exaggerate many of these conditions. Extra care is therefore taken in the conduct of the operation to control all sources of bleeding, handle tissue gently, and thoroughly irrigate the wound.

Faulty technique at the arterial or venous suture lines may compromise *blood supply* to the kidney, as no collateral vessels exist. When a kidney had been undergoing active diuresis in the operating room, but concern had existed regarding the vascular anastomoses (because of factors in host vessels, the recipient vessels, or technique), any sudden fall in urine output immediately postoperatively should arouse suspicion. Although duplex scanning or arteriography can confirm vascular problems, by the time the diagnosis is confirmed it may be too late to reverse the process. If the index of suspicion is high, the patient directly returns to the operating room in the hope of correcting the problem.

Arterial complications may also occur long after transplantation. When a patient has had good function for a period of weeks, months, or years and presents with new resistant hypertension, renal artery stenosis must be suspected. It may occur in patients who continue to have a normal serum creatinine and a normal radionuclide scan. Preliminary duplex sonography or scintigraphy before and after the administration of captopril may assist in the diagnosis, but arteriography is the only definitive test. If a lesion is found, it must be treated by balloon angioplasty or by operation.

Urinary complications account for most of the noninfectious problems (3% to 5%). During the early postoperative period, obstruction may occur from a blood clot or malposition of the ureter during implantation. Urinary fistulas may develop at the site of implantation in the bladder or because of ischemic necrosis of the ureter, now entirely dependent for its blood supply on the renal artery. Such problems require urgent surgical intervention. Obstruction may be treated by percutaneous insertion of a stent or by surgical reimplantation. Urinary fistulas usually require an operation, which may range from simple reinforcement of a bladder implant site to reconstruction of a sloughed ureter. A nephrectomy is sometimes the safest alternative. Ureteral obstruction, due to extrinsic compression by lymphocele or to scarring, may also occur months after transplantation. Treatment, as during the acute period, may be by percutaneous or open surgical means; it is important to investigate late rises in serum creatinine, rather than making an assumption that what is occurring is untreatable chronic rejection.

The development of a *lymphocele* must especially be considered after transplantation. The lymph may arise from lower extremity lymphatics disrupted during the operation or from the kidney. It may present as a mass, as extrinsic compression on the ureter causing an elevation in creatinine, pain, or sometimes fever. Once the fluid is confirmed to be lymph, drainage is necessary, which may be done internally into the peritoneal cavity by an open operation or laparoscopically. Less desirable is the insertion of an external drain, which must be left in for an extended period because it is a potential source of infection.

The diagnosis of most surgical problems at the transplant site, including those mentioned above, can usually be made with relative ease. Sonography, B-mode and duplex, provides clear visualization of the structures and of abnormal findings such as obstruction, collections, and occlusion. Radionuclide scanning offers additional help. Occasionally, the use of CT or magnetic resonance imaging (MRI) is required.

Specific Drug-Related Complications

Corticosteroids were responsible for most of the complications of transplantation in previous years, including changes in appearance (obesity, growth retardation, cushingoid habitus), aseptic necrosis of bone, cataracts, peptic ulcer disease, glucose intolerance, and hypertension. Many of these complications are dose-related and with low-dose steroid regimens the incidence is rapidly decreasing, although steroid-induced diabetes still occurs.

Azathioprine, if administered in excessive doses, causes nonspecific depression of the bone marrow, resulting in leukopenia, thrombocytopenia, and anemia. Because azathioprine is partially excreted by the kidney, a dose that is well tolerated by a patient with normal renal function may become excessive for a patient in rejection. It is sometimes necessary, therefore, to reduce the dose of azathioprine when rejection occurs. A late complication of azathioprine is hepatotoxicity, which appears chemically as obstructive jaundice; a liver biopsy reveals bile deposits in the canaliculi. Both of these complications are usually reversed with cessation of the drug. Some patients also experience transient alopecia.

Cyclosporine principally causes renal and hepatic dysfunction, both of which usually respond to a decrease of the dose. Minor complications are hirsutism, tremors, gingival hyperplasia, hypertension, hyperkalemia, neuropathy, and hypercholesterolemia. The unpredictability of absorption, common with the old formulation, is less of an issue with the newer microemulsion formulation (Neoral). It must be used cautiously with many commonly used therapeutic agents because of drug interactions.

Tacrolimus has adverse effects similar to those of CsA. Neurologic side effects are common, including headaches, tremors, and insomnia. Glucose intolerance also occurs, sometimes requiring insulin. On the other hand, hirsutism, gingival hyperplasia, and hypercholesterolemia are not commonly seen.

Both calcineurin inhibitors will generate a dose-related renal vasoconstriction that affects the afferent arteriole and decreases the glomerular ultra filtration coefficient. This vasoconstriction is initially reversible and may be severe in those treated with cyclosporine than with tacrolimus. However, chronic use is associated with irreversible nephrotoxicity and may account for a significant amount of CAD.

Sirolimus alone has not produced the same nephrotoxicity that has been seen in the calcineurin inhibitors, but when combined with calcineurin inhibitors, will potentiate their nephrotoxicity and cause a hypokalemia and hypomagnesemia. It does produce pancytopenia, with sometimes a more severe thrombocytopenia. Sirolimus also inhibits wound healing and causes hyperlipidemia. A noninfectious pneumonia has been associated with Sirolimus, and if it is believed to be the cause of the pneumonia, after ruling out all others, the Sirolimus must be stopped. In addition, patients on Sirolimus should receive an entire year of Bactrim prophylaxis for PCP pneumonia because of the fatal associated cases that have been described.

Mycophenolate Mofetil (MMF) is often associated with gastrointestinal side effects, including bloating, diarrhea, and vomiting. These symptoms may appear more often with higher doses. There has not been shown to be any significant difference in the gastrointestinal side effects of the enteric-coated formulation. A pancytopenia similar to that with azathioprine is also seen, and may improve with changing the dosage. MMF should not be used with azathioprine because of the increased risk for hematologic side effects. Cyclosporine has also been noted to decrease the concentrations of MMF in the bloodstream.

Muromonab CD3 (OKT3) causes the number of working T cells and cytokines from T cells to drop rapidly and severely, while releasing TNF, IL-2 and γ-interferon, causing a cytokine release syndrome. This syndrome includes fever and often, rigors, diarrhea, and a rapid pulmonary edema. As with all biologic agents, OKT3 can induce anaphylaxis. Development of antibodies to the mouse antibody also limits the prolonged or repeated use of the product. Because it is a powerful agent there is heightened susceptibility to infection, particularly of viral origin, during and shortly after its use. There is also a risk of lymphoproliferative disorder, especially a fatal B-cell lymphoma that is seen within the first few months after transplantation. EBV-negative patients who receive an EBV+ graft are particularly at risk.

Polyclonal antibodies will cause many side effects as the body is reacting against a foreign protein with symptoms such as chills, fever, arthralgias, and occasional anaphylaxis. Thrombocytopenia and leucopenia is seen, with leucopenia seen in up to half of the patients treated with Thymoglobulin. The dosage of Thymoglobulin should be adjusted according to the platelet and leukocyte count. The infectious complications are those seen with OKT3.

Intravenous immunoglobulin (IVIG) can cause some minor immediate reactions such as nausea, headache, and myalgia, all of which resolve when the infusion is paused or given at a slower rate. Aseptic meningitis can be seen in the first 72 hours after an infusion, but it resolves spontaneously and can be prevented by pretreating with nonsteroidal anti-inflammatories.

Basiliximab and daclizumab, the anti-CD25 monoclonal antibodies, have virtually no significant side effects. Basiliximab can cause a first-dose reaction of anaphylaxis, but there are no known long-term side effects for either.

Results of Renal Transplantation

Even after the failure of a kidney transplant, patients can continue to be sustained on dialysis, so the rate of graft survival and patient survival are not identical. The mean 1-year patient survival of all renal transplants is reportedly 96%, with the mean graft survival at 92%. Graft survival is dependent on several factors, including with the source of kidney and, as discussed before, histologic compatibility. In general, the 1-year graft survival rate for deceased donor transplants is 85%, while it improves to 98% for living transplants. Patient mortality after the first year tends to be related to their age or issues that were present before their transplant, such as cardiovascular disease. The 5-year graft survival rate is now approximately 82%, although some have continued to function nearly 30 years after transplantation.

Given that patients are able to survive on dialysis, the greatest advantage with renal transplantation is in the improvement of their quality of life. Patients who have been chronically ill are now able to experience a life of near normalcy. Women can regain fertility and bear normal children. Children, when transplanted early, are able to grow and develop alongside their peers, without the stigma or restrictions of a lifetime of dialysis. Despite the continued need for immunosuppression, most patients are able to return to a normal life.

Transplantation of Other Organs

While the majority of transplants continue to be renal, now almost 40% of the 430,000 transplants performed to date are of other organs. It is common for multiple organs to be obtained from most cadaveric donors for transplantation.

Heart

One of the most striking accomplishments of the past two decades has been the improvement in the results of cardiac transplantation, with the patient survival rates at 1, 3, and 5 years at 88%, 80%, and 72%, respectively. The typical heart transplant patient in the United States is male (75%), over 50 years old (57%), and Caucasian (78%); the primary indication for transplant is coronary artery disease or cardiomyopathy. It should be noted, however, that approximately 12% of all heart transplants have been performed in pediatric patients (less than 18 years old).

A patient becomes a candidate for cardiac transplantation if he can be fully rehabilitated by transplantation, has a life expectancy of less than 6 months without transplantation, and has no other treatment option available. The relative contraindications include severe diabetes mellitus, smoking, obesity, malignancy, age, and psychiatric problems. Pulmonary disease was previously considered a contraindication but may now serve as an indication for possible heart–lung transplantation. Patients accepted for transplantation, listed with UNOS by weight and blood group, are assigned to one of two status groups: status 1, patients hospitalized on life-supporting drugs or devices and status 2 (all other patients). Status 1 patients are given priority. In 2007, over 300 patients died while on the waiting list, almost all of them designated status 1.

Cadaver donor hearts are transported in cold storage to the transplant center where the recipient, on cardiopulmonary bypass, has been prepared by excision of the diseased heart. The new heart is transplanted orthotopically. Emphasis is placed on minimizing the ischemia time between donor cardiectomy and restoration of flow in the recipient. The usual time is 4 to 6 hours; longer periods of ischemia can adversely affect cardiac performance. Immunosuppression is similar to that for other organs (CsA, prednisone, and azathioprine). Posttransplant patients are monitored for rejection by percutaneous transvenous endomyocardial biopsies. Infection (40%) is still the most common cause of death after transplant, followed by cardiac complications (25%) and acute rejection (25%). Patients unresponsive to acute rejection therapy and those who experience accelerated coronary artery disease or chronic rejection must undergo retransplantation, their only alternative being death.

Lung

Lung transplantation remains a challenge, but is acknowledged as an effective treatment for many pulmonary diseases. Beginning in 1983, a new era in lung transplantation was initiated by the Toronto lung transplant group. Through careful patient selection, the use of CsA, and an omental wrap for the bronchial anastomosis, they reported improved results in 15 single lung transplant patients. Most patients achieved maximal aerobic capacity within 6 months after transplant. In addition, with the development of the *en bloc* double-lung transplant method, patients with end-stage cystic fibrosis and emphysema have undergone transplantation successfully. Since then the increasing knowledge of immunosuppressants that has improved survival in kidneys has improved the lives of those undergoing lung transplantation, with the current survival rate of patients at 1, 3, and 5 years at 83%, 62%, and 46%, respectively.

In cystic fibrosis or bronchiectasis patients, who have chronically infected lungs, bilateral lung transplantation can be performed, on or off bypass. Also, in some centers, living lobar transplants are now being performed as well, with the insertion of a right and left lobe inserted into the recipient from two different donors.

Heart–Lung

Cooley performed the first heart-lung transplantation in 1968, but it was not until 1981 that a heart–lung transplant actually induced long-term survival. The most common indications for heart–lung transplantation are primary pulmonary hypertension (31%) and congenital lung disease (40%), with the idea that patients who have pulmonary hypertension usually have cardiac problems as well, either as part of a syndrome or secondary to the pulmonary hypertension. This operation maintains the connection between the heart and lungs so preserves collaterals and improves anastomotic healing. However, it also increases the risk of bleeding and removes multiple organs from the supply at a time.

Relative contraindications for heart–lung transplantation include previous extensive thoracic surgery and impaired liver function. The 1-year survival rate is 84% with high early postoperative mortality, usually associated with inadequate hemostasis and prolonged cardiopulmonary bypass time. Infection is the most common cause of late death following heart–lung transplants. Tracheal anastomotic problems are avoided by withholding the use of steroids for the first 2 weeks after transplant. The diagnosis of rejection is difficult because endomyocardial biopsy is not a good monitor for pulmonary tissue. Chest radiography, although imprecise, is the established method for diagnosing rejection. Long-term graft failure from bronchiolitis obliterans and accelerated coronary artery disease occurs in 50% of patients. Consequently, the need for retransplantation is high.

Liver

Although technically demanding, LTX has evolved into a safe, predictable surgical operation. Still controversial are issues of patient selection, surgical strategies, immunosuppression, and retransplantation. The inadequate supply of organs and the problems encountered financing LTX add to the difficulties.

Adult candidates for LTX are patients with end-stage liver disease that is not expected to recur after transplantation. Included in this group are patients with primary biliary or alcoholic cirrhosis, Budd–Chiari syndrome, and primary sclerosing cholangitis. More controversial are patients with postnecrotic cirrhosis secondary to hepatitis B or C virus, because the viral infection may recur. It should be noted, however, that the most common liver disease among adults for which LTX is performed is hepatitis C, followed by alcoholic liver disease. Patients with liver cancer, especially hepatocellular carcinoma, may undergo transplantation successfully if the tumor is strictly confined to the liver. Gallbladder carcinoma or cholangiocarcinoma are relative, not absolute, contraindications for LTX.

Acute fulminant hepatic failure has emerged as a strong indication for LTX. The predominant causes of this form of liver failure are hepatitis C, hepatitis B, and unspecified fulminant hepatitis. Indications for emergency transplantation are relentless progression of hepatic failure, severe coagulopathy, cardiovascular instability, sepsis, and grade 3 to 4 encephalopathy. The results are equivalent to those for patients given transplants for chronic liver diseases, especially in the 10- to 40-year age group.

In the pediatric patient, biliary atresia is the most common indication for transplantation (54%), with inborn metabolic errors being next (13%). Because of particular difficulty finding pediatric donors, techniques have been developed that allow an adult liver to be utilized in a child. They include the "split liver technique" from cadaver livers and transplantation of segments of livers from living related donors. Extensive thrombosis of the portal, mesenteric, or splenic veins or multiple prior upper abdominal surgical procedures does not preclude LTX. Patients with bleeding esophageal varices may be better served by a liver transplant than a shunt procedure. The pool of potential recipients is increasing and LTX is increasingly becoming the treatment of choice, rather than a last-ditch attempt, for many conditions.

Deceased donor livers can be preserved for up to 24 hours, using the University of Wisconsin (UW) solution, allowing time for selection and preparation of the most appropriate candidate. The recipient's liver is removed, often the most challenging aspect of the operation; during the anhepatic phase, a venovenous bypass may be utilized, shunting the splanchnic and distal systemic venous blood into a major tributary of the superior vena cava. The donor liver has been removed *en bloc* with the vena cava, portal vein, and arterial supply, including a cuff of aorta. Grafts of donor iliac vessels are utilized to provide additional length when necessary or to convert multiple arteries into a single trunk while the liver is still "on the back-table" in cold preservation solution. The proximal and distal cut ends of the vena cava are then end-to-end anastomosed to the corresponding ends of the recipient vessels, and air is evacuated. The portal vein is then anastomosed and finally the arterial supply is restored. Release of vascular clamps may be accompanied by acidosis and circulatory instability due to sudden changes in volume. The biliary tract is reconstructed using a choledochocholedochostomy or a Roux-en-Y choledochojejunostomy.

The main causes of death during the early post-transplant period are primary nonfunction and coagulopathy. During the ensuing weeks, acute rejection and hepatic artery thrombosis become the most frequent causes of graft loss. Complications of LTX can result in a 15% to 30% graft loss and include nonfunction, technical problems, bleeding, infection, and acute rejection. In many of these cases, retransplantation is required. Bacterial infection secondary to staphylococci and gram-negative organisms is frequent. Viral infections are also common, especially with CMV and herpes simplex virus. Fortunately, an increasing number of antiviral agents (e.g., acyclovir, ganciclovir, and foscarnet) are available.

Acute rejection occurs with more than 50% of liver allografts, usually within the first 2 weeks. Accurate diagnosis is obtained by needle biopsy of the liver. The most common histologic findings are portal tract inflammation and edema and mononuclear cell involvement of portal vein branches and small bile ducts.

The 1-year graft survival rate has improved from about 50% prior to CsA to the present level of 85%. The best results are in patients aged 5 to 60 years. In many centers, the results of emergency liver transplants equal those of elective liver transplants. The 5-year survival rates now range from 40% to 70%, except for patients with liver cancer, who have only a 10% to 15% survival rate at 5 years. The future for LTX depends on better methods for the diagnosis and treatment of rejection and refinement of surgical techniques, which allows more frequent use of a single deceased donor liver for two or three patients (split liver technique). Furthermore, live donor liver transplants have been performed utilizing the left lobe. Both of these techniques allow for some alleviation of the greatest problem currently facing LTX: the serious shortage of organs.

Pancreas

Kelly and Lillehei performed the first clinical pancreas transplant in 1966, and while this was considerably later than other organs, was actually the first extrarenal organ transplanted from a living donor in 1979. The goals of pancreas transplantation are to provide physiologic replacement of insulin and prevent the secondary complications of diabetes mellitus. These goals may be achieved by either full pancreas or islet cell transplantation.

In general, the risks of immunosuppression outweigh the benefits for most juvenile-onset diabetics, who can regulate their glucose with exogenous insulin. Currently, pancreas transplantation is considered the standard of care for insulin-dependent diabetic uremics who will also need a renal transplant, which may, but does not need to, be performed simultaneously. Since these patients would require immunosuppression regardless, a simultaneous pancreas transplant induces little added risk. The same is true of those patients who have already undergone a kidney transplant. While it may seem to be unfavorable to perform two separate surgeries, a high-risk patient may be able to tolerate two smaller surgeries than one combined larger one. The last category of potential pancreatic transplantation candidates is nonuremic diabetics who have catastrophic complications of diabetes or are simply unable to control their glucose levels medically. These complications include frequent insulin reactions, neuropathies, atherosclerosis, and endothelial dysfunction.

All potential candidates for pancreas transplantation generally undergo cardiac evaluation in addition to the usual preparation required for a kidney transplant, because as diabetics, they are at high risk of also having coronary artery disease. Patient survival is markedly improved if significant cardiac disease, common in these patients, is diagnosed and treated before transplantation.

While the pancreas is usually obtained from a cadaver donor, combined pancreatic and kidney transplants from living donors have been successfully completed since 1994. The large number of patients who die waiting for a kidney, the rapidly increasing waiting list for a pancreas, and the increased morbidity and mortality of diabetic patients have all contributed to a growing trend toward exploring living donor options. Living donor transplants are associated with a high technical failure rate, however, and also carry the risk of future glucose intolerance in the donor, even when only the distal segment of the pancreas is removed.

The pancreas transplant is placed intraperitoneally in the iliac fossa. The recipient operation varies in the amount of pancreas transplanted, the site of revascularization, and management of the duct. The results are essentially the same, whether the whole pancreas or the distal segment is transplanted. The pancreas is usually revascularized by anastomoses of its blood supply to the external iliac artery and vein, but some surgeons prefer portal venous drainage. Exocrine pancreatic function can be managed by anastomosis (to the recipient's gastrointestinal or urinary tract) and less commonly by duct ligation or duct injection (with neoprene or proline). Bladder drainage has the advantage of allowing direct monitoring of pancreatic function by measuring urinary amylase. A decrease in urinary amylase precedes hyperglycemia by 24 hours, providing earlier diagnosis of pancreas rejection. Bladder drainage appears to be associated with a higher graft survival rate than intestinal drainage or duct injection. However, because of the increasing incidence of cystitis and other adverse events, more and more pancreas transplants are being drained into the bowel.

In addition to immunosuppression, exogenous insulin is given to maintain serum glucose levels at less than 150 mg/dL during the early postoperative period because chronic hyperglycemia has been shown to be detrimental to the islets. Anticoagulants are given to reduce the risk (12%) of thrombosis of the splenic vessels of the transplant. Serum glucose levels, C peptide, urinary amylase, and pH are monitored. Radionuclide flow scans are performed early to distinguish between thrombosis and pancreatitis. Significant postoperative complications include pancreatitis, wound infection, ascites, and fever of an unknown origin. Immunosuppression appears to prevent recurrence of the autoimmune type I diabetes mellitus in the transplanted pancreas.

A functioning pancreas transplant can lead to a normal metabolic state, with normal oral and intravenous glucose tolerance tests with the hemoglobin A1 C and C-peptide levels returning to normal. Information is limited regarding the effects of a pancreas transplant on the secondary complications of diabetes. Regression of the histologic lesions of diabetic nephropathy has been demonstrated after pancreas transplantation, and neuropathies have been shown to improve. While retinopathies or vascular disease does not, actual endothelial dysfunction and atherosclerosis will decrease.

The results have improved markedly over the past few years, primarily due to better immunosuppression and better preservation of the pancreas with UW solution. Living donor pancreas transplants that will be transplanted within an hour are usually flushed with Ringer's Lactate. As in renal transplant patients, tacrolimus and mycophenolate mofetil are now the mainstays for immunosuppression, with some patients tolerating a full withdrawal of steroids. Anti-T cell therapy and often anti-CD-25 antibodies continue to be used during induction. HLA matching appears to play a role in pancreas graft survival; DR matching has been noted to have a beneficial effect.

An alternative to pancreas transplantation is islet cell transplantation. Bollinger and Lacy performed the first successful animal islet cell transplant in 1972. It appears to be a safe, simple procedure that permits in vitro manipulation of the graft prior to transplantation. Despite the remarkable success of experimental studies, by the late 1990s, fewer than 8% were actually insulin-dependent after islet cell transplantation. In addition, there were the difficulties of preparing sufficient quantities of human islet tissue (multiple donors are required for a single recipient) and also the marked immunogenicity of these allografts. In 1999, however, the Edmonton protocol that focused on avoiding the use of corticosteroids and the use of sirolimus, tacrolimus, and anti-CD25 as the immunosuppressant regimen demonstrated marked improvement in graft survival, with now approximately 80% of islet cell transplant patients insulin-free at 1 year. This has only been applied to patients with brittle diabetes, and most require more than one transplant procedure to attain that insulin independence. Long-term success rates are still not sufficient; at 5 years, only 10% remain insulin-independent. It is not known whether this is from rejection or decayed function from the constant use of these islet cells. Research is still continuing to improve the long-term success of islet cell transplants.

Small Bowel

Small bowel is the most recent organ to be transplanted. Small bowel transplants have become an option for those patients who are dependent on total parental nutrition (TPN) due to either dysfunction or paucity of their small bowel. This can be due to either a congenital or acquired loss of absorptive capacity of the small intestine. Candidates for transplantation are those who suffer life-threatening complications of TPN dependence. Small bowel transplantation (SBTx) can obviate the significant morbidity of vascular access problems and cholestasis associated with TPN. SBTx was first attempted in 1901 by Carrel and Lillehei revived interest in the procedure in 1959. TPN dependence is also associated with liver failure, which is why so many patients die while on the waiting list. Combined liver and small bowel transplants were performed successfully for the first time in 2004.

While the profound impact cyclosporine had on transplantation has already been discussed, it was seen that cyclosporine did not seem to be as effective with small bowel transplants, with less than 20% of intestinal grafts surviving at 1 year. The use of tacrolimus improved graft survival and continues to be the current primary immunosuppressive agent after SBTx. In 1997, the University of Minnesota published guidelines for small bowel transplants, including the preference of the use of ileum to the jejunum because of its superior absorptive capacity, preserving the terminal ileum, ileocecal valve and cecum in the living donor, the use of only one artery or vein in the vascular pedicle, and restoration of bowel continuity with the creation of a distal ileostomy, to be taken 6 months after the transplant or after the last rejection episode. Approximately 1,560 have been performed to date. However, with small bowel transplants, there still remains a higher incidence of infection, rejection, and PTLD.

Some of the difficulty is because rejection will actually change the mucosa of the bowel itself, and endotoxins then translocate, augmenting the antigraft autoimmune response, but also causing infection. These grafts are constantly being exposed to bacteria and viruses, causing infections to be the most common cause of death after a small bowel transplant. Also, cells in the gut can serve as APCs, stimulating inflammation. In addition, since the small bowel contains so many mesenteric lymph nodes and lymphoid tissue seen in Peyer's patches, it is at very high risk for developing graft-versus-host disease (GVHD). This has been reported in 5% to 14% of small bowel transplant patients. Symptoms are nonspecific and diagnosis must be confirmed by tissue biopsy. Patients are then treated symptomatically and occasionally with steroid or increase tacrolimus administration to try to prevent the removal of the graft.

PTLD is seen more in intestinal transplants than in any other solid organ, largely because of the potent immunosuppression that is used. Oral ganciclovir is usually used as long-term prophylactic treatment, but there is still no consensus on the optimum treatment of PTLD.

Acute rejection has been reported to be as high as 78% or more. Unfortunately, many times patients will demonstrate no symptoms except for worsening diarrhea or increase in their ostomy output until late in the rejection.

There is still sparse literature regarding small transplantation, but it seems that about 200 cm of graft for an adult and 150 cm for a child is required to become independent from TPN. There are still no long-term results available.

While a great deal of work has been done recently toward the improvement of small bowel transplant, it remains a difficult organ to work with. Studies are continuing to optimize both the technical and immunosuppressive aspects of intestinal transplant management.

Bone Marrow

Most allogeneic bone marrow transplants have been performed using HLA-identical sibling donors. Attempts now have been made using partially mismatched donors. Bone marrow transplants are indicated for the following conditions: (a) hematologic malignancies such as acute lymphatic leukemia, acute and chronic myelogenous leukemias, and non-Hodgkin's lymphoma; (b) nonmalignant disorders such as severe aplastic anemia; and (c) hereditary disorders such as Fanconi's anemia, thalassemia, and severe combined immunodeficiency syndrome. The preparation of the recipient involves complete destruction of all functional lymphoid tissue by irradiation and chemotherapy. For this reason, there is little initial fear of acute rejection. The major early complication is GVHD. The major relative contraindications are age, sex, mismatch of the transplant, CMV infection, and neutropenic sepsis. Early immunosuppression is directed toward preventing GVHD. The future for bone marrow transplants includes the use of unrelated matched and mismatched related bone marrow donors. Better immunosuppression and anti-T cell monoclonal antibodies may improve the results. In addition, growth factors are being evaluated to improve the engraftment rate in mismatched situations or after T cell depletion.

XENOTRANSPLANTATION

Although great strides have been made in the immunobiology of transplantation, the number of human organs available has limited clinical transplants for the ever-growing number of potential recipients. Among the other options explored are organs from animals of different species. These organs, called *xenografts,* have the advantage that they act similarly to the recipient's own organ and do not need to be replaced unless rejection occurs. There are many barriers before xenotransplantation becomes a viable option. One of the major barriers is hyperacute rejection, which occurs between "discordant" organs (e.g., pig to baboon). This is thought to occur because of the binding of xenoreactive antibodies of the recipient to the blood vessels in the donor organ leading to activation of the complement system and the intrinsic susceptibility of the graft to injury by the heterologous complement. Another major barrier is acute cellular rejection, or "delayed xenograft rejection." In "concordant" species (e.g., baboon to human), hyperacute rejection does not occur, but the graft is then subjected to severe acute cellular rejection. The mechanism of this reaction is not well delineated at this time. Ethical and moral issues arise as well. Concordant species (nonhuman primates) are sentient, have prolonged and limited gestation periods, and some are endangered. These factors override the fact that humans do not have a natural antibody against them.

Use of the pig overcomes these objections, as the pig breeds rapidly and the species is already in widespread use for food. However, the natural antibody must be overcome. Currently, swine herds are being bred that are genetically altered to avoid initiation of the complement cascade and thus avert hyperacute rejection. Xenotransplants will continue to be experimental until these issues have been convincingly resolved.

A final issue is specific to xenotransplantation: *zoonosis,* which is the transmission of disease from animals to humans. Although a relatively rare phenomenon now, it may be of concern if xenotransplantation is widely practiced. Specific concerns include the possible transmission into the human population of diseases not currently known and to which humans have no resistance. A related concern is if such infection does occur, it may have the potential of a pandemic. These issues have been addressed in depth by national panels, and the current policy is to proceed with caution, on an experimental basis, until knowledge is gained.

Conclusions

Advances in clinical transplantation have resulted in greatly improved short- and intermediate-term

TABLE 15.8   **One-Year Survival**

Organ	Survival (%)	
	Graft	Patient
Kidney (LRD)	95	98
Kidney (cadaver)	90	95
Liver	82	87
Heart	87	88
Heart–lung	75	75
Lung	82	84
Pancreas	86	95
Intestine	73	81

Source: UNOS OPTN/SRTR data as of May 1, 2007, based on UNOS OPTN/Scientific Registry data (11/09/08). LRD, living related donor.

allograft survival (Table 15.8). Today, transplant physicians have increased awareness that chronic immunosuppression is associated with significant problems, including increased risk of infection, malignancy, nephrotoxicity, and cardiovascular effects. With the continual exploration of transplant immunology, the field has undergone developments unforeseen. Immunosuppressive therapy has become more refined, allowing most organ transplant recipients a more normal life.

Improved outcomes have been accompanied by increased demand and a chronic organ shortage, in part ameliorated by expanded donor criteria. There has been a clear shift with the transplantation of older patients with older donors, thus expanding not only the pool of available organs but also the patients treated. However, the struggle remains. While studies are investigating other sources of transplantable tissue, society, and especially those in the medical profession, must do what they can to aid those 1,00,000 people on the waiting list, awaiting a chance at an active life.

GLOSSARY

Antibody—soluble protein that reacts to a specific antigen; produced by B cells

Antigen-presenting cells (APC)—cells that present antigen to initiate T cell activation; can be various cells, such as monocytes, dendritic cells

Autologous—graft that originates from the same individual who receives it

Azathioprine (Imuran)—immunosuppressive agent that acts by inhibiting cell division; often used with prednisone and CsA in "triple therapy"

B-lymphocytes—small white blood cells essential to immune defenses; derived from marrow; produce antibodies

CD (cluster of differentiation)—variety of cell surface molecules each with a different function (e.g., CD3 T cell antigen receptor; CD4 helper T cells, recognize MHC class I; CD8 cytotoxic T cells, recognize class II

Cellular immunity—immunity mediated by direct action of cells (in contrast to humoral immunity)

Chimera—cell populations from one organism surviving in another

Class I and II molecules—see MHC

Clone—groups of cells that are genetically identical

Cyclosporine (CsA)—immunosuppressive agent derived from fungal extract; prevents rejection by inhibiting production of IL-2; two oral formulations exist: the older Sandimmune and the newer Neoral

Cytotoxic cells—T lymphocytes that can kill certain target cells; usually carry CD8 surface marker

Dendritic cell—white blood cell found in lymphoid organs; presents trapped antigen to T cells

Haplotype—set of genetic determinants on a single chromosome

Helper cells—T lymphocytes activated early in the immune process; help generate cytotoxic T cells and stimulate B cells to form antibodies; usually carry CD4 surface marker

Heterologous—antigenic differences between species

Histocompatibility—ability to accept grafts between species

Human leukocyte antigen (HLA)—major histocompatibility genetic region in humans: self-markers

Homologous—of the same species

Humoral immunity—immunity through soluble factors (e.g., antibody)

Interferons—mediators of cell function with implications for immune response, infection, and cancer chemotherapy; IFNα produced by leukocytes; IFNβ by fibroblasts; IFNγ by T cells

Interleukins (IL)—agents involved in cell signals: IL-1, many effects, including activation of T cells to express IL-2 receptors; IL-2, released by activated T cells, necessary for T cells to proliferate; many other ILs

Lymphokines—soluble T cell products that regulate the activation, growth, and differentiation of many cell types

Major histocompatibility complex (MHC)—genetic region in all mammals, products of compatibility responsible for rejection of grafts between individuals

MHC class I molecules—expressed on all cell types, consists of heavy αchain, associated with light β chain

MHC class II molecules—expressed on B cells, macrophages, and activated T cells; have α and β chains, which may form a common binding site

Monoclonal antibody—homogeneous antibodies, derived from a single clone, with a specific action

Mycophenolate mofetil (MMF)—antiproliferative agent targeting lymphocytes. Actions similar to azathioprine; also known as CellCept

Natural killer (NK)—lymphocytes that recognize and destroy certain cells (e.g., virally infected, tumor)

Polyclonal antibody (ALG, ATG)—antibody usually generated against lymphocytes using horse, rabbit, or goat; action not restricted to lymphocytes

Tacrolimus (FK 506)—immunosuppressive agent; prevents rejection by inhibition of IL-2; structurally different from CsA but functionally similar; also known as Prograf

T lymphocytes—lymphocytes processed in the thymus; direct participants in immune response

Tolerance—specific immunologic unresponsiveness

Xenograft—graft between species (e.g., baboon to human, mouse to rat)

Zoonosis—disease of animals transmissible to humans

QUESTIONS

Select one answer.

1. Seven days after cadaver renal transplantation, a patient develops a fever to 101°F, pain, and tenderness over the incisional area, and oliguria. Serum creatinine has risen from 1.5 mg/dL to 1.9 mg/dL. Likely possibilities include:
   a. Acute rejection.
   b. Wound infection.
   c. Urinary leak.
   d. Wound dehiscence.
   e. All of the above.

2. The patient in Question 1 should:
   a. Be rushed to the operating room.
   b. Receive high doses of steroids immediately.
   c. Be investigated using ultrasonography, nuclear scan, or both.
   d. Receive broad-spectrum antibiotic coverage.
   e. None of the above.

Possible answers for Questions 3 through 6:
   a. IL-2.
   b. Interferon-2.
   c. T-helper cells.
   d. T cytotoxic cells.
   e. B cells.

3. These cells are usually CD8+ and recognize class I molecules.

4. Stimulated by antigen or other cells, these cells ultimately produce antibody that causes graft destruction.

5. Secretion that stimulates various antigen-activated cells to proliferate.

6. Normally resting, these cells are stimulated by antigens and macrophages to initiate the immune response.

7. For a through e, below, choose the best option from i through v (choice may be repeated).
   a. Blocks IL-1.
   b. Blocks IL-2.
   c. Inhibits cell division.
   d. Can depress bone marrow.
   e. Nephrotoxicity is a problem.

      i. Cyclosporine.
      ii. Azathioprine.
      iii. Corticosteroids.
      iv. Tacrolimus.
      v. Mycophenolate mofetil.

8. True or false:
   a. Because of high mortality, cardiac transplantation should be restricted to the terminally ill.
   b. Patient survival 1 year after kidney transplantation exceeds 90%.
   c. Cytomegalovirus infection is a common problem after all organ transplants.

   d. Liver transplantation should never be considered for acute hepatic necrosis.

9. In regard to transplant rejection:
   a. Acute rejection is irreversible and leads to loss of the kidney.
   b. There is no treatment for chronic rejection.
   c. Hyperacute rejection is precipitated by circulating humoral antibodies.
   d. a, b, and c are correct.
   e. b and c are correct.

10. The following statements are true *except*:
   a. Deep hypothermia sharply reduces cell metabolism.
   b. Oxygen-derived free radicals may be responsible for reperfusion injury.
   c. Cell swelling can be minimized by the addition of impermeable osmotic agents to the preservation/perfusion solution.
   d. Hypothermia prevents anaerobic metabolism.
   e. With the use of UW solution, preservation of abdominal organs more than 24 hours can be regularly achieved.

SELECTED REFERENCES

Annual data report 2006. United States renal data system. *Am J Kidney Dis* 2007;49:210–276.

Danovitch GM, ed. *Handbook of kidney transplantation,* 4th ed. Philadelphia: Lippincott Williams & Wilkins, 2005.

Langnas AN, Shaw BS Jr, Antonson DL, et al. Preliminary experience with intestinal transplantation in infants and children. *Pediatrics* 1996;97:443–448.

The 2006 SRTR report on the state of Transplantation. *Am J Transpl* 2007;7:1317–1433.

Terasaki PI, ed. *Clinical transplants 2006.* Los Angeles, California: Terasaki Foundation Laboratory 2007.

Todo S, Tzakis A, Reyes J, et al. Small intestinal transplantation in humans with or without the colon. *Transplantation* 1994; 57:840–848.

United Network for Organ Sharing Scientific Registry. Richmond: UNOS, 2008.

Thyroid and Parathyroid Disease

THYROID DISEASE

Embryology and Anatomy

The thyroid gland is formed by the proliferation of endodermal epithelial cells of the thyroid diverticulum arising from the foramen caecum, which is located at the junction of the anterior two-thirds and posterior one-third of the tongue. The parafollicular cells or C cells of the thyroid gland migrate from the neural crest and fuse with the ultimobranchial body (ventral portion of the fourth branchial pouch). The ultimobranchial body fuses with the developing thyroid gland diverticulum, dispersing the C cells throughout the thyroid gland. The pyramidal lobe of the thyroid gland is present approximately 50% of the time and is located in the superior midline above the isthmus. The blood supply to the thyroid gland is from the superior thyroid artery, a branch of the external carotid artery, and from the inferior thyroid artery, a branch of the thyrocervical trunk of the subclavian artery. The internal jugular vein provides drainage via the superior, middle, and inferior thyroid veins. The lymphatic drainage of the thyroid gland is into the central (level VI) and lateral nodal compartments (levels II, III, IV). The central compartment consists of the lymph tissue within the confines of the carotid arteries bilaterally, the sternal notch inferiorly, and the hyoid bone superiorly. The lateral compartment is composed of the lymph nodes along the internal jugular vein: upper jugular lymph nodes (II), middle jugular (III), and inferior jugular (IV). These neck levels are bounded by the lateral border of the sternohyoid muscle medially, the skull base superiorly, the clavicle inferiorly, and the posterior border of the sternocleidomastoid muscle posteriorly.

THYROID GLAND NEOPLASMS

Introduction

Thyroid gland tumors are the most common endocrine tumors of the body and comprise approximately 1% of all human neoplasms (1). Approximately 33,000 new thyroid tumors are diagnosed every year with approximately 1,500 deaths secondary to thyroid cancer (2).

Papillary Carcinoma

Papillary carcinoma is the most common malignancy of the thyroid gland, constituting 80% to 85% of well-differentiated tumors. Patients present at all ages with papillary carcinoma with the median age in the fourth decade of life. It is more common in women by a ratio of 3:1 (1). Radiation exposure is one of the proven risk factors for papillary carcinoma, especially in children. However, most patients who present with papillary thyroid carcinoma have no history of radiation exposure (1).

Histopathology of these tumors shows that most of them are mixed papillary-follicular variant tumors. Pure papillary carcinomas are rare with an incidence of 2%. Mixed papillary-follicular carcinomas are categorized with pure papillary carcinomas because of similar clinical behavior (3,4).

Serum thyroglobulin is used as a surveillance tumor marker for postoperative recurrence. It is highly sensitive after total thyroidectomy and radioablation of remnant tissue, as the level will be undetectable in patients who are free of disease. The American Thyroid Association (ATA) taskforce guidelines recommend measurement of serum thyroglobulin levels every 6 to 12 months after initial treatment (5).

Patients who have either less than total thyroidectomy or no radioablation after total thyroidectomy can be followed by the trend of serum thyroglobulin to determine disease recurrence; however, this is less reliable. The ATA task force also recommends that serum thyroglobulin should be measured after either withdrawal of thyroxine or injection of rhTSH (recombinant human thyroid-stimulating hormone) approximately 12 months after the ablation to verify the disease-free state. Diagnostic radioiodine scanning can also be used to verify that there is no evidence of disease.

Approximately 80% of papillary carcinomas are multicentric secondary to a rich intrathyroidal lymphatic network. The most common method of metastasis is by lymphatic channels. The relative 10-year survival rate for papillary carcinomas is 98%. Lymph node metastases have not been shown to change the survival rate in papillary carcinoma patients (6).

Follicular Carcinoma

Pure follicular thyroid carcinomas make up 10% of all thyroid malignancies (1). Seen in all age groups, they tend to occur more frequently in the elderly compared with papillary carcinomas. Hurthle cell cancer is a variant of follicular carcinoma, which was at one time thought to be an aggressive variant but has subsequently been shown to have similar biologic behavior of non–Hurthle cell follicular carcinoma (7).

The characteristic features of follicular carcinoma are capsular invasion and angioinvasion. The absence of characteristic cellular features of malignancy in this lesion limits the role of fine needle aspiration biopsy (FNAB) and frozen section as diagnostic tools. To demonstrate a follicular carcinoma, the patient must undergo a diagnostic thyroid lobectomy with comprehensive evaluation of the entire specimen to determine the presence or absence of capsular invasion or angioinvasion (8). In the majority of institutions, this requires permanent section analysis.

Primarily, follicular carcinomas metastasize hematogenously. The most common distant metastatic site is the lung (4). Other common sites are bone and the central nervous system. Lymph node metastases are seen in only 2% to 13% of the cases. The overall 10-year survival rate for follicular carcinoma is approximately 85% (9).

Medullary Carcinoma

Medullary carcinoma is the third most common malignancy, comprising 5% to 10% of thyroid neoplasms. It arises from the parafollicular or C cells of the thyroid gland. Seventy to eighty percent of the cases are sporadic in nature, with median age of presentation 51 years (6).

Only 20% to 30% of cases are associated with the hereditary disorders, multiple endocrine neoplasia (MEN) 2A, MEN2B, or familial medullary thyroid cancer (MTC), with median age of presentation 21 years (6). Thyroid cancers associated with the MEN syndromes and familial MTC are bilateral in nature. These are associated with a point mutation in the RET proto-oncogene. Serum calcitonin and serum carcinoembryonic antigen are used as preoperative indicators of the presence and extent of disease and as surveillance postoperative tumor markers for recurrence. Calcifications and amyloid deposits are characteristically seen in the histopathology (6).

The overall 10-year survival rate for medullary carcinoma patients is 80% (9). For the same stage there is no difference in the prognosis between the familial MTC group and the sporadic MTC group. However, since familial MTC is typically diagnosed earlier, it carries a better overall prognosis than sporadic MTC (10).

All patients with MTC including sporadic cases need genetic analysis, and those with RET proto-oncogene mutations should advise their family members to be tested as well (11). Studies by the European study group and Skinner et al (11) suggest total thyroidectomy before the age of 6 years in patients with familial MTC or MEN2A. Mutation of the RET proto-oncogene codon 918 is usually associated with MEN2B syndrome and considered to be aggressive; it is recommended that patients with this mutation undergo an early total thyroidectomy and lymph node dissection at diagnosis or at the age of 1 year (12).

Anaplastic Carcinoma

Anaplastic thyroid carcinoma is rare, comprising 2% of all thyroid cancers (9). It is generally diagnosed in the elderly with peak incidence in the seventh and eighth decades of life. It carries a dismal prognosis with a median survival rate of only 4 to 6 months. It accounts for 40% of all thyroid cancer deaths (9). Surgery cannot cure this tumor; therefore, the surgeon's role is to provide diagnostic tissue sampling and surgery for palliation only. There may be a role for palliative total thyroidectomy in some patients to prevent death by mass effect and asphyxiation. However, one must be very careful not to worsen the patient's condition by damaging a functional structure (such as the esophagus) while trying to operate on unresectable disease. Multimodal treatment with chemoradiation therapy after surgery may show modest improvement in survival rates (13).

Risk Stratification

There are multiple risk stratification systems available for differentiated thyroid tumors based on age, metastases, extent, size, nodal status, and completeness of resection. A few to mention are AGES (age, grade, extent, size), AMES (age, metastases, extent, size), TNM (tumor size, nodal status, metastases), and MACIS (metastases, age, completeness of resection, invasion, size). Patients are considered low risk if age is less than 45, tumor size is less than 1 to 2 cm, there is no extrathyroidal extension, and it is a well-differentiated tumor. Conversely, high-risk patients are older, with tumor size greater than 4 cm, or with extrathyroidal disease (6).

CLINICAL EVALUATION OF THE THYROID NODULE

Introduction

A thyroid nodule is defined as a distinct lesion within the thyroid gland, which is either palpable or radiologically identified. Thyroid nodules larger than 1 cm in size are generally considered clinically significant as they have a higher potential for malignancy and need further evaluation (14). A complete history and physical examination should be performed. History of radiation exposure and a family history of thyroid cancer are important. Physical signs pertinent to thyroid malignancy are (a) vocal cord paralysis, (b) lymphadenopathy, and (c) fixation of the lesion to surrounding tissues (14).

Measurement of Serum Thyroid-Stimulating Hormone

Serum thyroid-stimulating hormone (TSH) levels are obtained initially in patients with thyroid nodules of more than 1 to 1.5 cm in size. A hyperfunctioning gland will result in suppressed TSH levels, and a thyroid nuclear scan can be useful to determine if the entire gland is hyperfunctioning or if the condition is arising from a solitary nodule. Thyroid nodules in patients with normal or high TSH levels should generally be evaluated by ultrasound-guided fine needle aspiration cytology (14).

Thyroid Ultrasound

Thyroid ultrasound has a low pretest probability to diagnose malignancy and therefore cannot be used as a screening tool for thyroid cancer. However, ultrasound features thought to be associated with malignancy include microcalcifications, irregular margins, irregular shape, and solid and hypoechoic lesions (15). Still, none of these features is diagnostic of malignancy. Despite its limited role in detecting thyroid cancer, ultrasound remains a standard tool for evaluating the thyroid, particularly in a preoperative setting. Knowledge of the size, number of nodules, and presence of enlarged lymph nodes often help to guide intraoperative management.

Fine Needle Aspiration Biopsy

Fine needle aspiration biopsy is the single most reliable and highly accurate test available to evaluate benign versus malignant disease in thyroid nodules. The use of small-gauge needles for aspiration biopsy has minimized complications such as bleeding, hematoma, and nerve injury. On-site cytological evaluation of FNAB specimen adequacy improves the success rate. The sensitivity and specificity of an FNAB are in the range of 90% and 70%, respectively (14). FNAB is generally reported in four categories: (a) benign (negative), (b) malignant (positive), (c) suspicious, and (d) atypical. For nondiagnostic cytology or an inadequate specimen, FNAB needs to be repeated. In general, for a patient who is an acceptable surgical candidate, any FNAB result except "benign" should result in a recommendation for surgery. However, it should be noted that the finding of "follicular cells" without atypia does not necessarily mandate surgery. While it is true that a follicular neoplasm cannot be ruled out by FNAB, it is also true that normal thyroid tissue is composed of follicular cells. Therefore, the decision to remove a thyroid nodule that shows normal follicular cells on FNAB requires an intelligent appraisal of the characteristics of the nodule and the patient before recommending surgery.

Radionuclide Scanning

Radionuclide scintigraphy assesses the function of the thyroid nodule, comparing it to the surrounding thyroid tissues. The thyroid nodule is assessed as hot (hyperfunctioning), cold (hypofunctioning), or warm (euthyroid). Hot nodules are almost never malignant, whereas cold nodules possess a 5% to 8% malignant potential (14). The role of radionuclide scintigraphy is very limited in assessing malignancy.

Other Imaging Studies

Computed tomography (CT) scan and magnetic resonance imaging (MRI) are rarely used in the routine evaluation of thyroid nodules but can be useful for the assessment of substernal extension, invasion of structures such as the trachea, or evaluation of lymphadenopathy. Positron emission tomography (PET) scan is a common modality for evaluating various malignancies. Increasing use of PET scans has given rise to an increase in "incidentalomas" of the thyroid gland. There is a 15% to 30% risk of malignancy in these nodules (16).

SURGICAL TREATMENT

Surgery is the only curative treatment for thyroid cancers. For papillary carcinoma greater than 1 cm, total thyroidectomy has become a standard treatment. Sturgeon's analysis of the National Cancer Data Base in 2007 demonstrated a relative 10-year survival of 98.4% for total thyroidectomy and 97.1% for lobectomy ($p < 0.05$) for tumors greater than 1 cm in size—the first study to demonstrate a survival difference between the two approaches (17).

Proponents of lobectomy argue the following: (a) it has a nearly equivalent survival rate, (b) the risk of complications is reduced since only one recurrent laryngeal nerve is exposed and two parathyroid glands are left untouched, and (c) the patient is not rendered dependent on thyroid hormone (6).

Advocates of total thyroidectomy argue the following: (a) it facilitates the use of radioactive iodine (RAI) for postoperative ablation and subsequent surveillance for recurrent disease, (b) 80% of well-differentiated tumors are multicentric, (c) there are lymphatic drainage channels between the lobes, (d) several studies have shown no significant increase in complication rates, and (e) it may prevent conversion to anaplastic carcinoma (6). Thus, lobectomy may be appropriate for the rare case in which all of the prognostic indicators are favorable and there are no contralateral thyroid nodules. However, in most cases, a total thyroidectomy should be done.

A common scenario in thyroid surgery is the performance of a thyroid lobectomy, which is read as a follicular neoplasm on frozen section. This means that the pathologist cannot determine if the specimen is a follicular carcinoma or adenoma until the entire specimen is sectioned and carefully examined for any focus of angioinvasion or capsular invasion. Since only approximately 20% of these tumors will be carcinomas, it is generally recommended that a lobectomy alone is done. If permanent section reveals a malignancy, then a completion thyroidectomy should be performed. It is critical to discuss this algorithm preoperatively with the patient.

For patients with MTC with tumor size greater than 1 cm, total thyroidectomy with central compartment neck dissection is recommended (11). The role of surgery in anaplastic tumors is limited to palliative measures such as tracheotomy; rarely, total thyroidectomy is warranted to alleviate the mass effect of the tumor, if resectable (18).

Lymphadenectomy

The central compartment lymph nodes of level VI, which include pretracheal, paratracheal, and anterior mediastinal lymph nodes, are the most common site for metastatic papillary thyroid cancer. Jugular chain lymph nodes (levels II, III, IV) form the secondary drainage basin for the thyroid gland. Microscopic lymph node metastases are seen in 50% to 70% of patients with papillary thyroid cancer and in less than 10% of follicular cancers (6). In general, lymph node metastases have no impact on survival (17).

Indications for lateral lymph node dissection (lymphadenectomy of levels II, III and IV) for well-differentiated tumors of the thyroid gland include the presence of clinically palpable (or enlarged/suspicious by radiological criteria) cervical lymph nodes. However, central compartment neck dissection ipsilateral to the cancer has become standard practice even in the absence of clinically detectable disease (6). This is done to prevent the need for reoperation in the central compartment, which would put the recurrent laryngeal nerve at high risk of injury.

Medullary thyroid cancers greater than 1.5 cm in size have a 75% incidence of lymph node metastasis (12). There is controversy regarding management of the lymph node basins due to the lack of adequate scientific data to support one approach versus another. Recommendations for clinically detectable MTC range from hemithyroidectomy without neck dissection to total thyroidectomy with central and bilateral modified radical neck dissection (19,20). Additional prospective studies are needed to clarify the proper treatment for these patients.

NONSURGICAL THERAPY FOR THYROID TUMORS

Radiotherapy

There are two types of radiotherapy options available for thyroid tumors: (a) radioactive iodine remnant ablation with I-131 (RRA) and (b) external beam radiation. Usage of RRA after surgery is a controversial topic. Several studies have shown that RRA has no benefit in low-risk patients with tumor size less than 1 cm and favorable histology. In contrast, other studies have shown improvement in survival rates and decreased recurrence rates in groups where the tumor size is more than 1 cm and less than 4 cm, even though they are classified as stage I and stage II papillary and follicular carcinomas. ATA 2006 guidelines recommend RRA for stage I and stage II patients when the tumor size is more than 1 to 1.5 cm, as well as for stage III and stage IV patients (8). It should be noted that RRA is not entirely without side effects. Occasionally patients have significant xerostomia, and rarely a patient may have severe parotitis as a result of this treatment. Therefore, it should not be given to every patient who has had thyroid cancer without consideration of the risk of recurrence based on the pathological characteristics of the tumor. External beam radiation therapy has never been shown to improve survival or locoregional control, and thus is only used in cases of severe or unresectable disease (21).

There is no role for RRA in patients with MTC, as the tumor cells are not from thyroid epithelial cells and they do not trap I-131. External radiation therapy can be used as a palliative measure for patients with advanced disease, although no survival benefit has been shown.

Anaplastic thyroid tumors are resistant to I-131 therapy. External beam radiation therapy may be considered for these patients, as most of them are not surgical candidates. However, the use of radiation in patients with anaplastic carcinoma has not been shown to alter the course of the disease.

Chemotherapy

Chemotherapy has virtually no role in the treatment of thyroid tumors, except in anaplastic carcinoma. Anaplastic thyroid carcinoma shows a better response rate of 26% with doxorubicin and cisplatin compared with doxorubicin alone (response rate 17%) (22).

TSH Suppression Therapy

The principle behind TSH suppression is to prevent growth of thyroid tissue after thyroidectomy and ablation. It also serves to replace thyroid hormone function. There are retrospective studies that show benefit from TSH suppression therapy to levels less than 0.1 mU/L, especially in high-risk patients. The ATA and American Association of Clinical Endocrinologists recommend a goal of TSH less than 0.1 mU/L for high-risk patients and a TSH level of 0.1 to 0.4 mU/L for all other patients (8).

BENIGN THYROID CONDITIONS

Hyperthyroidism

The common causes of hyperthyroidism are Graves' disease, toxic multinodular goiter, and less commonly a single toxic nodule of the thyroid gland. Patients with these conditions may be asymptomatic, or they may present with signs and symptoms of hyperthyroidism. Patients who have thyromegaly or a thyroid nodule without any previous metabolic workup should have a TSH level to screen for a functional disorder. If this is abnormal then additional thyroid function tests (T3, T4) should be performed, and appropriate consultation should be obtained.

Options for treatment include medication, RAI treatment, or surgery. Medical treatments include the use of propylthiouracil or methimazole, both of which are antithyroid agents that block thyroid hormone synthesis. These agents do not cure the condition, but rather control it. Sometimes patients will have remission of their condition, in which case the medication can be discontinued. Alternatively, the disease may persist or worsen and require more definitive therapy.

In the United States, most patients with persistent hyperthyroidism are treated with RAI. This is an effective therapy, often rendering the patient hypothyroid. Contraindications include pregnancy and the inability (or unwillingness) of the patient to be separated from small children for a period of 2 to 3 days after treatment to avoid radiation exposure. There are reports of worsening Graves' ophthalmopathy after RAI treatment; therefore, surgery is generally preferred over RAI in patients with this condition. Finally, despite exhaustive explanation, some patients have a fear of radiation therapy and therefore prefer to have surgery.

Surgical treatment for hyperthyroidism is effective and safe. Preoperative workup in patients with a solitary nodule should include a diagnostic RAI nuclear scan to determine if the hyperfunctioning thyroid tissue is diffuse or limited to one lobe. If it is limited to one lobe, then a lobectomy can be performed to achieve a cure. If diffuse hyperfunctioning tissue is identified, then a total or subtotal thyroidectomy is appropriate.

Proponents of subtotal thyroidectomy argue the following advantages over total thyroidectomy for the surgical treatment of hyperthyroidism: (a) parathyroid tissue and its blood supply are more easily preserved by retaining a rim of thyroid tissue; (b) the recurrent laryngeal nerve can be better protected by retaining a rim of thyroid tissue; (c) the patient is not rendered completely dependent on thyroid hormone replacement since a small amount of thyroid tissue is preserved; and (d) in countries where the patient may not have guaranteed access to lifelong thyroid hormone replacement, a subtotal thyroidectomy is the only option. Proponents of total thyroidectomy argue the following: (a) since all thyroid tissue is removed, there is no chance of growth of the thyroid remnant with recurrent hyperthyroidism, (b) residual thyroid tissue may cause continued antibody formation to the TSH receptor, which is thought to be the cause of Graves' ophthalmopathy, and (c) parathyroid and recurrent nerve preservation should be consistently achievable in the hands of a well-trained surgeon.

Preoperative preparation with antithyroid medications and β-blockers is generally sufficient to prevent intraoperative or postoperative thyroid storm. However, the manipulation of the thyroid gland may place the patient at risk for thyroid storm postoperatively, and therefore these patients should be monitored closely.

Thyroiditis

Thyroiditis has many etiologies, the most common being Hashimoto's thyroiditis—an autoimmune disorder. Thyroid surgery in such patients is more difficult due to the inflammation and hypervascularity of the gland and should be avoided unless there is a concomitant thyroid mass requiring surgical intervention.

Thyroid Goiter

The term goiter means "mass of the thyroid." However, commonly the term is used to describe a markedly enlarged benign growth of the thyroid. Patients may present simply with thyroid enlargement or with symptoms such as dysphagia or dyspnea. Dyspnea may be constant, or it may be positional (generally worse in the recumbent position) or associated with exercise. On physical examination, a large thyroid may be apparent. Tracheal deviation may also be present if this mass is unilateral or markedly larger on one side. Occasionally, a patient may have a substernal goiter and a normal physical examination. Patients with tracheal compression may have a stridorous sound while breathing. Indications for surgery include a visibly enlarged thyroid gland, dyspnea, dysphagia, a concern for malignancy, or tracheal compression on imaging. However, most patients with benign, nontoxic thyroid goiters do not require surgery.

Workup should include a TSH level, and in many cases a CT scan or an MRI. If there does not appear to be substernal extension on physical examination then an ultrasound and chest x-ray may suffice. However, it is possible to have discontinuous thyroid tissue in the substernal region, and therefore, CT or MRI offers a more thorough examination for operative planning.

Total or subtotal thyroidectomy is appropriate for a diffusely enlarged thyroid goiter. An adequate incision is appropriate for excellent exposure, as identification and dissection of the recurrent laryngeal nerve can be challenging. Substernal thyroid goiters can almost always be removed through a cervical incision. On rare occasions a sternotomy may be required.

Oftentimes the surgeon is faced with the decision to perform a lobectomy versus a total or subtotal thyroidectomy for goiter. Occasionally, the goiter is limited to one lobe and the contralateral lobe is normal, in which case lobectomy of the enlarged lobe is the appropriate procedure. However, when one lobe is markedly enlarged and seems to be the cause of the patient's symptoms, but the other lobe is only moderately enlarged, the dilemma arises. Proponents of total thyroidectomy argue that the same physiologic process that caused the goiter of one side will likely cause continued enlargement of the contralateral side, requiring completion thyroidectomy in the future. Proponents of lobectomy in this situation argue that the operation is safer since only two parathyroid glands and one recurrent nerve are put at risk, and the patient is not rendered dependent on thyroid hormone.

Thyroid hormone suppression therapy to prevent or halt growth of a benign thyroid goiter has not been shown to be effective in most cases. Furthermore, addition of thyroid medication requires thyroid function test monitoring and can give rise to unwanted side effects. It may be indicated in patients who are poor surgical candidates.

Intraoperative Nerve Monitoring

Intraoperative recurrent laryngeal nerve monitoring requires the placement of a specialized endotracheal tube equipped with pressure sensors that are apposed to the vocal cords. Wires emanating from the sensors along the tube are then connected to a monitoring system that can alert the surgeon when the nerves are being stimulated, resulting in movement of the vocal cords. Such monitoring can be helpful to the surgeon, both in finding and tracing the nerve along its course. However, there have been no studies showing a statistically significant improvement in avoidance of nerve injury in cases where nerve monitoring is used. Furthermore, no paralytic agents can be used on the patients during surgery which can make the administration of anesthesia more difficult.

Postoperative Medical Management

Total thyroidectomy necessitates the administration of thyroid hormone replacement. Thyroid hormone should be started shortly after surgery for euthyroid patients, and 1 to 2 weeks after surgery for hyperthyroid patients. Levels should be checked and medication dosage should be adjusted 1 month after initiation. Calcium levels must also be checked after total thyroidectomy due to the possibility of hypoparathyroidism. Oral supplementation with calcium and vitamin D is almost always sufficient. As parathyroid function recovers and calcium levels normalize, medication can be discontinued. β-Blockers and antithyroid medications for hyperthyroidism can generally be discontinued within 1 to 2 weeks after surgery.

PARATHYROID DISEASE

Anatomy and Embryology

The parathyroid glands are small endocrine organs commonly located on the posterior surface of the thyroid gland in the neck. There are usually four parathyroid glands, each weighing approximately 35 to 40 mg. They are yellow to tan in color and can be difficult to distinguish from surrounding adipose tissue.

The superior parathyroid glands develop during embryogenesis from the fourth branchial pouch and migrate toward the posteromedial aspect of the thyroid gland near the tracheoesophageal groove. The inferior parathyroid glands originate from the third branchial pouch together with the thymus and migrate caudad to more variable locations than the superior glands; however, they are most commonly found on the posterolateral surface of the lower pole of the thyroid. Some of the most common ectopic sites are (in descending order of frequency) in the thyrothymic ligament, on the prevertebral fascia, in a retroesophageal, paraesophageal, or paratracheal position, in the carotid sheath, within the thyroid gland, and in the anterior or less commonly in the posterior mediastinum.

The inferior thyroid artery is the major arterial supply to both the superior and inferior parathyroid glands in 80% of cases. The parathyroid glands can also be vascularized by the superior thyroid artery and arteries of the larynx, pharynx, esophagus, trachea, and mediastinum. The superior, middle, and inferior thyroid veins provide venous drainage to the parathyroid glands. The lymphatics from the parathyroid glands drain with those of the thyroid gland (pretracheal, paratracheal, tracheoesophageal groove, mediastinal, and jugular lymph nodes).

The recurrent laryngeal nerve, a branch of the vagus nerve, is at risk for injury during thyroid and parathyroid surgery. On the right side, the nerve descends anteriorly to the right subclavian artery, crosses under the artery posteriorly, and then courses superiorly into the tracheoesophageal groove. The left recurrent laryngeal nerve descends anteriorly to the aortic arch, then crosses under the aorta posteriorly at the ductus arteriosus, and finally ascends to the larynx in the tracheoesophageal groove. On the right side, the nerve has an oblique course in the neck traveling more laterally near the thoracic inlet, whereas the left recurrent laryngeal nerve generally courses straight up the tracheoesophageal groove into the larynx.

Physiology

Parathyroid hormone (PTH), an 84 amino acid polypeptide chain, is secreted by the chief cells of the parathyroid gland. The entire polypeptide is referred to as intact PTH (iPTH) with a half-life of 2 to 5 minutes. Normal calcium homeostasis is regulated by a negative feedback mechanism directly on the parathyroid calcium-sensing receptors: an increase in serum calcium results in a decrease in PTH secretion. When the serum ionized calcium level falls, increased levels of PTH stimulate the resorption of calcium and phosphate from bone, decrease calcium excretion by the kidneys, and indirectly increase calcium absorption from the small intestine. PTH increases renal synthesis of $1,25(OH)_2D_3$, the hormonally active form of vitamin D, which augments absorption of dietary calcium from the intestine.

DISORDERS OF THE PARATHYROID GLAND

Primary Hyperparathyroidism

Hyperparathyroidism is a common endocrine disorder characterized by overproduction of PTH resulting in hypercalcemia. Hyperparathyroidism may be primary, secondary, or tertiary. Primary hyperparathyroidism tends to occur more frequently in women, affecting nearly 1 of 500 women and 1 of 2000 men per year. These patients are most often in their fifth, sixth, and seventh decades of life. Hyperparathyroidism is diagnosed by detection of elevated serum calcium and inappropriately elevated iPTH levels. The elevated PTH leads to excessive renal calcium resorption, phosphaturia, increased $1,25(OH)_2D_3$ synthesis, increased bone resorption, and enhanced absorption of intestinal calcium. In a systematic literature review of 20,225 cases by Ruda et al. (23), the causes of primary hyperparathyroidism were solitary adenomas (88.90%), multiple gland hyperplasia (5.74%), double adenomas (4.14%), and carcinomas (0.74%).

Because primary hyperparathyroidism is generally discovered by routine serum chemistry analysis showing elevated calcium levels, patients are usually asymptomatic at the time of diagnosis; however, they can have a wide range of signs and symptoms. The renal manifestations of primary hyperparathyroidism include calcium nephrolithiasis (most common complication of hyperparathyroidism), nephrocalcinosis (calcification within the parenchyma of one or both kidneys), and renal dysfunction. Associated signs and symptoms include flank pain, polyuria, polydipsia, hematuria, and passing of renal calculi. The classic skeletal presentation of hyperparathyroidism is osteitis fibrosa cystica, which is characterized as the combination of subperiosteal resorption of the distal phalanges, bone cysts, brown tumors of long bones, osteoporosis,

and fractures. Osteitis fibrosa cystica is now uncommon, occurring in less than 5% of patients. Although patients with primary hyperparathyroidism are now generally diagnosed long before the development of osteitis fibrosa cystica, many still demonstrate decreased bone mineral density on dual-energy x-ray absorptiometry, leading to bone pain and fractures. Nausea, constipation, peptic ulcer disease, and pancreatitis are some of the associated gastrointestinal disturbances. Neuromuscular abnormalities include complaints of weakness and fatigue. There are also a wide spectrum of neurological conditions associated with primary hyperparathyroidism (anxiety, depression, nervousness, psychosis, and cognitive dysfunction), some of which have been shown to improve after parathyroidectomy (24).

According to the National Institute of Health consensus conference established in 1990 and updated in 2002 (25), patients with overt complications of primary hyperparathyroidism (ie, renal stones, fractures, or significant gastrointestinal symptoms) should undergo parathyroid surgery. For asymptomatic patients, the indications for surgical intervention are controversial. A comparison of the old and new guidelines for surgical treatment is listed in Table 16.1. The current requirement for serum calcium elevation has been changed to 1.0 mg/dL above the upper limit of normal because this indicates susceptibility to the complications of the disease. Regarding bone mineral density, the latest recommendation for surgical intervention is bone density at the lumbar spine, hip, or distal radius that is more than 2.5 standard deviations below peak bone mass (t-score <−2.5). Nonsurgical management for those who do not meet the criteria for surgery includes biannual serum calcium levels, annual serum creatinine levels, and annual bone densitometry at three sites (lumbar spine, hip, and forearm). Traditionally, asymptomatic patients older than 50 years have not been offered surgery, reasoning that the risk of surgery outweighs the benefit. However, it is now recognized that many patients have subtle symptoms, such as neuropsychiatric disturbances, that can be elicited on detailed questioning. Furthermore, the risk and morbidity of surgery have decreased substantially with minimally invasive techniques. Therefore, it is quite acceptable to offer parathyroid surgery to elderly patients assuming a thorough risk and benefit analysis has been considered.

In a study by Silverberg et al. (26), a 10-year prospective study of 121 patients with primary hyperparathyroidism, parathyroidectomy resulted in normalization of biochemical values and increased bone mineral density (lumbar spine and femoral neck) in both symptomatic and asymptomatic patients. The results were similar between postmenopausal and premenopausal women. In asymptomatic patients who did not undergo surgery, no change was noted in the biochemical values or bone mineral density; however 27% of these patients developed at least one new indication for parathyroidectomy (marked hypercalcemia, marked hypercalciuria, and low cortical bone density). All symptomatic patients who did not undergo surgery had recurrent symptoms (kidney stones). This study suggests that symptomatic patients who are good surgical candidates should undergo parathyroid surgery, as well as asymptomatic patients with low bone mineral density at the lumbar spine and femoral neck at the time of diagnosis.

Surgical Management

The traditional operation for primary hyperparathyroidism has been bilateral neck exploration under general anesthesia with identification of all four parathyroid glands. With the introduction of minimally invasive parathyroidectomy, a more focused neck exploration with preoperative and/or intraoperative localization techniques is performed. Technetium-99m (^{99m}Tc) sestamibi scan is the best noninvasive modality for imaging hyperplastic parathyroid glands and adenomas; it has yielded sensitivity rates of approximately 90% in primary hyperparathyroidism. There is selective uptake of ^{99m}Tc-sestamibi by both the thyroid and parathyroid glands. This radionuclide is typically hyperconcentrated and retained longer in the hyperfunctioning parathyroid glands than in other tissues, providing three-dimensional localization when combined with single-photon emission computed tomography imaging (27). Ultrasonography, CT, and MRI are other noninvasive imaging tools with varying rates of sensitivity depending on the technique used and the experience of the examiner. Invasive preoperative localization studies include parathyroid arteriography, selective venous sampling for PTH, and ultrasound-guided fine needle aspiration of the parathyroid tumor. Aspirates of the parathyroid can be processed as a PTH assay, which can confirm the presence of parathyroid tissue by measuring extremely elevated PTH levels. Intraoperative handheld gamma probes can localize the gland concentrating ^{99m}Tc sestamibi, which is injected approximately 2 hours before surgery. Methylene blue has also been used intraoperatively as it is able to stain pathologically abnormal or supernumerary parathyroid glands. This technique is safe, cost-effective, and can significantly shorten operating time (28).

Parathyroid hormone has a very short half-life (2 to 5 minutes) in the circulation and is degraded by the liver and kidney. Before and after the abnormal parathyroid tissue is removed during minimally invasive parathyroidectomy, intraoperative PTH levels are measured. Many surgeons use a greater than 50% reduction from the highest PTH value (preincision or preexcision) 10 minutes after parathyroidectomy as the standard for operative success, whereas others simply recommend an absolute normalization of the PTH level, regardless of the preexcision value (29,30). If PTH levels remain elevated after excision of a lesion, then a four-gland exploration should be undertaken to identify additional parathyroid glands.

Secondary Hyperparathyroidism

Secondary hyperparathyroidism is most commonly associated with chronic renal insufficiency caused by decreased levels of $1,25(OH)_2D_3$, hyperphosphatemia, and hypocalcemia. Disorders of vitamin D (rickets, dietary absence, malabsorption, abnormal metabolism induced by drugs, liver disease), disorders of phosphate metabolism (malnutrition, malabsorption, aluminum toxicity), and calcium deficiency (postsurgical or congenital hypoparathyroidism, loss of calcium in the urine) can also cause secondary hyperparathyroidism. The diagnosis is made when PTH secretion is appropriately increased in the setting of low (or normal) serum calcium. The chronic hypocalcemic state causes a compensatory increase in parathyroid gland function and size; resected glands from patients with secondary hyperparathyroidism show diffuse and nodular hyperplasia on histologic examination (31). Patients with this disorder are usually asymptomatic; however, secondary hyperparathyroidism associated with chronic renal failure has been linked to renal osteodystrophy, hyperphosphatemia, pruritis, anemia, calciphylaxis, and coronary artery calcification. The manifestations of this disease require close observation because they are associated with an increased mortality rate in this patient population.

Medical management is the initial therapy for secondary hyperparathyroidism. Vitamin D replacement (lowers PTH) and phosphorus-binding drugs (reduce serum phosphorous without increasing serum calcium) are most commonly used. Another newer class of drugs, calcimimetics, directly inhibits PTH secretion by increasing the sensitivity of parathyroid calcium-sensing receptors to calcium. Surgery is reserved for patients with intractable disease that cannot be controlled medically and those with severe symptoms of hyperparathyroidism (bone pain or fractures, severe pruritus, persistent hyperphosphatemia, or calciphylaxis) (32). Because the underlying pathology in secondary hyperparathyroidism is hyperplasia, bilateral neck exploration with identification of all glands is the standard operation. Preoperative imaging is usually only indicated when a heterotopic or supernumerary gland is not identified at the first exploration. Both subtotal (three and one-half gland) parathyroidectomy and total parathyroidectomy with heterotopic autotransplantation (brachioradialis or sternocleidomastoid muscle) are acceptable alternative operative procedures.

Tertiary Hyperparathyroidism

Tertiary hyperparathyroidism occurs in patients with long-standing secondary hyperparathyroidism in which the hypertrophied parathyroid glands become autonomous, resulting in hypercalcemia. Virtually all patients with end-stage renal disease will develop secondary hyperparathyroidism due to their electrolyte (particularly phosphorous and calcium) imbalances. Many of these patients will progress to tertiary hyperparathyroidism and undergo total parathyroidectomy with autotransplantation or subtotal parathyroidectomy. Tertiary hyperparathyroidism is also characterized as a condition in which secondary hyperparathyroidism persists after successful renal transplantation due to the autonomous function of the parathyroid glands (33). Renal transplantation does not always reverse the effects of parathyroid hyperplasia, and hypercalcemia can persist in up to 50% of transplant recipients. However, in most of these patients, hyperparathyroidism gradually resolves within the first year of successful transplantation; therefore, less than 1% of transplant recipients require parathyroidectomy.

Multiple Endocrine Neoplasia

Formerly known as Wermer syndrome, MEN1 syndrome is an autosomal dominant disorder characterized by parathyroid hyperplasia, pancreatic endocrine tumors, and pituitary adenomas. A germline mutation in the *MENIN* gene located on chromosome 11 is associated with this syndrome. Hyperparathyroidism caused by multiglandular parathyroid tumors is the most common manifestation of MEN1 (>95%). Because patients with MEN1 develop multiglandular disease, the appropriate operative treatment is bilateral neck exploration and identification of all four glands (subtotal parathyroidectomy or total parathyroidectomy with heterotopic autotransplantation). Transcervical thymectomy is also performed at the initial operation because there is a high incidence of supernumerary glands (up to 20%). The optimal timing and extensiveness of surgical resection for patients with MEN1 remain controversial.

MEN2A (Sipple syndrome), caused by mutations in the *RET* proto-oncogene on chromosome 11, consists of MTC, pheochromocytoma, and primary hyperparathyroidism. Similar to MEN1, hyperparathyroidism in MEN2A is most commonly characterized by multiglandular hyperplasia. However, unlike MEN1, hyperparathyroidism is the least common manifestation of MEN2A (20–30%). Surgical management of hyperparathyroidism is similar to that described for MEN1.

Hypercalcemic Crisis

Hypercalcemic crisis is a life-threatening condition caused by extremely high serum calcium levels. The cause of this clinical syndrome is usually primary hyperparathyroidism or advanced malignancy (34). The most common symptoms involve the gastrointestinal tract and the central nervous system: nausea, vomiting, abdominal pain, constipation, fatigue, headache, weakness, lethargy, and coma. Renal symptoms include polyuria and polydipsia, and cardiac arrhythmias may also occur. Aggressive intravenous rehydration with normal saline (200–300 mL/hr) is the mainstay of treatment in severe hypercalcemia. Loop diuretics, calcitonin, glucocorticoids, and bisphosphonates can also be used to decrease serum calcium levels.

Parathyroid Carcinoma

Carcinoma of the parathyroid gland is extremely rare, and almost all cases are associated with severe hypercalcemia (>13 mg/dL). Several factors raise the suspicion for cancer: a palpable neck mass on physical examination, markedly elevated iPTH and alkaline phosphatase levels, and unambiguous symptoms of hyperparathyroidism (35). A parathyroid gland that is pale white, irregularly shaped, firm, and friable is also suggestive of cancer. Often there are no definitive histologic findings indicative of cancer; therefore, evidence of invasion or severe adherence to surrounding tissues should alert the surgeon to the possibility of this diagnosis. The treatment of choice is en bloc resection of the tumor and areas of potential local invasion, as well as resection of the ipsilateral thyroid lobe and central compartment lymphatics. The integrity of the parathyroid capsule should be maintained to prevent the spread of cancer cells; therefore, a frozen section incisional biopsy is not performed. The 5-year survival rate in patients with parathyroid carcinoma varies between 29% and 44%. Adjuvant external beam radiation and chemotherapeutic agents have been used with very limited success.

SURGICAL TECHNIQUES

The standard four-gland exploration is typically performed under general anesthesia while local anesthesia is commonly used for minimally invasive parathyroidectomy. Similar to thyroid surgery, a transverse cervical incision (Kocher) is made in the lower neck using a skin crease when possible. Once subplatysmal flaps have been created, the median raphe between the strap muscles is incised, allowing the strap muscles to be retracted laterally and the thyroid gland to be exposed. The thyroid gland is mobilized anteriorly and medially, and the middle thyroid vein is isolated and divided. The inferior thyroid artery and the recurrent laryngeal nerve are identified. The superior parathyroid glands are usually found on the posterolateral aspect of the superior pole of the thyroid lobe. The inferior parathyroid glands are more anterior than the superior glands and commonly adjacent to the inferior pole of the thyroid gland or within the thyrothymic ligament. If the abnormal parathyroid glands are not identified, further exploration is mandated. This may entail removing the thymic tissue on the side of the missing gland, palpation or intraoperative sonography of the thyroid for evidence of an intrathyroidal gland, careful exploration of variable and potential ectopic sites, and possible resection of the thyroid lobe ipsilateral to the missing parathyroid gland. If the missing gland is still not found, the operation is terminated, and the patient is reevaluated.

Subtotal parathyroidectomy involves resection of three or more glands, depending on the total number and size of the glands. A well-vascularized remnant of approximately 50 to 80 mg is preserved. The remnant can be marked with a titanium clip, which allows easier identification during reexploration for recurrent disease. One advantage of this procedure is that the well-vascularized remnant will continue to function while an autotransplanted gland will need several weeks to undergo neovascularization. However, the disadvantage of this technique is that in the event of recurrent disease, a reoperative neck exploration is required.

Total parathyroidectomy with autotransplantation identifies and removes all glands, and minced fragments of parathyroid tissue are placed in the brachioradialis muscle in the forearm or in the sternocleidomastoid muscle. The major advantage of the forearm implantation technique is that the residual parathyroid tissue can be easily accessed and resected under local anesthesia in the setting of recurrent disease. However, as mentioned previously, it takes several weeks for the parathyroid tissue to resume function, and patients need aggressive calcium replacement and monitoring during that time to avoid severe hypocalcemia. Autograft failure leading to hypoparathyroidism is another risk of this technique.

Minimally invasive video-assisted parathyroidectomy, pioneered by Paolo Miccoli, is one of the latest frontiers in parathyroid surgery (36,37). This procedure is performed under general anesthesia on patients who demonstrate a focal area of uptake on ^{99m}Tc sestamibi scan. Other eligibility criteria include no prior neck surgery and absence of concomitant thyroid nodules or significant thyroid enlargement. A 15-mm incision is made 1 cm above the sternal notch, and a 12-mm trocar is inserted between the strap muscles and the thyroid on the side of the lesion. Under direct vision, operative space is established by brief insufflation of carbon dioxide and then maintained by small external retractors. A 30-degree, 5-mm endoscope is used for visualization, and the dissection of the adenoma is performed with small instruments that are 2 mm in diameter. Small clips are used for vessel ligation. Intraoperative iPTH assay confirms the completeness of the surgical resection. The utility and true advantages of this technique are a subject of controversy.

THYROID DISEASE QUESTIONS

Select one answer.

1. Which one of the following is true about MTC?
   a. 70% to 80% of MTC cases are familial in origin.
   b. 70% to 80% of MTC cases are sporadic in nature.
   c. RRAI (radioactive iodine remnant ablation) is used to treat micrometastatic disease in MTC.

2. The following is not true about papillary thyroid cancer?
   a. Most common malignancy of thyroid gland.
   b. More common in men than women.
   c. Most commonly metastasizes by lymphatics.
   d. Lymphatic metastases have no effect on survival rate.
   e. True (pure) papillary cancer is rare.

3. The most common site for follicular carcinoma metastases is:
   a. Lung.
   b. Liver.
   c. Bone.
   d. Brain.
   e. Adrenal.

4. The following is not a characteristic feature of familial MTC:
   a. RET proto-oncogene mutation.
   b. Unilateral.
   c. Histopathology shows amyloid deposits.
   d. Serum calcitonin is used as a tumor marker.

5. Which of the following are true?
   a. 5% to 8% of cold nodules of the thyroid gland on iodine scintigraphy are malignant.
   b. 15% to 30% of incidentalomas of the thyroid gland on PET scan are malignant.
   c. Both are true.
   d. Neither one is true.

PARATHYROID DISEASE QUESTIONS

Select one answer.

1. What is the most common cause of primary hyperparathyroidism?
   a. Adenoma.
   b. Carcinoma.
   c. Hyperplasia.
   d. Chronic renal insufficiency.

2. All of the following are appropriate treatment options for secondary hyperparathyroidism except:
   a. Vitamin D replacement and phosphorus-binding drugs.
   b. Subtotal parathyroidectomy.
   c. Total parathyroidectomy with autotransplantation.
   d. Minimally invasive parathyroidectomy with preoperative technetium-99m sestamibi scan.

3. What percentage reduction in the PTH value from baseline indicates a successful operation?
   a. 40.
   b. 50.
   c. 60.
   d. Depends on the size of the resected parathyroid gland.

4. If the abnormal parathyroid glands are not found during bilateral neck exploration, all of the following measures are appropriate except:
   a. Inspect both thyroid lobes.
   b. Remove normal-appearing parathyroid glands.
   c. Remove the thymic tissue on the side of the missing gland.
   d. Explore common ectopic sites.

5. MEN1 is associated with:
   a. A mutation in the RET proto-oncogene.
   b. Medullary thyroid carcinoma.
   c. Only one standard surgical treatment.
   d. Multiglandular parathyroid disease.

REFERENCES

1. Sherman SI. Clinicopathologic and prognostic staging for thyroid carcinomas. *Thyroid Today* 2000;23(3)1–9.
2. American Cancer Society. *Cancer facts and figures 2008*. Atlanta, GA: American Cancer Society, 2008.
3. Carling T, Udelsman R. Thyroid tumors. In: DeVita VT Jr, Hellman S, Rosenberg SA, eds. *Cancer: principles and practice of oncology*, 7th ed. Philadelphia, PA: Lippincott Williams & Wilkins, 2005;1502–1519.
4. Braverman LE, Utiger RD, eds. *Werner & Ingbar's the thyroid: a fundamental and clinical text*, 8th ed. Philadelphia, PA: Lippincott Williams & Wilkins, 2000.
5. Roelants V, De Nayer P, Bouckaert A, Beckers C. The predictive value of serum thyroglobulin in the follow-up of

differentiated thyroid cancer. *Eur J Nucl Med* 1997;24: 722–727.

6. Tuttle MR, Leboeuf R, Martorella AJ. Papillary thyroid cancer: monitoring and therapy. *Endocrinol Metab Clin N Am* 2007;36(3):753–778.

7. American Cancer Society. *Thyroid cancer detailed guide*. http://documents.cancer.org/196.00/196.00.pdf. Accessed December 10, 2003.

8. Cobin RH, Gharib H, Bergman DA, et al. AACE/AAES medical/surgical guidelines for clinical practice: management of thyroid carcinoma. *Endocr Pract* 2001;7(3):202–220.

9. Hundahl SA, Fleming ID, Fremgen AM, Menck HR. A National Cancer Data Base report on 53,856 cases of thyroid carcinoma treated in the U.S., 1985–1995. *Cancer* 1998;83(12):2638–2648.

10. Machens A, Niccoli-Sire P, Hoegel J, et al. Early malignant progression of hereditary medullary thyroid cancer. *N Engl J Med* 2003;349:1517–1525.

11. Skinner MA, Moley JA, Dilley WG, Owzar K, DeBenedetti MK, Wells SA Jr. Prophylactic thyroidectomy in multiple endocrine neoplasia type 2 A. *N Engl J Med* 2005;353: 1105–1113.

12. Russell CF, Van Heerden JA, Sizemore GW, et al. The surgical management of medullary thyroid carcinoma. *Ann Surg* 1983;197(1):42–48.

13. Aldinger KA, Samaan NA, Ibanez M, Hill SC Jr. Anaplastic carcinoma of the thyroid: a review of 84 cases of spindle and giant cell carcinoma of the thyroid. *Cancer* 1978;41(6): 2267–2275.

14. Cooper DS, Doherty GM, Haugen BR, et al. Management guidelines for patients with thyroid nodules and differentiated thyroid cancer. *Thyroid* 2006;16(2):109–142.

15. Morris LF, Ragavendra N, Yeh MW. Evidence-based assessment of the role of ultrasonography in the management of benign thyroid nodules. *World J Surg* 2008;32(7):1253–1263.

16. King DL, Stack BC Jr, Spring PM, Walker R, Bodenner DL. Incidence of thyroid carcinoma in fluorodeoxyglucose positron emission tomography-positive thyroid incidentalomas. *Otolaryngol Head Neck Surg* 2007;137:400–404.

17. Bilimoria KY, Bentrem DJ, Ko CY, et al. Extent of surgery affects survival for papillary thyroid cancer. *Ann Surg* 2007; 246(3):375–381.

18. Goldman JM, Goren EN, Cohen MH, Webber BL, Brennan MF, Robbins J. Anaplastic thyroid carcinoma: long-term survival after radical surgery. *J Surg Oncol* 1980;14 (4):389–394.

19. Moley JF, DeBenedetti MK. Patterns of nodal metastases in palpable medullary thyroid carcinoma: recommendations for extent of node dissection. *Ann Surg* 1999;229(6): 880–887.

20. Dralle H, Scheumann GF, Proye C, et al. The value of lymph node dissection in hereditary medullary thyroid carcinoma: a retrospective, European, multicentre study. *J Intern Med* 1995;238:357–361.

21. Simpson WJ, Carruthers JS. The role of external radiation in the management of papillary and follicular thyroid cancer. *Am J Surg* 1978;136(4):457–460.

22. Shimaoka K, Schoenfeld DA, DeWys WD, Creech RH, DeConti R. A randomized trial of doxorubicin versus doxorubicin plus cisplatin in patients with advanced thyroid carcinoma. *Cancer* 1985;56(9):2155–2160.

23. Ruda JM, Hollenbeak CS, Stack BC Jr. A systematic review of the diagnosis and treatment of primary hyperparathyroidism from 1995 to 2003. *Otolaryngol Head Neck Surg* 2005;132:359–372.

24. Ahmad R, Hammond JM. Primary, secondary, and tertiary hyperparathyroidism. *Otolaryngol Clin N Am* 2004;37: 701–713.

25. Bilezikian JP, Potts JT Jr, Fuleihan GE, et al. Summary statement from a workshop on asymptomatic primary hyperparathyroidism: a perspective for the 21st century. *J Clin Endocrinol Metab* 2002;87(12):5353–5361.

26. Silverberg SJ, Shane E, Jacobs TP, Siris E, Bilezikian JP. A 10-year prospective study of primary hyperparathyroidism with or without parathyroid surgery. *N Engl J Med* 1999; 341:1249–1255.

27. Civelek AC, Ozalp E, Donovan P, Udelsman R. Prospective evaluation of delayed technetium-99 m sestamibi SPECT scintigraphy for preoperative localization of primary hyperparathyroidism. *Surgery* 2002;131:149–157.

28. Kuriloff DB, Sanborn KV. Rapid intraoperative localization of parathyroid glands utilizing methylene blue infusion. *Otolaryngol Head Neck Surg* 2004;131:616–622.

29. Inabnet WB. Intraoperative parathyroid hormone monitoring. *World J Surg* 2004;28:1212–1215.

30. Carneiro DM, Solorzano CC, Nader MC, Ramirez M, Irvin GL 3rd. Comparison of intraoperative iPTH assay (QPTH) criteria in guiding parathyroidectomy: which criterion is the most accurate? *Surgery* 2003;134(6): 973–981.

31. Llach F, Velasquez Forero F. Secondary hyperparathyroidism in chronic renal failure: pathogenic and clinical aspects. *Am J Kidney Dis* 2001;38:S20–S30.

32. Tominaga Y, Matsuoka S, Sato T. Surgical indications and procedures of parathyroidectomy in patients with chronic kidney disease. *Ther Apher Dial* 2005;9:44–47.

33. Schlosser K, Endres N, Celik I, Fendrich V, Rothmund M, Fernández ED. Surgical treatment of tertiary hyperparathyroidism: the choice of procedure matters! *World J Surg* 2007;31:1947–1953.

34. Ziegler R. Hypercalcemic crisis. *J Am Soc Nephrol* 2001; 12:S3–S9.

35. Wang C, Gaz RD. Natural history of parathyroid carcinoma. *Am J Surg* 1985;149:522–527.

36. Miccoli P, Berti P, Conte M, Raffaelli M, Materazzi G. Minimally invasive video-assisted parathyroidectomy: lesson learned from 137 cases. *J Am Coll Surg* 2000; 191(6): 613–618.

37. Miccoli P, Berti P, Materazzi G, et al. Minimally invasive video assisted parathyroidectomy (MIVAP). *Eur J Surg* 2003;29:188–190.

CHAPTER **17**

Jennifer Stableford
Alex Stone

Adrenal Surgery

ANATOMY AND EMBRYOLOGY

The adrenal glands are paired organs located at the superior pole of the kidneys, each weighing approximately 5 g. The left-sided gland is leaf shaped and lies in the retroperitoneum above the left renal vein. The right gland is pyramidal in shape and lies lateral to the vena cava with its medal surface wrapped around the vena cava. They receive arterial blood supply from three arteries: the superior adrenal which is a branch of the inferior phrenic artery, the middle adrenal artery which originates off the aorta, and the inferior adrenal artery which is a branch of the renal artery. Venous drainage is primarily via the central adrenal vein that empties directly into the vena cava on the right and into the renal vein on the left. The arterial supply is rarely a problem during surgery and is easily controlled. Most surgical misadventures involved the venous supply, especially the short right renal vein. This can easily be avulsed from the venal cava, resulting in bleeding which is difficult to control.

The adrenal gland is divided into two components: the outer cortex which constitutes 90% of the gland and is of mesodermal origin and the inner medulla which contains chromaffin cells derived from neuroectodermal origin and comprises the remaining 10% of the gland. The outer cortex is further divided into three histological zones. The zona glomerulosa is located just under the capsule and is responsible for mineralocorticoid production. The middle layer, the zona fasciculata, and the central zona reticularis are the site of cortisol production as well as the adrenal sex hormones. The adrenal medulla is located in the center of the organ and is the site of catecholamine synthesis, storage, and metabolism.

ADRENOCORTICAL TUMORS

Cushing's Syndrome

Cushing's syndrome encompasses a constellation of symptoms caused by an excess of glucocorticoids. Signs and symptoms include truncal obesity, moon facies, abdominal striae, supraclavicular fullness, glucose intolerance or frank diabetes, hypertension, and dyslipidemia (Table 17.1).

Cushing's syndrome results from either exogenous administration of steroids or endogenous overproduction of cortisol. Endogenous sources include pituitary overproduction of adrenocorticotropic hormone (ACTH) (Cushing's disease) leading to bilateral adrenal hyperplasia, adrenal production of cortisol from a benign adrenal adenoma or malignant adrenal adenocarcinoma, or a nonpituitary source of ACTH or corticotropin-releasing hormone such as in a paraneoplastic syndrome.

Diagnosis of Cushing's syndrome begins with measuring the serum cortisol level. The sensitivity and specificity is about 80%; however, drawing levels at 8:00 AM and 6:00 PM can improve the sensitivity, as the normal diurnal variation of plasma cortisol levels is lost in Cushing's syndrome. Urinary 17-OH corticosteroids and 24-hour urinary free cortisol are the most sensitive tests for Cushing's syndrome.

Biochemically, adrenal cortical hyperplasia is distinguished from Cushing's syndrome due to neoplasm by the Dexamethasone Suppression Test, the Rapid Dexamethasone Test, or the Metyrapone Test.

The Dexamethasone Suppression Test involves monitoring 24-hour urine content of 17-hydroxysteroids for 6 days (2-day control period, 2-day low-dose suppression period, and 2-day high-dose suppression

TABLE 17.1	Signs and Symptoms of Cushing's Syndrome

Moon facies	Osteoporosis
Truncal obesity	Edema
Hypertension	Diabetes
Plethora	Supraclavicular fat pad
Amenorrhea or impotence	Buffalo hump
Weakness and fatigue	Muscle wasting
Hirsutism	Emotional lability
Striae	Renal calculi
Ecchymoses	

TABLE 17.2	Treatment of Cushing's Syndrome

Adenoma
　Unilateral adrenalectomy
Carcinoma
　Unilateral adrenalectomy
Nodular dysplasia
　Bilateral adrenalectomy
Hyperplasia
　Pituitary surgery
　Pituitary irradiation
　Bilateral adrenalectomy

period). Low-dose dexamethasone (0.5 mg) is given every 6 hours for 48 hours and the urine cortisol and 17-OH corticosteroid levels are serially measured. Following this, high-dose dexamethasone (2 mg) is given every 6 hours. In the normal individual, low-dose dexamethasone provides a negative feedback loop, which will suppress the hypothalamic–pituitary secretion of ACTH and consequently decrease urine cortisol level, whereas in Cushing's syndrome, cortisol production is not suppressed by low-dose dexamethasone. High-dose dexamethasone will suppress cortisol production in patients with bilateral hyperplasia, based on pituitary feedback; however, Cushing's syndrome due to a cortical neoplasm will not suppress, since it is not pituitary dependent.

Since the Dexamethasone Suppression Test is quite tedious, requiring six 24-hour urine specimens, a simpler option is the Rapid Dexamethasone Suppression Test, which is based on serum specimens. A control specimen is drawn. The patient then takes 1 mg of dexamethasone in the evening, and a suppressed serum specimen is drawn in the morning. The results parallel that of the standard Dexamethasone Suppression Test.

The Metyrapone (metapyrone) Test also looks at the pituitary–adrenal axis feedback mechanism. Metyrapone stops 11-beta hydroxylation of cortisol, producing 11-deoxycortisol. This is not recognized by the pituitary as cortisol; hence, production of ACTH rises. Patients with hyperplasia then increase their steroid production in response to Metyrapone, whereas in patients with adrenal neoplasms, steroid production remains unchanged.

Following this, the adrenals should be imaged with a computed tomography (CT) scan. Patients with hyperplasia will have both adrenals diffusely enlarged, where as in patients with a neoplasm, a single lesion is visible with suppression of the remaining adrenal tissue as well as the contralateral gland.

Treatment of Cushing's syndrome caused by an adrenal adenoma or carcinoma is unilateral adrenalectomy. Cushing's syndrome due to hyperplasia can be treated by bilateral adrenalectomy or by pituitary ablation by either surgery or external beam irradiation (Table 17.2). At the present time, the majority of these patients are treated with pituitary irradiation.

Following unilateral adrenalectomy for adrenal neoplasm, patients are effectively Addisonian due to chronic suppression of the contralateral gland. They therefore require maintenance corticosteroids until the pituitary–adrenal axis recovers. This recovery is stimulated by the gradual tapering of the corticosteroids, a process which can take from several months to more than a year. Following bilateral adrenalectomy, patients will require life-long maintenance steroids. In cases where pituitary ablation is pursued, patients will require steroid maintenance as well as replacement of other pituitary hormones.

Aldosteronoma (Conn's Syndrome)

Hyperaldosteronism results in hypertension and hypokalemia, and although less than 1% of all patients with hypertension have hyperaldosteronism, it should be investigated in anyone with hypertension who has hypokalemia and/or an adrenal mass. Although most are asymptomatic, some patients have complaints related to hypokalemia and elevated total

Primary Hyperaldosteronism

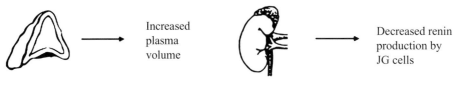

Secondary Hyperaldosteronism

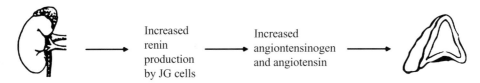

FIGURE 17.1. Hyperaldosteronism.

body sodium such as headache, polyuria, muscle weakness, cramps, and paresthesias. Severe hypokalemia may lead to electrocardiographic changes and cardiac arrhythmias.

Since patients with hypertension develop secondary hyperaldosteronism, these patients must be separated from those with primary hyperaldosteronism. This is done with laboratory evaluations of serum aldosterone and renin levels. A plasma aldosterone level of more than 15 ng/dL, plasma renin level of less than 1 ng/dL, and a plasma aldosterone/renin ratio of more than 30 are all highly sensitive for primary hyperaldosteronism. An elevation of both the plasma aldosterone and renin levels suggests the patient has secondary hyperaldosteronism (Fig. 17.1). Spironolactone may lead to a false-positive result and must be held prior to testing.

Infusion of 2 L of normal saline over 4 hours should suppress serum aldosterone levels to less than 10 ng/dL in normal individuals, whereas in the case of hyperaldosteronism, the serum aldosterone level remains elevated. Renal artery stenosis can lead to a false positive in this test. Administration of captopril, an angiotensin-converting enzyme inhibitor, has results similar to that of the saline infusion with a failure to suppress aldosterone levels seen in those with hyperaldosteronism.

Eighty percent of patients with hyperaldosteronism have an adrenal adenoma, whereas up to 20% have primary adrenal cortical hyperplasia. Once the diagnosis of hyperaldosteronism is confirmed, it is important to identify whether the patient has an adenoma or hyperplasia, because only those with adenomas will benefit from unilateral adrenalectomy. If there is no adenoma seen on CT or magnetic resonance imaging (MRI), then it is beneficial to measure serum 18-hydroxycorticosterone levels. This aldosterone precursor is known to be elevated (>100 μg/dL) in patients with adenomas, whereas the levels are normal in those with hyperplasia. Aldosteronomas can vary in size but, in general, are smaller in diameter than other adrenal tumors such as a pheochromocytoma or Cushing producing tumor and are therefore more difficult to image.

Finally, selective venous sampling, which measures aldosterone levels in the right and left adrenal veins, is extremely useful in localization an adenoma prior to surgery. In fact, many surgeons will perform this even in cases with a clearly identified adenoma on imaging. A recent study demonstrated that when selective venous sampling was performed on patients with an adenoma seen on CT imaging, 18% demonstrated hypersecretion of aldosterone from the normal appearing contralateral gland and 9% demonstrated bilateral aldosterone secretion, suggestive of bilateral adrenal hyperplasia. Overall, selective venous sampling altered management in 27% of patients with hyperaldosteronism and a single adrenal adenoma seen on CT imaging.

Treatment of hyperaldosteronism resulting from an adenoma is unilateral adrenalectomy. Hyperaldosteronism caused by primary adrenal cortical hyperplasia is usually treated with targeted pharmacotherapy, although in refractory cases, bilateral adrenalectomy may be indicated. Unlike cortical neoplasms, which produce cortisol, aldosteronomas do not suppress the contralateral adrenal. Therefore, steroid replacement therapy is not needed after unilateral adrenalectomy for aldosteronoma.

Adrenogenital Syndrome

Adrenogenital syndrome in children results from a deficiency in an enzyme required for the production of cortisol, leading to an excess production of sex hormones. The two most common deficiencies are 21-OH and 11β-OH.

In adults, the adrenogenital syndrome is most commonly virilizing and therefore clinically evident only in women. Patients develop amenorrhea, increased muscle mass, male pattern hair loss, decreased female secondary sexual characteristics, and clitoral enlargement. Typically, this syndrome is caused by an adrenal adenoma or adenocarcinoma. Although these tumors have a higher incidence of malignancy than other endocrine-secreting cortical tumors, they are still quite rare.

Adrenocortical Carcinoma

Adrenocortical carcinoma is rare, with an incidence of 1 to 2 per million. There is a 2:1 female predominance and it most commonly presents in the fourth and fifth decades. Adrenocortical carcinoma spreads by both hematogenous and lymphatic routes and up to 40% of patients present with metastatic disease at the time of initial diagnosis. The most common sites of metastases are the lung, liver, bone, and brain. Local invasion into adjacent organs such as the kidney, liver, diaphragm, pancreas, spleen, and vena cava is also common at presentation. The 5-year survival for stage I is approximately 60%, whereas stage IV has a 0% 5-year survival.

Up to 60% of patients present with a hormonally active tumor, with Cushing's syndrome being the most common. Virilizing or feminizing tumors are also a common presentation. Although hypoaldosteronism can be seen, this is a rare presentation.

Primary treatment of adrenocortical carcinoma is surgery, as it provides the only hope for cure. Aggressive local resection should be attempted whenever possible. When a complete resection is not possible, debulking should be attempted as this may provide symptomatic relief for excess hormone production and has been associated with an improved overall survival. Mitotane is used for unresectable disease, incomplete resections, or metastatic disease. As it is cytotoxic to adrenocortical cells, resulting in necrosis of zona fasciculata and zone reticularis, side effects include adrenal insufficiency.

Metastatic Disease to the Adrenal

The most common malignant tumor of the adrenal gland is metastatic disease. In fact, the adrenal gland is the fourth most common site of metastasis from other primary tumors. Malignancies which frequently metastasize to the adrenal include lung, breast, melanoma, renal, thyroid, and colon.

Incidentaloma

The term "incidentaloma" refers to a tumor of the adrenal gland discovered on an imaging study performed for another indication. The frequent use of CT imaging has resulted in an increase in the number of incidentalomas identified. The approach to an incidentaloma must include an assessment of whether it is a functional tumor, the risk of carcinoma, as well as the possibility that it is metastatic disease.

A detailed history and physical examination may identify signs or symptoms of a functional adrenal tumor; however, most incidentalomas are asymptomatic. Hormonal screening for Cushing's syndrome, aldosteronoma, and pheochromocytoma should be included in the workup.

An incidentaloma discovered in a patient with a history of another malignancy may represent metastatic disease. Tissue biopsy by fine needle aspiration or surgical approach should be obtained only if the results would alter treatment.

The incidence of malignancy in adrenal cortical tumors is directly related to size. Carcinoma is extremely rare in patients with lesions smaller than 3 cm, whereas the incidence of malignancy is high in lesions greater than 6 cm. Incidentalomas greater than 5 cm in size should be removed, as the incidence of carcinoma is significant in this population. Those less than 4 cm should be followed with serial imaging and removed if they increase in size. Incidentalomas between 4 and 5 cm have been observed in the past; however, with the increasing use of the less invasive laparoscopic adrenalectomy, many surgeons are now recommending an adrenalectomy for any incidentaloma greater than 4 cm.

ADRENAL MEDULLARY TUMORS

Pheochromocytoma

Pheochromocytoma is a rare tumor arising from chromaffin cells of neuroectodermal origin. They have an incidence of 2 to 8 per million and typically present in the fourth or fifth decade with no gender predilection. Classically, they follow the "rule of 10s," where 10% of pheochromocytomas are malignant, 10% bilateral, 10% hereditary, 10% seen in children, and 10% extra-adrenal (paraganglionoma).

Pheochromocytomas most often secrete norepinephrine, epinephrine, and dopamine; however, they have been reported to also secrete peptides such as ACTH, vasoactive intestinal peptide, enkephalins, IL-6, neuropeptide Y, and serotonin.

The typical presentation is that of classic "spells," which include headache, palpitations, and diaphoresis with hypertension. These spells can last from 30 seconds to 24 hours and may be precipitated by strenuous activity. Only 50% of patients remain hypertensive outside of a spell (Table 17.3).

The diagnosis of pheochromocytoma requires the identification of elevated levels of catecholamines or their metabolites in the urine or plasma. The most

common test employed is the measurement of 24-hour urinary levels of vanillylmandelic acid (VMA), metanephrines, or fractionated catecholamines. This has a sensitivity of 99% and is more specific than the measurement of plasma levels. Since 24-hour urine collection is tedious, patients can be screened using serum specimens. Patients with pheochromocytoma have geometric increases in catecholamine levels. If a positive value is found, the diagnosis still must be confirmed by 24-hour urine collection.

Once the diagnosis has been confirmed, the pheochromocytoma must be localized. CT scan is the most appropriate first imaging study to employ with an accuracy of 90%. Pheochromocytomas will enhance on T2-weighted MRI, so this modality is a useful study in patients who cannot tolerate intravenous contrast as well as in those with extra-adrenal lesions. I-123 metaiodobenzylguanidine (MIGB) scans have a reported sensitivity of up to 90% and also may be useful in finding extra-adrenal lesions as well as identifying synchronous lesions or metastatic disease.

Surgery is the primary treatment of pheochromocytoma, and appropriate presurgical preparation is essential. Patients are severely volume contracted secondary to the chronic catecholamine secretion and are prone to hemodynamic instability during general anesthesia. Preoperative α-adrenergic blockade for 1 to 4 weeks with phenoxybenzamine, metyrosine, or prazosin is essential and must precede any β-blockade, as β-blockade alone will lead to unopposed α-receptor stimulation and malignant hypertension. Intraoperatively, patients will have labile blood pressure, particularly during manipulation of the tumor. Intra-arterial blood pressure monitoring is essential and anesthesia must have intravenous drips prepared to treat both hypertension and hypotension.

Although the majority of pheochromocytomas are sporadic in nature, they can be associated with a familial genetic syndrome such as MEN2a (Sipple's syndrome), MEN2b, neurofibromatosis (von Recklinghausen's), and von Hipple–Lindau's disease. In the past, it was recommended to perform bilateral adrenalectomy in patients presenting with a pheochromocytoma in the setting of a familial syndrome; however, given the risk and overall morbidity of adrenal insufficiency after bilateral adrenalectomy, this practice is now being questioned, as it has been shown that only 50% of patients who undergo unilateral adrenalectomy for a familial pheochromocytoma go on to develop a second pheochromocytoma in the contralateral adrenal. Current recommendation is to

TABLE 17.3	Symptoms of Pheochromocytoma

Alpha symptoms
  Hypertension
  Gluconeogenesis
  Pallor
  Smooth muscle contraction
  Platelet aggregation
Beta symptoms
  Tachycardia
  Diaphoresis
  Hypotension

perform a unilateral adrenalectomy in patients with a macroscopically normal contralateral gland with serial follow-up to screen for the development of a second pheochromocytoma. Treatment for patients with a sporadic pheochromocytoma remains unilateral adrenalectomy.

ADRENAL INSUFFICIENCY

Primary adrenal insufficiency is a failure of the adrenal gland to produce sufficient levels of corticosteroids. The most common cause of primary adrenal insufficiency is autoimmune adrenal atrophy (Addison's disease). Other causes include infection, adrenal hemorrhage, metastases, and surgical removal (bilateral adrenalectomy). Waterhouse–Friderichsen syndrome describes the condition of adrenal hemorrhage associated with meningococcal sepsis.

Secondary adrenal insufficiency results from a deficiency in the secretion of ACTH at the level of the pituitary or hypothalamus. The most common cause of secondary adrenal insufficiency is glucocorticoid administration.

SURGICAL CONSIDERATIONS

Surgical options for adrenalectomy include open anterior transabdominal, flank, or thoracoabdominal approaches and the transperitoneal or retroperitoneal laparoscopic approach. Several nonrandomized studies have demonstrated a reduction in morbidity, mortality, and length of stay in patients undergoing laparoscopic adrenalectomy when compared with open surgery. Even after adjusting for confounding factors, the 30-day mortality has been demonstrated to be much higher in patients undergoing open adrenalectomy, so that laparoscopic adrenalectomy is becoming the standard of care, with the open procedure being reserved for large, bulky, or malignant tumors.

QUESTIONS

Select one answer.

1. Which of the following statements is incorrect?
   a. The right superior adrenal artery is a branch of the superior phrenic artery.
   b. The left middle adrenal artery is a direct branch of the aorta.
   c. The left adrenal vein drains into the renal vein.
   d. The right adrenal vein drains into the vena cava.
   e. The right inferior adrenal artery is a branch of the renal artery.

2. All of the following are true regarding the adrenal gland except
   a. The zona glomerulosa is responsible for mineralocorticoid production.
   b. The outer cortex comprises 90% of the gland.
   c. The inner medulla contains chromaffin cells of mesodermal origin.
   d. The inner medulla is the site of catecholamine synthesis, storage, and production.
   e. Cortisol is produced in the zona fasciculata and zona reticularis.

3. Which of the following statements about Cushing's disease is true?
   a. Treatment involves unilateral adrenalectomy.
   b. High-dose dexamethasone will cause suppression of cortisol production.
   c. It is often associated with a malignancy.
   d. Unlike in other forms of Cushing's syndrome, patients demonstrate diurnal secretion of cortisol.
   e. Pituitary irradiation is contraindicated in Cushing's disease.

4. All of the following are true regarding the Dexamethasone Suppression Test except
   a. It involves measuring 17-hydroxysteroids in 24-hour urine samples for 6 days.
   b. Low-dose dexamethasone is 2 mg.
   c. A normal individual will have suppression of cortisol production by low-dose dexamethasone.
   d. Cortisol production by a cortical neoplasm will not be suppressed by either low- or high-dose dexamethasone.
   e. Cortisol production by a pituitary adenoma will be suppressed by only high-dose dexamethasone.

5. All of the following are expected laboratory results in a patient with primary hyperaldosteronism except
   a. Elevated plasma aldosterone/renin ratio.
   b. Hypokalemia.

   c. Elevated plasma renin level.

   d. Plasma aldosterone level of more than 15 ng/dL.

6. Which of the following is true regarding adrenocortical carcinoma?

   a. It is common in adrenal masses 4 cm in size.

   b. It is the most common malignant tumor found in the adrenal gland.

   c. It spreads by both hematogenous and lymphatic routes.

   d. Only 20% of patients demonstrate metastatic disease at the time of presentation.

   e. The 5-year survival of stage I disease is 90%.

7. All of the following are true regarding pheochromocytomas except

   a. 10% are malignant.

   b. 10% are seen in children.

   c. 10% are hereditary.

   d. 10% are seen in females.

   e. 10% are extra-adrenal.

8. All of the following are genetic syndromes which include pheochromocytoma except

   a. MEN 2b.

   b. von Recklinghausen.

   c. MEN 2a.

   d. von Hipple–Lindau.

   e. von Gierke.

9. All of the following are elevated in a patient with pheochromocytoma except

   a. Urinary VMA.

   b. Urinary metanephrines.

   c. Urinary 17-OH corticosteroids.

   d. Urinary fractionated catecholamines.

10. Which of the following statements is true about surgery for pheochromocytoma?

   a. Patients should receive preoperative α-blockade for 1 to 4 weeks prior to surgery.

   b. The adrenal vein should be taken only after the arterial supply is isolated and ligated.

   c. Intravenous fluids should be restricted until the tumor is removed.

   d. Preoperative β-blockade should precede any α-blockers to avoid the precipitation of malignant hypertension.

   e. Bilateral adrenalectomy should be performed for patients with MEN2a.

SELECTED REFERENCES

Ditzhuijsen CIM, van de Weijer R, Haak HR. Adrenocortical carcinoma. *Neth J Med* 2007;65:55–59.

Elamin MB, Murad MH, Mullan R, et al. Accuracy of diagnostic tests for Cushing's syndrome: a systematic review and meta-analysis. *J Clin Endocrinol Metab* 2008;93(5): 1553–1562.

Lairmore TC, Bull DW, Bailin SB, et al. Management of pheochromocytoma in patients with multiple endocrine neoplasia type II syndrome. *Ann Surg* 1993;217:595–603.

Lee J, Mahmoud ET, Schifftner T, et al. Open and laparoscopic adrenalectomy: analysis of the national surgical quality improvement program. *J Am Coll Surg* 2008;206:953–961.

Lee JA, Kebebew E. Adrenocortical tumors. In: Current surgical therapy. 9th ed. Philadelphia, PA: Mosby Elsevier, 2008:583–592.

Schwab CW, Vingan H, Fabrizio MD. Usefulness of adrenal vein sampling in the evaluation of aldosteronism. *J Endourol* 2008;22:1247–1250.

Stifelman MD, Feneg DM. Work-up of the functional adrenal mass. *Curr Urol Rep* 2005;6:63–71.

Thompson GB, Grant CS. Pheochromocytoma. In: *Current Surgical Therapy*. 9th ed. Philadelphia, PA: Mosby Elsevier, 2008:592–597.

Udelsman R. Adrenal. In: Norton JA, Bollinger RR, Chang AE, et al. *Surgery Basic Science and Clinical Evidence*. New York: Springer, 2001:897–917.

Head and Neck Cancer and Salivary Disease

HEAD AND NECK CANCER

Squamous Cell Carcinoma of the Head and Neck

Squamous cell carcinoma (SCC) of the head and neck is a relatively common disease that is complicated by the rich lymphatic and vascular supply to the region. This necessitates an investigation of lymph node involvement for all but the smallest of primary tumors. Most SCC in the head and neck occurs either in the mucosa of the upper aerodigestive tract (HNSCC) or on the skin (cutaneous SCC). These two entities vary significantly in their risk factors and appropriate treatment.

HNSCC is the most common malignancy of the upper aerodigestive tract. Despite significant advances in imaging, radiation technology, and chemotherapeutic treatment strategies, there has been little to no improvement in the overall survival of this disease over the past 30 years. This has led to numerous clinical trials using new combinations of chemotherapy, radiation technology, and surgery. Recent attention has also been given to the genetic profiling of tumors in an attempt to predict aggressiveness and response to treatment.

Epidemiology and Classification

In 2007, an estimated 47,560 new cases of HNSCC were diagnosed in the United States, and 11,260 died of the disease, accounting for approximately 3% of adult malignancies (1). Although tobacco use and alcohol consumption are the leading risk factors, several others have also been identified (Table 18.1). Males seem to be at a much higher risk of developing HNSCC, as do African Americans. Although rare in the United States, nasopharyngeal carcinoma is quite

problematic in other parts of the world. In fact, it is the leading cause of cancer-related death in young men in southern China and Taiwan.

Overall 5-year survival rate for head and neck cancer is less than 40%. Advanced stage, which is defined by the presence of invasiveness and metastasis, suggests poorer prognosis. Mortality is largely due to failure of locoregional control, with fewer patients succumbing to metastatic disease (15% to 25%) or second primary tumors (10% to 15%). The presence of regional nodal disease is the strongest predictor of prognosis for HNSCC, which may decrease survival rate by up to 50%.

HNSCC is classified according to the staging criteria published by the American Joint Committee on Cancer (AJCC). The current sixth edition from 2002 uses the TNM staging system that identifies the primary site (T), the presence of cervical lymph node involvement (N), and distant metastasis (M) (2). These are used to stratify patients between stages I and IV. The lip and oral cavity TNM criteria are given as an example of staging in Table 18.2.

HNSCC is further characterized by its location within the head and neck. The major sites of HNSCC include (a) nasal cavity/paranasal sinuses, (b) pharynx, (c) lip and oral cavity, and (d) the larynx. Within each of these sites are subsites to further classify tumors according to their location (Table 18.3), such as the supraglottis, glottis, and subglottis of the larynx.

Cervical lymph nodes are classified as levels 1 to 6 according to their location within the neck (Table 18.4). These levels are defined by bony, muscular, and nerve landmarks in the neck. Each tumor site has typical lymphatic drainage patterns to specific lymph node levels that guide treatment of the neck.

TABLE 18.1	Risk Factors for HNSCC	
Tobacco	Plummer–Vinson syndrome	Leukoplakia
Alcohol	Radiation exposure	Erythroplakia
Nickel	HPV	Poor oral hygiene
Wood dust		

Presentation and Evaluation

The diagnosis of HNSCC can be particularly elusive in the early stages of disease when patients may present with nonspecific symptoms in the head and neck region that could be attributable to a less worrisome cause. These may include a sore throat or odynophagia, ear pain, loose teeth, hoarseness, dysphagia, or epistaxis. Alternatively, HNSCC may present as an isolated asymptomatic neck mass. Given the variability and nonspecific nature of these signs and symptoms, a diagnosis often requires astute attention to the identification of risk factors and a thorough physical examination with a low threshold to proceed with additional workup in the form of tissue sampling and imaging.

The initial evaluation of a patient with a suspected malignancy in the head and neck requires a thorough examination in the office. This includes the inspection of the oral cavity and oral pharynx with the assistance of headlight illumination and tongue depressors. Finger palpation of the base of tongue and floor of mouth should also be performed. Otoscopy, nasal endoscopy, and flexible laryngoscopy should also be included, with a thorough and systematic examination of each subsite of the upper aerodigestive tract. The neck should be carefully palpated for adenopathy along with a full cranial nerve examination.

TABLE 18.2	T Staging of Lip and Oral Cavity Tumors
T1	2 cm or less
T2	>2 cm but <4 cm
T3	>4 cm
T4 lip	Invades through cortical bone, inferior alveolar nerve, floor of mouth, or skin of face
T4a oral cavity	Invades adjacent structures (cortical bone, deep muscles of tongue [genioglossus, hypoglossus, palatoglossus, or styloglossus], maxillary sinus, skin of face)
T4b oral cavity	Tumor invades masticator space, pterygoid plates, or skull base and/or encases internal carotid artery

In the case of a suspicious mass, the appropriate next step is typically a biopsy. In the oral cavity and some easily accessible oropharyngeal tumors, a small incisional biopsy may be performed with a cupped forceps in an office setting. If bleeding or airway compromise is considered a possibility given the nature of the tumor, then a biopsy should be done in the operating room. Alternatively, a biopsy of the neck mass can be done easily and safely via fine needle aspiration (FNA) for histological evaluation, which has a very high sensitivity and specificity. If the FNA is nondiagnostic, an incisional or excisional biopsy may be necessary.

Most patients with a suspected or biopsy-proven HNSCC should undergo a formal evaluation in the operating room prior to the initiation of treatment. This includes a bimanual palpation of the floor of mouth, base of tongue, and assessment of cervical lymph node involvement under anesthesia. Furthermore, a laryngoscope, bronchoscope, and esophagoscope

TABLE 18.3	Sites and Subsites of the Upper Aerodigestive Tract			
Site	Nasal Cavity/ Paranasal Sinuses	Pharynx	Lip and Oral Cavity	Larynx
Subsites	Nasal cavity	Nasopharynx	Lip	Supraglottis
	Ethmoid sinuses	Oropharynx	Tongue	Glottis
	Maxillary sinus	Hypopharynx	Buccal mucosa	Subglottis
			Gingiva	
			Retromolar trigone	
			Hard palate	

| TABLE 18.4 | Anatomic Boundaries of the Cervical Lymph Node Levels |

Lymph Node Level	Anatomic Boundaries
Level IA (submental)	lymph nodes bordered by the anterior belly of the digastric muscles and the hyoid bone
Level IB (submandibular)	lymph nodes bordered by the anterior belly of the digastric muscle, the stylohyoid muscle, and the body of the mandible
Levels IIA and IIB (upper jugular)	lymph nodes bordered by the skull base superiorly, the inferior aspect of the hyoid bone inferiorly, the stylohyoid muscle medially, and the posterior aspect of the sternomastoid muscle laterally. Level IIA nodes are located anterior to the vertical plane defined by the accessory nerve, while level IIB are located posterior to this plane.
Level III (midjugular)	Lymph nodes bordered by the inferior aspect of the hyoid bone superiorly, the inferior aspect of the cricoid cartilage inferiorly, the lateral border of the sternohyoid muscle medially, and the posterior aspect of the sternomastoid muscle laterally
Level IV (lower jugular)	Lymph nodes bordered by the inferior aspect of the cricoid cartilage superiorly, the clavicle inferiorly, the lateral border of the sternohyoid muscle medially, and the posterior aspect of the sternomastoid muscle laterally
Levels VA and VB (posterior triangle group)	Lymph nodes bordered by the convergence of the sternomastoid and trapezius muscles superiorly, the clavicle inferiorly, the posterior border of the sternomastois muscle medially, and the anterior border of the trapezius muscle laterally. Level VA is separated from VB by a horizontal marking the inferior aspect of the cricoid cartilage.
Level VI (anterior compartment group)	Lymph nodes of the central compartment bordered superiorly by the hyoid bone, inferiorly by the suprasternal notch, and laterally by the common carotid arteries.

Robbins KT, Clayman G, Levine PA, et al. Neck dissection classification update. Revisions proposed by the American Head and Neck Society and the American Academy of Otolaryngology–Head and Neck Surgery. *Arch Otolaryngol Head Neck Surg* 2002;128:751–758.

("panendoscopy") can be used to thoroughly and systematically examine the upper aerodigestive tract, as the incidence of concomitant tumors at diagnosis may be as high as 18% (3). Particular attention should be given to an accurate description of the exact boundaries of a given tumor. Lesions of the hypopharynx and larynx should be assessed specifically for vocal cord movement and subsite involvement.

Consideration should also be given at this time for prophylactic tracheotomy to protect the patient's airway. This is most pressing in the setting of advanced laryngeal cancer but may also have a role in large tumors of the pharynx. Impending airway compromise may not be evident at the time of initial evaluation, but it can occur with tumor growth before treatment is initiated. The tumor may also swell during radiation therapy resulting in interrupted and suboptimal treatment should airway management become an emergent issue.

It is not uncommon for a patient to present with a large neck mass that represents a metastatic lymph node in the absence of a detectable primary tumor. Conversely, a large primary tumor may surprisingly have no associated palpable cervical adenopathy. These two scenarios have generated much discussion on the treatment of "the unknown primary" and "occult metastasis," respectively.

Radiographic Imaging

Imaging is a standard component of both the initial workup and subsequent surveillance for most HNSCC. Computed tomography (CT) of the neck with intravenous contrast is most commonly used, as it allows for an accurate description of the primary tumor and the presence of suspicious or enlarged lymph nodes. Specific attention is given to the involvement of structures in the vicinity of the tumor, such as the thyroid cartilage in larynx cancer or the mandible in oral cavity cancer. Attention is also directed toward the identification of metastatic lymph nodes. This is most clinically relevant in the neck that is negative for metastasis on physical examination. The most consistent finding suggestive of lymph node metastasis on imaging is central necrosis within a node (4).

Recently, the use of positron emitted tomography (PET) and PET–CT fusion imaging has received significant attention in the workup of patients with HNSCC. These technologies assess metabolic activity, which allows the identification of the tumor and metastasis to lymph nodes or distant sites. The role of PET in the evaluation and treatment of HNSCC is still being defined, especially in early stage disease when the chance of cervical nodal involvement or distant metastasis is low. The lack of specificity of PET imaging has also led to some confusion in the interpretation of positive signals in atypical or unanticipated regions that may or may not represent metastasis.

Ultrasound technology is used extensively in Europe as an adjunct to, or substitute for CT imaging. Although the success and accuracy with ultrasound are largely dependant on the user, it can be used quite effectively for staging purposes and guiding FNA biopsies. Magnetic resonance imaging (MRI) can also be used to delineate soft tissue characteristics of the tumor and surrounding structures such as at the skull base or within the carotid sheath.

Pathology

SCC represents one end of a spectrum of mucosal aberrations of the upper aerodigestive tract. However, there is seldom a clinically apparent stepwise progression from normal mucosa to premalignancy to invasive cancer. Premalignant states include leukoplakia and erythroplakia (erythroplasia), with the former being much more common whereas the latter having a much greater propensity to become an SCC. Of note, leukoplakia is not a histological diagnosis but rather is a descriptive term for a white patch that is adherent to the underlying mucosa. Erythroplasia appears as red mucosa that is not ulcerated. It may have normal or roughened texture, and it is usually asymptomatic. Up to 90% of erythroplasia may progress to SCC.

Early SCC that is limited to the epithelial layer and has not penetrated the basement membrane is called *carcinoma in situ*. Once the carcinoma has penetrated the basement membrane it becomes *invasive SCC*. Some pathologists describe the entity "microinvasive" SCC if it has minimal extension (0.5 to 2 mm). Features such as hyperchromatism, mitotic activity, dedifferentiation, and host lymphocytic response may also be helpful in determining the aggressiveness of the tumor.

Human papilloma virus (HPV), most notably HPV 16 and 18, is implicated in several HNSCC, but its role seems strongest in the oropharynx. Specifically, the virus has a clear predilection for crypts within lymphoid tissue (Waldeyer's ring) and the subsequent development of tumors of the tonsil and base of tongue (5).

Treatment of HNSCC

Historically, the treatment of HNSCC was purely surgical. However, this paradigm has changed over the past several decades. HNSCC is now best addressed in a multidisciplinary team approach with medical oncologists, radiation oncologists, and surgeons. If opportunities allow, the inclusion of speech pathologists, counselors, research coordinators, and prosthodontists can positively impact patient outcomes as well.

The treatment of HNSCC must strike a balance between minimizing morbidity without sacrificing survival. Although most tumors can be treated successfully via several modalities, it is the physician's duty to select the modality that will give the best chance at survival without adding toxicity or morbidity associated with excessive treatment.

Treatment modalities generally fall into either single modality (namely surgery or radiation) for early stage disease or multimodality treatment (a combination of surgery, radiation, and/or chemotherapy), which is used for advanced stage disease. In addition to the primary tumor site, the cervical lymph node basin must be treated in the presence of cervical metastases.

In the absence of cervical nodal disease, however, the treating physician must consider the presence of "occult" cervical metastasis. This refers to the presence of microscopically metastatic disease that has not yet manifested on physical examination or imaging. In the absence of known cervical metastasis, each HNSCC primary tumor has a specific likelihood of occult metastasis. This is a function of the size of the tumor and tumor location. The consensus threshold to initiate treatment of cervical lymph nodes occurs if the risk of occult cervical metastasis is more than 15% to 20% (6).

In patients with early stage disease, the decision to treat with surgery or radiation is based on several factors. In general, oral cavity tumors are best treated with surgery both because of the favorable functional results and the relative resistance of the tissues to radiotherapy. Early nasopharynx, oropharynx, hypopharynx, and larynx tumors are generally treated with radiation to preserve function and because these regions are typically more radiosensitive.

Oral Cavity

The oral cavity is the most common site of all head and neck cancers, representing about 30% of cancers. The oral cavity extends from the lips anteriorly to the junction of the hard and soft palate superiorly and the circumvallate papillae inferiorly. There are several subsites within the oral cavity. The lips are the most common subsite for oral cavity cancer, of which a majority occurs on the lower lip (90%).

The oral tongue is the second most common location of oral cavity HNSCC. Among the other subsites, the retromolar trigone and alveolar ridge subsites have a tendency to invade bone earlier, necessitating extensive surgical resection of the involved bone and a poorer prognosis.

Verrucous carcinoma represents a variant of HNSCC. It often has a broader base and more keratotic appearance and mostly occurs on the buccal mucosa. Verrucous carcinomas are generally treated surgically and have a much more favorable prognosis.

The treatment of most oral cavity tumors is surgical, with the use of radiation postoperatively for close/positive margins or bony invasion. This is driven by the tongue's tremendous ability to compensate and "fill-in" resected defects, and the problematic nature of tongue movement during radiotherapy as well as the fact that oral cavity tumors are generally not very radiosensitive.

Large tumors of the tongue or floor of mouth often abut or invade bone, which is a poor prognostic factor for a complete response to chemoradiation, and require removal of the involved bone. If the lingual aspect of the mandibular periosteum is abutted, treatment of the primary site includes removal of the periosteum and the outer cortex of adjacent mandible (a marginal mandibulectomy). Conversely, if the periosteum is violated, the underlying bone must be removed in a bicortical fashion (segmental mandibulectomy). Reconstruction can vary from simple to complex. Most basically, the patient can be allowed to "swing" by simply reapproximating the mucosa and leaving the bony ends of the mandible unattached. Alternatively, a metal plate can be anchored between the bony remnants of the mandible with the additional recruitment of tissue from a regional (e.g., pectoralis major) or free flap (e.g., fibula).

Pharynx

Pharyngeal HNSCC consists of tumors in the nasopharynx, oropharynx, and hypopharynx. The location and confinement of the pharynx makes surgical access quite challenging for nearly all tumors of this region. A transoral approach can be used for small tumors of the oropharynx, but surgical access for most other tumors requires more extensive exposure such as through a mandibulotomy or lateral pharyngotomy approach. Experienced surgeons can remove some tumors of the pharynx endoscopically, but this technique is generally limited by visualization and instrumentation. Several institutions have recently begun using robotic technology to gain access to regions of the pharynx previously treated nonsurgically.

The nasopharynx lies superior to the soft palate and posterior to the choanae of the nasal cavity. Nasopharyngeal SCC is very distinct from other HNSCCs. The World Health Organization (WHO) has classified three types of nasopharynx tumors. WHO type I refers to a more classic keratinizing SCC. It carries a poor prognosis, as it is minimally radiosensitive. WHO type II, which is strongly associated with Epstein–Barr virus (EBV), refers to a nonkeratinizing SCC. It is more sensitive to radiation and carries a better prognosis. WHO type III, also associated with EBV and radiosensitive, does not have significant squamous features, but instead may represent lymphoepitheliomas.

The oropharynx is bounded anteriorly at the hard/soft palate junction and circumvallate papillae. The superior limit is the level of the hard palate, and the inferior boundary is the level of the pharyngoepiglottic folds. The tonsils are the most common site of oropharyngeal HNSCC.

The hypopharynx is the region bounded superiorly by the hyoid bone and inferiorly by the esophageal inlet. The pyriform sinus is the most common subsite for HNSCC. The postcricoid region is rarely a site of primary tumor. However, there is a strong association with postcricoid SCC and Plummer–Vinson syndrome, which is characterized by dysphagia, iron deficiency anemia, glossitis, and esophageal webs.

Larynx

The larynx represents the second most common location of head and neck malignancies. It consists of the supraglottis, glottis, and subglottis. The supraglottis includes the region from the tip of the epiglottis to the apex of the laryngeal ventricle. Subsites include the epiglottis, aryepiglottic folds, arytenoids, and false cords. Patients with tumors in this region typically present with sore throat or hemoptysis, which often does not occur until the tumors are very large and at an advanced stage. The subglottis begins 1 cm inferior to the apex of the ventricle and extends to the level of the cricoid cartilage. Tumors of this region are very rare and have a poor prognosis.

The glottis is the most common subsite of the larynx for HNSCC. Its superior limit is the apex of the ventricle and extends inferiorly 1 cm, which includes the vocal folds. Patients typically present with hoarseness, which develops very early in the course of disease. As such, many patients are identified at an early stage of disease. Similarly, anatomic barriers such as the vocal ligament and conus elasticus prevent the spread of many glottic tumors.

Surgery is often used in the treatment of early stage laryngeal HNSCC of the glottis and supraglottis. Conventional treatment would include endoscopic laser resection of the tumor or an open partial laryngectomy with preservation of laryngeal function. Alternatively, radiation therapy can be used, which has equivalent cure rates for early larynx cancers. Deciding between these two modalities is typically determined by weighing the surgeon's experience with endoscopic resection against the expected side effects of radiation.

The treatment of advanced staged laryngeal cancer was historically surgical by means of total laryngectomy. However, a landmark study performed by the Department of Veterans Affairs in 1991 (7) showed that many patients with advanced stage laryngeal SCC could be treated with chemotherapy and radiation therapy without sacrificing survival. This introduced "organ-sparing" protocols for most advanced larynx cancer, and surgery is now reserved for "salvage" in the case of persistence or recurrence with few exceptions.

Nasal Cavity/Paranasal Sinuses

There are several types of tumors that can develop in the paranasal sinuses, such as adenocarcinomas, adenoid cystic carcinomas, melanomas, sinonasal undifferentiated carcinomas, and olfactory neuroblastomas. The most common type of malignancy in the sinonasal tract is SCC, which most often involves the maxillary sinus and, secondly, the nasal cavity. In general, radiation is not a curative treatment for most sinus cancers, thus one must weigh the chance of cure with surgery against the morbidity of surgery. If the chance for cure is low and the morbidity is high with surgery, then radiation may be preferable.

"Unresectable" HNSCC

Although a tumor's "resectability" can be debated amongst surgeons, a tumor is generally considered "unresectable" if it invades the base of skull, preverte-

bral fascia, mediastinum, or the subdermal lymphatics. This means that controlling tumor margins surgically is not feasible. Carotid artery involvement is a relative contraindication to surgery, as it can be sacrificed if contralateral flow is sufficient as determined preoperatively via a balloon occlusion test and electroencephalography. However, most tumors that require carotid artery sacrifice have an extremely poor prognosis given the extent of disease.

Cervical Lymph Nodes

As with treatment of the primary tumor, cervical metastases have historically been addressed surgically. Now, radiation is often employed in the absence of clinically positive nodes for possible occult metastasis. A neck with N1 disease can typically be treated with either radiation or surgery, but is sometimes treated with both if extracapsular invasion is seen on histology. A neck with N2 or N3 disease is typically treated with surgery, radiation therapy, and chemotherapy. The surgical removal of cervical nodes is also employed when the surgical treatment of the primary tumor involves accessing the neck. This most commonly occurs for tumors of the oral cavity and less commonly for laryngeal tumors. A neck dissection is also indicated when there is an incomplete response to radiation or chemoradiation at the primary tumor or cervical nodal basin.

Cervical lymph node dissections are performed in specific formats according to tumor site and staging. There is essentially no circumstance in which adequate and oncologically sound surgical treatment consists of "cherry picking" a metastatic lymph node. Instead, all lymph nodes in a particular level should be removed when that level is at risk.

In the presence of cervical nodal metastasis, certain pathologic features on the specimen portend an even poorer prognosis. These include extracapsular spread from a lymph node or more than three metastatic cervical lymph nodes. In such circumstances, the addition of chemotherapy to postoperative radiation is usually included. Furthermore, the presence of metastasis to the lower cervical lymph nodes (levels IV and V) is also correlated with worse survival.

Radical Neck Dissection

A radical neck dissection includes the removal of all nodal levels (unilateral) as well as the spinal accessory nerve, sternocleidomastoid muscle, and internal jugular vein. It represents the most aggressive form of surgical treatment of nodal metastasis and leaves the patients with significant morbidity (e.g., shoulder drop, hypoesthesia of neck and periauricular region, potential for facial edema from venous insufficiency, and cosmetic deformity). It is reserved for scenarios in which the sternocleidomastoid, spinal accessory nerve, and internal jugular vein are involved with tumor.

Modified Radical Neck Dissection

In contrast, a modified radical neck dissection still removes all nodal levels but spares the accessory nerve, internal jugular vein, and/or accessory nerve. Although technically more difficult, this type of dissection can be performed when any of the three structures are not involved and has significantly less deformity and associated morbidity.

Selective Neck Dissection

A selective neck dissection addresses only nodal levels at high risk based on the primary tumor size and location. Subtypes of selective neck dissection include a supraomohyoid neck dissection, lateral neck dissection, and a posterior lateral neck dissection. A supraomohyoid neck dissection removes levels I to III and is indicated for many oral cancers in an N0 or N1 neck. Lateral neck dissection involves the removal of levels II to IV and is indicated for supraglottic, oropharyngeal, and hypopharyngeal cancers. Posterior lateral neck dissection removes levels II to V and is indicated for later staged oropharyngeal and hypopharyngeal cancers as well as for some posterior scalp cancers.

Radiation Therapy

External beam radiation for HNSCC can be in the form of electron or photon energy. It can be given preoperatively, postoperatively, or in lieu of surgery. It is typically administrated as fractional dosing, meaning that the dose of radiation is given in several smaller doses over days or weeks instead of all at once. There are several methods of fractionation.

A standard conventional fractionation regimen would consist of daily radiation treatments of approximately 2 Gy (1 Gy = 100 rads) 5 days per week for a total of 62 to 70 Gy. Fractionation can be modified in several ways in an effort to increase effectiveness and minimize radiation side effects. *Hyperfractionation* increases the rate of treatments, whereas *accelerated fractionation* involves increasing the dose during each treatment with a corresponding decrease in the number of treatments. *Boost fractionation* increases the dose as treatment progresses.

A relatively new technique of delivering external beam radiation is intensity-modulated radiation therapy (IMRT). A computer generates a 3D image of the tumor on the basis of the size and location, and radiation is applied in various intensities from several different beam directions. This technique has the benefit of focusing the radiation on the tumor while sparing nearby uninvolved structures such as the eye and brachial plexus.

Complications of radiation therapy vary significantly in severity. Most mildly, skin erythema or thickening and fibrosis of the overlying tissue may occur. More bothersome is the associated xerostomia secondary to damage to the acinar units of the salivary glands, which may result in dental caries. This side effect is intensified in the presence of chemotherapy. Chemoradiation-induced xerostomia and possibly mucositis can be in part limited by the concurrent intravenous administration of amifostine.

More problematic, osteoradionecrosis (ORN) of the mandible can occur from months to years following radiation treatment. The likelihood of developing ORN is related to the cumulative radiation dose. It is more likely to occur in the anterior portion of the mandible, owing to its less robust blood supply. A significant risk factor to this seems to be carious teeth, prompting most radiation oncologists to have dental consultation and appropriate extractions prior to therapy.

Radiation therapy has also been identified as a causative factor in cancers such as sarcomas, thyroid cancers, and leukemias.

Chemotherapy

Chemotherapy is not used as a single modality treatment with intent for "cure" in HNSCC. It is mostly used in combination with radiation as a form of primary treatment for advanced stage disease. Alternatively, chemotherapy can be used for palliation during end-stage disease to slow progression and prolong life expectancy. The common chemotherapeutics are listed in Table 18.5.

There are several techniques of administering chemotherapy. *Induction chemotherapy* (neoadjuvant) is the sequential chemotherapy given before the local treatment modality, whether that is surgery or radiation or even chemoradiation. It has the theoretical advantage of improving drug delivery to the tumor prior to surgery or radiation. It can also decrease tumor bulk, potentially enabling a surgical resection. *Concomitant chemotherapy* is given during the course of radiation. This has the

TABLE 18.5	Common Chemotherapeutics in HNSCC	
Name	**Mechanism**	**Common Side Effects**
Cisplatin Carboplatin	Alkylating agent	Nephrotoxicity, peripheral neuropathy, ototoxicity, electrolyte disturbances
5-Fluorouracil	Antimetabolite in thymidine pathway (S-phase)	Myelosuppression, cardiac toxicity, mucositis, diarrhea
Methotrexate	Antimetabolite to DHFR	Bone marrow suppression, GI disturbances, mucositis (Leucovorin: Rescue agent)
Paclitaxel Docetaxel	Microtubular organization	Neutropenia, alopecia, mucositis
Cetuximab	Anti-EGFR monoclonal antibody	Rash, fever, hypomagnesia

DHFR, dihydrofolate reductase; EGFR, epidermal growth factor receptor.

advantage of giving simultaneous therapies that may synergistically maximize their therapeutic effect. This has been shown to improve survival and locoregional control in advanced HNSCC (8,9). Unfortunately, adding chemotherapy to radiation treatment significantly increases the side effects of mucositis, infection, and malnutrition. *Adjuvant chemotherapy* is given after the primary treatment modality (surgery or radiation) to help control microscopic disease. There has been significant debate regarding the efficacy of adjuvant chemotherapy, but it appears that it offers a significant survival advantage in high-risk HNSCC with extracapsular spread or microscopically positive margins at the time of surgery (10).

There has been interest in chemopreventative strategies for use in individuals at high risk for the development of HNSCC. Most attention has been directed at retinoids, which have been shown to decrease the transformation rate of premalignant lesions to malignancies and also to decrease the risk of the development of second primary, with no survival advantage in the latter group. Similarly, the toxicities from treatment have limited the long-term use of this strategy (11).

Summary of HNSCC

HNSCC is a complex disease that requires a thorough evaluation of both the primary tumor and the cervical lymphatic bed. Treatment of advanced disease is usually multimodality, and should be customized to the patient and the tumor burden. This is best performed in a multidisciplinary tumor board setting with medical oncologists, radiation oncologists, and surgeons with experience in the head and neck region.

Novel approaches for the management of HNSCC, such as with HPV vaccination for oropharynx cancer or tumor markers that portend susceptibility to radiation or specific chemotherapeutics, will likely be at the forefront of research in this field. In the meantime, risk reduction through smoking and alcohol cessation combined with aggressive measures to detect early disease remain the best chance at success with this disease entity.

Cutaneous Head and Neck Squamous Cell Carcinoma

Cutaneous SCC is the second most common skin malignancy of the head and neck after basal cell carcinoma (BCC). Risk factors include Fitzpatrick skin types I and II; history of UV-B exposure, childhood sunburns, immunosuppression such as in transplant recipients, actinic keratosis, and HPV infection.

There is a small but not insignificant risk of nodal metastasis associated with cutaneous SCC. Such nodes may lie in the superficial lobe of the parotid gland (for lesions of the upper face and anterior scalp) or in the cervical lymph node region.

Treatment of cutaneous SCC is generally surgical. Margins should be 4 to 6 mm for small cancers and 1 to 2 cm for larger tumors. Mohs micrographic surgery can be used to minimize the amount of healthy tissue resected in anatomically complex regions such as the eyelid, nose, or perioral region. Radiation therapy is usually reserved for patients with close surgical margins in which further surgery would leave significant dysfunction or disfigurement, or if the patient is a poor operative candidate. Unlike upper aerodigestive tract SCC, there seems to be very little role for chemotherapy in cutaneous SCC.

The current concept in treating lymph node metastasis is rather basic. Namely, lymph node dissection, either in the form of superficial parotidectomy or a variant of a standard neck dissection, is only performed in the setting of clinically positive nodes. Scant attention has been given to the depth of invasion or degree of cytologic atypia of the primary tumor in determining the need for treating lymph nodes, whether that is surgical or with radiation.

Basal Cell Carcinoma of the Head and Neck

BCC represents the most common cutaneous malignancy in the head and neck. Risk factors include sun exposure, family history, ionizing radiation, immunosuppression, and genetic disorders such as xeroderma pigmentosa and Gorlin syndrome. UV-B seems to play a greater role than UV-A in the development of BCC. BCC tends to spread in a lateral or peripheral fashion as opposed to a vertical fashion, in part owing to its very low predilection for metastasis. BCC can also develop in the context of Gorlin syndrome (basal cell nevus syndrome), an autosomal dominant disorder in which patients have numerous BCCs, odontogenic keratocysts, frontal bossing, bifid ribs, and scoliosis.

Several subtypes of BCC exist, including superficial, morpheaform, pigmented, nodular (noduloulcerative), and micronodular. These subtypes are treated similarly, but require an astute dermatopathologist because determining margins may not be clearly evident, especially in the sclerosing variant. Of note, morpheaform BCC may require wider margins given its propensity for recurrence. Nodular subtype represents the most common type of BCC.

The management of BCC can take the form of surgery, radiation, or chemotherapy. Surgery remains the most common treatment of BCC, with most being treated via curettage with electrodessication, and the wound bed is allowed to heal by secondary intention. In the head and neck, this treatment modality is not generally used, as the risk of recurrence is significant and the associated scarring is cosmetically not acceptable. Instead, surgical excision is typically performed with sharp technique to obtain at least a 4-mm margin. Excision can also be performed with Mohs technique, which has the highest success rate of clearance (96%).

In patients who do not want surgery or are poor surgical candidates, topical chemotherapy with 5-fluorouracil or imiquimod cream can also be very effective, especially if the tumor is small. External beam radiation can also be used in poor operative candidates or in regions not easily reconstructed.

SALIVARY GLAND DISEASE

Anatomy and Physiology

On average, a person secretes almost 1 L of saliva daily. The major salivary glands include the parotid, submandibular, and sublingual glands. Nearly 1,000 minor salivary glands are distributed throughout the upper aerodigestive tract. The salivary gland secretory unit is a complex network of components. Lobules of acini produce serous (parotid gland), mucinous (submandibular and minor glands), and seromucinous (sublingual gland) saliva.

Epidemiology

One to four per 100,000 people per year develop salivary gland tumors, which comprise 6% to 10% of all head and neck cancers (12). There is no overall gender predilection and the usual age of onset is in the seventh and eighth decades of life. About 75% of adult salivary tumors are benign, although 6,000 new malignant cases are diagnosed each year. In children, the malignancy rate in salivary tumors is considerably higher at about 60%. About 80% of salivary gland tumors arise in the parotid gland (88% are in the superficial lobe), 12% in the submandibular gland, 6% in the minor salivary glands, and less than 1% in the sublingual gland (13,14). About 20% of parotid gland tumors, 40% of submandibular gland tumors, and more than 50% of sublingual and minor salivary gland tumors are malignant (15). Currently, the WHO describes 17 subtypes of malignant lesions, most commonly mucoepidermoid and adenoid cystic carcinoma.

Benign Salivary Gland Tumors

Pleomorphic Adenoma

The most common benign tumor of both major and minor salivary glands is the pleomorphic adenoma

(16,17). These are generally asymptomatic until a painless mass is detected. A distinctive fibrous capsule surrounds a proliferation of myoepithelial and epithelial cells (18). The hypocellular variety of this lesion is the most likely to recur because of the presence of pseudopodia, which are finger-like tumor extensions present outside the thin pseudocapsule (12,17). Pleomorphic adenomas account for 60% of all parotid gland tumors, 50% of submandibular and minor gland tumors, and only 25% of sublingual gland neoplasms (16,17). Of the minor salivary gland variety, 55% arise in the palate, 25% in the lip (usually upper), and 10% in the buccal mucosa (17). With the presence of extracapsular foci, there is an increased likelihood for recurrence (16). A recurrence in the parotid poses tremendous difficulty in adequately excising the remaining mass due to the mandate to preserve the facial nerve and the likely discovery of numerous tumor rests. There exists a 1% to 3% risk for malignant transformation into a carcinoma ex-pleomorphic adenoma (13,17). This remains one of the important reasons why surgical excision is recommended in virtually all patients with a presumed pleomorphic adenoma.

Monomorphic Adenoma

Monomorphic adenomas have a variety of growth patterns—the two most common types are the basal cell and canalicular adenomas (17). Basal cell adenomas tend to be smaller and more firm than the pleomorphic variety (16,18). With a predilection for men in their 60s, these tumors are well encapsulated and often include cystic spaces containing a brownish fluid (17). Canalicular adenomas are found primarily in minor salivary glands, with about 80% occurring in the upper lip (16,17). With an affinity for women older than 50 years, this tumor arises as a single, painless mass, which is firm, yet freely moveable (16). Excision with negative margins is deemed adequate treatment (16).

Myoepithelioma

Similar in behavior to the basal and canalicular adenomas, the myoepithelioma is a rare, benign salivary neoplasm. This well-circumscribed, painless, and firm mass occurs equally among men and women. Often confused with a pleomorphic adenoma on cytology, the tumor must be composed of less than 5% ducts and glands to be diagnosed as a myoepithelioma (16). Myoepithelioma is cured by surgical excision.

Papillary Cystadenoma Lymphomatosum (Warthin's Tumor)

Considered to represent a hamartoma as opposed to a true neoplasm, this slow-growing lesion is composed of cystic salivary ductal elements and an abundance of normal lymphoid tissue (16). It is believed that at some point along their generation, lymph nodes incorporate salivary gland tissue. Warthin's tumors are commonly found bilaterally and have a doughy consistency when palpated over the angle of the mandible (16). Because of their potential for multicentricity, Warthin's tumors are preferably treated by lobectomy. If the diagnosis has been established with FNA biopsy, it is considered acceptable to manage certain patients—particularly the elderly and high risk—with observation alone.

Oncocytoma (Oxyphilic Adenoma)

Oncocytomas are uncommon salivary tumors that are slow growing and found in older populations (16). When present, oxyphilic adenomas are found in the parotid as well-circumscribed lesions with a brown lobular surface. Histologically, these lesions are comprised of oncocytes with abundant mitochondria surrounded by a fibrous capsule (17,19). Lobectomy with nerve preservation is the treatment of choice (16).

Osseous Tumors

Salivary tumors can also arise from heterotopic salivary gland inclusions in the bony structures of the oral cavity, namely the maxilla and mandible. Although extremely rare, these tumors are most commonly mucoepidermoid carcinoma. In addition, acinic cell and clear cell carcinomas as well as myoepithelial carcinoma within pleomorphic adenomas, have all been found within the jaws (16). Depending on the size and extent of the lesions, marginal or segmental resection is the standard of care.

Malignant Salivary Gland Tumors

Rapid tumor growth, pain, facial paralysis, or a sudden increase in growth of a chronic mass are signs of malignancy. Salivary gland tumors in children have a higher overall rate of malignancy.

Mucoepidermoid Carcinoma

Mucoepidermoid carcinoma is the most common malignant tumor of the parotid gland and the second most common malignant tumor of the submandibular and minor salivary glands. Almost 80% to 90% of mucoepidermoid carcinomas occur in the parotid (16,20). The tumor has a tendency to appear during the fourth to sixth decades of life. The tumor is usually seen in the superficial lobe of the parotid as a well-defined focal nodule that is often mobile (17).

The low-grade lesions have numerous mucous cells and cystic spaces and a limited potential for local invasion or metastasis. Most low-grade lesions present in a manner indistinguishable from a pleomorphic adenoma. The majority are treated by lobectomy without postoperative radiation resulting in a 5-year survival of more than 90% (16,17,19,20). High-grade tumors may resemble an SCC with marked anaplasia and a higher epidermoid to glandular cell ratio (17). These lesions have margins that may be less distinctive and therefore a propensity for invasion or metastasis. As many as 25% of patients will have facial paralysis and half will develop cervical metastases (20). The 5-year survival rates range between 75% and 90% for stage I and II lesions and 25% and 40% for stage III and IV lesions (16,17,19,21).

The management of mucoepidermoid carcinoma must be tailored to its location and grade of malignancy. A mucoepidermoid carcinoma of the parotid is treated with a lobectomy with postoperative radiation therapy indicated for high-grade lesions. In the palate, low-grade tumors can be treated by wide local excision, whereas high-grade tumors are treated with a palatectomy or partial maxillectomy (16). High-grade lesions of the tongue carry the worst prognosis of all intraoral sites for this lesion (17). Partial or hemiglossectomy is the standard of care in this circumstance (17,22).

A cervical node dissection is performed when regional nodes are palpable. However, an elective neck dissection for high-grade lesions is controversial, because most patients will receive postoperative radiation, which includes the neck in the field (22,23). If neither radiation therapy nor an elective neck dissection is performed for high-grade lesions, recurrence has been seen in approximately 75% of cases (17,23).

Adenoid Cystic Carcinoma

Adenoid cystic carcinomas comprise 25% of malignant salivary gland neoplasms. It is found in both major and minor salivary glands, and it is the most frequently occurring malignancy of the submandibular gland. The most common intraoral site for this lesion is the palate where it may appear as an ulcerated nodule (17). The peak incidence is in the fifth and sixth decades of life. There are three histologic subtypes based on appearance: cribriform, tubular, and solid. The cribriform pattern consists of tumor islands surrounded by multiple prominent microcytic spaces lending to the classic "Swiss cheese" or "honeycomb" appearance on histology (17). The tubular variety has a trabecular pattern with a more glandular architecture and has the best prognosis (18,19). The solid pattern displays sheets of cells with little or no luminal spaces and has the worst prognosis (19).

It is difficult to determine the actual extent of an adenoid cystic carcinoma because it often extends well beyond its primary location, usually by tracking along nerves. Distal spread to bone or lung tissue is more common than nodal disease, with nearly 40% of patients developing metastases (16). About 20% of patients may present preoperatively with paresthesias and 30% with partial or total facial paralysis, due to nerve invasion (20).

In the major glands, resection with adequate margins is acceptable. Submitting frozen sections of the surrounding nerve bundles is recommended for confirmation of the adequacy of resection (18). Because of the propensity for local recurrence, surgical resection is often followed by a full course of radiation therapy (17).

Acinic Cell Carcinoma

Acinic cell carcinoma accounts for 10% of salivary gland tumors and mainly occurs in the parotid gland (16). The minor salivary glands of the buccal mucosa and lips are more commonly affected than those of the palate. After mucoepidermoid carcinoma, it is the second most common malignant salivary gland tumor of the parotid (17). Until 1953, it was classified as a benign adenoma until sufficient follow-up led to the recognition of its malignant behavior (20). There appears to be no age predilection with equal frequency of occurrence in patients throughout the second to seventh decades (17,19,20). Although considered to be low grade there is a possibility of metastasis, with a propensity for lung and bone (20). Excision with adequate margins is the standard of care.

Polymorphous Low-Grade Adenocarcinoma

Polymorphous low-grade adenocarcinoma is an indolent malignant lesion and is more frequent in the minor salivary glands of the palate and buccal mucosa

(17). Most of these tumors are found in the sixth to eighth decades of life. Although perineural invasion is characteristic of this lesion, local recurrence and distant metastasis are rare. Infiltration is often visualized histologically just beneath the surface epithelium in a whorled or targetoid arrangement without encapsulation (16). Surgical excision including adequate margins is the treatment of choice.

Squamous Cell Carcinoma

True squamous cell primaries are rare and must be differentiated from metastatic carcinomas or high-grade mucoepidermoid carcinomas (20). The patient must be questioned for a prior facial or scalp skin cancer that was previously excised. Squamous cell lesions of the submandibular or minor salivary glands are more likely to represent metastasis from adjacent sites. The stage of the disease will ultimately determine the survival and prognosis.

Malignant Mixed Tumor

Three different neoplasms have been included under the generic term malignant mixed tumor (18). The first is histologically benign but is considered a metastasizing pleomorphic adenoma. The second of these tumors has both a malignant epithelial and myoepithelial component. This lesion is a true carcinosarcoma. The third and most common type, known as carcinoma ex-pleomorphic adenoma, represents the malignant transformation of a pre-existing pleomorphic adenoma. It is important to distinguish that in this latter form, only the epithelial component metastasizes. The risk of this malignant transformation increases with the age of the pleomorphic adenoma and rises from around 2% within the first 5 years to almost 10% after 15 years (20). Malignant mixed tumors comprise 12% of submandibular gland malignancies with a 25% incidence of lymph node metastases, and a 30% incidence of distant metastases (20).

Nonepithelial Tumors

Lymphomas of the major salivary glands can arise within the intraglandular lymphoid tissue and are characteristically of the non-Hodgkin type. (Muscle, fibrous tissue, and nerves within the parotid region also have malignant potential.) Non-Hodgkin lymphoma accounts for about 10% of all malignant tumors that occur in the major salivary glands with disease in the parotid gland accounting for nearly 80% of cases.

Immune-Mediated and Reactive Lesions

Benign Lymphoepithelial Lesion (Myoepithelial Sialadenitis)

Benign lymphoepithelial cystic disease of the parotid presents as bilateral, firm parotid masses most commonly in HIV positive patients. Definitive diagnosis can be made by CT scan or MRI. Most lesions respond to low-dose radiation (16). Surgery is rarely necessary.

Salivary Retention Lesions

A mucocele is composed of pooled mucous that extravasates into the connective tissue from a severed or ruptured excretory duct (16). An inflammatory reaction ensues with the development of fibrosis. The minor salivary glands of the lower lip are most prone to this condition from trauma to the mucosa (16,17). Although local excision removes these collections, care must be taken not to further transect additional ducts thereby creating a potential for recurrence (17). When the ducts of the parotid, or less frequently of the submandibular gland, are affected, the extravasation is known as a sialocele. Although rare, the subcutaneous collection at these locations can thin the overlying skin and create a fistula (17).

Ranulas are mucoceles that occur in the floor of the mouth, often from a severed sublingual duct. A plunging ranula occurs when enough fluid pressure accumulates that the mucocele herniates beneath the mylohyoid muscle into the submental space. These types of ranulas are of concern for potential airway compromise (17). Removal of the fibrous capsule treats most simple ranulas whereas more extensive ranulas may require the excision of the entire gland from which it arises (16,17).

Sialolithiasis

Sialoliths are calcifications found within salivary gland ducts and have no known predisposing condition nor are they associated with hypercalcemia. The submandibular gland is most commonly affected due to the viscous, glycoprotein consistency of its secretions and the upward course of the duct making it more prone to retrograde bacterial invasion and stasis (16,17). The affected gland and distended ducts can fill with purulent exudates. The degree of acinar necrosis and lobular fibrosis will determine the recoverability and regenerative capacity of an obstructed gland.

Sialoliths are not always visible on plain radiographs. Early in their development, they are quite small and not adequately mineralized to be visible radiographically. Even after they are fully formed, about 40% of parotid and 20% of submandibular sialoliths are radiolucent (24). These radiolucent sialoliths can be visualized indirectly by the imaging defect they produce on sialography or directly through sialoendoscopy. Noncontrast CT has at least a 10-fold increased sensitivity over plain films (25). Noncalcified sialoliths are best seen on a sialogram, but small faintly calcified stones can be obscured by contrast. MRI is less sensitive than plain films and CT in detecting sialolithiasis. However, MRI can delineate differing soft tissues clearly with high-contrast resolution.

Accessible stones may be removed directly followed by sialodochoplasty to repair the injured duct (26). Sialoendoscopy with interventional techniques to destroy and remove stones is also possible (24,26). When the stones are deeply embedded or there is suspicion of a tumor or chronic recurrence of the stones, excision of the entire gland is indicated.

Diagnosis

Examination

Clinical examination is important when evaluating a patient with salivary gland disease. Bimanual palpation of both the gland and the course of its duct, visual confirmation of diminished or absent salivary flow, and assessment of the consistency of ductal discharge are essential. Palpation assists in determining fluctuant and soft swellings (usually benign) from indurated and fixed lesions (often malignant). Infectious and obstructive lesions are often accompanied by pain, whereas neoplastic and immunologic disorders are often painless. However, the presence or absence of pain does not definitively distinguish benign from malignant (13). Facial paralysis on presentation indicates malignancy and a poor prognosis that occurs in less than 15% of parotid carcinomas (14). Xerostomia can be idiopathic, drug or radiation induced, or the manifestation of Sjogren syndrome—an intense T lymphocyte–mediated autoimmune process of the salivary and lacrimal glands, which also presents with xerophthalmia (23). Tumors of the deep lobe of the parotid can grow undetected until large enough to displace the soft palate as well as structures of the lateral pharyngeal space, such as the ipsilateral tonsil.

Radiology

Plain films including occlusal, frontal, lateral, lateral-oblique, and panoramic views are usually only diagnostic for benign, obstructive lesions. Salivary scintigraphy is a radionuclide scan that can identify glandular masses greater than 1 cm and produce a dynamic, objective, and quantitative measurement evaluating the effect of the obstruction on glandular dynamics and function (25,27). Ultrasonography is only useful in determining location relative to key landmarks but is otherwise nondiagnostic. CT scan helps in identifying parenchymal or extraparenchymal masses that can cause obstruction by pressure or ductal invasion (25). CT scan shows bone invasion much better than MRI, whereas MRI is better at distinguishing a neoplasm from inflammatory tissue. A chest radiograph or chest CT scan may be appropriate to diagnose metastases in a patient with a known salivary malignancy.

Biopsy

Although some still argue that salivary masses should be resected without preoperative biopsy, there are many circumstances in which a biopsy may obviate the need for surgery or alter the surgical plan. For example, the parotid gland may harbor enlarged intraparotid reactive lymph nodes or lymphoma. Warthin's tumors or benign pleomorphic adenomas might be observed particularly in elderly or high-risk patients. Knowledge of a malignant lesion preoperatively may warrant a more extensive workup and will prepare the surgical team for a potentially more aggressive resection.

Refinements in sampling techniques and specimen preparation, as well as improvements in cytologic interpretation, have made FNA the first step in the evaluation of most salivary masses. The use of FNA biopsy is particularly useful in differentiating between neoplastic and nonneoplastic masses, such as inflammatory and lymphoid lesions (28,29). The specificity of the procedure ranges from 88% to 100% and the sensitivity is 85% to 95% (13,20,28,29). If a malignancy is present, an FNA may be able to determine if the lesion is primary to the salivary gland or metastatic from another site.

Intraoperatively, frozen section is beneficial in evaluating the nature of the lesion as well as the surgical margins (18). Core needle biopsy is not performed in the parotid given the risk of facial nerve injury.

Operative Techniques

Parotid Gland Surgery

Thorough knowledge of the anatomy of the parotid gland is essential for a successful surgical outcome. Injury to a branch of the facial nerve can lead to facial muscle paresis or paralysis; corneal exposure and ulceration may ensue if the temporofacial branch is affected (27). The parotid gland's borders lie posterior to the masseter muscle, inferior to the zygomatic arch, and anterior to the sternocleidomastoid muscle, with the medial aspect abutting the lateral pharyngeal space (27,30). The duct of the parotid, known as Stenson's duct, penetrates the buccinator muscle and enters the oral cavity through the buccal mucosa at the level of the maxillary second molar. The terms superficial (lateral) and deep (medial) lobes simply refer to the tissue superficial and deep to the facial nerve as there is no anatomic plane between the "lobes" (12). Within the parotid, the facial nerve divides into the temporofacial and cervicofacial branches. The temporofacial branch gives rise to the frontal and zygomatic branches whereas the cervicofacial branch yields the marginal mandibular and cervical branches. The buccal branch has been found to arise from either or both. Careful identification of the nerve during dissection is essential, and the use of a nerve stimulator and monitor may be beneficial—particularly in revision cases (12,16). The tympanomastoid fissure is a reliable landmark in locating the main trunk of the facial nerve. Its average distance to the main trunk is 2.7 mm (31). The tragal cartilage pointer has also been shown to be a reliable landmark located less than 1 cm from the nerve's main trunk (31). The main trunk is found deep to the tissue between the pointer and the digastric's posterior belly attachment on the mastoid. The more proximal posterior auricular, stapedial, and chorda tympani branches of the facial nerve are not in the operative field in parotid gland surgery (12). The auriculotemporal segment of the trigeminal nerve lies in close proximity to the superficial temporal artery in the superior aspect of the parotid and is generally not visible at surgery (30). If severed during surgery, Frey syndrome (gustatory sweating) may develop as these gustatory nerves grow into the sweat glands of the skin—when salivation occurs, the patient sweats over the parotid region.

For early stage or low-grade parotid tumors, a superficial parotidectomy is performed. Lesions of the deep lobe, which invade the parapharyngeal space may require a mandibulotomy for access (30). For invasive T4 tumors, a radical parotidectomy may include resection of nerve, skin, muscle, bone, and the external auditory canal. The facial nerve should never be sacrificed during parotidectomy for benign lesions (30).

If the facial nerve is intact prior to surgery, it should be spared even if the malignancy is high grade. However, if the facial nerve is involved preoperatively, and the tumor is otherwise resectable, it should be sacrificed with immediate nerve grafting. Elective modified radical neck dissection may be added to the procedure for staging or to prevent the need for postoperative neck irradiation (22,23). Therapeutic neck dissections should be performed in patients with palpable or radiographically demonstrable cervical metastasis.

Submandibular Gland Surgery

The parotid and submandibular glands are separated by the stylomandibular ligament. The submandibular gland lies in the submandibular triangle, superior to the anterior and posterior bellies of the digastric muscle (30). The facial vessels run through the submandibular triangle and are crossed superficially by the mandibular branch of the facial nerve. Wharton's duct tracks deep to the lingual nerve prior to entering the floor of the mouth. It is important to note that with advancing age, the normal position of the gland becomes lower in the neck (30). Benign tumors of this gland and low-grade malignancies without nerve involvement are resected by en-bloc excision of the gland and the accompanying submandibular nodes. More extensive lesions may require partial mandibulectomy. A neck dissection should be performed if there is evidence of cervical lymph node involvement (12,22,23).

Sublingual Gland Surgery

The sublingual gland is the smallest of the major salivary glands and lies atop the mylohyoid muscle. Tumors of this gland are treated in a similar manner to those of the floor of the mouth. Benign tumors in this region should be treated with simple transoral excision. The hypoglossal and lingual nerves are nearby and should be spared with careful dissection (30).

Minor Salivary Gland Surgery

Minor salivary glands must be evaluated and treated according to the size, location, and extent of the tumor. Salivary retention lesions and pleomorphic and monomorphic adenomas of the lip, buccal mucosa, or other accessible sites are treated by local excision. Small tumors of the hard palate, whether benign (pleomorphic adenoma) or low-grade malignant (mucoepidermoid carcinoma), may be resected transorally (16). A palatectomy is indicated in the treatment of more invasive low-grade malignant tumors, such as the infiltrative polymorphous low-grade adenocarcinoma. When the underlying palatal bone is invaded by a malignant tumor, a partial or complete maxillectomy is warranted depending on the pathology and extent of the tumor (16).

Adjuvant Therapy

Current indications for adjuvant radiation include high-grade T3 or T4 lesions, unresectable cancers, or instances where tumor spillage occurred during surgery. Radiation therapy should also be considered when close or positive margins have been obtained, or for recurrent disease. The reported overall incidence of metastatic cervical lymphadenopathy of major and minor salivary gland malignant tumors is 15%. The most common site from which metastatic lymph node involvement occurs is the parotid gland in 18% to 25% of cases (32). A neck dissection is warranted in a clinically positive neck and if there is extensive disease, radiation therapy should be performed as well (22,23). A neck dissection should include levels I, II, and III at the minimum (22). Chemotherapy is generally limited to investigational and palliative roles.

HEAD AND NECK CANCER QUESTIONS

Select one answer.

1. What upper aerodigestive site has the highest association between SCC and HPV?
   a. Larynx
   b. Hypopharynx
   c. Oral cavity
   d. Oropharynx

2. The landmark Veterans Affairs paper regarding larynx cancer established what treatment paradigm?
   a. Advanced stage larynx cancer should mainly be treated with surgery.
   b. Chemotherapy and radiation result in a lower should replace surgery for treatment of most advanced larynx cancers.
   c. Failure of chemotherapy and radiation leaves patients with no options.
   d. Chemotherapy and radiation result a lower quality of life than surgical treatment for advanced stage larynx cancer.

3. Primary tumors of what site in the aerodigestive tract are most consistently treated surgically?
   a. Nasopharynx
   b. Oral cavity
   c. Oropharynx
   d. Larynx

4. The most common cutaneous malignancy of the head and neck is
   a. Squamous cell carcinoma
   b. Basal cell carcinoma
   c. Melanoma
   d. Merkel cell carcinoma

5. In HNSCC, even if no cervical lymph nodes are clinically or radiographically evident, prior to treatment one must consider the presence of
   a. Distant metastasis
   b. Occult cervical metastasis
   c. Wrong diagnosis
   d. Radioresistant primary tumor

SALIVARY DISEASE QUESTIONS

Select one answer.

1. The following statements are true EXCEPT
   a. Pleomorphic adenomas have a very small risk of malignant transformation.
   b. Warthin's tumor is also known as papillary cystadenoma lymphomatosum.
   c. Basal cell and canalicular adenomas are varieties of pleomorphic adenoma.
   d. Oncocytoma is also known as oxyphilic adenoma.

2. The malignant salivary tumor most likely to invade surrounding nerve tissue is:
   a. Mucoepidermoid carcinoma
   b. Acinic cell carcinoma
   c. Adenoid cystic carcinoma
   d. Squamous cell carcinoma

3. The following lesion(s) has potential for distant metastasis to the lungs and bones:
   a. Polymorphous low-grade adenocarcinoma
   b. Adenoid cystic carcinoma
   c. Acinic cell carcinoma
   d. All of the above

4. A plunging ranula occurs when the mucocele herniates beneath which muscle into the submental space?
   a. Genioglossus
   b. Mylohyoid
   c. Geniohyoid
   d. Platysma

5. All of the following statements are TRUE except
    a. The auriculotemporal segment of the trigeminal nerve lies in close proximity to the superior aspect of the parotid and is generally not visible at surgery.
    b. The facial nerve should always be sacrificed during parotidectomy for malignant lesions.
    c. The tympanomastoid fissure is a reliable landmark in locating the main trunk of the facial nerve.
    d. Within the parotid, the facial nerve divides into the temporofacial and cervicofacial branches.

REFERENCES

1. Jemal A, Siegel R, Ward E, et al. Cancer statistics. *CA Cancer J Clin* 2008;58(2):71–96.
2. Greene FL, Compton CC, Fritz AG, Shah JP, Winchester DP, eds. *AJCC cancer staging atlas.* New York, NY: Springer, 2007.
3. Guardiola E, Chaigneau L, Villanueva C, Pivot X. Is there still a role for triple endoscopy as part of staging for head and neck cancer? *Curr Opin Otolaryngol Head Neck Surg* 2006;14(2):85–88.
4. van den Brekel MW. Lymph node metastases: CT and MRI. *Eur J Radiol* 2000;33(3):230–238.
5. Ragin CC, Taioli E. Survival of squamous cell carcinoma of the head and neck in relation to human papilloma virus infection: review and meta-analysis. *Int J Cancer* 2007; 121(8):1813–1820.
6. Weiss MH, Harrison LB, Isaacs RS. Use of decision analysis in planning a management strategy for the stage N0 neck. *Arch Otolaryngol Head Neck Surg* 1994;120(7): 699–702.
7. The Department of Veterans Affairs Laryngeal Cancer Study Group. Induction chemotherapy plus radiation compared with surgery plus radiation in patients with advanced laryngeal cancer. *N Engl J Med* 1991;324(24): 1685–1690.
8. Cooper J, Pajak TF, Forastiere A, et al. Postoperative concurrent radiotherapy and chemotherapy for high-risk squamous-cell carcinoma of the head and neck. *N Engl J Med* 2004;350:1937–1944.
9. Bernier J, Domenge C, Ozsahin M, et al. Postoperative irradiation with or without concomitant chemotherapy for locally advanced head and neck cancer. *N Engl J Med* 2004;350:1945–1952.
10. Bernier J, Cooper JS, Pajak TF, et al. Defining risk levels in locally advanced head and neck cancers. *Head Neck* 2005; 27(10):843–850.
11. Wrangle JM, Khuri FR. Chemoprevention of squamous cell carcinoma of the head and neck. *Curr Opin Oncol* 2007; 19(3):180–187.
12. Silver CE, Levin RJ, Greenstein B, et al. The parotid and submandibular glands. In: Silver CE, Rubin JS, eds. *Atlas of head and neck surgery,* 2nd ed. Philadelphia, PA: Churchill Livingstone, 1999:315–342.
13. Califano J, Eisele DW. Benign salivary gland neoplasms. *Otolaryngol Clin North Am* 1999;32:861–873.
14. Spiro RH, Huvos AF, Strong EW. Cancer of the parotid gland: a clinicopathologic study of 288 primary cases. *Am J Surg* 1975;130:452.
15. Spiro RH. Salivary neoplasms: overview of a 35-year experience with 2,807 patients. *Head Neck Surg* 1986; 8:177.
16. Marx RA, Stern D. *Oral and maxillofacial pathology: a rationale for diagnosis and treatment.* Carol Stream, IL: Quintessence, 2003.
17. Sapp JP, Eversole LR, Wysocki GP. *Contemporary oral and maxillofacial pathology,* 2nd ed. St. Louis, MO: Mosby, 2004.
18. Westra WH. The surgical pathology of salivary gland neoplasms. *Otolaryngol Clin North Am* 1999;32:919–943.
19. Regezi JA, Sciubba JJ, Pogrel MA. *Atlas of oral and maxillofacial pathology.* Philadelphia, PA: WB Saunders Co., 2000.
20. Rice DH. Malignant salivary gland neoplasms. *Otolaryngol Clin North Am* 1999;32:875–886.
21. Gold DR, Annino DJ Jr. Management of the neck in salivary gland carcinoma. *Otolaryngol Clin North Am* 2005; 38:99–105.
22. Medina JE. Neck dissection in the treatment of cancer of major salivary glands. *Otolaryngol Clin North Am* 1998;31: 815–822.
23. Rice DH. Chronic inflammatory disorders of the salivary glands. *Otolaryngol Clin North Am* 1999;32:813–818.
24. Capaccio P, Cuccarini V, Ottaviani F, et al. Comparative ultrasonographic, magnetic resonance sialographic, and videoendoscopic assessment of salivary duct disorders. *Ann Otol Rhinol Laryngol* 2008;117:245–252.
25. Rabinov JD. Imaging of salivary gland pathology. *Radiol Clin North Am* 2000;38:1047–1057.
26. Capaccio P, Torretta S, Ottaviani F, Sambataro G, Pignataro L. Modern management of obstructive salivary diseases. *Acta Otorhinolaryngol Ital* 2007;27:161–172.
27. Haller JR. Trauma to the salivary glands. *Otolaryngol Clin North Am* 1999;32:907–918.
28. Cotrim AP, Mineshiba F, Sugito T, et al. Salivary gland gene therapy. *Dent Clin North Am* 2006;50:157–173.
29. Elagoz S, Gulluoglu M, Yilmazbayhan D, et al. The value of fine-needle aspiration cytology in salivary gland lesions, 1994–2004. *ORL J Otorhinolaryngol Relat Spec* 2007;69: 51–56.
30. Sinha UK, Ng M. Surgery of the salivary glands. *Otolaryngol Clin North Am* 1999;32:887–906.
31. Cannon CR, Replogle WH, Schnek MP. Facial nerve in parotidectomy: a topographical analysis. *Laryngoscope* 2004; 114:2034–2037.
32. Carlson ER. The comprehensive management of salivary gland pathology. *Oral Maxillofac Surg Clin North Am* 1995; 1:387–430.

Thoracic Surgery

CHEST WALL

Pectus Excavatum

Pectus excavatum is a congenital malformation that presents as posterior displacement of the sternum distal to the angle of Louis. A large depression on the right side is frequent, and displacement of the heart is variable. Patients with this condition may have frequent respiratory infections and decreased exercise tolerance. These symptoms are usually alleviated after correction. Corrective surgery, done ideally before 7 years of age, consists of removing the deformed cartilages and lifting the sternum, which can be accomplished by performing a posterior osteotomy followed by insertion of a bone wedge at the osteotomy site.

Other sternal defects are less common. Among them is pectus carinatum, which is forward protrusion of the sternum. Superior, distal, and complete sternal clefts are rare malformations that are often associated with multiple chest wall abnormalities.

Chest Wall Tumors

Primary tumors of the chest wall are unusual and originate equally from the soft tissues and the skeletal structures: bone and cartilage. Metastatic tumors of the chest wall are more common than primary tumors and are frequently multiple. They can result from direct extension of breast, lung, or pleural tumors, although these tumors also metastasize by the usual hematogenous and lymphatic routes. Other primary tumor sites include kidney and prostate. An interesting group of tumors originating in the kidneys and thyroid can produce metastasis in the sternum, which present clinically as a palpable pulsatile mass.

Solitary chest wall tumors can be metastatic or primary with about the same frequency. More than half of the primary tumors are malignant. Usually they are painful, although some small rib tumors are asymptomatic. The anatomic location of the tumor is important when considering a possible preoperative diagnosis; for example, fibrous dysplasia is found in the posterior aspect of the chest wall. Cartilaginous tumors are located anteriorly, at the costal cartilages. Sternal tumors are almost always malignant, particularly if they are more than 4 cm in diameter. Radiographic evaluation of a chest wall tumor is helpful: sharp delineation and intact cortical margins are characteristic of benign tumors. Malignant tumors are poorly defined with frequent cortical disruption, usually with tumor-specific features. Computed tomography (CT) is helpful for defining possible invasion of the pleura, lung, and mediastinum.

Benign Tumors

Benign chest wall tumors are less frequent than malignant tumors. The most common benign tumors are chondroma, osteochondroma, and fibrous dysplasia. Benign neurogenic tumors such as neurofibroma and neurilemoma (also known as schwannoma) also occur in the chest wall. Desmoid tumors are rare and arise from intercostal muscles and grow to the surface of the chest wall. Occasionally, these tumors grow internally and are detected only with chest radiography. Desmoid tumors are not malignant but locally are highly invasive. Resection should be of a radical nature, avoiding injury to major structures. Local recurrence should be treated by wide reresection. All benign rib tumors should be excised along with segments of the ribs from which they originated. Osteochondromas can be excised flush to the rib, as they present as exostoses.

Primary Malignant Tumors

Soft tissue sarcomas comprise 70% of chest wall primary malignant tumors. They are classified as fibrosarcomas, malignant fibrous histiocytomas, rhabdomyosarcomas, angiosarcomas, neurosarcomas, synovial sarcomas, and others.

General Principles of Treatment

Before treatment is initiated, a tissue diagnosis is made with an open biopsy to obtain sufficient tissue for accurate diagnosis, which is often not feasible with a needle biopsy. Radical surgical excision with wide margins of normal tissue (at least 4 cm) is necessary for the treatment of most malignant tumors. Previous biopsy sites should be included. For sternal tumors the uninvolved side may be left in place to preserve the balance of the chest wall. When the tumor is situated in the posterior chest, beneath the scapula, three or four ribs may be removed without the need to reconstruct the chest wall.

Anteriorly, extensive reconstruction is necessary for large defects. Reconstruction has been accomplished with Marlex mesh as a composite with methylmethacrylate or with a sheet of 1 to 2 mm Gore-Tex. Soft tissue reconstruction can be accomplished with free or transposed grafts such as deltopectoral cutaneous, thoracoabdominal cutaneous, and myocutaneous flaps of latissimus dorsi.

Chondrosarcoma

Chondrosarcomas constitute 15% of primary malignant tumors of the chest wall and are found at the costochondral junction or at the sternum. Often exceeding 4 cm at presentation, they may involve cartilage, ribs, muscle, pleura, and sometimes directly invade lung. Symptoms are mostly represented by tenderness, redness, and rib fixation. Radiographs demonstrate a large lobulated mass associated with bone destruction. Treatment should be wide surgical excision, which results in a 70% 5-year survival. Inadequate resection often results in early local recurrence.

Osteosarcoma

Osteogenic sarcomas are seen in all age groups and are not as frequent as chondrosarcomas. Radiographs demonstrate a typical "sunburst"-like appearance. These tumors metastasize early. Treatment consists of wide local surgical excision followed by chemotherapy. When there is direct pulmonary invasion, the involved lung is resected at the time of the initial operation, preferably as a wedge resection. Despite all therapeutic efforts, 5-year survival is only 15%.

Ewing's Sarcoma

The typical onionskin calcifications seen in Ewing's sarcoma are produced by periosteal elevation. These tumors occur more commonly in adolescents. Surgical resection is not sufficient and should be followed by chemotherapy. When there is no response to chemotherapy, radiotherapy may be helpful.

Eosinophilic Granulomas

Eosinophilic granulomas are rare and usually multiple. They typically produce fever and leukocytosis.

Thoracic Outlet Syndrome

Thoracic outlet syndrome includes a variety of symptoms resulting from compression of the neurovascular bundle at the thoracic outlet. The brachial plexus, subclavian artery, and subclavian vein may be compressed between the first rib and the clavicle. Other structures causing potential compression are the scalenus anterior muscle, situated between the subclavian artery posteriorly and the subclavian vein anteriorly, and the scalenus medius, situated posteriorly and laterally to the neurovascular structures.

Cervical ribs, often accompanied by congenital fibromuscular bands, may also cause thoracic outlet compression. Symptoms vary depending on the presence or absence of vascular or neurologic compression. Most patients complain of symptoms related to brachial plexus compression. Neck pain spreading to the ear, jaw, forehead, and posterior neck suggests compression of C5 and C6 roots. When lower roots are compressed, pain is experienced in the scapular area and the ulnar nerve distribution. Other neurologic symptoms include paresthesias, motor weakness, and tenderness over the scalenus muscle.

Atrophy of the interosseous muscles in the hand is found in neglected cases. When the subclavian artery is compressed, symptoms of distal ischemia similar to those of Raynaud syndrome may be present and are manifested by coldness, claudication, or even necrosis of the digits. Subclavian vein compression can result in edema and cyanosis of the extremity and proliferation of collateral veins. Venous compression can also lead to acute axillosubclavian venous thrombosis or "effort thrombosis."

Diagnostic Tests

Several tests have been proposed to demonstrate the presence of clinically significant thoracic outlet narrowing. Maneuvers intended to obliterate the radial pulse (Adson's maneuver) are not reliable and may be positive in a large number of normal subjects. Radiography is necessary to diagnose the presence of cervical ribs, elongated cervical vertebral transverse processes, and other bony abnormalities such as clavicular fractures. Ulnar nerve conduction velocity across the thoracic outlet is 72 m/sec in normal individuals and may be less than 57 m/sec in patients who exhibit neurogenic thoracic outlet syndrome. However, these results are not universally reproducible. When there is clinical suggestion of subclavian artery compression, arteriography is useful. Phlebography can be diagnostic when the clinical impression is subclavian vein compression or thrombosis. The symptoms of nerve compression resulting from thoracic outlet syndrome are sometimes difficult to differentiate from carpal tunnel syndrome and cervical disc compression.

Treatment

Uncomplicated cases of thoracic outlet syndrome do not require surgery. Surgical intervention is indicated only when the patient is symptomatic with severe pain, neurologic deficits, or symptoms of significant subclavian artery or vein compression. Conservative treatment consists of physical therapy with posture control. Poor shoulder position results in a decrease of space between the clavicle and the first rib, which aggravates the compression. Patients should also avoid carrying loads such as grocery bags. With conservative management, improvement is seen in 50% to 90% of patients with neurogenic thoracic outlet syndrome.

Surgical procedures are designed to eliminate compression of the anatomic structures that traverse the thoracic outlet. The most commonly recommended procedure is a first rib resection, frequently performed via a transaxillary approach. When neurologic symptoms result from compression of C5 or C6 roots, an anterior scalenectomy may be sufficient decompression. Cervical ribs and fibromuscular bands should also be resected when present. Although good outcomes can be obtained in up to 95% of patients with neurogenic thoracic outlet syndrome, suboptimal results are obtained when these bands are not recognized and divided. Insufficient decompression may also exacerbate the symptoms because of scar tissue growth.

Vascular complications of thoracic outlet syndrome may present unique challenges. Significant arterial compression may result in aneurysmal degeneration of the subclavian artery and arterial reconstruction may be required in addition to thoracic outlet decompression. Acute axillosubclavian venous thrombosis is usually treated with thrombolysis followed by thoracic outlet decompression, usually with first rib resection.

TRAUMA

Sternal Fractures

Sternal fractures result from severe blunt trauma and are often associated with steering wheel injuries. If displacement with separation of the fragments occurs, reduction and fixation may be required. Observation is sufficient for nondisplaced fractures. Evaluation for possible cardiac contusion with serial electrocardiograms and cardiac enzymes is required. Mortality rates of 20% to 45% are reported, almost always due to the severity of the associated injuries.

Isolated Rib Fractures

Isolated rib fractures may be associated with pneumothorax or hemothorax that requires chest tube drainage. Thoracotomy may occasionally be necessary to control bleeding or repair air leaks. Analgesics should be administered in sufficient doses to prevent splinting and atelectasis.

Flail Chest

Flail chest can occur when multiple ribs are fractured, especially if there are double fractures on ribs or the fractures are associated with costochondral separations. The resultant mechanical dysfunction of the chest wall manifests as limited expansion during inspiration and paradoxical movements of parts of the chest wall. Poor ventilation is associated with intrapulmonary shunting.

The immediate treatment for patients in respiratory distress who do not improve with face mask oxygen is endotracheal intubation with mechanical ventilation. Some believe that most patients with flail chest also have significant pulmonary contusion and recommend adding fluid restriction and physiotherapy to the ventilatory support. Endotracheal intubation and mechanical ventilation should be considered for patients with a room air $PO_2 < 60$ mm Hg or with a $PO_2 < 80$ mm Hg with oxygen administered by face mask.

Weaning from ventilatory support follows the same guidelines as in other circumstances. If the patient requires prolonged ventilatory support for treatment of flail chest and has no other serious injuries, internal fixation of the fractured ribs can be considered. This option allows early ambulation, avoiding the usual complications that result from prolonged bed rest and prolonged artificial ventilation.

MEDIASTINUM

Mediastinal Tumors

The mediastinum is divided into anterior, middle, and posterior portions. A tentative diagnosis, including the probable histologic type of a tumor, can be assigned on the basis of the location of the tumor. Tumors arising in the thyroid and parathyroid glands are most frequently found within the superior mediastinum.

The relative tumor frequency varies with patient age. In children, 50% of mediastinal tumors are neurogenic, 20% are lymphomas, and 20% are cysts; whereas in adults, the tumors are represented equally: 20% neurogenic tumors, 20% thymomas, 20% lymphomas, and 20% cysts.

Neurogenic tumors are mostly found in children younger than 4 years. Germ cell tumors such as seminomas, teratomas, choriocarcinomas, embryonal cell carcinomas, and yolk sac tumors found in the anterior mediastinum comprise 10% of mediastinal tumors and are found primarily in adolescents and adults. Thymomas and endocrine tumors are rarely seen in children.

Symptoms are present in 50% of patients with malignant mediastinal tumors and in only 10% of those with benign tumors. The most frequent symptoms are pain, cough, dyspnea, respiratory infections, and dysphagia. Rarely, superior vena cava compression or invasion may occur. Horner syndrome due to involvement of the stellate ganglion is also rare. Even less common is spinal cord compression. Some mediastinal tumors secrete endocrine substances that are capable of producing metabolic alterations. Hypercalcemia may be found in patients with parathyroid adenomas. Hypertension due to a neurogenic tumor and thyrotoxicosis due to an intrathoracic goiter are not uncommon. Myasthenia gravis and red blood cell aplasia are associated with thymomas.

The evaluation of patients with mediastinal tumors includes chest films, followed by CT scan, in some cases magnetic resonance imaging (MRI), and occasionally angiography. Tissue diagnosis can be obtained by needle biopsy, transcervical standard or extended mediastinoscopy, or anterior mediastinotomy (Chamberlain procedure). Often specialized studies are indicated. MRI is useful for clarifying intraspinal extension of neurogenic tumors. Radioisotope scanning with I_{131} is useful for evaluating a possible mediastinal thyroid.

MRI is helpful for defining mediastinal masses. Anterior mediastinal exploration through a Chamberlain procedure is indicated for evaluation and biopsy of a lesion situated in that location. Differentiation between thymomas, lymphomas, and seminomas may be difficult on frozen section.

Neurogenic Tumors

At least 50% of unilateral paravertebral masses in children are malignant, whereas in adults most masses in this location are benign. Chest pain produced by bony erosion or nerve root compression is the most frequent symptom. Dyspnea due to tracheal compression is sometimes present. Intraspinal extension of a tumor with compression of the cord may produce a neurologic deficit. Hypertension is present when the tumor is a catecholamine-secreting pheochromocytoma. Vanillylmandelic acid can be produced by ganglioneuromas and neuroblastomas and cause clinical symptoms such as diarrhea, flushing, and diaphoresis.

The most common neurogenic tumor is the neurilemoma (schwannoma), which arises from the nerve sheath. It presents as a well-circumscribed lesion that may advance into the intervertebral canal. Less frequently seen are neurofibromas. These poorly circumscribed tumors may be part of generalized neurofibromatosis. Patients with Von Recklinghausen disease occasionally have a posterior mediastinal meningocele. Neurilemomas and neurofibromas can undergo malignant degeneration to malignant schwannomas, which are highly invasive tumors. Ganglioneuromas arise from sympathetic ganglia, are well encapsulated, and grow to a large size. Their malignant counterparts, ganglioneuroblastomas, may metastasize widely. Neuroblastoma is the most undifferentiated neurogenic tumor and is highly malignant. Often when first diagnosed it has already metastasized to brain, bone, and liver. Fever, cough, and sometimes diarrhea are the presenting symptoms.

Pheochromocytomas are rarely seen. Even less common are paragangliomas, which arise from the chemoreceptor tissue located at the aortic arch.

The treatment for neurogenic tumors is surgical resection. When there is intravertebral extension the intravertebral component should be excised synchronously with the intrathoracic tumor. To obtain sufficient exposure, the skin incision is placed over the laminectomy site and extended into a posterolateral thoracotomy. Neuroblastomas may be unresectable at the time of presentation. When complete resection is not possible, adjuvant chemotherapy and radiotherapy are utilized. These tumors have a better prognosis when located in the mediastinum than in other sites.

Thymoma and Parathymic Syndromes

Thymomas are the most common anterior mediastinal tumor in adults older than 30 years. About 5% of patients who present with red blood cell aplasia and 10% with myasthenia gravis have associated thymomas. Myasthenia results from the destruction of acetylcholine receptors located at the neuromuscular endplate by thymic antibodies.

The Masaoka staging system is utilized for determining prognosis and therapeutic recommendations.

Stage I—Macroscopically encapsulated. Microscopically, may invade into, but not through capsule
Stage II—Microscopic transcapsular invasion. Macroscopic invasion into surrounding fatty tissue or mediastinal pleura
Stage III—Macroscopic invasion into surrounding organs (pericardium, lung, and great vessel)
Stage IVa—Pleural or pericardial dissemination
Stage IVb—Lymphatic or hematogenous metastases

Histologically, thymomas are classified as epidermoid, spindle cell, or mixed. Lymphocyte content in these tumors is variable. The presence of a thymoma is indication for surgery. Noninvasive tumors have a 10-year survival approaching 90%, whereas the 10-year survival for invasive tumors is only 20%. In the presence of severe myasthenia, plasmapheresis prior to surgery is recommended to remove acetylcholine receptor antibodies. Perioperative use of steroids has proven beneficial. Patients with generalized myasthenia without an obvious thymoma should undergo thymectomy.

Resection of the thymus may be accomplished via a number of approaches: mediasternotomy, transcervical, and thoracoscopic. Although superiority of one method has not been proven, some surgeons have combined the transcervical and thoracoscopic approaches.

In 50% of patients the symptoms of myasthenia remit during the first year after surgery, and almost 90% of patients improve within 4 to 5 years after surgery. When the tumor is invasive, radiotherapy is recommended. Neoadjuvant chemotherapy has improved the resectability rate for some lesions believed to be unresectable.

Lymphoproliferative Diseases

Primary mediastinal lymphomas, observed mostly in young adults, are usually confined to the middle and anterior mediastinal lymph nodes. Hodgkin disease is the most frequent type, representing two-thirds of primary mediastinal lymphomas. As with other mediastinal tumors, cough, chest pain, and fever are the most common symptoms. When the tumor is bulky it may compress mediastinal structures, including the superior vena cava and trachea. Surgery is commonly limited to the acquisition of tissue samples for a pathologic diagnosis and can be done through an anterior mediastinotomy (Chamberlain procedure) or cervical mediastinoscopy. Treatment usually consists of radiotherapy and chemotherapy.

Giant lymph node hyperplasia or pseudolymphoma is also known as Castleman disease. It is associated with markedly enlarged lymph nodes in the mediastinum, which may measure up to 700 g.

Germ Cell Tumors

Mediastinal germ cell tumors are found in the anterior mediastinum. Although rare, this location is second only to the gonads, where 95% of these tumors are found. Similar to other mediastinal tumors, they manifest as cough, pain, and shortness of breath. When invasive, tumors may erode into a bronchus, the pericardium, or the pleural cavity. The most common germ cell tumor is the teratoma, composed of several embryologic layers that may be cystic or solid. They are mostly benign. The radiologic presence of calcifications makes identification straightforward. These tumors should be resected for both diagnosis and treatment. Sometimes resection is difficult due to adhesions and the intimate relationship of the tumor to intrathoracic structures. Teratocarcinomas are the malignant counterparts and are highly invasive, producing metastasis early.

Malignant mediastinal germ cell tumors are classified as seminomas and nonseminomatous tumors. Seminomas occur almost exclusively in men 20 to 40 years old. Nonseminomatous germ cell tumors are further classified as embryonal cell carcinomas, choriocarcinomas, yolk sac tumors, and mixed forms. These tumors produce increased titers of β-human chorionic gonadotropins and α-fetoprotein. They are highly malignant tumors found in young men, commonly with early metastatic spread.

Although seminomas respond well to chemotherapy alone, this is not the case for the nonseminomatous tumors. If residual tumor is found following chemotherapy and tumor markers return to normal titers, surgery is indicated followed by radiotherapy and chemotherapy. Pathology of the residual tumor can be active cancer, scar tissue, and benign teratoma. The role of adjuvant therapy is currently under investigation.

Benign Tumors

Benign mediastinal tumors are usually asymptomatic when they do not compress a vital structure such as an airway. Superior mediastinal tumors are mostly thyroid in origin. They may descend into the chest and produce symptoms based on size and occasional compression of major vessels and/or the trachea. When the thyroid pedicle is insinuated between the esophagus and the vertebral bodies, dysphagia may result because of compression of the esophagus. Removal of an upper anterior mediastinal thyroid gland can usually be accomplished through a cervical incision. If the thyroid is large and cannot be removed via the cervical incision, a partial sternotomy and rarely a thoracotomy may be necessary.

Other benign mediastinal tumors are generally asymptomatic and include lipomas, fibromas, myomas, or angiomas. When symptoms are present one must suspect the presence of malignancies such as liposarcoma, etc.

Mediastinal Cysts

Cysts represent 20% of mediastinal tumors in all age groups. The most frequently diagnosed cysts are bronchogenic and esophageal cysts, which are malformations derived from the primitive foregut.

Bronchogenic cysts are found close to the tracheal bifurcation and have an inner lining of ciliated respiratory epithelium. Esophageal cysts, also known as enteric or duplication cysts, are situated in close association with the esophagus. They may be found inside the muscular layers of the esophagus. Neuroenteric cysts are associated with anomalies of the vertebral bodies and may communicate directly with the dural space.

Two frequently diagnosed mesothelial cysts are pericardial and pleural cysts. Pericardial cysts are usually found in the right pericardiophrenic angle. Because they contain clear fluid, they are known as clear water cysts. Less frequently seen are thymic cysts, found in the anterior mediastinum. These cysts can become acutely symptomatic if they rupture. Cysts may be accurately diagnosed with CT and MRI scans. Resection is indicated if symptoms are present. Malignant degeneration is extremely rare.

Pneumomediastinum

The most frequent cause of pneumomediastinum is the forced passage of air alongside pulmonary vascular and bronchial structures toward the hilum of the lung and then into the mediastinum. This situation is seen sometimes in patients being ventilated with high airway pressures, but it can happen also in otherwise healthy patients. Treatment is usually supportive. In rare cases when excessive air is present and produces discomfort and pressure, some surgeons recommend that an incision may be made above the sternal notch deep to the pretracheal fascia to decompress the air trapped in the mediastinum.

Less frequently air is introduced into the mediastinum when the trachea or bronchus is ruptured because of deceleration during a motor vehicle accident. Spontaneous esophageal rupture (Boerhaave syndrome), foreign body perforation or iatrogenic injury also permit air to enter the mediastinum. Rarely, a ruptured posterior wall of the duodenum is responsible for passage of air into the retroperitoneal tissues, from where it insinuates upward, entering the mediastinum. Treatment for these various conditions is directed at the initial pathology.

Mediastinitis

Mediastinitis is produced by bacterial contamination of the mediastinum. Proper treatment includes drainage, the use of organism-specific antibiotics, and identification of the source of contamination to prevent continuous soilage. When mediastinitis is due to esophageal rupture or perforation, the esophageal defect is closed at the same time the mediastinum is cleaned and drained. Antibiotics are used as necessary.

Mediastinitis occasionally results from extension of a pharyngeal abscess or perforation of the piriform sinus or hypopharynx proximal to the cricopharyngeus during traumatic intubation. Fibrosing mediastinitis is rare and usually idiopathic. It may also be secondary to Histoplasma or tuberculous infection of the mediastinal lymph nodes. When advanced, it can result in compression of the superior vena cava, trachea, or esophagus, producing the symptoms and signs, respectively, of superior vena cava syndrome, dyspnea, or dysphagia. Surgery is directed at decompression of the involved structures.

TRACHEA

Tracheal Tumors

Primary tracheal tumors are rare. Sixty percent of these tumors are squamous cell carcinomas and adenoid cystic carcinomas (also known as cylindromas). Almost half of malignant tracheal tumors have mediastinal or pulmonary metastases at the time of initial diagnosis. Benign tumors are rare and include fibromas, leiomyomas, and chondromas. Secondary tumors may invade the trachea by direct extension and include esophageal tumors (which may grow through the posterior membranous wall of the trachea) and tumors of the larynx, bronchus, and thyroid.

Symptoms, which are generally due to airway obstruction, include shortness of breath, wheezing, and cough. Voice changes and hoarseness may also be present when the recurrent nerve is invaded or when the vocal cords are directly involved.

The thoracic surgeon should be prepared to deal urgently with a patient who comes to the emergency department with tracheal obstruction. A rigid pediatric bronchoscope can be used to provide an interim airway and may be maneuvered to dilate the airway sufficiently to permit intubation with a small-caliber endotracheal tube. After emergency treatment, surgery should be considered. Even when unresectable for cure, the lumen can be opened endoscopically and the tumor debulked with biopsy forceps and suction. Bleeding is generally not a critical problem in such cases and a stent may be placed to maintain patency. No advantage is seen with the use of laser.

Tumor resection can usually be accomplished through an anterior cervical approach combined with a median sternotomy if necessary. Distal tracheal tumors can be approached with improved exposure through a right thoracotomy. Up to 50% of the tracheal length can be resected and the distal and proximal trachea can be approximated by keeping the head flexed during the end-to-end tracheal anastomosis. This flexion should be maintained postoperatively to prevent suture disruption. It may be necessary to suture the patient's chin to the chest. Results are satisfactory for benign tumors and for malignant tumors confined to the tracheal wall. Adenoid cystic carcinomas can infiltrate the trachea at an area remote from the original tumor, making complete resection difficult.

Tracheal Stricture/Tracheostomy

Tracheal stricture results from prolonged endotracheal intubation with injury produced by endotracheal balloon cuffs. Modern low-pressure cuffs have significantly reduced the incidence of this complication.

Stricture may also occur from contracture of a tracheal stoma following tracheostomy. Tracheostomy must be performed at the appropriate level to avoid complications. Tracheostomy is performed via a longitudinal incision through the second and third tracheal rings. For optimal exposure, the thyroid isthmus is divided if necessary. Tracheostomies performed at a lower level have the potential to injure the innominate artery, which may produce delayed and massive bleeding occurring several days after the initial procedure. Tracheostomies performed at a higher level may be associated with injuries to the cricoid cartilage with subsequent development of subglottic stenosis. The sides of the tracheal wall can be secured with long stitches taped to the skin so as to be able to reintubate the trachea if the tracheostomy tube is inadvertently dislodged during the immediate postoperative period.

Tracheal Disruption

Blunt chest trauma, deceleration injuries, or falls from heights can produce partial or complete tracheal disruption. Complete tracheal disruption is almost always fatal. Intubation can be difficult, as a large amount of blood obscures the vision of the endoscopist. If possible, a cervical incision and "fishing" of the distal trachea with a tracheostomy hook may be the only way to direct the endotracheal tube into the disrupted airway. Once the airway is secured, the patient is taken to the operating room for controlled repair of the trachea.

Incomplete disruption of the trachea or the major bronchi is heralded by hemoptysis and the presence of air in the mediastinum near the site of disruption.

Treatment options include observation or repair of the disruption.

PLEURA

Pneumothorax

In the absence of adhesions between the visceral and parietal pleura, pneumothorax develops when air enters the pleural cavity. Ruptured bullae, damage to the lung by fractured ribs or penetrating injuries, and esophageal perforation or rupture are all potential causes of pneumothorax.

Spontaneous pneumothoraces commonly occur in two distinct groups. The first is composed of tall, slender young men and women in their 20s. The second is comprised of mostly elderly patients. In the young adults, the pneumothorax is associated with sudden rupture of a congenital pulmonary bulla or a subpleural bleb. In older patients with emphysema, rupture of acquired bullae is usually the cause of pneumothorax.

Symptoms of spontaneous pneumothorax are of variable intensity and consist of sudden chest pain associated with dyspnea and tachypnea. When there is a ball-valve effect at the site where the lung ruptured, it is possible for a large volume of air under pressure to build up inside the pleural space, creating a tension pneumothorax. This dangerous clinical situation manifests as diaphoresis, tachypnea, and dyspnea associated with decreased breath sounds in the involved hemithorax. The position of the mediastinum, including the cardiac apex and trachea, may shift. Immediate relief of the tension is accomplished by draining the hemithorax with a needle or catheter. If not diagnosed and treated, this situation can rapidly evolve to cardiac arrest. Radiologic studies delay treatment and are not indicated. Treatment in all cases of spontaneous pneumothorax is directed to re-expanding the lung, which is accomplished by inserting a small-caliber chest tube connected to an underwater seal and suction system. The chest tube may be introduced into the second interspace at the midclavicular line or at the midaxillary or anterior axillary line where it intersects the xiphoid line. The latter approach is preferred in female patients, who may be concerned with cosmesis and scars. During insertion of the chest tube care must be taken to avoid injury to the lung. Unless the lung is detached from the chest wall or totally collapsed as seen on chest films, the pleural space should be identified before inserting the chest tube.

Surgery is indicated for an air leak that persists for 48 hours, recurrent pneumothorax, or a patient with previous contralateral pneumothorax. Treatment should include bullectomy and abrasion of the parietal pleura (pleurodesis) to create adhesions between the two layers of pleura. The procedure can usually be accomplished via thoracoscopy. Pleurodesis, undertaken to avoid surgery on patients with spontaneous pneumothorax, is indicated only when surgery is excessively risky and when there is no radiologic evidence of bullae. Attempted pleurodesis will fail when the lung becomes only partially attached to the chest wall, thereby creating multiple noncommunicating compartments in the pleural space.

Pleural Tumors

The visceral and parietal pleura can be invaded by tumors originating in the lung or breast, which are the most frequently encountered pleural tumors. Often, large pleural effusions result and require supportive treatment that includes drainage and pleurodesis to obliterate the pleural. Talcum powder is the most effective substance used for pleurodesis, although doxycycline and bleomycin have also been used successfully. Radiotherapy or chemotherapy can also decrease the size of the pleural effusion. A percutaneously inserted catheter is also an option for patients who are able to care for the device at home.

The most common primary tumor of the pleura is mesothelioma, which is frequently associated with asbestos exposure. Until recently, asbestos was used in the production of a large number of items of daily use, including insulating materials, brake linings, and so forth. Approximately 3,000 new cases of mesothelioma are diagnosed each year in the United States. Two types are recognized: localized benign and diffuse malignant. The localized form can attain a large size (up to several pounds), is pedunculated, and is surgically resectable. The diffuse form can be histologically classified as epithelial, sarcomatous, or mixed. Median survival of the patient with the malignant form is only 8 to 12 months. Unlike other malignancies, mesotheliomas are lethal because of local, uncontrolled growth. Surgical treatment has generally been discouraging. Two types of surgical treatments are available: pleurectomy and extrapleural pneumonectomy. Pleurectomy suffices when the tumor is in the parietal pleura, and there are no attachments between the visceral and parietal pleura. When there are attachments with obliteration of the pleural space, an extrapleural pneumonectomy is an option for selected patients. Some surgical series report survivals of up to 14 to 20 months, but this observed increase in survival may be due to patient selection rather than any benefit attributable to surgery. Other series comparing surgery with chemotherapy or radiotherapy alone do not show any improvement in survival, although minor improvement was noted when a combination of these modalities was used.

LUNG

Bronchogenic Carcinoma

Approximately 210,000 new cases of bronchogenic carcinoma were diagnosed in 2008. Lung cancer is the most common cause of cancer death in both men and women and remains a significant public health problem. Although cigarette smoking is well established as the causative agent in most cases, up to 25% of the U.S. adult population continues to smoke cigarettes.

Non–small cell lung cancer represents 80% of bronchogenic tumors. Adenocarcinomas and squamous cell carcinoma account for 45% and 35% of cases, respectively. The remainder are classified as large cell, mixed histology, and poorly differentiated. Small cell lung cancer comprises 15% of lung tumors, although the incidence (for reasons which are not known) appears to be decreasing. These tumors behave more like a systemic disease than other tumors and have a predilection for early spread to other organs. Carcinoid tumors constitute 2% to 3% of lung tumors. Serotonin and other endocrine substances can be secreted by these tumors. The majority are classified as "typical."

Symptoms

Intraparenchymal tumors with a size of less than 3 cm are usually asymptomatic. As the tumors enlarge, cough or hemoptysis may result. Airway obstruction is associated with atelectasis and pneumonia. Hoarseness may result from recurrent laryngeal nerve invasion and occurs more frequently with left lung tumors because of the course of the recurrent nerve as it loops around the aortic arch. The right recurrent nerve is involved less frequently because it is positioned around the innominate artery and is less vulnerable to pulmonary pathology. When the phrenic nerve is compromised, paralysis and elevation of the hemidi-aphragm occurs, producing basal atelectasis of the lower lobe and dyspnea.

Superior sulcus (Pancoast) tumors invade the structures at the apex of the chest. Horner syndrome (ptosis, miosis, anhydrosis) results from invasion of the stellate ganglion. The lower roots of the brachial plexus and upper ribs are commonly invaded, producing unrelenting shoulder and arm pain.

Obstruction of the superior vena cava manifests as edema of the head, neck, and upper extremities followed by the appearance of collateral veins in the upper chest. The esophagus can also be compressed by a lung tumor or enlarged mediastinal lymph nodes, causing dysphagia. Pericardial effusion due to metastatic disease may occur. Commonly, the chronicity of the process permits the pericardium to stretch slowly to accommodate large amounts of fluid. Cardiac tamponade may or may not be evident.

Rarely, symptoms result from the production of hormone-like substances. Squamous cell carcinoma can produce a parathyroid hormone–like substance, whereas adrenocorticotropic hormone, and antidiuretic hormone are sometimes produced by small cell carcinoma. Other hormonal substances are responsible for pulmonary osteoarthropathy manifested by clubbing and pretibial pain due to periosteal proliferation. Frequently, the initial symptoms of lung cancer are caused by distant metastases commonly located in the brain or bones. Liver metastases are also frequent, but often remain asymptomatic.

Solitary pulmonary nodules in patients younger than 30 years are malignant in only 1% to 2% of cases. Most of the benign solitary lesions in this age group are hamartomas and granulomas related to tuberculosis, histoplasmosis, or sarcoidosis. In older patients, and particularly in smokers, solitary lung lesions are likely to be malignant.

Evaluation

The initial step in the evaluation of a pulmonary nodule should be a review of the previous chest radiographs. A nodule that has remained unchanged for many years is likely benign. If the tumor was not seen on previous films or if growth is demonstrated, the presumptive diagnosis is malignancy. CT scan provides detailed anatomic information regarding the primary tumor and also permits assessment of the mediastinal lymph nodes, liver, and adrenal glands. Positron emission tomography (PET) is indicated in every patient with suspected lung cancer to identify metastatic disease. False-positive scans can occur, and suspected metastases should be biopsied. Brain MRI and bone scans are indicated to evaluate symptoms localized to these sites.

Sputum cytology may be diagnostic but is rarely obtained. Bronchoscopy is useful for assessing the extent of central tumors. Although a histologic diagnosis of a suspicious nodule is not necessary prior to excision, some physicians will routinely perform bronchoscopy or percutaneous needle biopsy. The role of mediastinoscopy remains controversial. Certainly, patients with enlarged or PET-avid mediastinal node should undergo biopsy to evaluate the presence of metastatic disease.

Pulmonary function tests are routinely performed prior to surgery. Predicted postoperative FEV_1 (forced expiratory volume in 1 second) or DLCO (diffusion capacity of the lung for carbon monoxide) of less than 40% is associated with increased morbidity and mortality. Surgery should be avoided when the predicted postoperative FEV_1 is less than 0.8 L. Split function ventilation/perfusion scans are sometimes utilized to determine the extent to which the affected lung contributes to overall ventilation. Oxygen consumption with exercise of below 15 cc/kg/min is also associated with increased morbidity. Cardiac evaluation is performed as necessary.

Staging

Lung cancer staging is based on the TNM classification, the most recent modification of which was in 2009. Although the staging system can be utilized for both non–small cell and small cell lung cancer, the latter are usually categorized as "limited" (confined to the hemithorax) or "extensive" (disease outside the hemithorax). The current classification is given in Tables 19.1 and 19.2.

Treatment

Surgery is indicated for patients with clinical stages I and II. The minimum preferred operation is lobectomy, as lesser resections are associated with increased local recurrence. Pneumonectomy is necessary is approximately 10% of patients. Mortality following lobectomy is 2% and following pneumonectomy 6%. Survival rates following resection of stage I, II, and IIa non–small cell lung cancer approximate 60%, 40%, and 25%, respectively. Adjuvant chemotherapy should be offered to patients found to have nodal involvement and improves survival by approximately 5%.

TABLE 19.1	Stage Grouping AJCC		
Stage	**T**	**N**	**M**
Occult carcinoma	TX	N0	M0
Stage 0	Tis	N0	
Stage IA	T1a,b	N0	M0
Stage IB	T2a	N0	M0
Stage IIA	T2b	N0	M0
	T1a,b	N1	M0
	T2a	N1	M0
Stage IIB	T2b	N1	M0
	T3	N0	M0
Stage IIIA	T1a,b T2a,b	N2	M0
	T3	N1, N2	M0
	T4	N0, N1	M0
Stage IIIB	Any T	N3	M0
	T4	N2	M0
Stage IV	Any T	Any N	M1

Controversy exists regarding the best treatment for patients with N2 disease identified prior to surgery. Two large phase III trials have failed to identify a survival benefit for patients with N2 disease treated with neoadjuvant followed by surgery when compared with chemotherapy and radiotherapy alone. Selected patients with solitary brain metastases may benefit from resection of both the primary lung cancer and the brain lesion. Patients with Pancoast tumors are treated with radiotherapy and chemotherapy prior to resection. Carcinoid tumors are treated similarly to non–small cell lung cancer.

Limited small cell lung cancer is generally treated with chemotherapy and radiotherapy, whereas extensive disease is commonly treated with chemotherapy alone. Small cell cancer rarely presents as a solitary nodule and an accurate diagnosis is generally not made prior to excision. If a solitary nodule is established as small cell lung cancer, recommended treatment is resection followed by chemotherapy.

Lung Abscesses

The most common sites for lung abscesses are the superior segments of the right and left lower lobes. There is a slight preponderance on the right side due to anatomic characteristics, as there is a more direct line between the trachea and the right main bronchus. It is also of note that the carina is situated more to the left of the midline. Frequently involved (but less often than the superior segments of the lower lobes) is the posterior segment of the right upper lobe.

TABLE 19.2	**Definitions of the TNM Categories**

Primary tumor (T)

T0   No evidence of primary tumor.

TX   Primary tumor cannot be assessed, or tumor proven by the presence of malignant cells in sputum or bronchial washings but not visualized by imaging or bronchoscopy

Tis   Carcinoma in situ.

T1   Tumor 3 cm or less in greatest dimension surrounded by lung or visceral pleura, without bronchoscopic evidence of invasion more proximal than the lobar bronchus (i.e. not in the main bronchus)

T1a   Tumor 2 cm or less in greatest diameter

T1b   Tumor more than 2 cm but not more than 3 cm in greatest diameter

T2   Tumor more than 3 cm but not more than 7 cm; or tumor with any of the following features:
– involves main bronchus, 2 cm or more distal to the carina
– invades visceral pleura
– associated with atelectasis or obstructive pneumonitis that extends to the hilar region but does not involve the entire lung

T2a   Tumor more than 3 cm but not more than 5 cm in greatest dimension

T2b   Tumor more than 5 cm but not more than 7 cm in greatest dimension

T3   Tumor more than 7 cm or one that directly invades any of the following: chest wall (including superior sulcus tumors), diaphragm, phrenic nerve, mediastinal pleura, parietal pericardium; or tumor in the main bronchus less than 2 cm distal to the carina but without involvement of the carina; or associated atelectasis or obstructive pneumonitis of the entire lung or separate tumor nodule(s) in the same lobe as the primary.

T4   Tumor of any size that invades any of the following: mediastinum, heart, great vessels, trachea, recurrent laryngeal nerve, esophagus, vertebral body, carina; separate tumor nodule(s) in a different ipsilateral lobe to that of the primary.

Nodal involvement (N)

N0   No demonstrable metastasis to regional lymph nodes.

N1   Metastasis to lymph nodes in the peribronchial or ipsilateral hilar region (or both) including direct extension.

N2   Metastasis to ipsilateral mediastinal lymph nodes and subcarinal lymph nodes.

N3   Metastasis to contralateral mediastinal lymph nodes, contralateral hilar lymph nodes, ipsilateral or contralateral supraclavicular lymph nodes.

Metastasis (M)

M1   Distant metastases

M1a   Separate tumor nodule(s) in a contralateral lobe; tumor with pleural nodules or malignant pleural or pericardial effusion

M1b   Distant metastasis

M0   No distant metastases

Lung abscesses may result from aspiration of foreign bodies, including teeth or dental caps. They are also associated with tooth and gum infections. Some alcoholic patients aspirate while intoxicated, and the aspirated material drains into the most dependant portions of the airways. Pulmonary abscesses may also result from necrotizing pneumonia and usually occur in the basal segments of the lower lobes. Less frequently seen are cavitating carcinomas, which mostly occur in the upper lobes and have a different clinical presentation. On CT scans, necrotizing carcinomas

have a thick, irregular wall. A diagnostic biopsy can be obtained by bronchoscopy.

The conservative treatment for abscesses of infectious origin consists of physiotherapy, postural drainage, and broad-spectrum antibiotics. Abscesses due to aspiration frequently have a mixed flora including anaerobes. Bronchoscopy is indicated for both diagnosis and treatment. An obstructing foreign body can be found, which can continue to prevent adequate drainage of purulent material if not removed. Percutaneous drainage of lung abscesses, as initially described by

Monaldi and subsequently abandoned, is again a first-line treatment. When adhesions do not exist between the two pleural layers, the lung may collapse when punctured for drainage, resulting in soiling of the pleural space and giving rise to an empyema. This complication may also occur spontaneously as abscesses can rupture into the pleural space. A more frequent complication is soiling of the lung resulting from drainage of the abscess contents into the bronchial tree with spillage into other areas including the contralateral lung.

If the abscess is 6 cm or larger and does not respond to conservative treatment, resection is indicated. If possible, the abscess contents are percutaneously drained before surgery. A double-lumen endotracheal tube is used to prevent soiling of the dependent lung when the patient is placed in the lateral decubitus position for thoracotomy.

Empyema

Empyema is present when there is pus in the pleural space and may occur in a number of situations. It may follow an episode of pneumonia, be secondary to a ruptured lung abscess, or result from penetrating trauma produced by stab wounds or gunshot wounds leading to an infected hemothorax.

The initial empyema fluid is thin, and there are no adhesions between the two pleural surfaces. At this early stage, simple chest tube drainage is adequate treatment. In the later stages, adhesions form and large amounts of fibrin are deposited on the lung surface, preventing re-expansion. The lung becomes immobilized by this fibrinous casing and is virtually trapped and unable to distend when the chest wall expands during inspiration. At this stage, treatment with chest tube drainage is insufficient, and decortication is necessary to free the contracted lung from under the fibrinous layer.

In a patient with a contraindication for thoracotomy who can tolerate the reduced lung volume available for gas exchange, an alternative treatment is open drainage. An Eloesser flap requires resection of one or two lower rib segments, followed by suturing a flap of skin based on the upper side of the incision to the parietal pleura. This procedure creates a skin valve that permits the release of purulent material from inside the pleural space. Antibiotics are given according to the results obtained from cultures of the empyema.

In the surgical patient, postpneumonectomy empyema can result from a bronchopleural fistula caused by disruption of the bronchial closure. Pedicle flaps using the intercostal or pectoralis muscles are options for reclosure of the bronchus. Rarely, thoracoplasty is required as a space-reducing procedure for the treatment of this surgical complication.

Pulmonary Sequestration

Pulmonary sequestration is a congenital malformation in which the sequestered part of the lung receives its blood supply through an anomalous branch of the aorta that frequently originates below the diaphragm. Sequestrations are located in the basal region of the right or left lower lobe. The artery supplying this anomalous part of the lung may be of large caliber and is located in the inferior pulmonary ligament, making inadvertent injury difficult to repair.

Two types of sequestration are found: the extralobar form is covered by its own visceral pleura and does not communicate with the air spaces in the lung. The intralobar form is not separated and communicates freely with the air spaces in the lung. It does not have a separate visceral pleura layer. Because of this communication with pulmonary air spaces intralobar sequestrations can become infected and develop a clinical picture identical to that of a lung abscess. The key to the diagnosis of pulmonary sequestration is the position of the abscess in the lower portion of the lung. This is different from other lung abscesses, which are usually in the superior segments of the lower lobes. An angiogram is indicated when a basal segment abscess suggests the possibility of intralobar sequestration. Treatment consists of ligation of the arterial branch arising from the aorta and resection of the accessory lung tissue.

QUESTIONS

Select one answer.

1. Which predicted FEV_1 value contraindicates pulmonary resection?
   a. Above 0.8 L.
   b. Below 0.8 L.
   c. Above 1.2 L.
   d. Below 1.2 L.

2. Seven days after insertion of a chest tube for a spontaneous pneumothorax, several attempts to reposition the chest tube did not decrease the air leak. What is the next step?
   a. Insert a new chest tube.
   b. Reposition the chest tube.
   c. Chemical pleurodesis.
   d. Surgically close the air leak plus pleurodesis.

3. The initial workup of a newly found lung mass in a 30-year-old man does not include
   a. Sputum cytology.
   b. Bronchoscopy.
   c. Review of old films.
   d. Open lung biopsy.

4. A 50-year-old female cigarette smoker was found to have a 3-cm lung mass not present 1 year before. Cytologic and bronchoscopic examination results were negative. The next step should be
   a. Radiotherapy alone.
   b. Radiotherapy and chemotherapy.
   c. Resection.
   d. Follow-up after 3 months.

5. A lung abscess measuring 4 cm in the superior segment of the right lower lobe is best treated with
   a. Antibiotics and physiotherapy.
   b. Percutaneous drainage.
   c. Resection.
   d. Chest tube drainage.

6. A postpneumonic empyema is best treated with
   a. Antibiotics and physiotherapy.
   b. Chest tube drainage and antibiotics.
   c. Decortication if more than 7 days old.
   d. Thoracentesis and pleural injection of streptokinase.

7. Small cell carcinoma is different from other bronchogenic carcinomas in that
   a. It is always incurable.
   b. It is not seen in female subjects.
   c. It is has a predilection for early spread to other organs.
   d. It is not responsive to chemotherapy.

8. The presence of a thymoma
   a. Is always associated with myasthenia gravis.
   b. Is never associated with myasthenia gravis.
   c. Is indication for resection.
   d. Can be diagnosed by radiographic appearance only.

9. Treatment of an apical tumor with Horner syndrome is
   a. Radiotherapy.
   b. Surgery.
   c. Radiotherapy and chemotherapy followed by surgery.
   d. Radiotherapy and chemotherapy alone.

10. The initial treatment for a patient with multiple bilateral rib fractures and flail chest with CO, retention is
    a. Endotracheal intubation and positive-pressure ventilation.
    b. Surgical fixation of ribs.
    c. Chest wall immobilization with sand bags.
    d. Intercostal nerve blocks.

SELECTED REFERENCES

Edge SB, Byrd DR, Compton CC, Fritz AG, Greene FL, eds. *AJCC cancer staging manual,* 7th ed. New York, NY: Springer, 2010.

Grillo HC. *Surgery of the trachea and bronchi.* Hamilton, Ontario: BC Decker Inc, 2004.

Patterson GA, Cooper JD, Deslauriers J, et al. eds. *Pearson's thoracic and & esophageal surgery,* 3rd ed. Philadelphia, PA: Churchill Livingstone Elsevier, 2008.

Sellke F, del Nido PJ, Swanson S, eds. *Sabiston & Spencer surgery of the chest,* 8th ed. Philadelphia, PA: Elsevier Saunders, 2010.

CHAPTER

20

Patrick J. Greaney Jr.
Evan S. Garfein

Management of Burns

INTRODUCTION

Burn injuries represent a complex group of problems in a varied patient population. To develop a systematic approach to their management, a clear understanding of the pathophysiology and natural history is needed. Burn management can be divided into initial treatment and resuscitation, early excision and grafting, definitive closure of burn wounds, and secondary reconstruction. The purpose of this chapter is to provide a framework on which the care of the burned patient can be organized.

EPIDEMIOLOGY

According to the 2011 American Burn Association Fact Sheet, approximately 450,000 patients seek medical treatment for burns annually in the United States. Hospitalizations for burn injury total 45,000 including 25,000 admissions to hospitals with specialized burn centers. Estimates of burn injuries in this country have slowly been decreasing since the 1960s. Approximately 50 years ago, burn injuries in this country were estimated at two million annually.

Mortality from fires and burns numbers approximately 3,500 per year in the United States. Nearly 3,000 deaths result from residential fires while the remaining deaths result from various other causes including electrical burns, chemical burns, and motor vehicle accidents. More than one-third of admissions exceeded 10% total body surface area (TBSA) and 10% of admissions exceeded 30% TBSA. Overall 70% of burn injuries are sustained by males and 30% by females with the home being the most common place of occurrence (1).

According to the most recent Safe Kids USA national data from 2007, children sustain approximately 116,600 burn- and fire-related injuries annually. Of these, each year, approximately 528 children aged 14 years and under die from these injuries. Children at greatest risk of death include children younger than 4 years and children with disabilities. Scald burns caused by hot liquids or steam are the most common burns sustained by young children and account for 65% of hospitalizations for burn-related injuries for children aged 4 years and younger. Hot tap water accounts for nearly 25% of all scald burns and is associated with more deaths and hospitalizations than any other hot liquid burns. Meanwhile, contact burns caused by direct contact with fire are more common among older children.

In 2006, approximately 2,300 fireworks-related injuries among children younger than 15 years were sustained. Burns account for more than half of all fireworks-related injuries and primarily injure the hands and areas around the face and head. Sixty percent of fireworks-related injuries typically occur around July 4th holiday (2).

LOCAL AND SYSTEMIC RESPONSE TO BURN INJURY

Depending on the type and severity of the burn injury, any and all structures in the body may be affected. The skin, the body's largest organ, is the most frequently injured structure. Significant burns to the skin impair the body's ability to regulate temperature, regulate fluid balance, defend itself from microbial infection, provide neurosensory input about the environment, and maintain structural integrity. Burns can produce cosmetic deformities that have long-lasting and profound impact on the patient's life. The goal of burn management is to mitigate the damaging effects of burn injury by understanding their mechanisms and natural history and acting to counter them.

Although many burn patients can be managed adequately in a hospital setting, others require transfer to a specialized burn center. Burns covering more than 10% of TBSA in the very young or old or 20% TBSA in others meet these criteria. The same is true for patients with burns to the face, hands, perineum, or genitalia and those with inhalational injury, multitrauma, and multiple comorbidities.

ASSESSING BURN DEPTH AND ZONES OF INJURY

Burns are often described by degree (first degree, second degree, third degree) or by thickness (partial or full thickness). First-degree burns involve only the epidermis. Second-degree burns involve part of the dermis as well. Third-degree burns involve the entire dermis. Similarly, partial-thickness burns involve part of the dermis while full-thickness burns affect the entirety of both skin layers.

First-degree burns (e.g., sunburns) heal by themselves, usually within 5 to 7 days, and leave no scar. Superficial second-degree burns (hot water scald) take longer to heal (2 to 3 weeks) and are very painful, but usually heal without scarring and without requiring surgical intervention. Deep second-degree burns are more similar to third degree or full-thickness burns and should be treated as such. Full-thickness burns (exposure to open flame) are characterized by pale, dry, painless wounds. Full-thickness burns will heal with scarring and need to be excised and grafted.

ASSESSING BURN SIZE

The Lund–Browder chart is the most accurate method for estimating burn size. The more commonly used, "Rule of Nines," is simpler but less accurate. In this scheme, the head and neck and each upper extremity are estimated to be equivalent to 9% of the TBSA. The front of the torso, the back of the torso, and each lower extremity are estimated to be equivalent to 18% TBSA. The perineum is equivalent to approximately 1%. The palm is also roughly estimated as composing 1% TBSA.

PRIMARY SURVEY

Patients with significant burn injuries may present with other, potentially life-threatening issues. As with any trauma patient, the airway should be secured, breathing supported if necessary, and an assessment made of the circulatory status. The cervical spine should be examined and immobilized, if necessary, and the patient's mental status observed. Intravenous access is vital and should be central. A nasogastric tube and a Foley catheter are placed as well.

The airway is of special concern in the burn patient. Nasopharyngoscopy is the best method by which to examine the upper-most portion of the aerodigestive tract. Evaluation on initial presentation may be normal even in patients who have sustained injury as edema may not manifest for 6 to 8 hours. Physicians must maintain a high level of suspicion for airway compromise in the early resuscitative period. If stridor or respiratory distress are noted or if significant burns to the head and neck exist, the patient should be intubated immediately, given 100% oxygen, and transported to a burn center. Lower-airway injury can manifest itself with coughing, wheezing, bronchorrhea, shortness of breath, or impaired gas exchange. Any of these are indications for intubation.

SECONDARY SURVEY

The secondary survey of a burn patient involved an organized approach to history and physical examination that will guide both the initial resuscitation and the early management of the patient. A top-to-bottom approach is useful.

Neurological evaluation begins with assessment of possible trauma to the brain and spinal cord. This can be done radiographically in the patient who is sedated for pain control. Early evaluation of mental status can provide information on the efficacy of resuscitation and onset of complications such as sepsis.

Head and neck examination begins with evaluation of the eyes and specifically with assessment of visual acuity and corneal injury. A fluorescein test will demonstrate corneal abrasions. Ocular antibiotics and topical anesthetics are the treatment of choice for corneal injuries. Examination of the oral cavity and larynx yields information about the likelihood of inhalational injury. The presence of frank burns or carbonaceous sputum is an indication for endotracheal intubation. Finally, examination of the neck is performed as for all trauma patients, with radiographic evaluation of the integrity of the cervical spine.

Cardiac monitoring is routine in the early management phase. Elderly patients or those with preexisting coronary artery disease are prone to develop arrhythmias or ischemia due to the physiological stress of the injury. Monitoring cardiac output can provide information about the efficacy of resuscitation but is rarely indicated.

Inhalational injury can result in damage to the pulmonary epithelium and concomitant airway edema. If this is suspected, the plan for early bronchoscopy should be made as slough of tissue can lead to plugging of airways or of the endotracheal tube itself. In ventilated patients, elevated peak airway pressures above 40 cm H_2O may indicate the need for escharotomies of the chest. Escharotomies that extend to the abdomen may be indicated to permit adequate ventilation in patients with significant burns to the trunk.

Gastrointestinal injury is usually a concern with direct ingestion of caustic liquids. With other types of burn injuries, the important aspects of gastrointestinal management include ulcer prophylaxis and decompression of the stomach and proximal gastrointestinal tract with a nasogastric tube to prevent vomiting and aspiration.

Burned extremities require close attention during the early phase of evaluation. The major, devastating complication of burned extremities results from impaired perfusion of the distal limb due to circumferential constriction secondary to swelling. In this situation, axial escharotomies are indicated and must release constricting fascia. Escharotomies are successful when there is restoration of vascular flow to the distal extremity. Dressings that are loosely applied and are amenable to frequent replacement are required for examination of the wounds. Burned wrists, hands, fingers, and feet should be splinted in positions of function.

LABORATORY EVALUATION

Baseline laboratory values are important for a variety of reasons. An arterial blood gas gives information about the extent of damage to the pulmonary tree. Carboxyhemoglobin levels provide information about inhalation of carbon monoxide. Baseline electrolytes, urinalysis, and a complete blood cell count help guide resuscitative efforts.

Inhalation injury is managed by mechanical ventilation on 100% oxygen until carboxyhemoglobin levels fall to less than 10%. The half-life of carbon monoxide's binding to hemoglobin or carboxyhemoglobin falls

from 4 to 5 hours on room air to approximately 80 minutes on 100% oxygen. Prophylactic antibiotics for patients with inhalational injury have not been shown to be effective in preventing pneumonia and carry the risk of selecting resistant strains of bacteria.

CARBON MONOXIDE EXPOSURE

Carbon monoxide (CO) is a poisonous gas that is odorless, colorless, and tasteless. These characteristics contribute to carbon monoxide's insidious and deadly nature. Each year in the United States, carbon monoxide poisoning claims approximately 400 lives and leads to 20,000 emergency department visits (3).

Carbon monoxide results from the incomplete burning of hydrocarbon-containing substances such as wood, gasoline, and oil. Residential fires, unvented kerosene and gas space heaters, leaking chimneys and furnaces, back-drafting from wood stoves and fireplaces, gas water heaters, automobile exhaust, and tobacco smoke are all potential sources. When inhaled, CO displaces oxygen in the blood and forms carboxyhemoglobin, thereby depriving the body tissues of oxygen (4).

Initial symptoms of carbon monoxide poisoning may be fairly nonspecific and include headache, fatigue, nausea, disorientation, drowsiness, and dizziness. Chest pain may result in those with preexisting cardiac disease. Typically, symptoms occur more rapidly in those most susceptible, namely the very young or old or those with predisposing cardiopulmonary health problems. Smokers who already have elevated CO blood levels may also become symptomatic more rapidly. At moderate to high concentrations, angina, altered vision, seizures, and brain anoxia may result. Very high levels may be fatal (4,5).

Burn patients who present for medical care after being involved in a fire within an enclosed area must be carefully examined for signs of carbon monoxide poisoning. Because of vague symptoms, a high level of suspicion is paramount. The diagnosis can be confirmed by measuring the ratio of carboxyhemoglobin to the amount of hemoglobin in the patient's blood (6). The ratio of carboxyhemoglobin to hemoglobin molecules in an average person may be approximately 5% whereas smokers may have levels of up to 9% (7). Serious toxicity typically occurs with a carboxyhemoglobin to hemoglobin ratio greater than 25%.

After removal of the patient from a fire or carbon monoxide source, 100% oxygen is administered to the patient by means of a nonrebreather mask, which shortens the half-life of carbon monoxide. Typically, this treatment dramatically reduces the half-life from approximately 320 minutes (average on room air) to 80 minutes (8).

More recently, hyperbaric oxygen has been introduced as another method of treatment for carbon monoxide poisoning. Hyperbaric oxygen at three times atmospheric pressure can further reduce the half-life of carbon monoxide from 80 minutes with oxygen to approximately 23 minutes (9). Nonetheless, it remains controversial whether hyperbaric oxygen actually improves outcomes.

Additional treatment may be necessary for other complications of carbon monoxide poisoning. Antiseizure medications, fluid resuscitation, and cardiac dysrhythmias must be treated when present. Neurologic damage may require radiologic studies for confirmation and appropriate follow-up.

SPECIFIC TYPES OF BURNS

Chemical Burns

Chemical burns are characterized by often atypical presentation and underappreciated severity. Consequently, an accurate history and a high index of suspicion are vital to effective management. Thermal injury to tissues produces characteristic red, white, or charred appearance. Chemical injury often produces a brown or gray appearance. While thermal injuries affect superficial layers of skin followed by deeper layers, chemical burns can penetrate outer layers and produce deeper tissue damage or systemic toxicity with relatively minor superficial changes. The presence of persistent severe pain may indicate ongoing tissue destruction.

The initial management of the patient with chemical burn injury is the same as for thermal injury. History, including type, duration, and setting of chemical exposure, is critical. Irrigation of contacted skin with room temperature water is indicated. Sulfuric acid can cause full-thickness burns that produce a brownish gray appearance. Lime powder or concrete powder burns are often seen in construction workers. Initial treatment is with water irrigation. Hydrofluoric acid burns, usually to fingers, are characterized by extreme pain caused by leeching of calcium from tissues by fluoride ions. Treatment is with topical, intra-arterial, and/or subcutaneous calcium gluconate. Alkali burns produce tan or gray discoloration of the skin and are extremely painful. Initial treatment is again by irrigation with water. Phenol burns can cause significant systemic toxicity including cardiac and respiratory depression and hypothermia. Treatment is aimed at minimizing the surface area available for absorption. Large-volume irrigation with water or polyethylene glycol is indicated. Tar burns are treated by removing the adherent tar. Neosporin contains an emulsifier that is helpful in this regard.

Electrical Burns

Electrical burns are caused by the passage of electrical current through the body. The resistance of the tissue path transited by the current produces heat. Electrical burns have four components. The first is the injury caused by the current itself. The second component is caused by arcing, which occurs when air is ionized by a large voltage drop. Because it can produce heat up to 4,000°C, arcing can result in ignition of clothing. The third component is caused by a flash injury from the electrical source or from ignition of clothing. The fourth and final component is the traumatic injury caused by the resultant shock, muscle spasm, or fall.

Electrical injuries are classified as either high voltage (>1,000 V) or low voltage (<500 V). High-voltage burns produce tissue damage along the path of current and often cause cardiac and neurological injury. Low-voltage burns cause injury at the point of contact with the skin but not along its path through the body. Low-voltage injuries are associated with cardiac arrhythmias.

Frostbite

Frostbite refers to localized tissue injury caused by exposure to subfreezing temperatures. Histopathologically, it is characterized by intra- and extracellular formation of ice crystals. As with thermal injury, frostbite may be superficial or deep. Superficial frostbite presents as a grayish or whitish area of skin that is associated with a tingling, numb, or burning sensation. Deep frostbite is characterized by a larger area of cold, waxy, cyanotic tissue. The appearance of the tissue after thawing predicts prognosis. If large, fluid-filled blisters form, the prognosis tends to be better. Small blisters or absence of blisters altogether increases the likelihood of necrosis and gangrene. The cornerstone of frostbite management is rapid rewarming with water 104°F to 108°F. This process may be very painful and narcotics may be required. Loose dressings should be applied after rewarming.

FLUID RESUSCITATION

All patients with burns involving greater than 15% TBSA will require fluid resuscitation. The goals of resuscitation are hemodynamic stability, adequate urine output, normal acid–base balance, and normal mental status. Urine output guidelines vary by age. The urine output goal for infants is 1 to 2 mL/kg/hr, for children is 0.5 to 1.0 mL/kg/hr, and for adults is 0.5 mL/kg/hr. Similarly, the goal for systolic blood pressure varies between 60 and 70 mm Hg for infants and 90 to 120 mm Hg for adults.

Fluid resuscitation should be given through large-bore peripheral intravenous access. Lactated Ringer's solution is the solution of choice. The 4 cc/kg/%TBSA is a reliable estimate for total fluid requirements for resuscitation over the first 24 hours but increased amounts should be expected in young and old patients, those with inhalational injury, and patients who have sustained electrical burns. After calculating the fluid requirements for the first 24 hours, half of that volume should be administered in the first 8 hours after injury (not after presentation), 25% over the next 8 hours, and 25% over the final 8 hours.

INITIAL BURN MANAGEMENT

Following the primary and secondary survey, initiation of fluid resuscitation, and appropriate radiographic evaluation of the patient, wound management can commence. Initial steps are to remove constrictive clothing, clean wounds that may be contaminated, administer tetanus prophylaxis, and determine the depth of the burn injury.

Nutritional support of the burn patient must be tailored to the metabolic demands. Burn injury creates a hypermetabolic state and a concomitant catabolic state. Nutritional support is aimed at meeting the energy demands of the patient as well as his or her protein requirements. Research has established the so-called "ebb" and "flow" phases of burn injury in which there is an initial (12 to 24 hours) reduction in metabolic requirements followed by a phase of increased metabolism that may last for many weeks. The hypermetabolism of the "flow" phase is mediated primarily by increases in epinephrine, cortisol, and glucagons, resulting in depletion of glycogen and protein stores.

While enteral feedings are preferred over parenteral sources of nutrition, oral intake alone is often inadequate and nasogastric feeding tubes are usually necessary in patients with larger burns to administer adequate nutrition. When considering parenteral feeding, it is always important to consider that central line placement can be associated with many life-threatening complications including pneumothorax, hemothorax, retroperitoneal bleed, line sepsis, and endocarditis.

There are several formulas, which are useful to estimate the caloric nutritional needs of burn patients. The two most commonly used formulas include the Harris–Benedict equation and the Curreri formula. The Harris–Benedict formula determines the basal energy expenditure (BEE) in kilocalorie per day for male and female burn patients based on the following formulas (note: weight measured in kg, height in cm, and age in years)

Harris–Benedict Equation

Males: BEE (kcal/d) = 66.47 + (13.75 × Weight) + (5 × Height) − (6.76 × Age)

Females: BEE (kcal/d) = 655.1 + (9.56 × Weight) + (1.85 × Height) − (4.68 × Age)

These estimates are then multiplied by a stress/injury factor. For burns up to 20% TBSA, the factor is 1.0 to 1.5; for burns between 20% and 40% TBSA, the factor is 1.5 to 1.85; and for burns with a TBSA greater than 40%, the factor is 1.85 to 2.05. The Harris–Benedict formula takes into account that smaller burns result in less significant increases in metabolic rate while large burns may increase the metabolic needs of the human body over twice that of normal.

The Curreri formula is a simpler formula for estimating caloric needs of burn patients with burns up to 50% TBSA.

Curreri Formula

BEE (kcal/d) = (25 × body weight (kg) + 40 × % TBSA burned)

Although carbohydrates remain the major energy source for burn patients, glucose intolerance remains a major concern. Strict control of hyperglycemia is necessary for optimal patient care and patients often require supplemental insulin administration. It is important to note that excess carbohydrate feeding may also result in an increased respiratory quotient (RQ) causing increased production of carbon dioxide and difficulty in weaning from a ventilator. Many recommend that approximately 30% of nonprotein calories be derived from fat, both to provide essential fatty acids and to reduce the administered glucose load. Protein needs of the burn patient must also be addressed. While normal patients require approximately 80 g of protein daily, burn patients may catabolize more than 150 g daily. Protein needs typically increase with increasing burn size and measurement of nitrogen balance is frequently helpful. General recommendations are for 1.5 to 2.0 g of protein per kilogram daily for adult burn patients and up to 3.0 g/kg/d in pediatric patients (10,11).

Topical antimicrobials are frequently used in the treatment of burns that have yet to be excised or are small enough to not warrant excision and grafting. The most commonly used topical antimicrobial is silver sulfadiazine. Although it is painless and has a broad spectrum of activity and low risk of complications, it does not penetrate eschars well. Mafenide acetate, on the other hand, does penetrate eschars and is the agent of choice for burned ears. It can be associated with development of metabolic acidosis due to its activity as a carbonic anhydrase inhibitor, and it is painful on administration. Finally, silver nitrate solution is also a broad-spectrum antimicrobial and antifungal agent. Its major drawback is its tendency to produce systemic hyponatremia.

Excision and Grafting

Early removal of devitalized tissue has become the mainstay of initial management of burn injuries. This is often accomplished during the first postinjury week. Exceptions to early excision and grafting include burns involving the face, hands, feet, and genitals. Benefits of this approach include improved survival, decreased length of stay and treatment costs, and fewer dressing changes for the patient.

Face, Eyes, and Ears

Burns to the face vary in management and prognosis based on location. The skin of the face varies considerably in thickness from the cheek and nose to the eyelids. Many burns to the central face can be managed conservatively with topical antibiotics. Those that are clearly full-thickness can be excised and grafted with full-thickness skin grafts from the supraclavicular or retroauricular regions to maximize aesthetic matching. Burns to eyelids pose different and more difficult problems. Wound contracture of the burned eyelid can result in corneal exposure and ulceration. Release of the lid and grafting may be necessary to prevent this. Burned ears are treated with the topical application of mafenide acetate and pressure relief. The major complication from burned ears is suppurative chondritis, which can result in loss of significant portions of the cartilage framework of the ear.

Hands and Feet

Burns to the hands and feet can cause significant morbidity. Reducing this morbidity has become more important as overall survival continues to increase. Burns to hands are initially managed the same way as burns to other parts of the body. During the initial assessment, the burned hand is evaluated to assure uncompromised perfusion. If there is any concern about vascular perfusion, prompt escharotomies of the hand and digits are performed. Superficial burns are managed by splinting in the position of function, topical antibiotics, and passive range of motion physical therapy. More significant burns are managed by excision and grafting with sheet grafts. Open joints or compromised joints benefit from fixation with Kirschner wires to prevent contracture.

Perineum/Genitalia

Burns to the perineal area are most commonly treated conservatively with daily antibiotic dressing changes. The urethra is stented with an indwelling Foley catheter until local edema subsides and the wound demarcates. Thighs are placed in approximately 15 degrees of abduction using a wedge splint to minimize hip contracture. The burned area is allowed to demarcate and very often left to heal secondarily. Persistent, nonhealing wounds may be managed with skin grafting or local tissue flap mobilization from adjacent areas. Delayed Z-plasty release of perineal band deformities is sometimes necessary.

Complete loss of the male penis from burn injury is extremely rare, and reconstruction is performed in a delayed manner. Many methods for construction of a neophallus are available and include the use of rectus myocutaneous flaps, anterolateral thigh free flaps, and forearm osteocutaneous free flaps, amongst others (12).

COMPLICATIONS

Complications in the burn patient are varied. Neurological complications include delirium from metabolic disorder or anoxia, seizures from hyponatremia, and neuropathy from demyelinization, direct thermal injury, or compartment syndrome. Cardiovascular complications such as arrhythmias can arise in the acute setting in conjunction with electrical burns. Bacterial sepsis arising in the delayed setting can cause endocarditis. The most common pulmonary complication is pneumonia associated with either inhalational injury or prolonged intubation. Early hepatic dysfunction, acalculous cholecystitis, gastroduodenal ulceration, and pancreatitis are all relatively common. Neutropenia and thrombocytopenia may arise due to the systemic response to massive burns and may herald the onset of sepsis. Heterotrophic ossification is a process characterized by massive, uncontrolled growth of bone tissue, often in muscle beds or around burned joints.

OPERATIVE WOUND MANAGEMENT/RECONSTRUCTION

Initial operative wound management of deep second- and third-degree burns mandates excision of necrotic tissue. Small burns may be amenable to direct excision and primary closure or adjacent tissue transfer. More often, tangential excision, initially described by Janzekovic (13), is utilized for burn wound excision.

The concept of tangential excision involves the gradual removal of tissue down to a healthy wound base with copious punctate bleeding, over which split-thickness skin grafts can be applied. In cases of very deep wounds, fascial excision may be necessary. Popular instruments utilized for excision include the Watson and Goulian knives. To limit blood loss during excision, tourniquets, predebridement tumescence, epinephrine-soaked sponges, and topical thrombin may be used.

Skin grafts utilized for burn wound resurfacing are categorized as either split-thickness or full-thickness. Split-thickness skin grafts contain epidermis as well as a variable amount of dermis while full-thickness grafts contain the entire dermis. Full-thickness grafts retain all dermal elements and typically demonstrate greater initial (primary) contraction after harvest. However, the utility of full-thickness grafts is limited by the fact that donor sites must be closed primarily or grafted. Split-thickness grafts tend to result in greater delayed (secondary) wound contraction. Split-thickness skin grafts are by far the most common type of skin graft utilized in immediate burn reconstruction with the exception of areas such as the hands or face.

Donor sites for split-thickness skin grafts vary depending on the location and severity of the burn injury. Facial burns are best resurfaced with skin with a good color match obtained from supraclavicular or scalp areas. Smaller burns on other areas of the body are generally amenable to skin graft harvest from the less conspicuous upper thigh and buttock area. With larger body surface area burns, harvest from areas such as the back or torso become necessary with the ability to reharvest from the same area after several weeks of healing. A variety of methods are used to manage the donor site wound. Popular options include OpSite™, Tegaderm™, Xeroform, and Biobrane™.

Split-thickness skin grafts for burn resurfacing are typically harvested using a dermatome, and are often taken at an intermediate depth between roughly 0.012 and 0.018 inches. Split-thickness grafts may then be meshed to provide a greater surface area of skin coverage or merely "pie-crusted" with small incisions that allow for drainage of serous fluid during the healing process. Skin graft survival or "take" consists of three stages including plasmatic imbibition, inosculation, and revascularization. The first phase called plasmatic imbibition occurs during the first 24 to 48 hours during which the graft receives nutrients via diffusion by capillary action. During inosculation, the donor and recipient capillaries align to establish a vascular network. Finally, revascularization occurs with the ingrowth of new vessels into the graft from the wound bed.

The healing process after skin grafting often takes 12 months or longer for full maturation. Hypertrophic scar may become evident within 2 to 3 months of skin grafting. While still immature, burn scars may react favorably toward a number of interventions. Pressure therapy in the form of custom compression garments (Jobst garments), elastic bandages (Tubigrip™), and thermoplastic facial masks are frequently utilized. In addition, silicone inserts in combination with compression therapy often proves effective in combination with burn scar massage. Steroid-impregnated tape (Haelan tape) or steroid injections may also be considered. Dry, pruritic skin is also common and is ameliorated by frequent application of moisturizing agents.

Microvascular free flaps are at the peak of the reconstructive ladder and represent another option for burn reconstruction. Free tissue transfer is often considered for burn injuries to the extremities with exposure of vessels, nerves, tendons, and bone. While free flaps may be utilized in the acute setting for limb salvage, studies have demonstrated a much higher flap failure rate (24%) in free flaps performed for primary reconstruction versus those performed for secondary reconstruction (approaching 0%). Flap failures typically occurred between 5 days and 6 weeks after burn injury and were attributed to increased infection rate, intravascular thrombogenicity, and posttraumatic vascular damage. Despite the higher failure rate, acute performance of a free flap may be the only means of limb salvage feasible in certain patients (14).

SKIN REPLACEMENT PRODUCTS

Multiple skin replacement products are available to the clinician and many more are in development. Burn wounds represent just one indication for the use of skin replacement products with venous ulcers, diabetic wounds, and pressure ulcers comprising the other major indications. Bioengineered skin substitutes can be of human, porcine, or bovine origin, or autologously engineered products. These products can be bilayer products (replacing both dermis and epidermis), dermal, or epidermal. *Apligraf* is a bilayer skin replacement composed of human fibroblasts and keratinocytes. *Dermagraft* is a human dermal product made from fibroblasts. *TransCyte* is also a human dermal replacement that is composed of fibroblasts with a silicone sheet that acts as a temporary epidermal layer. *Integra*, a dermal replacement product, is made of bovine collagen and chondroitin. *AlloDerm* is another dermal matrix substitute processed from cadaver skin that is made acellular. Lastly, *Epicell* is an epidermal substitute engineered from the patient's own keratinocytes. While skin replacement products continue to evolve, the ideal skin replacement for the treatment of the seriously burned patient remains controversial (15).

QUESTIONS

Select one answer.
1. Burns characterized by painful blistering are best characterized as:
   a. First-degree burns.
   b. Second-degree burns.
   c. Third-degree burns.
   d. Fourth-degree burns.

2. The initial symptoms of carbon monoxide poisoning include:
   a. Fatigue.
   b. Headache.
   c. Disorientation.
   d. Lethargy.
   e. All the above.

3. Hydrofluoric acid burns are typically treated with topical, intra-arterial, and/or subcutaneous administration of:
   a. Calcium carbonate.
   b. Sodium bicarbonate.
   c. Calcium gluconate.
   d. Calcium phosphate.
   e. Potassium gluconate.

4. Burns to ears are best treated with what medication to prevent chondritis:
   a. Silver sulfadiazine.
   b. Mafenide acetate.
   c. Bacitracin.
   d. Silver nitrate.
   e. Chlorhexidine.

5. Split-thickness skin grafts typically are defined as "mature" after what period of time:
   a. 1 month.
   b. 3 months.
   c. 6 months.
   d. 9 months.
   e. 12 months or longer.

REFERENCES

1. American Burn Association. Burn incidence and treatment in the United States: 2011 fact sheet. December 2010. ABA. 29 December 2010. http://www.ameriburn.org/resources_factsheet.php. Accessed December 29, 2010.
2. Safe Kids USA. Burns and scalds safety fact sheet. September 2007. Safe Kids USA. 29 December 2010. http://www.safekids.org/assets/docs/ourwork/research/burn-scalds.pdf. Accessed December 29, 2010.
3. U.S. Fire Administration. Fire safety topics: carbon monoxide. November 2010. U.S. Fire Administration. 29 December 2010. http://www.usfa.dhs.gov/citizens/co/index.shtm. Accessed December 29, 2010.

4. United States Environmental Protection Agency. An introduction to indoor air quality: carbon monoxide. November 2010. EPA. 29 December 2010. http://www.epa.gov/iaq/co.html. Accessed December 29, 2010.

5. U.S. Department of Labor. OSHA carbon monoxide poisoning fact sheet. 2002. Occupational Safety and Health Administration. 29 December 2010. http://www.osha.gov/OshDoc/data_General_Facts/carbonmonoxide-factsheet.pdf. Accessed December 29, 2010.

6. Nelson LH. "Carbon monoxide". In: Goldfrank LR, Flomenbaum N, eds. *Goldfrank's toxicologic emergencies*, 7th ed. New York, NY: McGraw-Hill, 2002; 1689–1704.

7. Ford MD, Delaney KA, Ling LJ, Erickson T, eds. *Clinical toxicology*. Philadelphia, PA: WB Saunders Company, 2001; 1046.

8. Weaver LK. Clinical practice. Carbon monoxide poisoning. *N Engl J Med* 2009;360(12):1217–1225.

9. Raub JA, Mathieu-Nolf M, Hampson NB, Thom SR. Carbon monoxide poisoning-a public health perspective. *Toxicology* 2000;145(1):1–14.

10. Peck M. Practice guidelines for burn care: nutritional support. *J Burn Care Rehabil* 2001;22:59S–66S.

11. Waymack J, Herndon D. Nutritional support of the burned patient. *World J Surg* 1992;16:80–86.

12. Herndon D. *Total burn care*. Philadelphia, PA: Elsevier Health Services, 749–758.

13. Janzekovic Z. A new concept in the early excision and immediate grafting of burns. *J Trauma* 1970;10:1103–1108.

14. Sauerbier M, Ofer N, Germann G, Baumeister S. Microvascular reconstruction in burn and electrical burn injuries of the severely traumatized upper extremity. *Plast Reconstr Surg* 2007;119(2):605–615.

15. Garfein E. Skin replacement products and markets. In: Orgill D, Blanco C, eds. *Biomaterials for treating skin loss*. Boca Raton, FL: CRC Press LLC, 2009;9–13.

Ronald J. Simon
Salman Ahmad
Steven Blau

CHAPTER **21**

Surgical Critical Care

T he American Board of Surgery has placed increasing emphasis on the role of critical care in the education of the general surgeon. It is obvious that with a large amount of material germane to critical care, this chapter must be considerably less than complete. It is designed, instead, to stress those concepts with which the reader is probably already familiar and to reinforce the reader's bedside experiences and prepare for the board exam.

SHOCK

It has been more than a century since Samuel Gross defined shock as the "rude unhinging of the machinery of life." More "modern" definitions include: shock represents a point where tissue perfusion is inadequate for the needs of the cell, or the point at which inadequate oxygen is provided the cell. These modern definitions fail to consider shock as a dynamic state where there is an insult to an organ and a physiologic response to that insult. They are helpful, though, for focusing the initial discussion of shock on events that occur at the cellular level. In the simplest terms, the cell requires perfusion to deliver to it supplies of oxygen and energy substrate (to metabolize to produce energy) and as a means of ridding itself of waste products.

Cells exist bathed in interstitial fluids whose electrolytic constitution resembles that of plasma. Although the "outside" of the cell is characterized by high sodium (130 to 140 mEq/L) and low potassium (4 to 5 mEq/L) concentrations, the relation of the two cations is reversed within the cell. Intracellular sodium is low (only about 10 to 15 mEq/L) and potassium is high (about 100 mEq/L). This difference creates an electrical potential across the cell membrane. The cell requires adenosine triphosphate (ATP) energy to maintain this equilibrium and thus its own integrity. Normally, this energy is produced by the *aerobic* metabolism of glucose, which is converted to carbon dioxide and water. The metabolic pathways traversed include the Embden–Meyerhof glycolytic pathway (in which glucose is cleaved into two three-carbon fragments) and the Krebs tricarboxylic cycle. The net yield of this aerobic glycolysis of 1 mol of glucose is 38 mol of ATP (18 mol of ATP per three-carbon fragment in the Krebs cycle plus 2 mol of ATP for the production of pyruvate).

In shock, adequate oxygen is not provided to the cell, which must then metabolize glucose by an alternative pathway, namely *anaerobic* glycolysis. The end product of this metabolic pathway is lactate and yields a paltry 2 mol of ATP per mol of glucose. This deficiency of energy production leads directly to failure of the pump, with inflow of sodium and water and a decrease in the electrical potential across the cell membrane. Prolonged dysfunction of the "pump" leads to cell death or apoptosis via cell lysis, either immediately or upon reconstitution of effective perfusion. At a biochemical level, then, shock results in lactic acidosis, the byproduct of anaerobic metabolism. We will discuss the use of lactate in assessment of perfusion later.

Moving from shock at the cellular level to shock at the organism level, the clinician recognizes a number of shock states. Indeed, clinicians have become taxonomists of shock. Clinical signs of impending shock are listed in Table 21.1.

Shock may be categorized as a defect in a pump (the heart) or in a fluid-filled container (the intravascular space and fluid within it). Figure 21.1 demonstrates the types of shock and their etiologies. On the pump side, obstructive shock describes extrinsic obstruction of pump function, that is, tamponade, tension pneumo/hemothorax, positive pressure ventilation, ruptured diaphragm with intrathoracic

TABLE 21.1   Clinical Signs of Shock

1. Hypotension
2. Tachycardia
3. Pale, cool, clammy skin in vasoconstrictive shock
4. Warm, dry, red skin for vasodilatory shock
5. Tachypnea or hypoxemia
6. Mental status changes
7. Heart failure/ischemia
8. Metabolic acidosis
9. Oliguria/anuria

abdominal organs, thoracic compartment syndrome from circumferential burn eschar, or abdominal compartment syndrome. This could also include intrinsic obstruction from vascular lesions such as atherosclerosis or emboli. Cardiogenic shock is described as intrinsic pump failure due to ischemia/infarction, arrhythmias, traumatic injury or rupture, acidemia, preexisting heart failure, or a massive pulmonary embolus.

On the container side, the classifications all involve changes in the effective volume within the intravascular container. Causes of hypovolemic shock include blood loss and dehydration from vomiting/diarrhea or strenuous exercise. Hemorrhagic shock is discussed further later. Neurogenic shock stems from the loss of sympathetic vascular tone from a central nervous system (CNS) injury. Causes include spinal cord injury or epidural anesthesia. It results in vasodilatation (container expansion) and a drop in effective blood volume. Septic shock results from release of immune system mediators due to an infectious source. Endotoxins elaborated by gram-negative bacteria "turn on" a cascade of intrinsic mediators that ultimately affect the precapillary arteriolar sphincters, relaxing them and causing an increase of the intravascular space. The clinical clue that the patient is in septic shock is a reflection of this change

in vascular status: the skin is usually warm to touch, not cold and clammy as is the skin of the patient in hypovolemic or hemorrhagic shock. Anaphylactic shock can also be considered a form of septic shock in that similar inflammatory mediators are involved. Compressive shock, similar to obstructive shock on the pump side, describes extrinsic compression of the container's vasculature from processes such as the abdominal compartment syndrome.

Hemorrhagic shock may be subclassified into four states based on the degree of blood loss in a schema derived from the American College of Surgeon's Advanced Trauma Life Support (ATLS) course. This description also demonstrates the graded physiologic responses of the patient. The reader must note as well that these physiologic observations are consistent with those seen in otherwise healthy young adults, and that a less healthy or older patient may be unable to maintain an adequate blood pressure in the face of less severe blood loss. Concomitant organ dysfunction or concurrent medications may further blunt these homeostatic physiologic responses.

The patient with a *class I hemorrhage* has suffered a loss of about 10% of the intravascular volume (for a 70-kg man that is about 1 unit of whole blood). The patient is alert but may be a bit lightheaded. The blood pressure is normal, and the major organs are satisfactorily perfused as seen by a normal urine output. Less important vascular beds such as the skin have not been sacrificed. The patient has compensated for the blood loss by a tachycardia, that is, by increasing the heart rate.

As the blood loss increases to about 20% to 25% of the blood volume, the patient develops a *class II hemorrhage*. He or she is likely to be confused and combative. Although the mean arterial blood pressure is normal, the pulse pressure (systolic minus diastolic pressure) has narrowed. Urine output has decreased. The skin is cool and moist. The patient is manifesting further effects of

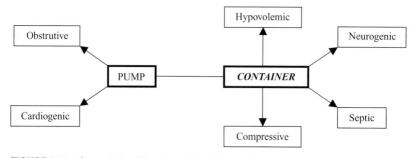

FIGURE 21.1   General classification of shock determined by etiology.

catecholamine release along with some degree of decreased perfusion. The mental status reflects in part the "flight or fight" reaction to sympathetic discharge and some degrees of cerebral hypoxemia. The change in pulse pressure is consistent with increased vasoconstriction, as with shunting of the available circulatory output from less critical vascular beds such as the skin.

The patient with a *class III hemorrhage* has lost about 35% to 40% of the blood volume and can no longer maintain his blood pressure. He has sought to maintain cardiac output by increasing the heart rate and increasing afterload. The mental examination demonstrates stupor. Urine output has decreased further. One of the important things to remember when resuscitating a hypotensive trauma patient is the fluid of choice, blood, either packed cells or preferably whole blood.

Additional bleeding brings the patient to a *class IV hemorrhage*, with coma and blood pressure incompatible with life. This patient requires prompt therapeutic intervention (i.e., stop the bleeding and replace the blood) for survival.

Treatment of Shock

Once clinical signs of impending shock are diagnosed, it is important to consider the source. This will determine which treatment pathway you will follow. One uses the history and physical exam, electrocardiography, chest X-ray (CXR), and laboratory studies including complete blood cell count, glucose, electrolytes, and an arterial blood gas.

Immediate life-threatening sources should be diagnosed quickly and treated accordingly. A tension pneumothorax causing obstructive pump shock should be decompressed. Abdominal compartment syndrome causing anuria and elevated peak airway pressures, which could soon result in a fatal cardiac arrhythmia, should be relieved. Neurogenic shock from spinal cord injury should be recognized by mechanism of injury and loss of rectal tone and treated with an α-receptor agonist vasoconstrictor (norepinephrine or Neo-Synephrine) to supplement disrupted vascular autonomic tone. The source driving septic shock should be isolated as soon as possible to facilitate an intervention to treat and/or remove it. This includes foreign bodies, infection, abscess, or other injury. Broad-spectrum antibiotics are critical first-line agents in the treatment of septic shock to reduce the physiologic insult driving the shock state. More on the treatment of septic shock will be discussed later.

The treatment for all forms of shock is resuscitation to improve perfusion. The "rude unhinging of the machinery of life" must be rectified. To that end, the essential components of early resuscitation include obtaining vascular access for volume administration and correction of hypothermia, electrolyte abnormalities, acidemia, and coagulopathy. Initial intravenous fluid administered should be isotonic to maximize effective intravascular volume and thus effective blood pressure. Although there have been decades of controversy over crystalloid versus colloid fluid resuscitation, the SAFE trial demonstrated no difference in risk or benefit.

The most accepted colloid is albumin. Another option is hetastarch (Hespan™) which has a 24-hour dose limit due to risk of coagulopathy. The role of the crystalloid, hypertonic saline (HTS), is expanding. It now has clear indications in people with brain injury. Its role outside of this indication is still being evaluated. Blood products should certainly be used if the hematocrit (HCT) is less than 30% or hemoglobin is less than 10 g/dL. Evidence now exists that discourages "supranormal" HCT goals for transfusion. This will be discussed in greater detail later.

All intravenous fluids should be warmed either within a warm storage container or through an active warming pump such as the Level 1 Transfuser. This insures correction of hypothermia which if untreated can attenuate the patient's own coagulation cascade. Coagulopathy, likewise, should be aggressively corrected to an INR of 1.0 using fresh frozen plasma (FFP) and/or cryoprecipitate. There is growing literature supporting the use of recombinant factor VII to quickly correct coagulopathy in patients suffering from massive hemorrhage and requiring more than 10 units packed red blood cells (PRBCs). It can also be used in patients with preexisting bleeding disorders suffering from shock. Keep in mind, however, that the only FDA-approved use for rFVII is in hemophiliacs. Our combat experience in recent conflicts overseas also supports a 1:1 PRBC:FFP transfusion ratio for massive transfusions (*expected* greater than 10 units PRBCs). Civilian experience has bolstered this recommendation.

Other adjuncts to resuscitation include modulators of the inflammatory response. In septic shock specifically, the use of activated Protein C (APC/Xigris™) has been shown to reduce mortality from severe septic shock with at least two organ systems failing. The controversy lies in the limited patient population that will benefit from it. Patients outside of this select group will not benefit from its use and may suffer from the increased bleeding risk associated with it. This is especially concerning in a trauma or postsurgical patient. Therefore, APC is mainly recommended in medical sepsis patients with severe multiorgan system failure.

Steroid use in shock has also been controversial over the past few decades. The most recent evidence on the use of steroids in septic shock demonstrates no added benefit. The latest guidelines for the treatment of sepsis by the Society of Critical Care Medicine states:

> Although corticosteroids do appear to promote shock reversal, the lack of a clear improvement in mortality—coupled with the known side effects of steroids, such as increased risk of infection and myopathy—generally tempered enthusiasm for their broad use. Thus, there was broad agreement that the recommendation should be downgraded from the previous guidelines.

There have been one or two trials that demonstrated benefit; however, the latest most definitive study (CORTICUS) failed to demonstrate any advantage to steroid use in septic shock. There are those who would still use them in the case of life-threatening shock refractory to all other treatments including fluids, vasopressors, and source control, although the evidence does not convincingly support this. Incidentally, determining whether patients are adrenocorticotropic hormone (ACTH) responsive or not did not differentiate between survivors and nonsurvivors.

Drugs and Shock

Pressors, or, more accurately, vasoconstrictors, are usually inappropriate as first-line drugs for shock because they improve the blood pressure at the expense of further decreasing perfusion of capillary beds. However, while the patient is being resuscitated with fluids for volume expansion, vasoconstrictors may be useful to support some regional vascular beds. Although autoregulation maintains cerebral perfusion as cardiac output declines because of vasodilatation consequent to increases in partial pressure of carbon dioxide (Pco_2), the cerebral circulation benefits from increases in blood pressure produced by vasoconstrictors. Renal perfusion does not benefit from vasoconstrictor-induced increases in blood pressure nor does perfusion of the mesenteric circulation. In practice, keep in mind that your initial goal should be to optimize cardiac filling pressure or preload before resorting to a vasoconstrictor. The use of a central venous pressure (CVP) measurements for this is currently recommended, though it must be understood that it is often the *trend* in CVP measurements, in response to fluids, that give information on volume status rather than the individual number. Forcing an empty heart to contract or an empty blood vessel to constrict only increases cardiac demand ischemia and strangulates end organs.

Norepinephrine (Levophed™) is a commonly used pressor in a hypotensive septic patient. Although mainly an α-agonist, it does have some beta properties. Drug administration is defined in micrograms per minute and doses of 5 to 10 μg/min are common. There are no maximal doses reported in the literature, and patients frequently require increased doses over time to maintain the same degree of vasoconstriction or to overcome the vasodilatation of sepsis. Neo-Synephrine is an alternative to norepinephrine, but it is a pure α-agonist vasoconstrictor and can easily choke blood supply to the very organs you are trying to perfuse. It may also be efficacious, in low doses, in neurogenic shock. Care must be taken to insure no hemorrhagic component coexists with neurogenic shock. Otherwise the patient's blood pressure may be normalized by an α-agonist while they continue to bleed.

Vasopressin (Pitressin™) is another vasoconstrictor used in septic shock. Early experience with unbridled use of vasopressin resulted in severe end organ and limb ischemia resulting in higher mortality. More recently, the only use for vasopressin recommended in the literature is for septic shock that is refractory to volume loading and initial vasoconstrictors like Levophed™. The dose is only 0.04 U/min or 2.4 U/hr. There is no titration; it is either on or off. This avoids the drastic consequences of titrating vasopressin past the point of no return resulting in limb and splanchnic ischemia. The physiology behind its use is a theoretical total body depletion of intrinsic vasopressin due to acute phase reaction to sepsis. Replacing this loss with extrinsic vasopressin allows the clinician to use lower doses of other vasoconstrictors and limit volume loading.

Although dopamine is still commonly used as an adjunct for management of shock, its use should be discouraged. This is due to increasing evidence of its deleterious effects on the neuroendocrine system. Dosages of this drug are always given in micrograms per kilogram body weight per minute. The drug has three broadly different effects depending upon the dose given. At low doses (3 to 5 μg/kg/min), the effect is stimulation of dopamine receptors along with some β-adrenergic activity. The cardiac rate is mildly increased, and there may be some augmentation of contractility. Splanchnic flow is maintained. Renal blood flow seems to be increased, and a net natriuresis ensues; however, this effect is not as prominent as once believed, and recent studies have shown that although diuresis may be maintained with it, the incidence of acute renal failure (ARF) is unchanged and as previously mentioned, there may be a significant downside to its use. As the dose of dopamine is increased, there is an increase in α-adrenergic effect but β-adrenergic activity predominates until the dose reaches about 10 to 15 μg/kg/min. Beyond that, the effect is nearly pure α-adrenergic, and dopamine offers little more than norepinephrine. It is important to note that the effectiveness of dopamine is decreased by acidosis. Although safe, some patients, especially those with decreased intravascular volumes, exhibit a profound tachycardia even at low doses. Patients in atrial fibrillation seem especially sensitive to dopamine, and increasing the ventricular rate may be dangerous.

Dobutamine seems to have greater effect on cardiac contractility than dopamine, and this effect is maintained even in the face of acidosis. The improved cardiac function, unfortunately, is associated with increased oxygen consumption by the myocardium. It may, however, decrease cardiac afterload via vasodilatation. Initially, the dose is 2.5 to 5.0 μg/kg/min, and it may be increased to 15 to 20 μg/kg/min.

Milrinone, a phosphodiesterase inhibitor, has come into increased use in the surgical intensive care unit (SICU). Like dobutamine, it is an inotropic agent and is indicated in patients who already have an increased filling pressure. Milrinone came into clinical practice later and avoids the antiplatelet problems of the earlier drug (amrinone); it has largely displaced the earlier version from hospital formularies.

Digoxin seems to improve cardiac contractility without significantly increasing the oxygen consumption of the heart. Its use for clinical shock states is equivocal because of questions about its rapidity of action. The drug is indicated in patients with obvious congestive heart failure, and a surprising number of patients have never taken this agent before coming to the SICU. Moreover, digitalizing the patient forces the clinician to be even more vigilant regarding electrolyte abnormalities. Rapid-acting cardiac glycosides are being developed, and they may have a role here.

Isoproterenol, a β-agonist, may be used to increase the heart rate, but its effect on the peripheral circulation (vasodilation) may be adverse to the needs of the patient. Epinephrine (another β-agonist with some α-agonistic properties) exhibits a two-phase response according to the infused dose, with β-adrenergic activity predominating at lower doses and α-adrenergic activity at higher doses. Although it enjoys fairly widespread use in children, the arrhythmogenic potential decreases its value in adults. I have used it occasionally as a pressor in concert with other agents, such as Levophed™ or Neo-Synephrine, especially when vasopressin has failed to stabilize the blood pressure.

Vasodilators may improve cardiac performance by decreasing cardiac work function (afterload reduction). Most of these drugs (which include nitroglycerin and nitroprusside) act by increasing circulating nitric oxide. Nitroprusside must be used with caution in patients with renal failure, as cyanide toxicity can occur.

Hemodynamic Monitoring

Good physicians always seek to verify the positive or negative effects of their treatments. Monitoring of patient performance is thus an important part of shock resuscitation. The goal of therapy for hemorrhagic or hypovolemic shock is restoration of tissue perfusion by optimizing cardiac output. A useful pneumonic for remembering the four factors that affect cardiac output is C.R.A.P., contractility, rate, afterload, and preload, each of which is discussed later.

The mean arterial pressure (MAP) is the most readily available and thus easiest marker of resuscitation. Ideally, it is obtained from an arterial line tracing which is integrated to obtain the area under the waveform to calculate the MAP. Most intensivists would agree that a minimum MAP of 60 is an adequate goal and *supranormal* pressures are not necessary and may in fact be harmful.

Physiologically, one must measure the preload to know what steps need to be taken in the patient in shock. The filling pressure of the heart can be assessed by a variety of increasingly invasive maneuvers: visual inspection of the neck veins, placement of a central venous line to assess CVP, and placement of a pulmonary artery (PA) catheter to estimate left ventricular end-diastolic volume.

Bedside inspection and examination of neck veins is simply not reliable enough in the setting of acute care and was long ago replaced by direct measurement of the CVP. Analogous to right atrial pressure, this in turn is a surrogate for right ventricular end-diastolic volume. The reliability of CVP measurements is affected by respiratory variations and positive end-expiratory pressure (PEEP). The CVP directly measures the filling pressure of the right heart and does not specifically indicate anything about the intravascular volume status. It is, however, a valuable *trending* tool during active resuscitation. A patient with continued blood loss may have a high CVP because the cardiac mechanism is incapable of pumping the little intravascular volume available. Likewise, high positive-pressure ventilation (i.e., airway pressure release ventilation [APRV] or high PEEP) may falsely elevate the CVP reading.

The "gold standard" for measuring the filling pressure of the heart is to measure the preload presented, not to the right ventricle, but to the left ventricle. Although in otherwise healthy patients without cardiopulmonary disease, the two filling pressures are nearly identical, the same cannot be said for patients with previous cardiac or pulmonary disease. Ventricular dysfunction secondary to myocardial infarction, for instance, may produce ventricles of different mechanical efficiency. Severe pulmonary disease with chronic cor pulmonary renders the right ventricle filling pressures (as determined by the CVP) of little value for assessing the filling of the less damaged left ventricle. PA catheters allow direct determination of right ventricle filling pressure, indirect measurement of left ventricle filling pressure, and the cardiac output. Because of its location, a venous blood gas from a sample drawn through the distal PA catheter port can also be used to obtain the mixed-venous hemoglobin oxygen saturation, or $S_{mv}O_2$.

The PA catheter is usually introduced via the subclavian vein into the right atrium of the heart and passed through the tricuspid valve into the right ventricle. It can be advanced safely via the internal jugular vein, but this approach makes a stable dressing more difficult and increases the risk of an infected line. It can also be advanced via the femoral vein, but this method seems more difficult and some clinicians have reported an increase in arrhythmias acutely and an increase in infection using this approach. Proper placement of the catheter is usually achieved by observing the pressure waves measured at its tip as it traverses the chambers of the heart. The chest radiograph obtained after placement is usually performed to determine the presence of a pneumothorax or to determine which pulmonary vasculature has been entered (important if the patient is to be placed in a lateral decubitus position in the operating room). The "balloon" is inflated with the catheter in the right ventricle, and the tip of the catheter is carried downstream along the pulmonary outflow track into the PA. The "wedge" pressure (technically, the pulmonary artery capillary wedge pressure [PCWP] or the PA occlusion pressure) is usually less than the PA diastolic pressure.

PA catheters may be indicated for the sicker patient in whom preexisting conditions render the CVP reading inaccurate. Some studies have shown that patients managed pre- and intraoperatively with PA catheters do better than those managed without them, especially if there is adequate time to optimize cardiac function. Their efficacy when placed postoperatively is more difficult to confirm. However, the decision to place a PA catheter should not be considered lightly. The risk of complications is greater than with CVP catheters. Neglecting the risks attendant on subclavian venous puncture (which are common to both), the patient has a markedly increased risk of cardiac arrhythmias during both placement and manipulation and so long as the catheter traverses two cardiac chambers. Valvular lesions have been reported with catheters that have been maintained for long periods. Catheters that have been wedged for long periods may produce pulmonary infarctions. The balloon may even tear the PA and cause fatal bleeding. This problem is demonstrated clinically by the acute onset of hemoptysis after balloon inflation; emergency surgery can sometimes be avoided by retracting the catheter and inflating the balloon to tamponade the bleeding site. The infectious risks of PA catheters may be greater than for CVP catheters (possibly because of their longer length), but the incidence of left-sided endocarditis is definitely increased. PA catheters do not by themselves improve patient outcome. Misinterpretation of the data obtained and therapeutic misadventures in response to that data can outweigh any potential benefits. Retrospective studies to assess the role of the PA catheter in clinical practice have suggested that these catheters, in use since the early 1970s, are not panaceas.

Cardiac output may be measured directly with the PA catheter in place by the dye dilution technique using the *Fick* principle or by thermodilution. The latter is performed far more commonly. With this measurement, "optimum" filling pressure may be determined. The Frank–Starling relation between end-diastolic fiber length and muscle contraction can be converted to the relation between the PCWP and the cardiac output.

The normal response demonstrates that increased wedge pressure increases cardiac output only to a point beyond which increases in filling pressure produce virtually no augmentation of the cardiac output. It is a mistake to assume that a given patient needs a certain filling pressure; the optimal filling pressure must be individualized for each patient.

The distal tip of the PA catheter should lie within a PA branch. The blood flowing passed it is mixed venous in that it contains venous blood mixed from both the systemic circulation and the coronary sinus. The mixed venous oxygen saturation ($S_{mv}O_2$) is a marker of both the adequacy of oxygen delivery and the extent at which oxygen is extracted. It therefore can be used to assess the balance between oxygen delivery and extraction. Normally, $S_{mv}O_2$ runs between 60% and 70%. If it is much lower, then the either supply of oxygen has been reduced secondary to a change in one of the factors influencing cardiac output, or oxygen consumption (demand) at the cellular level has increased.

Pulmonary Artery Catheter Controversy

Finally, there are at least two recent trials published in the literature within the last 5 years that put to rest the controversy of the PA catheter. In 2003, Richard et al. studied the use of PA catheters in the nonprotocolized treatment of septic shock, acute respiratory distress syndrome (ARDS), or both. They found no difference in mortality or any other endpoint between the 300+ patients randomized to use a PA catheter and the 300+ that did not. In 2006, the ARDSnet group published their results of the Fluid and Catheter Treatment Trial. Almost 1,000 patients with acute lung injury (ALI) or ARDS were randomized to receive a central venous catheter (CVC) only (487) or a PA catheter (513). The treatment strategy was protocolized. They found no difference in mortality but did find an increased incidence of non–life-threatening complications from PA catheter use (i.e., arrhythmias).

The PA catheter allows one to demonstrate the change in vascular dynamics by a number of means. It is important to remember, however, that these other means are only measurements and trends, not treatment goals. Maximizing cardiac output and mixed-venous oxygen saturation have been shown to be appropriate goals. The vascular resistance can be calculated in both halves of the circulatory circuit: the systemic vascular resistance (SVR) for the peripheral circulation and the pulmonary vascular resistance for the pulmonary circulation.

Care must be taken in these and subsequent calculations that the user remembers whether the cardiac output or the cardiac index (which normalizes cardiac output for surface area) is used. Although either number may be used, interpretations of the data are predicated on using the proper normals. SVR, for instance, is normally 1,200 to 1,400 dynes/sec/cm^{-5}, whereas an SVR index of 1,800 to 3,000 dynes/sec/cm^{-5}/M^2 is considered normal.

SVR is increased in conditions in which the vascular resistance would be expected to increase, that is, hypovolemic or hemorrhagic shock. It is decreased in septic shock and can be decreased in cirrhosis (where arteriovenous [A-V] shunts are open in the liver) and with aggressive overhydration where capacitance vessels are open to allow the increased fluid load. It is important to remember that the SVR is NOT a goal to treat, simply a marker of the hemodynamic state.

The opening of precapillary sphincters, in septic shock, shunts blood away from the arterial system to the venous system without feeding a nutrient vessel. This shunting is also reflected in another parameter, the A-V oxygen difference. The oxygen content of the radial artery is a measure of the most saturated blood in the body. With the catheter in the PA, one can calculate the oxygen content of the desaturated blood, which reflects the net effect of all tissues extracting oxygen from the blood. Measurements obtained by substituting central venous blood for mixed venous are not absolutely correct, but the differences are not sufficient to obscure the clinical picture. It should be remembered, incidentally, that central venous blood is not the most desaturated blood found in the body. Blood in the coronary sinus has the lowest oxygen saturation. This is where oxygen has been maximally extracted by the functioning heart muscle. Thus,

$$\text{Arterial oxygen content} = \text{saturation} \times 1.34 \times \text{hemoglobin (g/dL)}$$

$$\text{Mixed venous oxygen content} = \text{saturation} \times 1.34 \times \text{hemoglobin (g/dL)}$$

$$\text{A-V oxygen difference} = \text{arterial} - \text{mixed venous oxygen content}$$

where saturation is the fractional saturation of the blood gas (arterial or venous), 1.34 is a coefficient reflecting the oxygen-carrying capacity of 1 g of hemoglobin, and the hemoglobin is expressed in grams per deciliter. The A-V oxygen difference is normally 3 to 5 mL/dL.

The difference between the content of the arterial and venous bloods is, as mentioned earlier, a measure of both A-V shunting and the metabolic activity of the body. The A-V oxygen difference (extraction) is increased in conditions of inadequate tissue perfusion, wherein the tissue tries to extract as much oxygen as it can. It is decreased in patients in septic shock and in patients with cirrhosis and portal hypertension where either the blood flow is shunted away from the cells or the cells are so dysfunctional that they cannot extract oxygen.

The relation between oxygen delivery and consumption can be expressed as an "extraction ratio," where extraction ratio is equal to oxygen consumption/oxygen delivery. Normal extraction ratio is 25% to 35%. What can the surgeon do when the patient is extracting a higher percentage? Increasing oxygen delivery might improve the extraction ratio. This is done by increasing oxygen saturation, cardiac output (remember C.R.A.P?), or hemoglobin. The biggest bang for your buck is obtained with a hemoglobin or blood transfusion which increases the arterial oxygen content and may increase cardiac output by improving preload.

One cannot introduce the matter of oxygen consumption without discussing oxygen dissociation curve (Fig. 21.2). Most of the oxygen transported by the blood is attached to hemoglobin. The classic S-shaped oxyhemoglobin dissociation curve illustrates the variable binding of oxygen to hemoglobin. The

right side of the curve demonstrates that increases in the partial pressure of oxygen (Po_2) at high levels do not significantly increase oxygen saturation. Therefore, there is no reason to keep a patient's FIO_2 higher than that which produces more than 90% to 95% saturation. The left side of the curve indicates that the unloading of oxygen from hemoglobin becomes progressively more difficult at lower saturations.

The factors that affect the dissociation of oxygen from hemoglobin are all clinically relevant. High temperatures, high partial pressures of carbon dioxide, and acidosis aid in oxygen extraction. This is teleologically understandable because there are the local conditions one would expect to find in the neighborhood of an exercising muscle. Clinically, this is a caveat against the overzealous use of sodium bicarbonate in shock states because it would tend to decrease the available oxygen to the tissues in need. All these factors move the curve to the right (easier unloading).

More important, perhaps, is the role of 2,3-diphosphoglycerate (2,3-DPG) in oxygen transport. 2,3-DPG is a product of red blood cell (RBC) glycolysis. As the stored erythrocytes in the blood bank exhaust their supply of glucose, their intracellular content of 2,3-DPG decreases. The low levels of 2,3-DPG cause an increased affinity for oxygen by the hemoglobin molecule, rendering it less able to release oxygen to the tissues (curve shifts to the left). This clinical problem is posed to the physician by the blood bank anxious to release the oldest blood from the backmost shelves of its refrigerator. This blood is relatively easy to oxygenate but holds onto its oxygen tightly and may further embarrass the unloading of oxygen at the tissue level.

FIGURE 21.2. Classic oxygen dissociation curve.

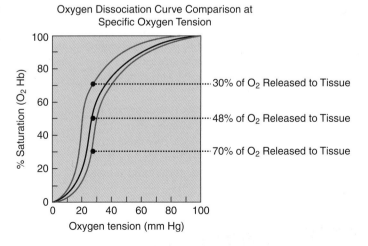

Regional Physiology

The classic teaching of septic shock as a hyperdynamic state with elevated cardiac output, decreased SVR, and decreased A-V oxygen difference is attainable only with optimum fluid replacement therapy and with a sound cardiac mechanism. The patient early in septic shock who has not yet received adequate fluids may not demonstrate a hyperdynamic state. Similarly, the patient in septic shock whose heart cannot meet the increased demand placed on it does not demonstrate the classic picture.

Lactic acidosis as a marker of shock entered the clinical world with the observations of the American physiologist Walter B. Cannon in the fields of France during World War I. The lactate level is predictive of the risk of death in some series and has been used as a guide for resuscitation of patients by many clinicians. An additional caveat to the emphasis on lactate as a marker of ischemia is that it may alternatively be produced by inhibition of pyruvate dehydrogenase, leading to the accumulation of pyruvate outside the mitochondria and thus production of lactate, a condition seen in experimental endotoxemia. Finally, lactate must be remembered as a cellular substrate that can be utilized by such tissues as heart (where it may be a preferred fuel) and brain.

Base deficit can be used as a surrogate for lactate in many instances. Care must be used, though, in patients with renal dysfunction. Base deficit will increase in these patients not because of anaerobic metabolism but due to build up of metabolic wastes.

At its best, the PA catheter can allow for measurement of global perfusion via $S_{mv}O_2$, but events may be occurring in one or another regional circulation that have clinical import but cannot be detected by this device. Global acidosis or lactic acidosis is a poor prognostic sign, but it may be observed too late to allow clinical manipulation of the patient and decrease the mortality associated with elevated lactate levels, for instance. The regional circulation of greatest concern at present is the splanchnic circulation because of the obvious concern for bacterial translocation. If acidosis or hypoperfusion in this region could be determined early, appropriate clinical intervention could be affected. At present, there is no good method for reliably measuring gut perfusion. Surrogates are being studied such as near-infrared. Near-infrared spectroscopy can measure local tissue perfusion and is being studied as a new way to assess regional hemodynamics.

NEUROENDOCRINE RESPONSE TO SHOCK

In addition to the physiologic responses to shock that serve to return the cardiac output to normal and the cellular perfusion to a satisfactory level, there are a number of neuroendocrine changes elicited by the shock state. They are both beneficial and harmful to the patient.

Trauma results directly in increased levels of ACTH and subsequently in increased levels of the glucocorticoids. Elevated cortisol results in an increase in circulating glucose and free fatty acids, thereby increasing the availability of energy substrate to the cells. Prolonged stimulation by ACTH can result in adrenocortical hyperplasia and persistence of these metabolic changes for weeks to months.

A decrease in renal blood flow stimulates the production of angiotensin, which acts directly on the adrenal cortex to cause the production of aldosterone. ACTH is a cofactor in this aldosterone production. Aldosterone then acts on the kidney to increase sodium reabsorption (and along with it water) and potassium excretion. The water retention favors amelioration of the cardiac output deficit. The body also produces an increase in antidiuretic hormone (ADH) secretion to further decease net water losses from the kidney.

Catecholamines are elaborated as described earlier to increase vasoconstriction and tachycardia. Metabolically, the catecholamines inhibit the release of insulin and oppose the effects of circulating insulin. This decreases the availability of glucose at the cellular level and favors the burning of fatty acids. It also forces an increase in muscle protein catabolism. Simultaneously, glucagon levels increase, further diverting energy utilization away from glucose. The catecholamine response seems beneficial to the patient when it is brief and progressively detrimental if catecholamine release is prolonged.

One therapy that has recently been shown to affect morbidity and mortality in the ICU is glycemic control. Van den Berghe and others published their results in the "New England Journal of Medicine" in 2001. They studied 1,548 patients in an ICU, mostly cardiac surgery postoperative patients, and randomized them to tight glucose control (80 to 110 mg/dL) versus liberal control. Using an insulin drip to maintain patient blood glucose levels within this tight range, they showed an improvement in mortality from 8% to 4.6%. The incidence of infection, hemodialysis for ARF, blood transfusions, polyneuropathy, ventilator days, and ICU lengths of stay were also reduced. Follow-up studies refined this protocol by showing an advantage only for sicker patients, that is, sepsis and prolonged ICU stays. More recent experience now cautions against such tight control due to the increased incidence of hypoglycemia. We use a more lax range of 90 to 140 mg/dL but still prescribe to the philosophy.

RESPIRATORY PHYSIOLOGY AND CARE

Basic Physiology

The basic principles of oxygen transport were described in some detail earlier. It is important to remember that at normal atmospheric pressure, nearly all oxygen is transported coupled to the hemoglobin molecule. Carbon dioxide, on the other hand, is transported dissolved in plasma. Oxygen affinity for hemoglobin is dictated by the oxyhemoglobin dissociated curve as discussed earlier.

Respiration is a property of all cells and is governed by oxygenation from the lungs. Ventilation is a mechanical process designed to move gas through the lungs and specifically refers to carbon dioxide clearance. Ventilation is maintained under close neurologic control and is modified as a consequence of acidosis and hypercapnia.

The patient's normal breathing produces a "tidal volume." The mathematic product of rate and tidal volume yields "minute ventilation." Maximum inspiratory effort produces a volume termed the "inspiratory capacity," which is the sum of the tidal volume and the inspiratory reserve. This inspiratory reserve demonstrates the fact that most patients are breathing at less than maximum volumes. Similarly, with maximal exhalation, patients are able to empty their "expiratory reserve volume." The patient is unable to empty the lungs of gas completely so there is always a "residual volume." It represents a physiologic dead space. The expiratory reserve volume and the residual volume constitute the function residual capacity.

Respiration and perfusion are closely linked in the intact patient. Blood is rapidly shunted away from areas of the lung that are not adequately ventilated (hypoxic vasoconstriction). Similarly, interruption of blood flow soon results in collapse of the alveoli. This association is destroyed in conditions of ventilation–perfusion mismatch. Anatomically, there normally exists some mismatch, with three "zones" identified within the lung that were apparently consequent to humans attaining an erect posture millions of years ago. The upper lung fields are somewhat better ventilated than perfused (zone I), and the lower (zone III) fields are better perfused than ventilated, and no surprise in zone II, perfusion and ventilation are well matched.

Alveoli remain distended because of the effects of pulmonary surfactant, a detergent produced by alveolar cells that serves to lower the surface tension. The absence of this substance in premature infants produces progressive alveolar collapse and a clinical condition known as hyaline membrane disease. Surfactant production is inhibited by high oxygen concentrations and in adults the ARDS. Alveoli also remain distended due to the different solubility coefficients of oxygen and nitrogen. Oxygen diffuses much more rapidly across the basement membrane into the vasculature than nitrogen, allowing nitrogen to stay behind and prevent alveolar collapse.

The goal of oxygenation of the patient is a Po_2 sufficient to maintain arterial saturations in excess of 90%. Oxygen is administered to patients at a given F_iO_2, and blood gases are expressed as the partial pressure of the gas, pO_2. The five most common causes of hypoxemia are decreased inspired F_iO_2, hypoventilation, V/Q mismatch, shunting, and diffusion abnormality at basement membrane.

Breathing and Ventilation

Breathing is a mechanical process unconsciously performed by patients outside the hospital. The diaphragm and intercostal musculature work in tandem to produce a negative pressure, and the tidal volume is inhaled. Exhalation is effected by elastic recoil of the lungs and chest wall. Difficulties with breathing (in contrast to oxygenation) may be caused by problems with neuromuscular control and coordination or mechanical factors.

Patients with CNS depression, whether intrinsic or secondary to the effects of sedation, may lose control of their breathing. This may occur because of destructive lesions in the brain stem but is more commonly an effect of narcosis, with the result that hypercapnia does not trigger increased ventilation.

The absence of medications may also serve to decrease breathing. Patients in pain soon "recognize" pleuritic components of pain or the effect of breathing deeply on peritoneal pain. This situation is seen in patients postoperatively and, along with the excessive sedation, is the principal cause of postoperative atelectasis.

Chest wall pain may also decrease the effectiveness of breathing in the presence of such conditions as chest wall contusion or rib fracture. Here, the patient splints the ribs by the action of the intercostals and therefore decreases the effective depth of ventilation. It also leads to some degree of ventilation–perfusion mismatch. Flail chest represents an even worse case in which ventilatory volumes are decreased due to pain, which exacerbates the adverse effects of the underlying pulmonary contusion on oxygenation. A pneumothorax also decreases the effective volume for ventilation.

Airway problems should not be overlooked as causes of inadequate breathing. Unconscious patients may occlude their airways with their tongue. Patients with facial or neck trauma may have upper airway obstruction from debris or laryngeal injury.

In general, changes in the Pco_2 represent changes in ventilation. Changes in the Po_2 reflect changes in V/Q mismatch or reflect barriers to the movement of oxygen from the alveolar space to the arterial space across the basement membrane; they include such conditions as ARDS and pulmonary edema. Although elevations in Pco_2 can occur with increased production of carbon dioxide, it is more likely to represent a decrease in minute ventilation.

Therapeutic Interventions

Management of the patient with inadequate ventilation requires first the physician's assumption of responsibility for breathing for the patient and the prompt recognition of the problems that have led to the situation. To ventilate the patient adequately, the physician must control the airway. Mechanical obstructions must be removed. The tracheobronchial tree may need to be approached emergently with cricothyrotomy (which has largely replaced tracheostomy as an emergency procedure in the field or in the emergency room [ER]). More commonly, the patient is intubated. Endotracheal intubation is easier, but nasotracheal intubation may be better tolerated by the patient. Although low-pressure, low-volume endotracheal tubes (ETTs) can allegedly be maintained for 3 to 4 weeks without adverse sequelae, tracheostomy is usually considered if the patient continues to require intubation for 10 to 14 days. The

timing of tracheostomy, however, continues to be controversial. Some studies have demonstrated a significant reduction in nosocomial pneumonia when tracheostomy is performed within the first 5 days of admission. Unfortunately, it is not always easy to predict which patients will need ventilatory support days in advance. The availability of bedside percutaneous tracheostomy may decrease the interval between the patient's needing the procedure and the surgeon performing it.

Mechanical Ventilation

The purpose of mechanical ventilation is to augment oxygenation and ventilation when the patient's own ability to do so is compromised. This may be due to a mechanical problem such as direct trauma or secondary injury. It may also be due to an indirect dysfunction caused by illness or injury in another part of the body. Of course, brain injury may also compromise respiratory function. Modern mechanical ventilators have been designed to offer increased flexibility to the clinician over the previous generation of machines. Microcomputer circuitry exposes the internal workings of the ventilator, so the physician caring for the patient can see just what the machine is doing.

When selecting a ventilator mode, one must decide whether you want to completely control all mechanical and spontaneous breaths (control mode) or just assist the patient's own spontaneous breaths (support mode). In the acute phase of critical illness, the wisest choice is the former: take complete control. Then the physician must decide if they want the ventilator to be controlled by volume or pressure goals. All new ventilators are designed to be able to deliver both volume-control and pressure-control modes of ventilation. The pressure-regulated modes deliver a flow of gas with the patient's compliance defining the volume of each breath. The machine continues to offer a flow of gas until the pressure in the circuit reaches the set maximum. One must be aware when using pressure-cycled ventilation that while the patient may initially be adequately ventilated, if the patient's compliance decreases, the machine may fail to deliver an adequate tidal volume. The physician is usually made aware of this by the ventilators alarms signaling the reduction in tidal volume or minute ventilation.

The other modalities in widespread clinical use are volume-controlled modes. With these, the physician sets the tidal volume (or minute ventilation and rate) and a pressure alarm limit. The machine then ventilates the patient with that preset volume up to the point where the pressure limit is exceeded. If the patient's compliance worsens, the desired tidal volume may not be given if the pressure needed exceeds the alarm limits, but again the clinician is apprised of the problem by the ringing of the appropriate alarms.

When using controlled ventilation, an awake patient, however, may be hyperventilated because every potentially small breath becomes a large breath. Anxious patients who are not adequately sedated frequently develop respiratory alkalosis. Management decisions to correct respiratory difficulties in such a patient include sedating patients so that their respiratory rates decrease or modifying the mode of ventilation to reduce the amount of support the patient is receiving.

In support mode (pressure support or continuous positive airway pressure [CPAP]), a preset pressure or volume support is set and the patient determines their own rate and tidal volume. Again, most important here is that the patient controls the inspiratory time and inspired volumes, not the ventilator. They decide when to terminate their breath. This mode should only be used on patients who have adequate ventilatory drive, as the mode does not deliver breaths unless the patient initiates it.

The other side of the ventilatory spectrum is when the patient essentially bypasses the ventilator, and the ETT is attached directly to humidified wall oxygen, usually via a T-piece. Here, the tidal volume and rate of ventilation are entirely under the control of the patient. This is not normal breathing, however, because the patient still has a narrow-lumen tube (instead of a relatively large trachea and hypopharynx), and there is no resistance to exhalation. This mode is primarily used as a test prior to extubation. If a patient is able to breath comfortably on a T-piece for 30 to 60 minutes, they have a good chance for a successful extubation. This is now often referred to as a spontaneous breathing trial.

The patient's tidal volume is usually set at 8 to 10 cm^3/kg body weight, but it may be decreased or increased as necessary to maintain adequate blood gases. Inadequate minute ventilation is usually reflected in an elevated Pco_2. These goals for tidal volume may not be appropriate in conditions where compliance is seriously compromised. These volumes may be associated with severe barotrauma, as the machine attempts to move this volume of gas through noncompliant lungs (i.e., ARDS). To avoid this situation, lower volumes (as low as 4 to 6 cm^3/kg) are cho-

sen and the consequent increase in carbon dioxide accepted. This is "permissive" hypercapnia and is acceptable, provided renal compensation for the respiratory acidosis is still available.

Patients breathing through closed mouth and nares are breathing normally against resistance. It is possible to emulate this condition by adding PEEP to the regimen. This resistance increases the chance that the patient's alveoli will not progressively collapse. A PEEP of 5 cm H_2O is physiologic in that it mimics the normal condition (0 cm PEEP is defined by the ETT alone); 5 cm H_2O is usually well tolerated, but increasing amounts of PEEP may embarrass the cardiac output by interfering with the heart filling because of the transmission of intrathoracic pressures.

Inverse ratio ventilation (IRV) allows the physician to change the inspiratory/expiratory (I/E) ratio. Normally, 25% to 33% of the respiratory cycle is devoted to inspiration for an I:E ratio of 1:3 or 1:4. With stiff lungs, it may not be possible to ventilate the patient during this time, and so the time for inspiration may need to be increased. The peak pressure developed during IRV ventilation is usually lower than that during normal ventilatory modes and therefore has been used in an attempt to reduce both barotrauma and volutrauma in patients with ARDS.

Another mode of ventilation used by some when the poor compliance associated with ARDS limits one's ability to safely ventilate a patient is APRV. This mode can be looked at as super IRV. With this mode, the physician selects the maximum pressure (P_{high}) the ventilator can develop, and the patient's compliance determines the tidal volume. The physician also selects the time (T_{high}) the lungs remain at this P_{high}. The time at this "high" pressure is usually around 5 seconds with a 1 second release followed by immediate return to the P_{high}. This process generally results in a higher mean airway pressure, a lower peak airway pressure, and improved oxygenation. Again, the cardiac effects of this mode of ventilation may limit its use in patients with intrinsic cardiac disease. It is a relatively new mode with few centers experienced in using it. However, it is becoming a good protective rescue mode for ARDS.

The goal of ventilatory support is eventually to remove patients from their need for mechanical ventilation. The decision to separate patients from the machine requires that they be able to deal with the mechanical aspects of breathing and oxygenation. The patient must be able to maintain satisfactory blood gases on an F_iO_2 easily administered by mask without marked tachypnea, manifesting a forced vital capacity of 10 to 12 cm^3/kg body weight. They should be able to generate a negative inspiratory pressure of 25 cm H$_2$O (as an adjunct to subsequent coughing).

Liberating a patient from the ventilator requires that the patient has met all other prerequisites for weaning: less than 50% F$_i$O$_2$, PEEP less than 8 cm H$_2$O, P$_a$O$_2$ more than 75 mm Hg, minute ventilation less than 15 L/min, and a pH 7.30 to 7.50. Testing the patient daily with a Spontaneous Breathing Trial has added to the success rate of extubations. As confirmed by clinical trials, a successful 30-minute trial on minimal ventilator settings of 0 or 5 mm Hg of pressure support (or T-piece) has greater than 90% sensitivity in predicting success of extubation.

Adult Respiratory Distress Syndrome

ARDS is a clinical condition characterized by profound hypoxemia, increased lung water, decreased functional residual capacity, and decreased pulmonary compliance; the reported mortality rate ranges from 60% to 100%. Recurrent sepsis and multiorgan failure are the most common causes for mortality in ARDS patients. Only 20% succumb to an inability to oxygenate or ventilate their lungs. ARDS is associated with a number of synonyms that commonly reflect its associated conditions (e.g., shock lung, posttraumatic pulmonary insufficiency), its historic trappings (DaNang lung), or the diseases it resembles (adult hyaline membrane disease).

We now know that high tidal volumes and pressures from positive pressure ventilation contribute to lung injury resulting in ARDS. This has been given the term "ventilator-induced lung injury or VILI." The primary pathway of injury involves activation of the C5 fragment of complement by direct damage to capillary endothelium and alveolar epithelium. Activated C5, cleared in the pulmonary circulation, is a chemotactic factor for neutrophils attracted to the pulmonary microcirculation. Anthropomorphically, these white blood cells arrive prepared to engulf bacteria, find nothing, but discharge their proteolytic enzymes nonetheless. The oxygen-free radicals damage the integrity of the endothelial–alveolar interface, which results in increased interstitial fluid and movement of proteinaceous fluid into the alveolus. The alveolar spaces fill and collapse. If the patient or animal survives long enough, it becomes the lattice for ingrowth of fibroblasts and deposition of collagen, resulting in pulmonary fibrosis. The above pathway seems to explain most of the experimental animal evidence and reflects much of the clinical picture. Unfortunately, it is probably incomplete.

The clinical picture begins with the increasingly hypoxic patient who manifests the tachycardia, tachypnea, anxiety, and restlessness observed with hypoxemia. The patient finally reaches the point where satisfactory blood gases cannot be maintained without intubation and ventilatory support and is intubated. Chest radiography may be normal at this point but invariably shows the effects of increased total lung water shortly. The hallmark diagnostic criteria for ARDS are as follows: acute onset of respiratory failure, bilateral infiltrates on frontal CXR, P$_a$O$_2$/F$_i$O$_2$ < 200, and PCWP < 18 mm Hg.

Mechanical ventilation is required for survival in all ARDS patients. For oxygenation, the patient's hypoxia must be reversed as rapidly as possible. The F$_i$O$_2$ is increased progressively and usually reaches 0.5 without significant improvement because gas diffusion is markedly decreased. The patient requires increasing application of PEEP, which is usually increased in 2- to 5-cm H$_2$O increments per half-hour. The PEEP is increased until the oxygenation improves or the cardiac output falls. If the patient cannot tolerate the high levels of PEEP because of the interference with cardiac filling, the PEEP is dropped to previously tolerated levels, the intravascular volume is increased, and the PEEP then is increased again.

For ventilation, a large multicenter ARDS network study clearly demonstrated a significant survival advantage to those patients who were ventilated with tidal volumes of 4 to 6 mL/kg of ideal body weight. Any higher would lead to volu/barotrauma and increased mortality. This leads to higher retained P$_{CO_2}$ but is tolerated as long as the pH is greater than 7.15 and is termed "permissive hypercapnia." Interestingly, oxygenation may in fact worsen with hypoventilation. However, the survival advantage from less barotrauma outweighs this apparent irony. APRV and IRV, as mentioned earlier, are ventilatory modes of choice in ARDS for patients without underlying chronic obstructive pulmonary disease (COPD). It is important to keep the plateau airway pressure below 35 to limit VILI. This is done by reducing the TV as needed to levels as low as 4 mL/kg.

In our practice, PEEP is increased up to the point that the F$_i$O$_2$ can be decreased. Once that point is reached, the patient often begins to recover, allowing a progressive decrease in the oxygen concentrations. The goal is to decrease the oxygen concentration to

0.5 or less. At this point, the oxygen toxicity seems to be tolerable.

Exogenous surfactant is now available and has been shown to improve the course in pediatric but not adult patients. Inhaled nitric oxide, which results in improved perfusion to the lung segments ventilated, should have solved the clinical problems of ARDS by abolishing the V/Q mismatch. Although effective in decreasing this mismatch, the studies have not yet demonstrated a consistent benefit in terms of patient survival.

With aggressive pulmonary manipulation, as described earlier, the diagnosis of ARDS does not seem equivalent to a death sentence. Moreover, the physician who can successfully care for a patient with ARDS proves his or her understanding of cardiopulmonary disease and the whole gamut of the ICU armamentarium.

FLUIDS AND ELECTROLYTES

Body Compartments

Water constitutes approximately 60% of the total body weight in young healthy men and about 55% of the weight in young women (consequent to their increased total body fat content). The average 70-kg man therefore contains about 40 L of fluid. This fluid is divided into three distinct compartments: intracellular, interstitial, and intravascular.

Intracellular fluid exists within the cells of the body and constitutes about two-thirds of the total body water (TBW). Interstitial fluid exists outside of both the cells and the intravascular space and includes such fluids as cerebrospinal fluid (CSF), lymph, and tissue fluids. Interstitial fluid represents about two-thirds of the extracellular fluid or about 20% of TBW. The smallest space is the intravascular fluid, which represents about one-ninth of TBW and about 7% of body weight. This space is filled with plasma and the formed elements of the blood.

Fluid movement between these compartments is dictated by a number of principles, all of which are clinically relevant. Fluid shifts between the intracellular space and the interstitial space are dictated by the electrical potential across the cell membrane. A charged ion moving into the cell is balanced by a similarly charged ion moving out of the cell. The critical control mechanism a cell uses to maintain the electrical potential is the Na-K-ATPase pump. This movement principle is valid only so long as the cell membrane retains its semipermeable integrity. When the pump fails due to lack of ATP, the cell can no longer regulate its electrolyte balance and thus its fluid balance and swells to the point of apoptosis.

Movement of fluid between the intravascular and interstitial fluid spaces is dictated by the Starling relation, which states that the hydrostatic forces moving fluid out of the capillary are opposed by oncotic and osmotic forces. Note that water can move freely within all three compartments. It is governed by both hydrostatic pressure and oncotic pressure. A change in osmolality of any compartment requires a net movement of water across the membranes to maintain iso-osmolality across all compartments.

The concepts of osmolality and tonicity should be addressed. Osmolality is simply the molar concentration of the osmotically active particles in a fluid, whereas tonicity describes the net force on water exerted by these particles along an osmolar gradient, also known as the oncotic pressure.

Water Balance

In addition to the movement of water between these body compartments, water moves into and out of the body. Intake is usually oral and averages about 2 L/day for the average adult. This figure includes not only fluids drunk but also the water absorbed from foodstuffs. The kidneys excrete most of the body's water (about 1.0 to 1.5 L), with additional water lost from the skin (as insensible loss) and in the stool (as rarely measured loss). The net water balance is usually zero because the patient neither gains nor loses water weight. Water intake is necessitated by the kidney's need to eliminate nitrogenous waste. An increase in water balance is usually the product of injudicious physician intervention. It may also occur as a consequence of chronic malnutrition with the loss of visceral protein mass or acute or chronic renal failure.

The clinical problems with water balance are usually secondary to excessive losses. Insensible losses increase as a function of the increase in the body's temperature. Vasodilation of cutaneous capillaries increases the rate at which water may be lost from the patient. Direct access to the tracheobronchial tree opens another surface for water exchange, and intubated patients who do not receive satisfactory humidification from a nebulizer experience drying of their respiratory epithelium and so lose fluid. The protective barrier of the keratinized layer of the skin protects against fluid loss, and the destruction of this layer with a burn injury, especially if the burn is moderate-to-deep second degree, is another area of fluid loss (areas of third-degree burns lose less fluid because of the reconstitution of a vapor barrier by the eschar formed).

Polyuria and diarrhea are other common sources of fluid loss that can be measured. Fluid may be lost directly from the intravascular space because of bleeding. Blood collected for diagnostic tests is another major source of water loss in the SICU. Loss of other body secretions such as nasogastric or ileostomy losses may decrease the fluid volume status. Note that these lost fluids are associated with the loss of other specific electrolytes and protein.

In addition to the fluid losses due to renal failure, there are a number of other neuroendocrine responses that affect water balance. ADH is released by the posterior pituitary in response to hypothalamic stimulation. It acts on the kidney's distal tubule to increase water reabsorption. This system is used for total body and intracellular dehydration in particular because free water can equilibrate with all three compartments. Patients with head injury may manifest a syndrome of inappropriate ADH levels (SIADH) and become progressively water intoxicated and hyponatremic.

Likewise, the renin-angiotensin-aldosterone system uses aldosterone to retain sodium and water using the Na-K-ATPase pumps in the collecting tubules. This system is activated when the kidneys perceive intravascular volume loss. By retaining sodium and drawing water with it, the system maintains intravascular volume via a feedback system using the macula densa in the glomerulus. Clinically, this becomes important in conditions such as cirrhosis, where high levels of aldosterone favor both sodium and water retention.

Cation Imbalances

Sodium

Sodium is the principal cation of the extracellular fluid space, and changes in sodium content usually follow logically from changes in water content. The serum sodium concentration is helpful in determining the total body volume status of the patient by contributing the majority of effective osmoles to the extracellular fluid and thus determining its osmolality. Thus, one must ask themselves whether the sodium imbalance represents hypo- or hypervolemia or if a pseudoelectrolyte imbalance exists due to the presence of another osmole, that is, glucose.

Clinical evaluation of the patient usually demonstrates the water problem directly, with dry mucous membranes and signs of hypovolemia in the patient who is hypernatremic. Neurologic signs of restlessness and delirium occur with hypernatremia but are probably secondary to volume contraction and the catecholamine responses.

Hypernatremia requires appropriate re-expansion of the vascular space with hypotonic fluids. One can estimate the presumed free water deficit with this formula:

$$\text{FW deficit} = (\text{target Na} - \text{current Na}) \times \text{TBW in liters}$$

where TBW is $0.60 \times \text{IBW (kg)}$.

This should be corrected slowly to prevent significant changes in brain water content, that is, cerebellar pontine myelinolysis. Do not correct sodium levels in either direction by more than 0.5 to 1 mEq/hr. All too commonly, iatrogenic hypernatremia results from over aggressive saline resuscitation, that is, "saltwater drowning." It may also be seen in hyperglycemic states, although the measured sodium level does not demonstrate it. For every 100 mg/dL increase in glucose, plasma sodium falls about 2 mEq.

The hyponatremic patient appears wet. CNS changes are demonstrable. The water-intoxicated patient is progressively hyperactive, even to the point of convulsions. These changes are usually encountered when the serum sodium has fallen to about 120 mEq/L.

Hyponatremia usually occurs as a consequence of water excess. It is generally iatrogenic, although abnormally high circulating ADH is responsible in a few patients (SIADH). It is usually a preventable condition but if it occurs, it should *not* be treated with infusions of isotonic or hypotonic fluids but with fluid restriction. Hyponatremia may also indicate significant volume loss as in persistent vomiting which depletes total body sodium. Treat this with iso-osmolar or isotonic fluid, that is, 0.9% NaCl along with 20 mEq KCl to replete potassium losses as discussed later.

Potassium

Sodium is the major *extra*cellular cation, and potassium is the major *intra*cellular cation. Although the body can conserve sodium if required, it cannot compensate for hypokalemia by decreasing its urinary losses. The major route of potassium excretion is the kidney, and most of the abnormalities associated with this ion impinge on renal sufficiency. The ion's most important function is to regulate the electrical potential across cell membranes, especially for controlling the automaticity of the pacemaker of the heart.

Hyperkalemia sufficient to cause electrical problems of the heart begins as early as a serum K^+ level of 6.0 mEq/L. The condition usually occurs in patients with renal failure but is also seen in patients with normal renal function who have increased tissue destruction, releasing potassium into the intravascular space. It is possible to kill a burn patient by the injudicious use of succinylcholine, which causes muscle cells to release a huge dose of potassium into the blood. Potassium may also be elevated as a consequence of excessive treatment with spironolactone to compensate for aldosterone excess because the body loses sodium in the urine and reabsorbs potassium. Electrocardiographic signs of hyperkalemia include high peaked T waves, widened QRS complexes, and eventually disappearance of T waves.

High levels of potassium may be life threatening. The solution is to eliminate the potassium ion from the intravascular space, which can be done by moving the ion into the cells or eliminating it entirely from the body. Potassium is a cofactor in the transport of glucose, and giving the patient a large glucose infusion along with insulin moves the ion into cells. Alkalosis also moves potassium into cells. Kayexalate™ is a cation-exchange resin that can bind potassium and carry it out of the gastrointestinal tract. Kayexalate™ may be introduced per rectum or via a nasogastric tube along with sorbitol. It is perhaps the best method of controlling hyperkalemia if the patient is in renal failure and diuretics are ineffective.

Hypokalemia is usually a consequence of body depletion of the ion. Diarrhea results in a large loss of circulating potassium, which is eventually replaced up to a point by movement of potassium out of cells. Large losses of gastric juice via a nasogastric tube may also produce hypokalemia, even though the potassium content of gastric juice is minimal. Here, the loss of potassium is secondary to the loss of chloride. The kidney, without adequate chloride, cannot reabsorb sodium. To compensate for the sodium loss, the aldosterone system secretes potassium as the sodium is reclaimed. Another clinical condition of hypokalemia is caused by the injudicious use of diuretics. Inadequate replacement of potassium during hyperalimentation may also produce hypokalemia. The clinical problem posed by hypokalemia is the rate at which potassium can be replaced. The limit seems to be somewhat shy of 40 mEq/hr, under close electrocardiography scrutiny.

Calcium

Calcium homeostasis involves balancing diet intake and storage in bone with GI and renal excretion. Vitamin D and parathyroid hormone (PTH) are the principle potentiators of serum calcium while calcitonin attenuates it. PTH stimulates osteoclast bone resorption, increased renal reabsorption, and enhances intestinal absorption via vitamin D or calcitriol. Calcium is principally found in bone in association with phosphate and carbonate. In serum, only about half of the calcium is ionized, and it is important for neuromuscular control. This ionized faction is a function of the protein level and the pH (acidosis increases ionization).

Hypercalcemia results from two relatively uncommon conditions: hyperparathyroidism and widespread osseous metastases. Clinical signs and symptoms of hypercalcemia are largely vague and include the classic complaint of "groans, moans, and stones" along with weakness and stupor. Treatment for acute hypercalcemia involves aggressive dilutional volume rehydration followed by a loop diuretic such as Lasix. Chronic conditions can be treated chemically with bisphosphonates and calcitonin which both take longer to work.

Hypocalcemia presents as marked hyperactivity, a positive Chvostek's sign, tetany, and carpopedal spasm. Clinically, it is commonly associated with acute pancreatitis and renal insufficiency. Questionably, it may occur in a consequence of massive infusion of large amounts of citrated blood. Intravenous calcium is the acute treatment of choice with longterm oral replacement in chronic conditions.

ACID–BASE BALANCE

Hydrogen ion concentration is usually defined in terms of pH (the negative logarithm). In the intact patient, its concentration is maintained within fairly tight limits by a combination of respiratory and metabolic compensatory mechanisms. Acid added to the extracellular fluid is buffered by a number of systems, especially the bicarbonate–carbonic acid system, with excretion of the acid by the lungs or the kidneys.

The bicarbonate buffer system is described by the Henderson–Hasselbalch equation, which states that

$$[H^+] = 24 \times ([P_{CO_2}]/[HCO_3^-]) \text{ or}$$
$$pH = 6.1 + \log (\text{bicarbonate}/[0.03 \times P_{CO_2}])$$

So long as the ratio between bicarbonate and carbonic acid remains 20:1, the pH remains normal.

When the system is working properly, adding acid decreases serum bicarbonate. Ventilation is increased to eliminate carbon dioxide and reestablish the 20:1 ratio. More slowly, the kidney eliminates the acid and reabsorbs additional bicarbonate.

Four abnormal states are recognized: respiratory acidosis, respiratory alkalosis, metabolic acidosis, and metabolic alkalosis. Each state may be associated with some degree of appropriate compensation. The diagnosis of acidosis is made with a pH less than 7.40. Elevated Pco_2 produces a diagnosis of respiratory acidosis, and the reverse is found with respiratory alkalosis. Similarly, the metabolic component is deduced from the level of the serum bicarbonate.

Respiratory acidosis is a common clinical result of inadequate alveolar ventilation with an elevated Pco_2. If it persists, the patient attempts to compensate by retaining bicarbonate and excreting acid in the urine. The change in pH from respiratory *acidosis* can be acute or chronic and is determined by this formula:

$$Acute: \Delta pH = -0.008 \times (\Delta Pco_2)$$
$$Chronic: \Delta pH = -0.003 \times (\Delta Pco_2)$$

Therapy must obviously be directed toward improving ventilation.

Respiratory alkalosis is commonly seen in hyperventilated, anxious, tachypneic patients, but COPD and morbid obesity are the most common chronic causes. The alkalosis forces a movement of potassium into cells and forces the kidney to retain acid. Again, an acute versus chronic respiratory *alkalosis* can be delineated by these formulae:

$$Acute: \Delta pH = -0.008 \times (\Delta Pco_2)$$
$$Chronic: \Delta pH = -0.017 \times (\Delta Pco_2)$$

Treat the respiratory drive or in ventilated patients decrease the minute ventilation.

Metabolic acidosis is usually a consequence of the accumulation of acid, commonly lactic acid, and usually reflects tissue hypoperfusion. Measurement of the anion gap usually points to elevated lactate levels even if they are not measured directly. Nonanion gap acidosis includes hyperchloremic metabolic acidosis. It may also result from the kidneys' inability to excrete acid and retain bicarbonate. The expected respiratory compensation on Pco_2 for metabolic *acidosis* is given by this formula:

$$Pco_2 = 1.5 \times [HCO_3^-] + 8$$

Therapy again is directed against the underlying causes of hypoperfusion. Correction of metabolic acidosis with exogenous bicarbonate may only exacerbate the acidemia by converting the bicarbonate to carbon dioxide and water via carbonic anhydrase. The increased CO_2 load burdens an already taxed respiratory system.

Metabolic alkalosis is commonly seen in association with hypovolemia in a state known as contraction alkalosis, which is usually a result of excessive loss of gastric secretions as seen in patients with pyloric outlet obstruction. Chloride is lost in large quantities into the nasogastric fluid. The kidneys are unable to absorb sodium without the anion, and sodium and water are lost. The kidney attempts to correct this imbalance by exchanging potassium and hydrogen ions for sodium. The alkalotic patient thus produces a paradoxical aciduria. The expected respiratory compensation on Pco_2 for metabolic *alkalosis* is given by this formula:

$$Pco_2 = 0.9 \times [HCO_3^-] + 15$$

Therapy requires re-expansion of the vascular space with isotonic saline along with appropriate infusions of potassium chloride. Severe alkalosis may require infusion of hydrochloric acid.

BLOOD AND BLOOD COMPONENT THERAPY

Blood Banking

Today's blood bank represents a compromise between the surgeon's impression of the needs of the patient and the hospital's need for efficiency and cost containment. When blood bank technology was in its infancy, blood banks were run by surgeons. Now, we merely wait in line, frequently behind internists, oncologists, and obstetricians. Fresh whole blood is virtually impossible to obtain in any hospital today. It should be noted, however, that current military experience has demonstrated the superiority of whole blood transfusion for combat-related injuries. The technology of component therapy has evolved to the point that a given unit of donated blood is divided and redistributed to a number of patients. The RBCs may be centrifuged and infused into one patient, the plasma frozen and available for another, and the platelets given to a third.

Risks of blood component therapy include acute versus delayed hemolytic reactions (1/250,000 to 1/1 million vs. 1/1,000), anaphylaxis (1/150,000), transfusion-related acute lung injury (1/8,000), and febrile reactions (1/100 to 1/200). Infectious risks include hepatitis B (1/60,000 to 1/200,000), hepatitis C (1/800,000 to 1/1.6 million), and HIV (1/1.2 to 1/2.4 million).

Red Blood Cells

Erythrocytes are indicated for the replacement of lost blood, but only to the point that the patient's hemoglobin content is adequate for the needs of oxygen transport. There is no need to transfuse the patient back to a premorbid hematocrit of 45% when a hematocrit of 30% or lower can suffice. Remember, too, that fully saturating these 10 g of hemoglobin provides better tissue oxygen delivery than poorly saturating a large mass of hemoglobin. The most complete study of transfusion thresholds (TRICC Canadian Study) established the safety and survival advantage for conservative (hemoglobin 7 g/dL) threshold for transfusion in younger patients without ongoing cardiac ischemia.

RBCs infused for these purposes are commonly delivered as packed RBCs. These cells are stored in the refrigerator of the blood bank in citrate–phosphate–dextrose, and the shelf life (defined as 70% of infused cells surviving 24 hours after transfusion) is about 28 to 35 days. In the refrigerator, the cells metabolize the glucose to lactate. Older units of blood contain increased amounts of extracellular potassium and decreased amounts of intracellular 2,3-DPG (see "Shock," above).

Blood is usually crossmatched prior to transfusion, but in urgent situations, type-specific blood (matching only ABO group and Rh factor) may be employed. In emergency situations, the infusion of type O Rh-negative blood may be lifesaving. Even the most careful crossmatching may miss some of the minor histocompatibility antigens and produce a mild hemolytic reaction. Reactions to mismatched blood may be dramatic, with fever and chills, tachycardia, hypotension, and brisk intravascular hemolysis. The patient under general anesthesia may not manifest these signs, but the surgeon can diagnose the hemolytic reaction by the diffuse oozing in the operative field.

Therapy for transfusion reactions must include immediate cessation of the infusion, returning the infusate and a sample of the patient's blood to the blood bank. The released hemoglobin may precipitate in the renal tubules and lead to ARF. This situation is best prevented by volume loading followed by a brisk dieresis, alkalinizing of the urine is controversial. Other causes of fever, chills, and hypotension (e.g., bacterial contamination of the line) should also be considered and sought.

Blood transfusions are also infusions of extracellular fluid. As stated earlier, old blood may have high levels of potassium, which could be a problem in patients with renal insufficiency. Ammonia tends to accumulate as well. Rapid infusion of cold blood may lead to hypothermia. Citrate accumulation and consequent hypocalcemia is probably rare, but the risks increase with massive transfusion and in patients with poor hepatic function due to drugs or toxic injury or because of immaturity, as in neonates. The addition of intravenous calcium is therefore somewhat controversial. It is only indicated for hypoperfused patients with liver or cardiac failure that manifest citrate toxicity. Anecdotal evidence exists of rebound hypercalcemia.

Micropore filters are probably indicated during massive transfusions to decrease the infusion of RBC aggregates and cellular debris. These particles, if infused, are capable of producing pulmonary insufficiency. Blood should not be infused through small-caliber needles and probably should not be administered through narrow cannulas such as those in Swan–Ganz catheters. Blood warmers should be employed whenever available.

Clotting Factors

Patients who have bled and been transfused with significant volumes are at risk of developing a washout coagulopathy because the transfused blood contains neither clotting factors nor platelets. There is growing evidence as mentioned in the shock section that massive transfusion (>10 unit of PRBCs) is accompanied by dilutional coagulopathy, thereby justifying a 1:1 PRBC:FFP transfusion ratio.

Clotting factors are also indicated in patients with coagulopathies who have not bled. Factors VII, IX, X, and XI may be found in pooled plasma. Factor V replacement requires the use of FFP. Factor VIII is available in FFP or in factor VIII concentrates. Cryoprecipitate contains not only coagulation factors VIII and XIII but also the circulating opsonic protein fibronectin.

Platelets

Platelet deficiency is rarely the cause of clinical bleeding unless the platelet count is less than 50,000/mm³.

Use this threshold for transfusion with ongoing bleeding. Otherwise an absolute threshold of 10 to 20,000/mm^3 can be used without evidence of bleeding. In the massive transfusion setting, a unit of pheresed platelets should be transfused for every unit of PRBCs. Care must be taken not to filter the platelet preparation because the platelets then end up in the filter, not in the patient.

Acute Renal Failure

Acute renal insufficiency is a common observation in the surgical patient in the ICU. It is defined by acute oliguria or less than 0.5 mL/kg/hr of urine output or less than 400 mL in 24 hours for adults or less than 1.0 mL/kg/hr in children weighing less than 10 kg. Fortunately, most of these patients do not require the services of the nephrologist (though many are called in for consultation) or need hemodialysis. These patients do require, however, an early diagnosis and appropriate management. The patient with decreased urine volumes may be suffering from a prerenal, renal, or postrenal problem. Remember, an occluded Foley catheter should be the first diagnosis ruled out. Table 21.2 helps to guide diagnosis of the causes of ARF.

Prerenal oliguria is consequent to a decrease in renal perfusion. Cardiac output is directly related to renal blood flow, as the renal arteriolar system cannot change its vascular resistance, so prerenal oliguria is usually associated with any conditions that decrease cardiac output, especially hypovolemia. It is also associated with drugs that increase vascular resistance, either globally (e.g., norepinephrine) or locally (e.g., angiotensin-converting enzyme inhibitors). Patients with prerenal disease usually have an elevated blood urea nitrogen (BUN)/creatinine ratio (>20:1) and restrict excretion of sodium to compensate for the real or apparent decrease in intravascular volume. Spot urine electrolyte assays usually demonstrate a sodium level of less than 20 mEq/L. Fractional excretion of sodium (FE$_{Na}$), as described later, is usually less than 1%.

$$FE_{Na} = (urine\ [Na^+]/plasma\ [Na^+])/(urine\ [creatinine]/plasma\ [creatinine]) \times 100$$

Therapy is relatively straightforward and includes reduction of hypovolemia and maintenance of cardiac output.

Intrinsic causes of ARF are most often acute tubular necrosis (ATN) and nephritis, the latter being drug related. The urinary sodium concentration is increased in these conditions because of tubular injury and consequent leak of sodium into the urine beyond that which the body would otherwise excrete. The urinary sodium level is greater than 40 mEq/L in most conditions. FE$_{Na}$ is more than 3%, as the body is better able to control creatinine excretion than sodium. The cause of ATN is often hypoperfusion, which usually indicates intraoperative hypovolemia in major cases or decreases in cardiac output from other causes. Initial management is correction of cardiac output. Management of drug-induced nephritis is removal of the drug. Examination of the urinary sediment, a process virtually unknown to house officers today, frequently demonstrates white blood cell casts in drug-induced nephritis.

A more controversial management practice for the patient with ATN is increasing the urine output to convert an anuric or markedly oliguric picture to a less oliguric one. The data suggest that patients whose urine output is 30 mL/hr or more do better, which suggests a role for pharmacologic intervention to achieve the higher urine output and the better clinical outcome. These data are scarce. The initial therapies advanced to produce this end include diuretics (usually furosemide) at increasing doses and then other agents such as bumetanide (Bumex), diuretic drips, and finally renal-dose dopamine. Furosemide (Lasix) drips

TABLE 21.2	Assessment Strategies for Determining the Etiology of Renal Dysfunction			
	Prerenal	**Renal**	**Mixed**	**Postrenal**
Volume	Decreased	Normal	Decreased	Normal
Urine sodium	<20 mEq/L	>40 mEq/L	Between 20 and 40	Usually >40 mEq/L
Fractional excretion of Na	<1%	>3%	Between 1 and 3	Usually >3%
Appearance of collecting system	Normal	Normal	Normal	Dilated

increase urine output better than bolus therapy in some, but not all, patients. Dopamine, because of its effect on renal blood flow, increases urine output and produces a natriuresis, but it has not been shown to improve outcome. In the setting of decreased cardiac output, it must be used carefully because of its arrhythmia potential and the risk of worsening tachycardia as well as its known adverse effects on the neuroendocrine system.

Additional support for the patient must include anticipating hemodialysis and preventing further injury. Acidosis should be avoided. Potassium should be removed from all intravenous fluids and the serum potassium carefully observed. Water balance must be maintained as tightly as possible, as the excess water infused today must disappear tomorrow. Nutrition must be carefully adjusted to minimize volume by concentrating formulae, eliminating potential toxins and electrolytes, and controlling for protein retention, that is, BUN. Note, however, that patients progressing to hemodialysis actually require protein supplementation due to the actual amount of protein lost during the dialysis process. Boluses of glucose, insulin, and bicarbonate can transiently lower the serum potassium by moving potassium into cells. Kayexelate™ enemas or per nasogastric tube decrease the potassium load rather than merely moving it around. As the patient develops profound renal insufficiency, other adjuncts include erythropoietin to maintain erythrocyte mass, DDAVP to treat the coagulopathy associated with uremia, and appropriate nutritional support.

Absolute indications for hemodialysis include severe water intoxication (worsening congestive heart failure), hyperkalemia, acidosis, and drug or toxin clearance. Severe azotemia (BUN >100 mg/dL) is a relative indication. The newer machines and increased experience of the nephrologists have decreased the acute hemodynamic consequences of hemodialysis (which is available even on Sundays and holidays now). Moreover, A-V hemofiltration and continuous venovenous hemofiltration are adjuncts that aid in water balance and azotemia.

An often preventable cause of renal failure is myoglobinemia. It is seen in patients with severe rhabdomyolysis, commonly after lengthy vascular procedures with inadequate peripheral perfusion. The diagnosis requires spectrochemical demonstration of myoglobin in the urine, but the test is rarely performed in the hospital, must be sent to an outside laboratory, costs too much, and takes too long. A useful alternative is a urine analysis. If the urine is positive for blood but on microscopic analysis is devoid of RBCs, then the likelihood is that there is myoglobin present in the urine. Acute muscle damage leading to myoglobin is usually associated with a markedly elevated serum creatine phosphokinase level. Treatment for both myoglobin and hemoglobin excess is the same. First, anticipate further production of the chemical if the underlying cause is hypoperfusion (myoglobin) or hemolysis (hemoglobin). Second, induce prompt diuresis in an attempt to clear the material before it precipitates in the urine. Mannitol or a similar osmotic diuretic is generally used here along with volume infusion. Alkalinization of urine with sodium bicarbonate may decrease the precipitation of these chromogens, but this point remains controversial.

Postrenal causes of ARF include obstruction to urine flow from the kidney. Serum creatinine is used as marker of renal function. It can distinguish prerenal from renal causes because of the increased BUN/creatinine ratio in the former. The serum creatinine level must be used with caution in the elderly and in those with extensive muscle wasting. (Creatinine is derived from muscle.) Serum creatinine declines normally with age, as reflected in the formulas below for estimating creatinine clearance.

Creatinine clearance (males)
$$= [(140 - \text{age in years}) \times \text{weight (kg)}]/72 \times \text{creatinine (mg/dL)}$$

Creatinine clearance (females) = 0.85 × above

In ill patients, creatinine clearance is better determined directly, most accurately with a 24-hour urine sample and less so with a 2- or 6-hour specimen.

Infectious Problems in the SICU

The infectious disease problems seen in the SICU could fill up another chapter by themselves. Three areas of interest have arisen during the past few years, and questions in these areas are likely to appear on the board examination.

We will focus our discussion on infections that arise in SICU patients after being treated for their primary disease, that is, trauma, abdominal catastrophe. Once those causes have been treated, the onset of new occult infection is perhaps the single biggest contributor to SICU morbidity and mortality.

Signs of new infection include fever and leukocytosis with left shift. They may also include local symptoms such as infiltrates and purulent sputum, cloudy or foul smelling urine, abdominal pain or ileus versus obstruction, and local wound infections manifesting as hot, red, indurated, swollen, and painful wounds. Mental status changes and tachycardia or tachypnea may also herald a new infection. Always suspect infection when a patient suddenly develops glucose intolerance.

Systemic signs of worsening infection can be described as the systemic inflammatory response syndrome or SIRS. This is characterized by fever, tachycardia, tachypnea, and leukocytosis. If the source is a bacterial infection, then the condition can be described as sepsis or SIRS with bacteremia. Note that not all sepsis can be traced back to an identifiable organism. These conditions can quickly degrade to septic shock with the onset of systemic hypoperfusion; oliguria, hypotension, lactic acidosis, and mental status changes. If not treated early, patients can proceed to multiorgan dysfunction syndrome, which predicts poor prognosis. Your job as a critical care physician is to prevent this progression.

In November 2001, Emanuel Rivers, an ER physician from Detroit, published his landmark study in the "New England Journal of Medicine" on "Early goal-directed therapy for severe sepsis and septic shock." He demonstrated a significant improvement in survival and early markers of perfusion for those patients diagnosed with severe sepsis or septic shock in his ER that were randomized to receive early goal-directed protocolized therapy (see Fig. 21.3).

Note that only a CVC was used to deliver fluid, blood, and pressors according to the guidelines. The catheter also used central venous oxygenation as marker of perfusion. The important lesson learned is that the patients were treated while still in the ER and demonstrated improved outcomes with definitive treatment in an ICU setting. If they did not receive this protocol, then no amount of "catch up" therapy benefited the patients.

Nosocomial pneumonia is a major problem in the critically ill, and it may lead directly to pulmonary insufficiency. Temporally, the lung is usually the first organ to succumb to multiple organ failure. Although the incidence of nosocomial pneumonia is increased in the most seriously ill patients (those with the highest APACHE II scores) and in patients who are intubated, it occurs in less sick, nonintubated patients as well.

Ventilator-associated pneumonia (VAP) mortality is as high as 30%. Current thinking places the cause of VAP as translocation of oral bacteria down the ETT to colonize the bronchial tree. Aspiration is certainly one of the potential causes of VAP; however, there are no data supporting bacterial translocation from the stomach resulting from acid suppression. Duration of mechanical ventilation is the single greatest predictor of VAP onset. Other contributors include trauma, sepsis, burns, and direct or indirect ALI. The Centers for Disease Control and Prevention criteria for suspicion of VAP include signs of inflammation (i.e., fever or leukocytosis), infiltrate on CXR, purulent sputum, and hypoxemia. There are no gold standards to diagnosing VAP. Most recently, studies have shown that both a deep ETT suction sputum sample or a formal bronchoalveolar lavage (BAL) have the same outcomes in diagnosing and treating VAP.

The critical point in treating VAP is starting the right antibiotic at the right time. A sputum sample should be obtained as soon as one suspects VAP. Broad spectrum antibiotics should be started immediately thereafter. They should cover the most common flora at one's SICU. Keep in mind that the organisms most likely to be responsible for VAP depend on the ventilator days. Less then 5 days on the ventilator predicts community-acquired flora, whereas greater than 5 days now predicts nosocomial flora and likely multidrug-resistant organisms. The antibiotics spectrum should treat the respective organisms suspected. On the third day of treatment, one should reevaluate the culture results and the patient's response to determine if in fact their infection is caused by VAP or another source. If VAP is the source, antibiotics should be narrowed and the course determined: 7 days for all organisms (including MRSA) except *Pseudomonas* or *Acinetobacter*, which are treated for 14 days. Onset of new multidrug-resistant organisms should prompt a collective decision on course.

When early signs of sepsis are detected, aggressive measures to diagnose and treat the source are warranted. Mortality increases for every hour without appropriate antibiotics. Culture and imaging must be obtained concurrently with initiation of broadspectrum antibiotics. De-escalation is equally as important once results start trickling in.

Other common sources of infection in the SICU include catheter-related bloodstream infections (CR-BSIs). Despite antibiotic coatings, one must remain diligent when assessing catheter sites as potential sources for bacteremia. Infections are now thought to start externally and colonize the catheter on their way into the bloodstream. Certainly, catheters can become

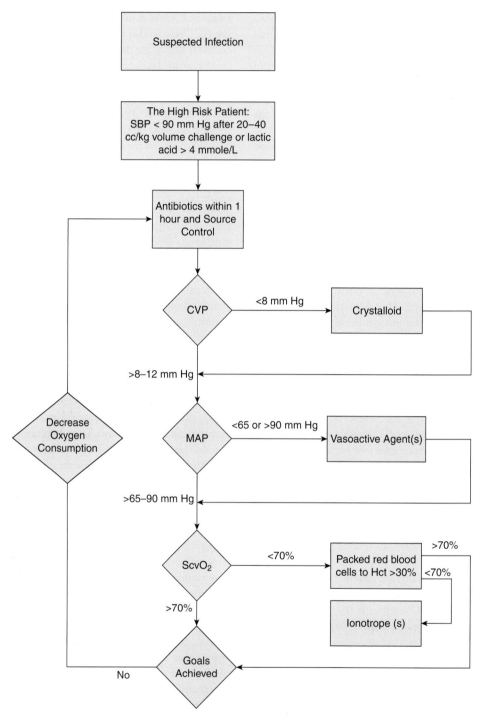

FIGURE 21.3 Protocol designed by Rivers et al. to treat a patient with presumed sepsis.

secondarily colonized as well, but if they are the source, they must be removed immediately and antibiotics should be started to cover likely skin flora, that is, *Staphylococcus aureus*/MRSA. One method to differentiate catheter-related infections from bacteremia colonization is the time-to-sensitivity test. If the blood culture from the catheter (not usually drawn) returns positive before a peripheral culture, the catheter is likely the source. We no longer advocate routine scheduled line changes, as these practices may in fact increase the incidence of CR-BSIs. Rather a pragmatic approach to new onset of infection should be used, that is, physical exam and number of catheter days at that point in time.

Urinary tract infections are also common in the SICU with indwelling bladder catheters in every patient. If a urinalysis is positive, many would consider simply exchanging the catheter to facilitate drainage of the infection. Antibiotics should also be chosen based on unit-specific susceptibilities.

Prevention of infection in the SICU is more likely to derive from better designed invasive devices and even more so by the prudent use of the devices we already have. Closed urine collection systems decreased the incidence of urinary tract infections. Today, we have silver-impregnated and antibiotic-coated catheters, which may help decrease the problem further. Similar coatings on CVCs have not always decreased the incidence of infection, which may be better prevented by judicious aseptic technique. The length-of-stay issue for central lines has been resolved in favor of not removing them routinely at a certain time after insertion. PA catheters, though, clearly must be removed in a timely fashion or replaced. The large, flexible, more frequently manipulated introducers must be removed as well. Finally, arterial catheters, for which there are no guidelines for length of use, must be remembered as possible sources of bloodstream infection.

Neurosurgical Critical Care

Probably no aspect of surgical critical care has undergone as abrupt a change as has that of the head-injured or general neurosurgical patient. Concepts, biases, and manipulations that seemed so logical in the past are being abandoned and replaced with new ideas, some of which remain untested.

The physiology of the head-injured patient rested on the Monro–Kellie doctrine that there were three volumes held together within a rigid barrier called the skull: brain, blood, and the CSF space. Increases in intracranial pressure (ICP) were not tolerated well by the brain,

and all interventions were predicated upon reducing this pressure. The brain's autoregulation, a system that allows the brain to increase its "share" of the cardiac output as the latter fails, had to be managed to decrease this perfusion because cerebral edema had to be prevented. The cornerstone of management, then, after placing a ventriculostomy or an ICP bolt, was hyperventilation to decrease the vasodilatation so as to prevent edema. There were two problems with this concept. First, it would not work for long because the difference in carbon dioxide tension between blood and tissue would equilibrate within 24 hours, and hypocarbia causes cerebral vasoconstriction, which starves the brain. This would be analogous to treating the edema consequent to a fractured femur by ligating the femoral artery.

As a clinical intervention, it seemed to work, but only because there was nothing with which to compare it. Hyperventilation did decrease ICP, at least transiently, so the theory seemed sound, but the patients did not necessarily wake up, either in the SICU or afterward. The classic Cushing's phenomenon (hypertension and bradycardia), which was observed in patients with malignant increases in their ICP, was seen as representing an appeal by the brain to generate perfusion.

Replacing it now is the current concept of maintaining cerebral perfusion, thereby maximizing delivery of blood, oxygen, and nutrients to the brain. Cerebral blood flow is difficult to measure, either clinically or experimentally. Flow probes can be placed on the inflow vessels, but in an intact human that means two carotid arteries and two vertebral arteries. This is not clinically feasible. Xenon-CT scanning allows quantification of both total and regional blood flow, but this technique is not yet universally available. Alternatively, one can determine the adequacy of perfusion by measuring the decrease in oxygen content across the brain, which can be done by placing an oxygen sensor in the jugular bulb. Some clinical centers do use this technique, but it remains controversial and the data are questionable because of the alternative venous channels. Moreover, the A-V oxygen difference reflects a global picture, and the regional perfusion of the brain remains indeterminate.

Current clinical practice focuses on cerebral perfusion pressure (CPP) rather than blood flow. The ICP is routinely measured via an inserted device. The difference between MAP and ICP is the CPP. It must be kept above 60 mm Hg. To maintain this pressure, in patients with high ICPs, the use of vasopressors is often required to maintain CPP. Prior to starting pressors, the use of fluids and inotropes should be considered.

Prior to instituting measures to increase blood pressure, attempts to reduce ICP should be made first. The first step of maintaining adequate CPP is to diminish intrinsic ICP. This entails elevating the head of the to bed 30 degrees and sedating the patient. Propofol is a good choice as it can be quickly turned on and off to facilitate serial neurological exams. However, it does depress cardiac function. Analgesia and ventilator support to minimize excess effort is also important.

If this fails, and an intraventricular drain has been placed, then the drain is opened like a CSF release valve. The rate of drainage depends on its height relative to the head. The next options for reducing ICP are mannitol and HTS. The goal is to reduce cerebral edema via concentration and diuresis. If these methods fail, then a craniectomy to decompress the cranial vault can be considered; although many believe that this may save a life, it leaves a severely debilitated patient. Hyperventilation can be used to transiently reduce ICP while waiting for other methods of treatment to take effect.

If all else fails, one can consider a barbiturate coma, but this is rarely used because at this point in the patient's course, it demonstrates little, if any, survival benefit. This too severely depresses cardiac function and often an inotropic agent and pressors are needed.

QUESTIONS

Select one answer.

1. The net result of aerobic metabolism of 1 mol of glucose is
   a. ATP (18 mol), lactate.
   b. ATP (38 mol), carbon dioxide, and water.
   c. ATP (38 mol), lactate.
   d. ATP (2 mol), lactate.

2. An estimated blood loss of 35% of blood volume reflects
   a. Class I hemorrhage.
   b. Class II hemorrhage.
   c. Class III hemorrhage
   d. Class IV hemorrhage.

3. Swan–Ganz parameters include a PCWP of 12 mm Hg and a cardiac index of 2.7 L/min/m. The patient is
   a. Normal.
   b. Hyperdynamic.
   c. Hypodynamic.
   d. Requires more information to determine.

4. An arteriovenous difference of 2.0 mL is most consistent with
   a. Septic shock.
   b. Cardiogenic shock.
   c. Hemorrhagic shock.
   d. Spinal shock.

5. Cardiac output is NOT affected by
   a. Contractility
   b. Heart rate
   c. Hemoglobin
   d. Afterload

6. A patient in being mechanically ventilated on assist/control mode. His arterial blood gases are: pH 7.55, Pco_2 24, Po_2 79, saturation 92%. The set rate is 12 breaths per minute; the patient is breathing 20 times per minute. What should be done?
   a. Increase the Fio_2.
   b. Sedate the patient.
   c. Add dead space to the circuit.
   d. Increase the rate of ventilation.

7. Low levels of erythrocyte 2,3-DPG
   a. Increase oxygen affinity.
   b. Decrease oxygen affinity.
   c. Increase acidosis.
   d. Increase alkalosis.

8. Appropriate treatment of a septic patient includes the following except
   a. Fluid resuscitation.
   b. Narrow spectrum antibiotics.
   c. Appropriate cultures.
   d. Early institution of goal directed therapy.

9. A patient has ARDS. With an Fio_2 of 75% on 10 cm H_2O PEEP, the Po_2 is only 50 mm Hg, Pco_2 is 39 mm Hg, and pH is 7.28. What would you do?
   a. Increase the Fio_2 to 100%.
   b. Increase the PEEP.
   c. Increase the ventilatory rate.
   d. Give bicarbonate.

10. A postoperative patient has a platelet count of 50,000/mm^3 and no clinically apparent bleeding. You would
    a. Transfuse 6 units HLA-matched platelets.
    b. Transfuse 6 units of banked platelets.

c. Do not transfuse unless the platelet count falls to 20,000/mm^3.

d. Administer cryoprecipitate.

SELECTED REFERENCES

Finfer S, Bellomo R, Boyce N. A comparison of albumin and saline for fluid resuscitation in the intensive care unit. *N Engl J Med* 2004;350:2247–2256.

Fulkerson WI, MacIntyre N, Stamler J, et al. Pathogenesis and treatment of the adult respiratory distress syndrome. *Arch Int Med* 1996;156:29–38.

Hebert PC, Wells G, Tweeddale M, et al. Does transfusion practice affect mortality in critically ill patients? Transfusion requirements in critical care (TRICC) Investigators and the Canadian critical care trials group. *Am J Respir* 1997;155 (5):1618–1623.

Marik PE, Pastores SM, Annane D, et al. Recommendations for the diagnosis and management of corticosteroid insufficiency in critically ill adult patients: consensus statements from an international task force by the American College of Critical Care Medicine. *Crit Care Med* 2008;36(6): 1937–1949.

Marino PL. *The ICU book*, 3rd ed. Baltimore, MD: Williams & Wilkins, 2006.

Moore FA, Haenel JB. Ventilatory strategies for acute respiratory failure. *Am J Surg* 1997;173:53–56.

Parrillo JE, Dellinger RP. *Critical care medicine—principles of diagnosis and management in the adult*. Philadelphia, PA: Mosby, 2008.

Richard C, Warszawski J, Anguel N, et al. Early use of the pulmonary artery catheter and outcomes in patients with shock and acute respiratory distress syndrome: a randomized controlled trial. *JAMA* 2003;290:2713–2720.

Rivers E, Nguyen B, Havstad S, et al. Early goal-directed therapy in the treatment of severe sepsis and septic shock. *N Engl J Med* 2001;345:1368–1377.

Sachdeva RC, Guntupalli KK. Acute respiratory distress syndrome. *Crit Care Clin* 1997;13:503–521.

Sprung CL, Annane D, Keh D, et al. Hydrocortisone therapy for patients with septic shock. *N Engl J Med* 2008;358: 111–124.

Thadhani R, Pascual M, Bonventre JV. Acute renal failure. *N Engl J Med* 1996;334:1448–1460.

Van den Berghe, Wouters P, Weekers F, et al. Intensive insulin therapy in the critically ill patients. *N Engl J Med* 2001;345: 1359–1367.

Wheeler AP, Bernard GR, Thompson BT, et al. Pulmonary-artery versus central venous catheter to guide treatment of acute lung injury. *N Engl J Med* 2006;354:2213–2224.

CHAPTER **22**

James Tait-Goodrich
Alexandre M. Scheer

Neurosurgery

HEAD INJURY

Epidemiologic Aspects

Despite significant government-guided improvements in head protection, head injuries remain the leading cause of death in the 2- to 42-year-old age group and account for significant morbidity in the United States. Each year, 10 million Americans sustain a head injury for which medical attention is sought. The incidence of head injury is 300 per 100,000 per year (0.3% of the population), with a mortality of 25 per 100,000 in North America. The majority (70%) of head injuries result from injuries sustained in motor vehicle accidents. In reviewing emergency room admissions, those patients with multiple injuries, the head remains most commonly involved area. A review of the records of fatal road accident victims showed that 75% were found to have significant injury to the central nervous system (CNS) (i.e., brain and spinal cord) at autopsy.

Types of Head Injury

Although head injuries could be classified in several different ways, the most practical categorizations are based on the mechanism of injury along with severity and morphology.

Mechanism

Although the words "closed" and "penetrating" are widely used to describe types of head injuries, they are not mutually exclusive. For practical purposes, the term *closed head injury* is usually associated with auto accidents, falls, and assaults, whereas *penetrating head injury* is most often associated with gunshot wounds and stab injuries.

Severity

The distinction between patients with severe head injury and those with mild-to-moderate head injury is distinguished with the Glasgow coma scale (GCS). Patients who open their eyes spontaneously, obey commands, and are oriented score a total of 15 points, whereas flaccid patients who do not open their eyes or talk score the minimum of 3 points. A GCS score of 8 or less has become accepted as a definition of a comatose patient. Head-injured patients with a GCS score of 9 to 13 have been categorized as "moderate," and those with a GCS score of 14 or 15 have been designated "mild." These distinctions are important, as the GCS score will often determine how aggressive the neurosurgical resuscitation measures will be.

Morphology

The advent of computer tomography (CT) and magnetic nuclear resonance (MR) scanning has revolutionized the classification and management of head injury. Head injuries may be broadly classified into two types: skull fractures and intracranial lesions.

The following sections outline the types of head trauma, specify the major types of injury that can occur, and summarize their neurosurgical management.

Blunt Head Injury

Contact

Contact injury results when an object strikes the head with sufficient force to cause tissue damage. The surface area of the object that comes into contact with the head is typically relatively small (e.g., a lead pipe or baseball bat). Often, the object is accelerating as it meets the skull, and as a result, there may also be shearing damage to the scalp. Most tissue damage is local: scalp laceration or avulsion, skull fracture, epidural hematoma (EDH), and, in more severe impacts, brain contusion underlying the area of impact.

Deceleration

The area of impact is larger with a deceleration injury than with a contact injury, as when the head's motion is stopped suddenly by a car windshield or concrete sidewalk. Brain tissue damage, for the most part, is due to sudden dissipation of forward momentum and/or shearing forces, resulting in intracranial injuries such as subdural hematoma, coup/contrecoup contusion, or, even worse for the patient, diffuse axonal shearing.

Penetrating Head Injury

Penetrating head injuries are typically more devastating than blunt injuries. The pathologic injuries to the brain tend to vary with the type of penetrating object: knife, ice pick, screwdriver, bullet (low vs. high velocity), and so on. The depth of penetration and the structures injured along the trajectory will determine both outcome and prognosis.

Gunshot Wounds

Firearm-related deaths are the second leading cause of deaths due to trauma in the western world with the United States leading with the highest frequency of firearm-related deaths. Handguns are the firearms most frequently used in fatal injuries in civilian trauma. The annual incidence of firearm-related head injury deaths in the United States is 2.4/100,000 or approximately 6,000 deaths per year. The switch from the low-power, low-velocity bullets of the "Saturday night special" to the high-power, high-velocity bullets of the 9-mm rapid repeating weapon has significantly increased the severity of gunshot injuries. The injury caused by a bullet depends more on its *velocity* than on its mass. The shock wave spreading out from the bullet often transiently elevates the intracranial pressure. The damage due to a gunshot wound includes not only direct traumatic effects as the bullet passes through brain but also the *ricochet* potential of the bullet traveling inside the skull. Hematomas often form as a result of torn blood vessels, adding to morbidity and mortality. The bullet or missile often causes additional brain injury from fragmentation and penetration of the brain by bone fragments from the skull (Fig. 22.1).

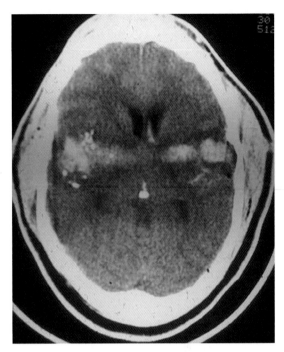

FIGURE 22.1.   A CT scan showing a gunshot wound to the head with a "through and through" injury with the bullet trajectory across the entire width of the brain. Bone fragments and blood clot can be seen along the trajectory; mortality and morbidity are exceptionally high in these types of injuries.

EXTERNAL TRAUMATIC FORCES AND THEIR EFFECTS ON THE SKULL AND ITS CONTENTS

Skull Fractures

Skull fractures are classified according to their *morphology* (e.g., linear, stellate, comminuted, depressed), their *location* (e.g., calvarial, basilar), and whether the overlying soft tissue is also involved (compound).

Linear Fractures

A linear fracture occurs whenever a hard object strikes the cranial vault with enough force to cause a temporary deformational change in the skull but without depression of the bone elements. Linear skull fractures are the most common fractures seen in children, accounting for more than two thirds of fractures. The parietal bone is the most common site of a skull fracture. A skull fracture typically involves more than one cranial bone in up to 48% of skull injuries. The most common sign is pain and swelling at the site of impact. Approximately 15% of fractures are contralateral to the external scalp lesion. Important to note is that 30% of infants and children will show no evidence of external trauma (e.g., scalp hematoma or laceration). Treatment of linear skull fractures, without adjacent injury, is almost always nonsurgical; however, reassurances need to be given to the parents or family that these fractures will usually heal well with time. However, if a linear skull fracture crosses the midline or a suture of the calvaria, these patients require further workup, and an underlying hematoma must be ruled out. Linear fractures of the calvaria are radiolucent and have well-defined margins. Linear fractures do not have sclerotic borders on skull x-ray, nor do they bifurcate (vascular grooves) as vascular structures do, this last occurs due to the overlying vessels grooving into the bone.

Depressed Fractures

Depressed skull fractures occur in roughly one quarter of all fractures. Once again, the parietal bone is the most common injury site. Compound fractures are more commonly seen in this group, with nearly half being contaminated fractures from road debris, helmet fragments among other foreign objects. EDHs (3%) and subdural hematomas (SDHs) (1%) are uncommon in these types of fractures. Most of these fractures are "greenstick" fractures, with the "ping-pong" type in infants being an excellent example. Only 15% of depressed skull fractures involve fragments that are separated from the skull. Dural lacerations are also uncommon, seen in approximately 10% of cases. External signs or findings of depressed skull fracture can be swelling and abrasions at the impact site. Scalp swelling can sometimes be large enough to actually hide the fracture from the examiner. Local pain can also limit the examination. If a fracture is suspected, a CT scan is warranted, if a CT is not available then a routine skull series can also be done. Other major problems associated with this type of fracture can also include lacerations of the dura mater and concomitant injuries of the underlying brain parenchyma which are uncommon (Fig. 22.2).

The rule of thumb in treatment of a skull fracture has been that if the fracture is depressed to a depth greater than the thickness of the skull, surgical elevation is often warranted. It used to be axiomatic that a depressed skull fracture should be elevated to reduce the possibility of pulsations of the growing brain against the depressed calvarial segment, which would

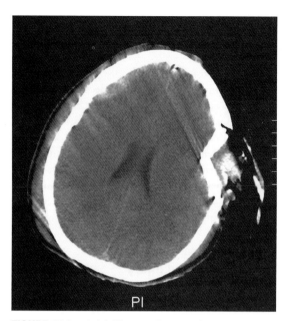

FIGURE 22.2.   Axial CT scan of a comminuted depressed skull fracture of the left fronto-temporal region resulting from an impact injury during a motorcycle accident.

likely cause underlying cortical damage. It has also been presumed that these cerebral pulsations could lead to an epileptogenic focus in the underlying injured brain. Other absolute indications for urgent elevation of depressed fractures include evidence of a dural tear, gross contamination of the wound, and evidence of a significant underlying intracerebral hematoma.

Basilar Fractures

Any of the bones that constitute the base of the skull—ethmoid (cribriform plate), frontal (orbital roof), sphenoid, temporal (squamous and petrous portions), and occipital bones—can be fractured. Most basilar skull fractures occur as a result of direct impact (occiput, mastoid, or supraorbital areas) or by energy transmitted from trauma to the mandibular or facial region to the skull base. The incidence of basilar skull fractures after head injury ranges between 3.5% and 24.0%.

Basilar skull fractures should be suspected when the clinical findings include cerebrospinal fluid (CSF) otorrhea or rhinorrhea, periorbital ecchymoses (raccoon eyes), periauricular ecchymoses (Battle's sign), and hemotympanum. Radiographic diagnosis can be difficult, and special imaging may be required to detect the fracture. Thin slice CT cuts through the temporal bones and cribriform plate are the studies most likely to yield positive findings. Intrathecal contrast dye may sometimes be needed to help determine where the CSF leak is originating from. However, even if the fracture cannot be found radiographically, this does not change the management of presumed basilar skull fracture. It also should be noted that this type of fracture is found more commonly in adults; in children, basilar skull fractures account for less than 10% of all childhood fractures.

Basilar skull fractures rarely require surgical intervention. If a CSF fistula is present, an indwelling lumbar spinal drain can be placed as the first line of treatment (typically in place for 7 to 10 days) to divert CSF away from the leak site. If spinal drainage fails, surgical intervention to repair the site of leakage is required. For basilar skull fractures that involve the temporal bone and petrous ridge, there can be also a facial nerve injury secondary to usually bone entrapment of the nerve from the fracture. Initial treatment can be the use of high-dose steroids, if there is no improvement then surgical decompression may be required to preserve the facial nerve.

Intracranial Hemorrhage

Intracranial hemorrhage types are listed in Table 22.1. The associated mortality is shown as well.

Subarachnoid Hemorrhage

Subarachnoid hemorrhage (SAH) is the most common form of intracranial hemorrhage following head injury, and it may occur as a result of trivial or severe trauma. SAH has little, if any, significance from a surgical standpoint with one exception. Blood in the subarachnoid space can interfere with the reabsorption of CSF, leading to a communicating type of hydrocephalus that may require treatment, such as ven-

triculoperitoneal shunting (see later). SAH occurs because of shearing or tearing of the plial vessels, allowing blood to diffuse throughout the subarachnoid space. Clinically, SAH may produce meningismus (i.e., stiff neck), photophobia, and headaches. In some patients, SAH can also be associated with bizarre and maniacal behavior.

Subdural Hematoma

After SAH, SDHs are the most common type of posttraumatic intracerebral hemorrhage. SDH result from a laceration or tearing of the "bridging" veins anatomically crossing between the cortex and the venous sinuses. SDH can occur as a result of a direct laceration of the cortical vessels, or contusion of the cortex with bleeding into the subdural space from torn pia–arachnoid membranes. These bleeds develop in the anatomic space between the inner layer of the dura and the arachnoid membrane.

SDHs are found in 9% to 13% of all severe head injuries. They may be classified as a simple SDH (i.e., hematomas not associated with brain injury) or a complicated SDH (those associated with laceration of the parenchyma and intracerebral hematomas). The mortality associated with simple SDH is about 22%, whereas for complicated SDH, it is 50% to 90%. Seventy percent of the intracerebral hematomas, lacerations, and contusions associated with SDH arise from contrecoup injuries; these are most commonly located in the temporal and frontal lobes, the areas most susceptible to this type of injury.

SDHs are also categorized according to the time period between injury and the appearance of the clinical symptoms.

Acute Subdural Hematoma

Acute subdural hematomas (ASDHs) are defined as those that produce symptoms within 48 hours of the injury. ASDHs are most commonly associated with a severe head injury. Frequently, the impact that produces the ASDH also causes severe injury to the underlying brain parenchyma. Unfortunately, an ASDH is also associated with high morbidity and mortality rates (60% in young patients and 90% in elderly patients).

The clinical presentation and course are determined by two factors: the severity of the injury at the time of impact and how rapidly the hematoma develops. The quality of consciousness varies from sustained loss of consciousness (17%), to fluctuations

TABLE 22.1	Mortality from Intracranial Hemorrhage
Type of Hemorrhage	**Mortality (%)**
Acute subdural hemorrhage	50–90
Acute intraparenchymal hemorrhage	30–60
Acute epidural hemorrhage	10–20
Acute subarachnoid hemorrhage	20–50

from lucidity to unconsciousness (17%), impaired consciousness with lucid intervals (13%), and unimpaired consciousness (29%). Clinical findings can include anisocoria (dilation of the pupil), contralateral hemiparesis, abducens palsy, hemiparesis, decerebration, aphasia, and seizures. Anisocoria and contralateral hemiparesis are referred to as Kernohan's sign, and in 85% of patients, they indicate the site of the hematoma (i.e., the side on which anisocoria appears) (Fig. 22.3).

The radiographic appearance of an ASDH on CT scan is that of a hyperdense crescentic mass adjacent to the inner table of the skull and overlying the affected hemisphere (Fig. 22.3). A significant midline shift and a mass effect on the brain hemisphere are commonly observed. For smaller hematomas with little mass effect, the gyral pattern of the brain can often be seen; this finding is very helpful to differentiate the subdural hematoma from the EDH. Although most commonly found over the convexity, ASDH may also be found in the interhemispheric space, layering along the tentorium, and in the posterior fossa, the last being a more ominous finding.

Early definitive treatment (i.e., surgical evacuation within the first 4 hours) has been shown to reduce mortality significantly. Patients who undergo operation within 4 hours have a mortality rate of 30% compared with 90% for patients in whom operation is delayed beyond 4 hours. If a CT scan is not available and the patient is deteriorating, the order of trephination placement starts on the side of the dilated pupil and follows this order (a) temporal, (b) frontal, and (c) parietal. If necessary, these burr holes can be connected to develop the "question mark" skin flap and craniotomy, a commonly used flap used in patients with trauma.

Subacute Subdural Hematoma

The subacute subdural hematoma (SSDH) produces neurologic deficits after more than 48 hours but less than 2 weeks after the injury. Typically, the patient has a history of trauma with or without loss of consciousness followed by gradual improvement but then neurologic deterioration, with findings that may include hemiparesis, cranial nerve deficits, and depressed mental status.

Evacuation of the hematoma is warranted if there is an impending risk of herniation or if midline shift is significant and cerebral compression is seen on the CT scan. Surgical treatment consists of a (a) formal craniotomy if the clot is solid or (b) trephination with external drainage if the clot has significantly liquefied. The gradual decrease in density of a SSDH on CT scan (Fig. 22.4) evolves over 10 to 12 days, with the hematoma becoming isodense with the brain parenchyma; this change can make the diagnosis of SSDH difficult. In these cases, the only clues to the presence of an SSDH may be obliteration of the sulci and a lateralizing shift of the ventricles (Fig. 22.4).

Chronic Subdural Hematoma

The chronic subdural hematoma (CSDH) presents more than 2 weeks after the injury. Its incidence is estimated to be 1/100,000 to 2/100,000 per year. Most patients are elderly or of late middle age. Typically, 20% to 50% of the patients have no history of

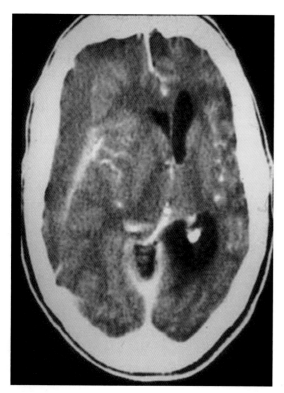

FIGURE 22.3.   Axial CT scan of a patient seen in the emergency room after a fall down a flight of stairs. A subdural hematoma is seen as a high signal bright area between the skull and brain. The bright high density layering against the brain is due to fresh blood that has accumulated in the subdural space. There is significant life-threatening right to left brain herniation (also called falcine and/or cingulate herniation). The right frontal ventricle is severely compressed and shifted, the occipital horn cannot be identified due to mass effect.

trauma. Predisposing factors for CSDH include alcoholism, epilepsy, shunting procedures for hydrocephalus, and anticoagulation therapy.

Approximately 7 to 10 days after bleeding into the subdural space, a semipermeable membrane forms around the clot. Fibroblasts migrate in from the surrounding meninges and establish a thin inner and a thick outer membrane around the hematoma. How the hematoma expands is unclear. One hypothesis states that as red blood cells and hemoglobin molecules break down, the osmotic pressure increases, leading to inflow of CSF through the semipermeable membrane and causing the hematoma to increase in size. In some studies in which the albumin/γ-globulin and albumin/total protein ratios in subdural fluid, serum, and the hematoma have been examined, the results indicate that the osmolality of the hematoma does not change with time. It is likely that albumin diffuses across the membrane, and that recurrent bleeding into the clot accounts for the enlargement of the CSDH.

The clinical presentation of a CSDH may be variable. The more typical picture is of slowly progressive symptoms, such as hemiparesis (45%), hemianopsia (7%), oculomotor palsy (11%), and impaired consciousness (53%), which develop 3 to 4 weeks after the injury.

The CT scan appearance of a CSDH is that of an isodense lesion, often lenticular in shape. Commonly, there can be a mixture of hypodense and hyperdense areas, indicating recent hemorrhage into CSDH (Fig. 22.5).

If a CSDH becomes symptomatic, the treatment of choice is surgical evacuation. Craniotomy, burr holes, and twist drill craniotomies have all been used successfully. The most commonly used surgical treatment is twist drill trephination over the site of maximal clot thickness. After drainage, external catheters are left in place for 24 to 48 hours to assist in the removal of any residual fluid. The patient is kept supine to decrease the likelihood of hematoma

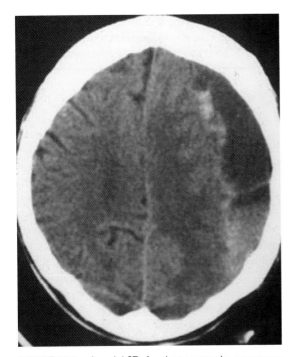

FIGURE 22.4. An axial CT of patient sent to the emergency room from a nursing home because of a recent altered state of consciousness after a fall from a bed. The CT findings are of a chronic subdural with an isodense collection between the skull and bone causing shift and mass effect on the brain. The gyral pattern of the brain can be seen abutting the subdural collection.

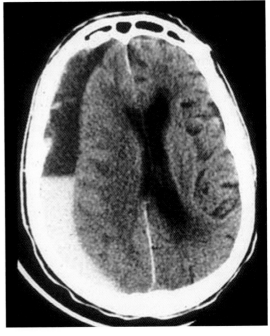

FIGURE 22.5. An axial CT scan of a mixed chronic and acute subdural hematoma. An isodense lesion can be seen between the brain and skull along with a hyperintense component layering out below. The darker image is the chronic subdural and the bright white hyperintense signal is fresh blood that has bled into the chronic SDH.

reaccumulation. Because of the natural atrophy of the brain with aging, this fails to re-expand allowing reoccurrence in the dead space; this has been reported in up to 45% of patients; however, about 75% of these patients are able to return to their premorbid status even when a residual hematoma remains.

Subdural Hygroma

Subdural hygromas represent about 10% of all traumatic intracranial mass lesions. Hygromas are collections of a clear, xanthochromic, or slightly bloody fluid in the subdural space. They are thought to arise from tears in the arachnoid membrane that allow escape of CSF into the subdural space. Most patients are asymptomatic. Those patients who become symptomatic present with symptoms similar to those of an ASDH or CSDH. The CT scan, the diagnostic study of choice, shows crescentic areas of hypodensity with a density signal similar to that of CSF. In contrast to a CSDH, there are no membranes and no enhancement after contrast infusion. Patients who are symptomatic undergo trephination or twist drill craniotomy. Because recurrence is common, the patient requires frequent follow-up.

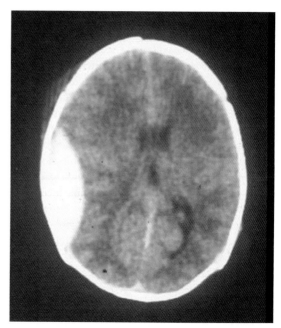

FIGURE 22.6. An axial CT scan showing a large acute epidural hematoma in the typical "lens-shape" appearance. The increased brightness is due to acute bleed in the epidural space. The smooth place of the clot against the dura is what differentiates this from a subdural hematoma.

Epidural Hematoma

The epidural hematoma (EDH) is defined anatomically as a collection of blood between the skull's inner table and the dura mater. The incidence of EDH is low (0.4% to 4.6%) compared with that of an ASDH (50%). The source of bleeding is arterial in 85% of the cases and venous in 15%. The middle meningeal artery is the most common source of bleeding in middle fossa EDH. About 70% occur laterally over the hemispheres with the pterion as the epicenter. The remaining 30% have a frontal, occipital, or posterior fossa location.

In the "textbook" presentation of an EDH (which occurs in only 10% to 30% of cases), there is (a) brief loss of consciousness following the injury, (b) restoration of consciousness (the so-called *lucid interval*), and then (c) progressive obtundation, hemiparesis, anisocoria, and coma. It must be remembered that a lucid interval can also occur in such conditions as SDH, though it is more commonly associated with an EDH. The appearance of the lucid interval depends on the rate at which the expanding clot enlarges. Other clinical presentations include headaches, emesis, seizures, and hyperreflexia.

Approximately two-thirds of the patients have anisocoria (85% ipsilateral to the EDH) and contralateral hemiparesis secondary to midbrain compression from a herniated uncus (temporal lobe). *Kernohan's phenomenon* (a dilated pupil contralateral to the EDH and ipsilateral hemiparesis) occurs in about 15% of patients. These clinical findings result from compression of the opposite cerebral peduncle against the tentorial notch by the expanding hematoma. CT scans show a high-density lenticular (biconvex) area adjacent to the skull that rarely cross the skull suture lines (Fig. 22.6).

Only those patients with EDH whom become symptomatic are treated. A large craniotomy is performed to expose and control the bleeding site and then evacuate the hematoma. The mortality rate, even with surgical treatment, varies between 15% and 45%. Mortality rates are low in children (5%) and much higher in the elderly (35% to 45%). Patients who have had periods of wakefulness before surgery have a better prognosis; those who are decerebrating or in a coma at presentation have a mortality greater than 50%.

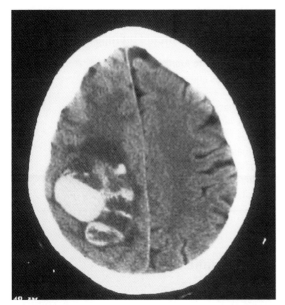

FIGURE 22.7. Axial CT scan of a patient who sustained a baseball bat injury to the left skull region. The CT reveals an acute cerebral contusion injury in the left posterior temporal region with acute intraparenchymal blood (hyperintense region) with surrounding edema.

Cerebral Contusion

Like contusions elsewhere in the body, those affecting the cerebrum are composed of areas of hemorrhage, necrosis, and infarction. Contusions occur in brain areas underlying the site of an external impact (coup lesion) but also commonly on the side of the skull opposite from the site of impact (contrecoup lesion). The temporal poles and undersurfaces of the frontal lobes are the most frequent sites of contusion. The CT scan shows areas of increased density mixed with areas of hypodensity, indicating hemorrhage and edema, confirming the diagnosis (Fig. 22.7). Small or deep

lesions are managed conservatively. Large lesions with mass effect are often removed surgically. The mortality rate varies from less than 5% to 60%, depending on the size of the contusion, its location, and the associated injuries. Contusions of the brain stem are seen after a shear-type injury and carry a significantly worse prognosis in terms of functional recovery.

Shaken Baby Syndrome/Nonaccidental Injury Syndrome

One of the most difficult situations that can occur in an emergency room is that of reaching a diagnosis for the child presenting with a head injury whose history is inconsistent with the historical findings. Most states now require the reporting of any suspected cases of child abuse. Recently, pediatric neurosurgeons have described clinical findings that might help identify the child who has been subjected to a nonaccidental injury (NAI), the terminology currently preferred for the entity formerly referred to as "shaken baby syndrome" (Table 22.2).

Depressed Skull Fracture in the Young Child

When is a skull fracture likely to result from abuse? When a fracture occurs on the front or side of the head, the examiner must carefully obtain a history, as these locations are suggestive of an abuse injury. Children have a primitive protective reflex, the Moro reflex, so when they fall forward, the outstretched hands tend to break the fall. A fracture on the back of the head is usually not due to abuse. When the young child falls backward (e.g., out of a crib), no protective reflex comes into play. In the infant, the typical fractures are of the "ping pong" type, that is, a depression in the bone that resembles a dent in a ping pong ball. Again the key point is that it is always vitally important that the clinical history makes sense and matches

---

TABLE 22.2	**Identifying the Child with a Nonaccidental Injury— Current Criteria**

1. Uncertain history or one that seems to be at odds with the physical findings
2. New onset of seizures associated with (a) retinal hemorrhage (due to sudden elevation intracranial pressure, subhyaloid bleed); (b) intradural surface hemorrhages on CT or MR.
3. Additional findings of new or healing fractures of long bones, in particular rib fractures (usually pathognomonic for NAI). Bruise marks and/or fingernail marks on the upper area of the child are potential sings of abuse.
4. Long-term findings: enlarging head, slowed development, failure to thrive, hyperirritability, and increased muscle tone.

the mechanism of injury. Other associated injuries commonly seen in NAI are listed in Table 22.2.

Radiographic Findings of Nonaccidental Injury

A finding that was once commonly categorized as benign external hydrocephalus has recently become recognized as a sequela to NAI. In a brain that has been "shaken" (i.e., subjected to repeated rapid acceleration–deceleration cycles), the plial and dural bridging vessels are torn and so bleed. As the blood is resorbed, the CSF circulating pathways can be partially occluded, and with time the brain atrophies and pulls away from the skull. As a result of the lack of CSF resorption, the skull continues to enlarge, and these children typically have a head circumference in the greater than 95% category. These radiographic findings are best revealed by CT or magnetic resonance imaging. For lack of a better term, it has been called the "shriveled walnut sign" (Fig. 22.8). The developmental outcome in these children is extremely poor. Their development is often moderately to severely delayed, and they often require long-term chronic care.

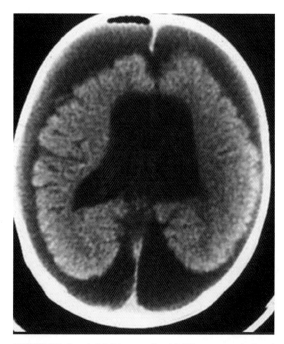

FIGURE 22.8. Axial CT scan of a child that was a victim of a NAI. The "shriveled walnut sign" is present here with the very generous subarachnoid spaces due to the traumatic brain atrophy and the brain atrophying and pulling away from the skull.

TABLE 22.3	Posttraumatic Syndrome— Clinical Findings

Headache (mild to excruciating)
Neck stiffness and cervical muscle spasm
Irritability
Forgetfulness (memory loss)
Postural vertigo (dizziness)
Enuresis
Disturbance in sleep patterns
Episodic aggressive behavior
Decline in school performance (impaired concentration, easily distracted)

Posttraumatic Syndrome

Often forgotten in long-term management of head injury is the posttraumatic syndrome, a common sequela in a patient who has lost consciousness as the result of a head injury. Table 22.3 lists the conditions commonly seen with posttraumatic syndrome. These findings may be immediate or may not develop for several days. With aggressive pain management and physical therapy, and in some cases psychological therapy, posttraumatic syndrome can usually be adequately treated.

MANAGEMENT OF HEAD INJURY

A detailed discussion of the cerebral dynamics and physiologic responses after a head injury is beyond the scope of this chapter, but certain basic principles must be kept in mind when managing the head-injured patient. In addition, the treatment of head injury and in particular the bedside management of increased intracranial pressure has undergone some significant changes in recent years. A critical parameter for adequate brain function and survival after an injury is blood flow to the neurons and supporting glial structures. Depending on the facility, cerebral blood flow (CBF) can be difficult to quantitate without recourse to invasive monitoring. But having said that, the cerebral perfusion pressure (CPP), which is directly proportional to the CBF, can be easily calculated at the bedside:

$$CPP = MAP - ICP$$

MAP is the mean arterial pressure, and ICP is the intracranial pressure. This is a simple but fundamental

TABLE 22.4	General Principles for Managing the Head-Injured Patient

Mannitol (0.25–1.00 g/kg maintaining a serum osmolality of 300–325 mOsm)
Hyperventilation (pCO2 30–35 mm Hg)
Barbiturates—used only in refractory patients that have failed other modalities
Ventriculostomy for CSF removal
Steroids—no longer used

concept in the management of head injury. The CPP in a normal adult is higher than 50 mm Hg. The therapeutic endpoint is simply that of maintaining an adequate perfusion pressure of the brain, typically in the head injured greater than 60 mm Hg (recently revised down from the earlier criteria of 70 mm Hg). With head injuries, the variable that compromises CPP is an increase in ICP. The treatment of elevated ICP is logically aimed at manipulating the three major components that make up the cerebral compartment: brain parenchyma, CSF volume, and blood volume.

In the case of elevated ICP, the brain parenchyma can be manipulated therapeutically by means of osmotic diuretic agents, which dehydrate cells (by removing free water) and thus reduce cerebral volume. Typically, mannitol is used in the range of 0.25 to 1.0 g/kg; the dose is repeated every 6 hours until a serum osmolality of 300 to 325 mOsm (exceeding 325 mOsm is counterproductive) is reached (Table 22.4). Historically, mannitol was routinely used in head injury but guidelines have now changed. The current view is that mannitol should be used only in cases where there is impending brain herniation or progressive neurologic deterioration. Diuresis is not recommended in patients without signs of significantly increased ICP. Furosemide can also be used with mannitol. Blood electrolytes must be closely monitored during diuresis to avoid rapid or extreme alterations. When diuresis is used, the blood volume and pressure must be kept up (i.e., euvolemia) to maintain adequate brain perfusion, which is always the end goal. Agents to keep blood pressure up (e.g., pressors) and hence provide better cerebral perfusion are routinely used in the management of head injury. A Foley catheter must be in place to monitor fluid output and especially if diuresis is being untaken.

Placing an external ventricular drain via a ventriculostomy and removing CSF can also manipulate the CSF volume and reduce ICP. ICP can also be adjusted by giving furosemide (Lasix), which is thought to decrease CSF production by interfering with chloride transport at the choroid plexus level.

Hyperventilation (via endotracheal intubation) can be used to decrease the size of the intracranial blood volume compartment, thereby reducing ICP (Table 22.4). Respiratory alkalosis produces a reflex vasoconstriction of the cerebral vasculature, reducing the total blood volume. A distinct disadvantage, and one that must be kept in mind, is that the blood volume can be so lowered that adequate perfusion of the brain is compromised, a condition called iatrogenic cerebral ischemia. Like the use of mannitol, the present recommendations for hyperventilation are to maintain a tidal volume and respiratory rate that maintain the Pco_2 within 35 to 40 mm Hg. In cases of acute decompensation, hyperventilation can be used to reduce ICP by bringing the end tidal Pco_2 down to 30—but only for short periods, as a too much can lead to vasoconstriction and a decrease in adequate CBF. The response of the brain to hyperventilation is rapid, but the effect ceases after 48 to 72 hours, when the kidneys adjust the blood pH to normal levels.

Steroids (glucocorticoids) were once commonly administered to head-injured patients (and unfortunately are still used by some physicians). Several large randomized trials have provided clear evidence that steroids exert no beneficial effect on morbidity and mortality in head-injured patients, as a result of these studies steroids are no longer routinely used by major academic centers in their treatment protocols for the head-injured patient.

Other measures that can be used in the management of head injury patients are sedation, muscle paralysis, head elevation, and control of systemic hypertension (i.e., driving up the arterial blood pressure to increase cerebral perfusion). The use of barbiturates (induced coma) is reserved only for patients with severe head injury who have become refractory to all other medical and surgical management; its aim is to provide cerebral protection by decreasing the cerebral metabolic rate ($CMRO_2$). Once commonly used for head injury, barbiturates are now reserved for patients with severe injury with an intractable high ICP and low GCS scores (Table 22.5).

In summary, the initial evaluation of a head injury includes a careful history, physical examination, and a neurologic evaluation. The protocol and prognostic factors are outlined in Table 22.6.

TABLE 22.5	Intracranial Pressure (ICP) Levels	
CP Level	**mm Hg**
Normal	1–10
Slightly increased	11–20
Moderately increased	21–40
Severely increases	>40[a]

[a]Head-injured patients that present with ICP >40 mm Hg have an extremely poor prognosis even with aggressive management.

SPINAL CORD INJURY

Epidemiology

Spinal cord injury most commonly affects the young, with the victims mostly male and in their second or third decade. The most common etiology remains motor vehicle accidents, followed by falls, sporting injuries, and more recently in the urban areas, penetrating gunshot injuries. The most common injury site is the mid to lower cervical spine. The outcomes of such injuries can be devastating and are evenly

TABLE 22.6	Summary of the Initial Evaluation of a Head Injury

1. Provision for adequate airway and ventilation
2. Observations of vital signs: evaluate for associated injuries (e.g., cervical and spine)
3. State of consciousness
4. Neurological examination
5. GCS evaluation
6. History of trauma
   a. Mechanism of injury
   b. Loss of consciousness (immediate? and how long)
   c. Progression of symptoms (lucid interval?)
   d. Evaluate for rug and alcohol use or other medical history (which might contribute to altered neurological findings)
7. Associated injuries: cervical spine radiographs or CT to rule out fractures or injury with evaluation of C1 to C7-T1
8. Prognostic factors: better outcomes seen with the following:
   a. High GCS scores (>13)
   b. Younger age
   c. Good pupillary response to light
   d. Normal intracranial pressure
   e. Brainstem reflexes present
   f. Epidural ≫ subdural > intraparenchymal injury

divided between quadriplegia and paraplegia. The mortality rate can be as high as 40% in quadriplegics.

Definitions

Incomplete Spinal Injury

With an incomplete spinal cord lesion, some residual motor or sensory function remains below the level of the lesion. Possible residual findings include sensation or movement of the extremities, voluntary rectal sphincter contraction, or voluntary toe movement. The three types of incomplete lesion include the Brown-Séquard syndrome (cord hemisection with ipsilateral motor loss and contralateral sensory loss below the lesion), central cord syndrome, and the anterior cord syndrome.

Complete Spinal Cord Lesions

A complete spinal cord lesion is one in which no motor or sensory functions are preserved below the level of the lesion. With time as many as 5% of these patients can progress to incomplete lesions, but most patients recover no function.

Spinal Shock

Often, there is confusion between spinal and neurogenic shock. Spinal shock refers to the loss of motor, sensory, and reflex functions below the level of the lesion that occurs immediately following the injury and spontaneously resolves 6 to 16 weeks later. Resolution does not mean improvement of neurologic function, but, rather, a change from a lower motor neuron lesion to an upper motor neuron lesion with concomitant hyperreflexia, hypertonia, and spasticity. By definition, spinal shock is associated with a complete lesion. Neurogenic shock refers to the condition of the patient who presents in a sympathectomized state with bradycardia, hypotension, and hypothermia.

Stability of the Cervical Spine

Cervical spine stability can be understood by dividing the spine into three functional columns or components: an anterior column made up of the anterior longitudinal ligament and anterior half of the vertebral body and disk; a middle column made up of the posterior longitudinal ligament and the posterior half of the vertebral body and disk; and a posterior column composed of the bony arch along with all associated ligaments: ligamentum flavum, supraspinous and interspinous ligaments, facet joints, and capsular ligaments. It is generally considered that a spine is stable if only one column is disrupted and unstable if two or three columns are damaged. A three-column injury is considered extremely unstable and always required external stabilization (e.g., cervical collar, stretcher board) until surgical correction and stabilization can be accomplished.

Types of Cervical Spine Injury

Atlantooccipital Dislocation

Atlantooccipital dislocations make up 1% of spinal injuries; they are also known as craniocervical injuries. These injuries can be immediately fatal or present with minimal neurologic deficits. Most fatalities result from anoxia secondary to a low bulbar/high cervical injury that affects the respiratory center causing a cessation of spontaneous breathing.

Atlas (C1) Fractures

Also known as Jefferson fractures (Fig. 22.9), atlas (C1) injuries comprise about 15% of cervical fractures. The ring of C1 is broken in at least two places, with the mechanism of injury most commonly axial loading. Because of the large capacity of the spinal canal at this level, these patients uncommonly present with neurologic deficits. The anteroposterior "open-mouth" view shows lateral displacement of the lateral masses of C1.

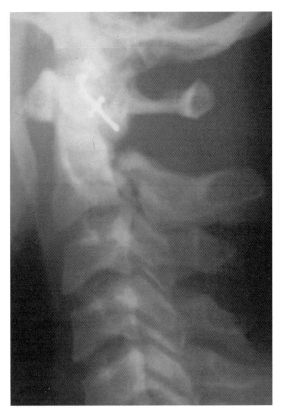

FIGURE 22.10. Lateral spine radiograph from the base of the skull to C5. A hangman's fracture of C2 can be seen. The radiographic clues are the widened interspinous distance between C1 and C2, and a fracture that can be seen in the lamina of C2 with downward disarticulation of the C2 lamina.

Axis (C2) Fractures

Hangman's Fracture

The hangman's fracture is through the pedicles of C2 (Fig. 22.10) at the pars interarticularis. The usual mechanism of injury is hyperextension. As with C1 fractures, neurologic deficits are rare (with exception of an intentional hanging). This injury is diagnosed with plain films or CT scans.

Odontoid Fractures

Fractures through the body or the dens of C2 (Fig. 22.11) are classified as type I, II, or III odontoid fractures (Table 22.7). These injuries are usually caused by hyperflexion with resultant displacement of C1 on C2. Because of the generous subarachnoid space around the cervical spine at this level, most patients have no neurologic deficit but do complain of severe neck pain.

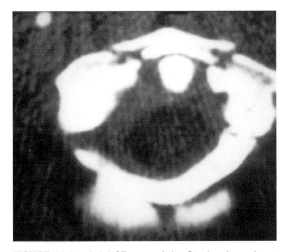

FIGURE 22.9. Axial CT scan of the C1 showing a burst fracture (Jefferson fracture) that occurred during a motor vehicle accident where an unbelted passenger was thrown directly forward into the windshield. There are multiple fractures present, typically referred to as a "burst-type" fracture of the ring of C1.

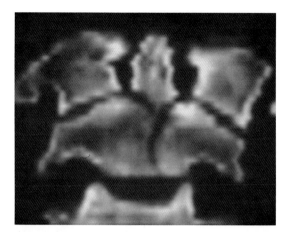

FIGURE 22.11. CT reconstruction of a type III odontoid fracture. There is a fracture through the base of the dens extending into the body of C2.

Subaxial Fractures

Several fracture patterns affect the cervical spine. The most commonly affected area is the C5 to C6 level, as this region has the greatest mobility in the cervical spine. Injuries include burst fractures of the vertebral body, teardrop fractures, subluxations, locked (or jumped) facets, and fractures of spinal processes (spinous or transverse). Cervical spine stability can be assessed by the use of dynamic spinal films (flexion–extension) and by looking for movement between the vertebral bodies (Fig. 22.12). Lower cervical injuries are associated with a higher rate of neurologic damage because the spinal cord/spinal canal ratio is less than that at higher cervical levels.

Management

Field Management

1. Immobilization of any patient suspected of having a spinal cord injury is imperative. It may be accomplished with the use of a hard collar (e.g., Philadelphia) or sandbags.

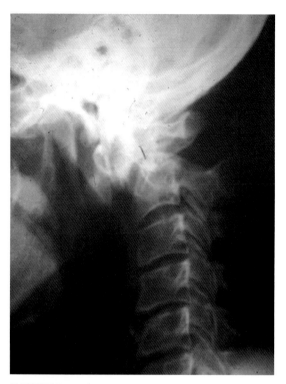

FIGURE 22.12. Lateral cervical spine radiograph revealing a subluxation fracture of C1 on C2. The diagnostic clue here is the lack of alignment of the edges of C1 on C2. The space between the lamina of C1 and C2 is also increased implying ligamental injury. Flexion/extension views would most likely show this malalignment even more dramatically. In doing flexion/extension films, they should always be supervised by a physician in an awake patient monitoring for any change in pain or new neurological complaints. In the obtunded patient flexion/extension views, in most cases, should be avoided. A rapid acquisition CT scan can also be used.

2. Systemic blood pressure must be maintained to prevent further injury secondary to ischemia. Pressors and intravenous fluids are used as necessary.
3. Adequate oxygenation must be maintained. If endotracheal intubation is necessary, caution is

TABLE 22.7	Odontoid Fractures		
Type	**Location**	**Stability**	**Treatment**
I	Tip of dens	Stable	Rarely required
II	Through the base of the dens	Unstable	Surgical fusion
III	Extending through body of C2	Stable/unstable	Halo immobilization

taken not to hyperextend the neck. In some cases, a fiberoptic intubation might be indicated.

Hospital Management

1. Immobilization is continued.
2. A thorough neurologic examination is performed.
3. A nasogastric tube is inserted to decompress the stomach and prevent functional ileus.
4. A Foley catheter is placed, as urinary retention is common in spinal cord injury.
5. In the past, a series of studies indicated a beneficial effect of very high dose corticosteroids (methylprednisolone) in spinal cord injury. Recent studies have indicated that this is not the case, so the recommendation now is to avoid the use of high dose steroids—this decision though still remains at the discretion of the treating physician.

Atlantooccipital dislocation is treated by means of stabilization and surgical fusion. Monitoring for apnea during the first 48 hours should also be considered. Treatment of Jefferson fractures and C2 fractures requires halo immobilization for 8 to 16 weeks. The outcome can be gratifying in most cases. Depending on the level and type of fracture, unstable fractures may be treated with skeletal traction (e.g., Gardner-Well tongs) or weights, halo immobilization, or surgical fusion (e.g., plates, screws, or wiring).

Decompressive surgery is reserved for patients with incomplete injuries who demonstrate external compression and those who, after reduction and alignment, still show (a) progression of neurologic deficits; (b) complete block; (c) presence of bony fragments or soft tissue/hematomas in the spinal canal, causing cord compression; or (d) compound fractures or penetrating trauma.

Contraindications to surgical treatment include a clinical presentation of a complete spinal cord injury after 24 hours, medical instability, and central cord syndrome. Patients should be studied with plain films, CT scans, and MRI. The recent development of soft tissue software for rapid CT acquisitions and CT 3-D reformatting of the images have been extremely helpful in sorting out various spinal injuries.

BRAIN TUMORS

Epidemiology

In almost 25% of all patients with cancer, the brain and its coverings are affected at some time in the clinical course. The average mortality from brain tumors ranges between 6/100,000 and 8/100,000 per year in the United States. Analysis of mortality rates for primary brain neoplasms indicates that the age-specific curve rises to a maximum during the seventh and eighth decades. The overall age-adjusted mortality rate is higher for men and for Caucasians.

Classification

Historically, classification of brain tumors has been based on their histologic features. A classification based on the embryonic origins of neural tissues is presented in Table 22.8. Table 22.9 shows the approximate incidence of each type of tumor.

Clinical Presentation

The clinical findings associated with brain tumors reflect their anatomic location and their effect on brain function. A "progressive" neurologic deficit is the most common presentation (68%) of brain tumors. These deficits can be caused by any of several mechanisms: (a) direct compression of neural tissue; (b) direct destruction or invasion of brain tissue by tumor cells; or (c) alteration of normal regional blood supply by the tumor. Other common clinical findings include headaches (54%), seizures (26%), and motor weakness (45%). Typically, signs and symptoms of progressive and generalized increased ICP are detected: decreased or cloudy mentation and consciousness, papilledema, vomiting, and Cushing's triad or phenomenon (bradycardia, systemic hypertension, and irregular respirations). Increased ICP may result from an increase in tumor size or from hydrocephalus secondary to obstruction of CSF circulation pathways. Cerebral edema (of the vasogenic type), associated with many brain tumors, is also a common cause of increased ICP (Fig. 22.13).

Although the clinical presentation of supratentorial tumors holds to the pattern described earlier, the presentation of infratentorial tumors varies in that seizures are rare. Most posterior fossa tumors present with signs and symptoms of increased ICP, headache, nausea, vomiting, gait ataxia, vertigo, diplopia, and lower cranial nerve (VII, VIII, IX, X, and XI) deficits. These findings are caused by compression of the pons and medulla and their respective cranial nerves (Figs. 22.13 and 22.14).

TABLE 22.8	Classification of Brain Tumors

Origin	Tumor Type
Neural tube derivatives	
Glial cell	
Astrocytes	Astrocytoma
	Anaplastic astrocytoma
	Glioblastoma multiforme
Oligodendrocytes	Oligodendroglioma
Ependymocytes	Ependymoma
	Choroid plexus papilloma/carcinoma
Neurons	Medulloblastoma (primitive neuroectodermal tumor)
Neuro crest derivatives	Ganglioma
	Ganglioglioma
Schwann cells	Schwannoma (acoustic neuroma)
	Neurofibroma
Archnoid cell	Meningioma
Melanocyte	Primary CNS melanoma
Other cells	Pituitary adenoma
Adenohypophyseal cells	
Vascular cells	Hemangioblastomas
Notocord	
Adipose cell	Chordoma (clivus or sacral)
Germ cell	Lipoma
Other	Germinoma
	Craniopharyngioma
	Teratoma

TABLE 22.9	Frequency Distribution of Brain Tumors in Adults and Children

Tumor	%
Adults	
Glioblastoma	52.0
Meningioma	16.0
Astrocytoma	10.0
Pituitary adenoma	7.0
Neurolemona	1.5
Medulloblastoma (PNET)	1.3
Ependymoma	1.2
Children	
Medulloblastoma/astrocytoma	24.0
Brain stem (glioma)	9.0
Glioblastoma	20.0
Ependymoma	8.0
Craniopharyngioma	5.6
Meningioma	1.5
Pinealoma (germ cell tumor)	2.0

Diagnosis

The state-of-the-art method for brain tumor diagnosis remains the MRI, usually with contrast (gadolinium) enhancement. CT scanning is also valuable, especially for assessing bony involvement and planning the surgical approach. Cerebral angiography has become less important with the introduction of CT angiograms and MR angiograms. The use of SPEC and PET scans has become more and more important in the preoperative diagnostic workup, though rarely affects the surgical planning. Depending on tumor location and histologic makeup, serum endocrine levels (prolactin, growth hormone, cortisol, luteinizing hormone [LH], follicle-stimulating hormone [FSH], triiodothyronine [T_3], and thyroxine [T_4]) and tumor markers (human β-chorionic gonadotropin, carcinoembryonic antigen, and α-fetoprotein) may be measured to aid in diagnosis. But having said that most patients end up going to surgery for both definitive diagnosis and surgical decompression.

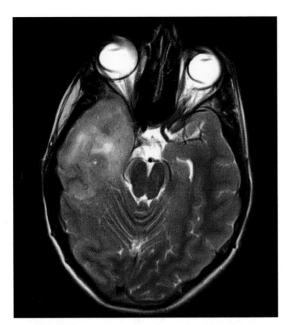

FIGURE 22.13. Axial MR (T-2) scan of a 14-year-old male that presented with 2 weeks of progressively severe headaches, aura that he described as a burning rubber taste. This MR reveals findings of a right temporal lobe infiltrating and intra-axial brain tumor. In the left temporal region, there is clear loss of normal brain architecture when compared with the left side. An anaplastic astrocytoma was found at surgery.

Management: Clinical Classification and Treatment

Astrocytoma

Astrocytomas are the most common primary intraaxial brain tumor, presenting with about 12,000 cases per year in the United States. Various classifications have been proposed for grading astrocytomas. The Kernohan system divides astrocytomas into grades I to IV, based on histologic findings, with grade I being the most benign and grade IV the most malignant. At present, a three-category system is more frequently used: low-grade astrocytoma (Kernohan grades I and II), anaplastic astrocytoma (Kernohan grade III), and glioblastoma multiforme (Kernohan grade IV). This classification is based on the degree of anaplasia, cellular pleomorphism, and number of mitoses—also called "mitotic index," neovascularity, and necrosis (Fig. 22.15).

For certain types of astrocytoma (childhood cystic cerebellar astrocytoma and pilocystic astrocytoma), surgery is the principal mode of treatment, with gross total surgical resection ideal. For most other astrocytomas, surgery is only part of the treatment: radiation

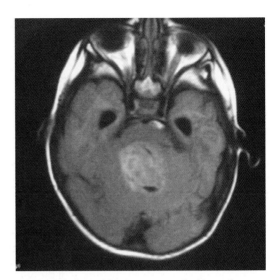

FIGURE 22.14. A child that presented with ataxia, severe headaches, and a sixth nerve palsy. This MR scan revealed a high-density lesion in the midline in the cerebellum. The pons has been compressed and flattened secondary to the tumor. The ventricles are dilated, causing hydrocephalus secondary to the fourth ventricle being occluded by the mass effect of the tumor. At surgery, this lesion was found to be a fourth ventricle ependymoma.

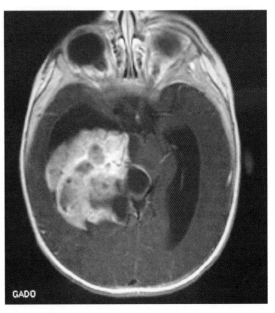

FIGURE 22.15. Axial MR (T1) scan demonstrating a contrast-enhancing lesion in the right temporal region with surrounding edema, multiple cystic structures, tumor necrosis, mass effect, and shift secondary to the tumor. Surgical diagnosis revealed this to be a glioblastoma multiforme.

therapy and chemotherapy are also administered. Glioblastomas have the worse prognosis, with a 1-year survival of 30% compared with 60% for anaplastic astrocytomas. The 5-year survival rate of patients with malignant astrocytomas remains at less than 5%.

Meningioma

Meningiomas account for 15% to 20% of primary intracranial tumors, with a peak incidence at 45 years and a female/male ratio of 2:1. Approximately 25% of adolescent patients with neurofibromatosis also develop meningiomas. These tumors are slow growing and arise from arachnoid cells. Meningiomas are parasagittal in 20%, over the convexity in 15%, in the sphenoid bone in 30%, and in the midline falx cerebri in 10% (Fig. 22.16). Commonly associated with meningiomas is an overlying hyperostosis of the bone, best seen on CT scan. These tumors are extra-axial and with rare exception (i.e., those with sarcomatous changes <5%) are histologically benign.

The extent of surgical removal is the most important factor in determining long-term outcome; complete excision implies cure, but this is not always possible. Incompletely resected tumors are reported to

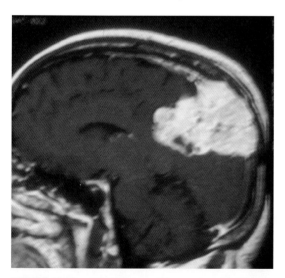

FIGURE 22.16. MR (T1) scan with contrast of a 55-year-old man who presented with visual loss and severe headaches occurring over several months. A large parafalcine meningioma is present on this MR scan causing significant compression of the occipital lobes bilateral and leading to the visual loss. This enhancing lesion can be seen to be clearly arising from the meninges of the falx, there is also clearly invasion of the overlying skull.

recur at rates of 37% to 85%. However, the 5-year survival rate for patients with meningioma is high, with 90% to 92% typically reported, indicating an excellent prognosis. Focus beam irradiation (e.g., Gamma knife) may be used as an adjunctive treatment for incompletely removed meningioma.

PITUITARY TUMORS

As with other CNS tumors, a number of classifications have been used to systematize pituitary tumors. Light-microscopic classification divides them into acidophils (prolactin, growth hormone, or TSH producers), basophils (ACTH, LH, FSH producers), and chromophobes (typically a nonsecreting tumor). Pituitary tumors can be separated into functional (secreting) and nonfunctional tumors. More specifically, they can be categorized according to the hormone they produce (e.g., prolactinomas). Their clinical presentation is either as an endocrinologic disturbance (e.g., Cushing's disease) or a mass effect (e.g., visual field deficits due to compression of the optic chiasm) (Fig. 22.17).

Clinical Presentation

Cushing's Syndrome

Cushing's syndrome is caused by hypercortisolism due to excessive ACTH production. Patients typically have centripetal obesity, moon facies, hirsutism, buffalo hump, striae, hypertension, and diabetes mellitus. The diagnosis is normally based on a positive dexamethasone suppression test and appropriately elevated hormones.

Acromegaly

Acromegaly results from excessive production of growth hormone. The patient presents with increased hand and/or foot size, frontal bossing, prognathism, macroglossia, hypertension, sometimes a carpal tunnel syndrome, and soft tissue swelling.

Pituitary Apoplexy

Pituitary apoplexy refers to the abrupt onset of neurologic deterioration, usually associated with headaches, visual deterioration or loss, ophthalmoplegia, and decreased mental status. It is caused by an abrupt hemorrhage within the tumor or by necrosis of the tumor with swelling. Pituitary apoplexy has a rather high association with pregnancy in that pregnant women with previously undiagnosed pituitary tumors

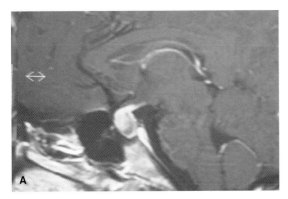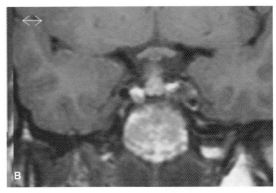

FIGURE 22.17. **A:** Sagittal MR of a pituitary tumor; in this case, a pituitary nonsecreting adenoma enlarging the sella turcica causing upward compression of the optic chiasm—the typical visual loss is a bitemporal visual field loss. **B:** Coronal MR of same patient showing a cross-section of the pituitary tumor, the optic chiasm can be seen tented over the enhancing tumor in the midline.

can present with pituitary apoplexy secondary to a sudden hemorrhage during pregnancy.

Progressive Visual Loss

With a pituitary tumor, progressive visual loss is caused by a mass effect of a tumor that extends above the sella to encroach on the optic chiasm. The most common visual loss is progressive bitemporal hemianopsia resulting from compression of the medial retinal fibers in the chiasm. This finding is easily demonstrated with a gross (finger-based) visual fields examination.

Treatment

Secreting pituitary tumors can be treated pharmacologically using dopamine agonists (bromocriptine), somatostatin analogs (octreotide), serotonin antagonists, and anti-inflammatory drugs (dexamethasone). Surgical treatment is indicated for Cushing's disease, prolactinomas (prolactin level over 500 ng/mL), acromegaly, large tumors causing mass effect, and pituitary apoplexy. Radiation therapy is not routinely recommended postoperatively. Patients should be followed yearly; and if after reoperation, a recurrence cannot be resected and the tumor continues to grow, focus beam radiation therapy is indicated.

CONGENITAL MALFORMATIONS

Hydrocephalus

CSF is normally produced in the adult at a rate of 500 mL/day. If CSF resorption or flow is blocked, hydrocephalus results. Its estimated prevalence is 1.5% with an incidence of 2/1,000 live births. Hydrocephalus is classified as communicating (malabsorption of CSF at the arachnoid villi) or noncommunicating (blockage of CSF circulation proximal to the arachnoid granulations). The etiologies of hydrocephalus include congenital conditions such as stenosis of the aqueduct (also called aqueductal stenosis) (38%), Chiari II malformation/myelomeningocele (29%), and Dandy–Walker malformation. Acquired conditions such as meningitis, intraventricular/SAH (e.g., bleeding from an aneurysm), intraventricular hemorrhage due to prematurity, or tumors blocking CSF pathways can also cause hydrocephalus (Fig. 22.18).

For the most part, hydrocephalus is a surgical condition, although in certain situations, patients with hydrocephalus can be managed medically until normal CSF resorption resumes. For this purpose, the carbonic anhydrase inhibitor acetazolamide (Diamox) is used. Multiple spinal taps are performed routinely in low-birth-weight infants with posthemorrhagic hydrocephalus with significant success. In those patients who do not clear their hydrocephalus go on to require a diversionary shunting of CSF. For most types of hydrocephalus, a ventricular shunt to the peritoneum, cardiac atrium, or pleural cavity is placed. Ventriculoperitoneal shunting is the preferred mode of shunting. Plural and atrial terminus shunts are reserved for patients where the peritoneum cannot be used. If hydrocephalus is caused by a tumor blocking CSF pathways, tumor removal to allow normal circulation usually results in resolution of the problem and symptoms. An alternative treatment for hydrocephalus is the third ventriculocisternostomy, a procedure whereby an endoscopic hole is made in the

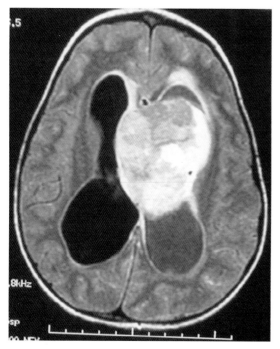

FIGURE 22.18. An axial MR (T1) of a 5-year-old child that present with lethargy and severe headaches. A large midline bright intraventricular tumor can be seen causing obstruction of the third ventricle and foramen of Monro leading to a second obstructive hydrocephalus. The severe ventricular dilatation can be clearly seen in this study. The tumor turned out to be a low-grade astrocytoma.

floor of the third ventricle, this is done to bypass an obstruction in the third and fourth ventricle.

Spina Bifida

Spina bifida occulta is defined as congenital absence of the spinal vertebral elements (spinous process and lamina). The defect is covered with normal skin and often presents as an incidental finding on spine radiographs. Spina bifida occulta occurs in approximately 15% to 20% of the US population, so it is not rare. Spina bifida aperta (also called myelomeningocele) refers to the condition in which, in addition to maldevelopment of the vertebral elements, the overlying skin and subcutaneous tissue fail to close, exposing the underlying spinal cord and related neural elements.

Meningocele

Meningocele refers to a skin- or membrane-covered cystic midline mass that is typically found in the lumbodorsal region in 10% of patients with spina bifida. The dorsal halves of the vertebrae are missing at one or more levels. The contents of the sac comprise CSF and meninges; no neural elements are present. The prognosis and end results are excellent after surgical treatment.

Myelomeningocele

Myelomeningocele represents the most common form of neural tube defect, with an incidence of 2/1,000 to 3/1,000 live births (Figs. 22.19 and 22.20). But having

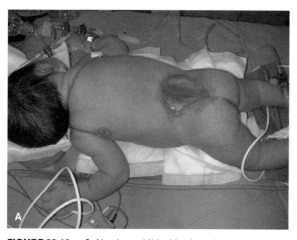
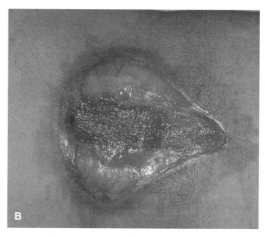

FIGURE 22.19.   A: Newborn child with a large lumbosacral myelomeningocele with an open myelomeningocele sac and neuroplacode seen in the middle of the defect. **B:** A close up view of the neuroplacode with the open neural defect clearly seen and the exposed spinal cord.

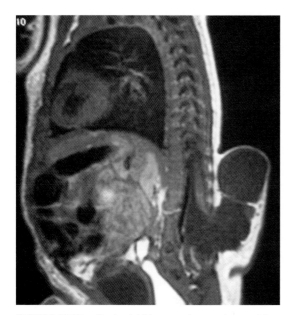

FIGURE 22.20. Sagittal MR scan of a newborn with a myelomeningocele. The spinal cord can be seen coming down the spinal canal and entering the fluid-filled meningeal sac has herniated out through the spina bifida defect.

said that the recent recommendations regarding the nutritional importance of folic acid given during pregnancy has definitely reduced the incidence of myelomeningocele substantially, the numbers are likely in the range of 2/3,000 births in developed countries. In addition, the regular use of prenatal ultrasound has also reduced the number of live births in countries where abortion are allowed.

Myelomeningocele is a condition representing failure of the posterior neuropore to close. The clinical findings vary with the level of the lesion. The most severe and debilitating forms are myelomeningoceles at the thoracic level; the least severe are located at the low lumbar and sacral levels.

The neurologic examination discloses sensory and motor changes below the level of the lesion. Varying degrees of anesthesia, weakness, or paralysis of the lower extremities are common, as are urinary and fecal incontinence and orthopedic abnormalities (clubfoot, scoliosis, hip dislocation). The coincidence of hydrocephalus with spina bifida is high, ranging from 75% to 90%. Treatment involves surgical closure of the defect with a lifetime of follow-up care to deal with multiple problems regarding ambulation, bladder care, orthopedic problems, and so on.

Encephalocele

Encephaloceles make up a group of congenital anomalies that produce varying degrees of protrusion of neural tissue through a cranial bone defect. The pathogenesis reflects failure of the anterior neuropore to close and fuse on about the 25th day of gestation. In the United States, the most common location is the occipital area, but other locations include the frontal, parietal, and frontonasal bones. Frontoethmoidal and basal encephaloceles are found less often in the United States and are more common in Mexico and the Indo-China areas.

The clinical presentation of an encephalocele is a bulging lesion in any of the aforementioned locations that may be apparent at birth. Lesions at the anterior cranial base rarely offer evidence of their presence at birth but, rather, do so later in life by obstructing airway passages or by the development of hypertelorbitism or unexplained meningitis from communication with the nasal passageway.

Treatment consists in surgical removal and closure. The prognosis depends on the size of the lesion (i.e., amount of brain involved) and its location. Posterior encephaloceles, those that occur in the posterior fossa and occipital region, have a high incidence of associated hydrocephalus, ranging from 30% to 60%.

Dermal Sinus Tract

The dermal sinus tract typically begins at the skin surface and communicates internally with the subarachnoid space. It is lined with epithelium or sometimes with sebaceous and hair material. The lesion is most commonly found at either end of the neural tube, along the midline. The three most frequent locations are the nasion, inion, and the lumbosacral region, typically always in the midline. Although innocent in appearance, their potential for producing meningitis is high; indeed, such tracts should never be probed or injected with contrast, as it may precipitate an infection. Lumbosacral lesion, often called "sacral dimples" can be confused with the pilonidal sinus, but because the latter lesion does not communicate with the subarachnoid space, it does not cause meningitis. Most true sacral dimples that communicate with the subarachnoid space appear above the gluteal cleft, whereas the pilonidal sinus is typical within the gluteal cleft and not visible unless the gluteal cleft is spread open.

Treatment requires complete surgical excision. The lesion must be surgical followed until intrathecal and any associated dermoid lesion along the tract are also removed.

VASCULAR DISORDERS

Cerebral Aneurysms

As in any other part of the body, an aneurysm of a cerebral vessel represents a weakening of the vessel wall leading to dilatation and possible rupture. The most common site is at an arterial bifurcation. In the United States, approximately 28,000 cerebral aneurysms rupture per year and are associated with high morbidity and mortality rates. About 90% to 95% of cerebral aneurysms are located in the carotid system and 5% to 15% in the vertebrobasilar system. The etiology may be congenital (berry aneurysms), atherosclerotic, embolic, infectious, or associated with other medical conditions such as polycystic kidney disease, fibromuscular dysplasia, connective

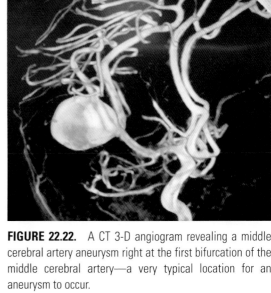

FIGURE 22.22.   A CT 3-D angiogram revealing a middle cerebral artery aneurysm right at the first bifurcation of the middle cerebral artery—a very typical location for an aneurysm to occur.

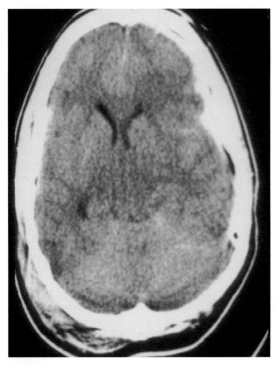

FIGURE 22.21.   Axial CT scan of a 37-year-old woman who suddenly developed the "worst headache of my life," fell to the group sustaining a hematoma over the left occipital region. She arrived in the emergency room with a stiff neck and photophobia and over a period of an hour became obtunded. The CT shows a picture of diffuse subarachnoid hemorrhage with blood throughout. An angiogram revealed a large posterior communicating artery aneurysm.

tissue disease (e.g., Ehlers–Danlos syndrome, Marfan's) coarctation of the aorta, and the like. Aneurysms most commonly present with an SAH and a severe, sudden, explosive headache (commonly described as the "worst headache of my life") along with photophobia and meningismus. Aneurysms can be diagnosed by lumbar puncture (presence of fresh blood—though this is a less common technique today), CT scan looking for subarachnoid blood, MRI, and angiography (Figs. 22.21 and 22.22). With the recent advances in software for CT and MR, the use of CT and MR angiograms has become the more common diagnostic choice than the cerebral angiogram. Surgical treatment includes isolating the neck of the aneurysm and applying a surgical spring aneurysm clip. In recent years, the introduction of endovascular approaches to aneurysms has led to a significant increase of treatment with placement of stents and coils within the aneurysm and thereby obliterating the aneurysm sac. The decision as to whether to coil or clip an aneurysm is a mutual decision made by the consulting neurosurgeon and interventional neuroradiologist. Cerebral aneurysms that occur secondary to infection, referred to as mycotic aneurysms, are typically treated first with antibiotics and in most cases resolve. If the aneurysm persists despite antibiotics, then surgical clipping may be required.

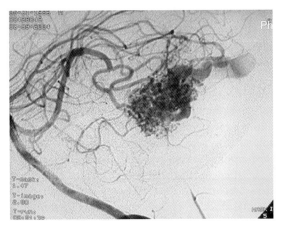

FIGURE 22.23. A lateral cerebral angiogram showing the nidus of a large posterior fossa, intracerebellar AVM being feed primarily by the superior cerebellar artery with venous drainage going to the transverse sinus.

Arteriovenous Malformations

Arteriovenous malformations (AVMs) form as a result of failed development of a capillary bed between the arterial and venous circulations. Clinical presentation is most commonly due to hemorrhage (e.g., SAH) or an intracerebral clot and associated neurologic deficit.

Seizures are not uncommon and are thought to be due to chronic ischemia caused by blood flow "steal." Diagnosis is made by cerebral angiogram, CT angio, or MR angio; in recent years, the CT and MR have become more commonly used but this very much depends on the equipment available at the respective hospital or clinic (Fig. 22.23).

Treatment of a ruptured AVM involves evacuation of the clot (if clinically significant) and surgical excision of the AVM. Endovascular obliteration of small AVMs is also sometimes possible. In smaller (typically <2.5 cm) AVMs that occur in deep eloquent areas of the brain, Gamma knife radiation (or other types of focused beam radiation) can also be used as an adjuvant therapy.

INFECTIONS

Brain Abscess

Brain abscesses are loculated infections found within the brain parenchyma (Fig. 22.24). They are approximately twice as common in men. At present, acquired immunodeficiency syndrome (AIDS) has become the most significant factor in the development of a brain abscess. The clinical presentation is nonspecific and

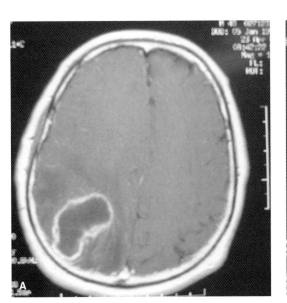
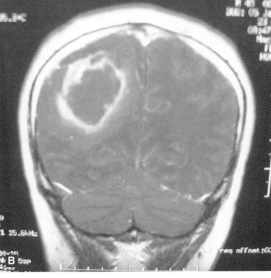

FIGURE 22.24. **A:** MRI (T1) with contrast showing an irregular necrotic ring-enhancing lesion in the left parietal occipital region. Patient presented with a week-long history of increasing headaches and visual changes. Subsequent workup revealed the patient had an endocarditis. **B:** MR coronal view with contrast of same patient again showing the typical ring enhancement that is irregular and with a necrotic center which is pus.

mostly related to the increase ICP (headaches, nausea, vomiting, lethargy). *Streptococcus* is the most frequent pathogen (30% to 50%). Multiple organisms can be cultured up to 80% of the time and typically include anaerobes. In AIDS patients, *Toxoplasma* is the most common cause of brain abscess. Pathophysiologic mechanisms include (a) hematogenous spread (lung abscess, cyanotic and congenital heart disease [left-to-right shunt]), pulmonary arteriovenous fistulas, endocarditis, empyema, and bronchiectasis; (b) contiguous spread from nearby infected nasal or mastoid sinuses; (c) dental extractions; and (d) introduction of organisms as a sequel to penetrating cranial trauma or from neurosurgical procedures.

Treatment depends on the age of the abscess. Early in the infection (<2 weeks) and in the cerebritis stage, antibiotics alone may be used. If there are signs of elevated ICP, neurologic findings, or the abscess is close to the ventricles (an ominous sign because of the possibility of rupture), surgical evacuation is the treatment of choice in conjunction with intravenous antibiotics for 6 to 8 weeks.

Subdural Empyema

The subdural empyema is a very serious infection of the CNS. The infection forms in a preexisting space whose lack of barriers allows easy spread. Such a space permits only poor penetration of antibiotics. The subdural empyema occurs in the subdural space, not within the brain substance, as seen with an abscess. The subdural empyema commonly starts within the paranasal sinuses (60% to 75%) or from the mastoid sinuses (15%). Patients typically present with fever (>90%), focal neurologic deficits (80% to 90%), meningismus (80%), headaches, and seizures. The severe inflammatory reaction with resulting thrombophlebitis of cerebral veins often leads to a high morbidity and mortality.

Subdural empyema is a neurosurgical emergency, and surgical evacuation with irrigation is the treatment of choice, along with a prolonged course of intravenous antibiotics. Once neurologic deficits occur, their reversal is rare, and a mortality rate of 20% is found even today despite early aggressive intervention.

Spinal Epidural Abscess

The spinal epidural abscess is an infection localized to the spinal canal, found mostly in the epidural space; it

occurs with an incidence of 1/10,000 hospital admissions. The thoracic level is the most common location, followed by lumbar and cervical levels. Hematogenous spread accounts for up to 50% of cases. Foci of infections include the skin, abdominal contents, endocardium, urinary tract, lower respiratory tract, and pharynx or oral cavity. Another mechanism is local extension of infections such as decubitus ulcers, psoas abscesses, abdominal wounds, mediastinitis, and pharyngitis.

Patients with a history of diabetes, intravenous drug use, or AIDS are the groups at highest risk for a spinal abscess. *Staphylococcus aureus* is cultured in more than 50% of cases. The patients typically present with severe back pain over the involved segments, bowel and bladder dysfunction, motor weakness, sensory changes, and abdominal distension.

Treatment consists in surgical evacuation with intravenous antibiotics. Patients with marked neurologic deficits rarely improve.

QUESTIONS

Select one answer.
1. The lesion most likely to cause neurologic injury and permanent sequelae is
   a. Basilar skull fracture.
   b. Subdural hematoma.
   c. Epidural hematoma.
   d. Brain stem shear injury.

2. Subdural hygromas:
   a. Are common following head injury.
   b. Are made up of a blood collection.
   c. Show as hyperdense lesions in a CT scan.
   d. Are treated with burr holes or twist drill trephination.

3. A complete spinal cord lesion is seen in which of the following?
   a. Anterior spinal syndrome.
   b. Central cord syndrome.
   c. Brown-Sequard syndrome.
   d. Spinal shock.

4. Jefferson fracture is a fracture of the
   a. Odontoid process.
   b. Ring of C1.
   c. Pedicle of C2.
   d. Pars interarticularis of C3.

5. Which of the following is the most common brain tumor in an adult?
   a. Ependymoma.
   b. Low-grade astrocytoma.
   c. Glioblastoma multiforme.
   d. Pituitary adenomas.

6. Cushing's disease is associated with an increase of which of the following hormones?
   a. Somatostatin.
   b. ACTH.
   c. TSH.
   d. GnRH.

7. Hangman's fracture refers to a fracture of which of the following?
   a. Odontoid process.
   b. Ring of C1.
   c. Pedicle of C2.
   d. Pars interarticularis of C3.

8. Which of the following is the most common type of myelodysplasia?
   a. Encephalocele.
   b. Dermal sinus tracts.
   c. Myelomeningocele.
   d. Meningocele.

Indicate whether each statement is true or false.

9. Neurogenic shock and spinal shock are the same clinical entity.

10. Tachycardia is associated with Cushing's phenomenon.

11. Meningiomas are usually benign tumors.

12. Subdural empyemas need to be treated urgently.

13. Type III odontoid fractures usually do not need surgical stabilization.

14. Chronic subdural hematomas are usually treated with craniotomy and evacuation.

15. Subarachnoid hemorrhage is the most common form of hemorrhage following head injury.

SELECTED REFERENCES

Brain Trauma Foundation. Guidelines for the management of severe traumatic brain injury. *J Neurotrauma* 2007;24 (suppl 1):S1–S106.

Bullock R, Chestnut R, Chajar J, et al. Guidelines for the surgical management of traumatic brain injury. *Neurosurgery* 2006;58:S21–S262.

Burger PC. Classification and biology of brain tumors. In: Youmans JR, ed. *Neurological surgery*. Philadelphia, PA: W.B. Saunders, 1990;2967–2999.

Goodrich JT. Acute repair of penetrating nerve trauma. In: Loftus C, ed. *Neurosurgical emergencies*. New York: Thieme Medical Publishers, 2008:305–317.

Goodrich JT, Blum KS. Management of scalp trauma. In: Mclone D, ed. *Pediatric neurosurgery. Surgery of the developing nervous system*. 4th ed. Philadelphia, PA: W.B. Saunders, 2001:565–572.

Goodrich JT, Staffenberg DA. Plastic surgical aspects of large open myelomeningoceles. In: Ozek M, Cinalli G, Maizner WJ, eds. *The spina bifida: management and outcome*. Milan, Italy: Springer Verlag, 2008:197–202.

Gordon D, Goodrich JT. Intracranial vascular malformations. In: Fisher M, Aldermann E, Kriepe R, et al., eds. *Textbook of adolescent health care*. New York: Mosby, 2008.

Keating RF, Goodrich JT. Congenital malformations repair techniques. In: *Plastic techniques in neurosurgery*. 2nd ed. New York: Thieme Medical Publishers, 2004.

La J, Marmarou A, Choi S, et al. Mortality from traumatic brain injury. *Acta Neurochir* 2005;95(suppl):281–285.

Okazaki H. *Fundamentals of neuropathology*, 2nd ed. New York: Igaku-Shoin, 1989:95–114.

Schoenberg BS. *Neurobiology of brain tumors*. Baltimore, MD: Williams & Wilkins, 1991:3–18.

Seiff ME, Goodrich JT. Postoperative considerations in pediatric brain tumors. In: Keating RF, Packer R, Goodrich JT, eds. *Tumors of the pediatric nervous system*. New York: Thieme Medical Publishers, 2001:477–501.

Young W, Ranshoff J. Injuries to the spinal cord. In: The Cervical Spine Society Editorial Committee, ed. *The cervical spine*. Philadelphia, PA: JB Lippincott, 1989:464–525.

Paul T. Haynes
David Kaye
Alok Sharan

CHAPTER 23

Orthopaedic Surgery

T he objective of this chapter is to provide a condensed overview of the major areas of orthopaedic surgery including trauma, adult orthopaedics, and pediatric orthopaedics for the general surgery resident. Significant advances have been made in orthopaedic surgery and any overview greatly simplifies areas of controversy, and in those instances the effort is made to present the most widely held opinions. Areas where the orthopaedic surgeon and general surgeon overlap, especially within the management of polytraumatized patients are stressed. The remainder is intended to provide a method of quick and easy review of specific entities within orthopaedics.

TRAUMA

Polytrauma

Management of the polytraumatized patient represents an area of medicine in which a multidisciplinary approach has had a significant impact on the outcome. In 2005, the number one cause of death for patients in their first four decades was unintentional injury with motor vehicle accidents accounting for most deaths. Unintentional injuries rank fifth in the top 10 most common causes of death in the United States. This equates to 160,000 deaths out of a total of 50 million injuries. The cost to society is staggering: more than 400 billion dollars in total with more than 80 billion in medical costs and more than 320 billion in productivity losses.

Most deaths during the first hour after injury are due to head injury and shock. It is estimated that at least one-third of these deaths are potentially preventable. Early orthopaedic intervention in the management of polytraumatized patients has the greatest impact on that group of patients who survive after the first few hours but are nonetheless seriously injured. The two greatest causes of death late in the management of polytraumatized patients are adult respiratory distress syndrome (ARDS) and infection. The management of the patient's orthopaedic injuries can have a significant impact on these entities. Beginning in the early 1980s, it became clear that stabilization of pelvic fractures and long bone fractures led to distinctly improved outcome for polytraumatized patients.

Starting in the 1980s, the trauma community began to realize that early fracture stabilization of the polytraumatized patient resulted in lower incidences of pulmonary complications. In 1989, Bone et al. demonstrated in a prospective randomized trial that delayed fracture stabilization (after 48 hours) in patients with a femur fracture and other multiple injuries (head and thoracic injuries) resulted in an increased incidence of complications. This delay resulted in higher incidences of ARDS, fat emboli syndrome, pneumonia and a longer hospital stay and intensive care unit stay. There was a statistically significant increase in hospital costs for delayed fracture stabilization. Brundage et al. demonstrated in a retrospective study in 2002 that in patients with femur fractures and concomitant head and/or thoracic injuries, early femur stabilization (within first 24 hours) resulted in lower incidences of acute respiratory distress syndrome, pneumonia, a decreased hospital length of stay and intensive care unit length of stay (Fig. 23.1).

Recently, "Damage Control Orthopaedics" has gained generalized approval and momentum. Damage control orthopaedics focuses on stratifying polytrauma patients into groups that range from those with isolated orthopaedic injuries to those with multiple injuries. Early fracture care versus temporary fracture stabilization with delayed definitive fracture

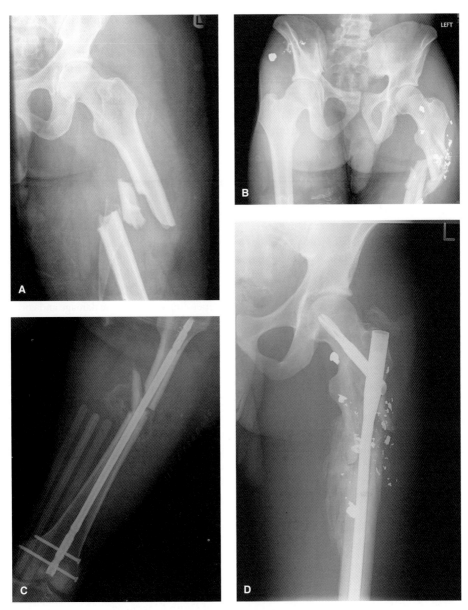

FIGURE 23.1. A 25-year-old male after multiple gun shot wounds to the pelvis and hip. **A:** Comminuted subtrochanteric femur fracture resulting from gunshot wound. **B:** Contralateral iliac wing fracture. **C:** Long cephalomedullary device placed. **D:** Three months postoperatively.

care in patients with multiple injuries is a clinical decision facilitated by a multidisciplinary approach. As shown above, work by many different authors have shown that early treatment of orthopaedic injuries in patients with multiple injuries is associated with reduced risk of pulmonary complications. But, as recently proposed and implemented, not all patients benefit from early definitive fracture treatment such as intramedullary nailing for femoral fractures. The main tenet for damage control orthopaedics is to achieve provisional fracture stabilization (often with an external fixator), control hemorrhage, and address soft tissue injuries to avoid or lessen the so-called second hit to the multiple injured patient. The definitive fracture care is planned and performed when the patient is adequately resuscitated. For a patient with an open femur fracture with a major head and/or chest trauma, application of an external fixator will stabilize the fracture and allow for soft tissue treatment and rest while lessening the additional insult of the procedure itself. As shown by Scalea et al., Taeger et al., and Seibel et al., operative time, blood loss, and physiologic stresses to the patient are decreased with this approach, and there is no increased rate of procedure-related complications. The definitive treatment of intramedullary nail fixation is planned when the patient has an improved physiologic status. In a prospective randomized trial by Pape et al. the operative burden of the second-hit phenomenon was studied by measuring the levels of IL-6 and IL-8. They concluded that early (<24 hours) fracture stabilization with intramedullary nail fixation resulted in a sustained inflammatory response but not with the use of damage control orthopaedics.

Not only does early operative intervention lead to a decrease in ARDS, it makes mobilization of the patient substantially easier. It is easier to transport the patient for tests and makes achievement of an upright posture possible. This, of course, leads to benefits such as lower incidences of pneumonia, urinary tract infection, and decubitus ulcer. Finally, the ability to mobilize a patient makes it substantially easier to meet his or her nutritional needs, leading to further reduction in the late death rate.

Open Fractures

Commonly, patients with serious trauma also have open fractures. Early management of the open fracture involves basic concepts: irrigation and debridement of the open wound and stabilization of the soft tissue envelope, which may involve closure by secondary intention, by skin graft, or by muscle flap. Recreation of the soft tissue envelope leads to an environment more conducive to bone healing and protects against infection. Preoperative treatment includes immediate sterile irrigation, sterile wound coverage, and splinting. Tetanus booster is provided. Antibiotic treatment is instituted immediately with a cephalosporin for Gram positive coverage–Gram negative coverage is added depending on the degree of contamination; penicillin is added for gross contamination to cover clostridium and barn yard infections. Ideally, the formal irrigation and debridement occurs within the first 6 hours. In addition, fracture stabilization via intramedullary nailing, plate osteosynthesis, or application of external fixator is performed after irrigation and debridement. Depending on soft tissue damage and contamination, an open fracture may be indicated for a "second-look" or second irrigation and debridement at 24 to 48 hours.

The classification of open fractures by the Gustilo method has prognostic significance (Table 23.1). Open fractures that are of a low-energy type with a small wound in general do well. These fractures have much the same prognosis as closed fractures. A grade I fracture is a fracture with a low-energy fracture pattern (i.e., very little comminution, little or no soft tissue loss, and a wound opening of 1 cm or less). A grade II open fracture is a fracture that may have mild comminution of the fracture site; there may be a small amount of soft tissue loss, and the wound shows an opening of 1 to 5 cm in the skin. There is little or

TABLE 23.1	Gustilo and Anderson Classification of Open Fractures
Fracture Type	**Description**
Type I	Wound ≤ 1 cm; clean; usually an inside-out wound; fractures are simple transverse or short oblique; unlikely comminution
Type II	Wound 1–5 cm; extensive soft tissue damage with some crush component; fractures are simple transverse or short oblique; minimal comminution
Type III	Extensive soft tissue envelope damage; usually high-energy injuries; often with severe crushing component
Type IIIa	Extensive soft tissue wound but with adequate bone coverage; fractures are often segmental; minimal periosteal stripping
Type IIIb	Extensive soft tissue wound with periosteal stripping and bony exposure; will require soft tissue procedure for closure; usually contaminated wounds
Type IIIc	Extensive soft tissue wound with a vascular injury necessitating repair

no crush injury component to the soft tissue injury. Grade III fractures, which are subdivided into subtypes A, B, and C, show a high-energy fracture pattern, usually with marked comminution on the radiograph. There may be moderate to severe tissue loss and a significant element of crush. The wound is, in general, 5 cm or more. A type III-A fracture has no exposed bone at the end of the irrigation and debridement procedure. Type III-B has exposed bone remaining, and type III-C has an associated vascular injury.

The likelihood of complications such as infection and nonunion increases with each grade, although most complications are seen with type III-B and III-C fractures. Early management of these fractures via the methods stated above leads to improved outcome of the specific fracture, positively benefiting management of the patient as a whole.

REGIONAL TRAUMA

A variety of fractures in locations throughout the body are discussed briefly. Emphasis is on general forms of management and specific complications that can be expected in any particular area. The concept of acceptability of fracture position is involved in the management of most diaphyseal fractures. Although the position may not be anatomic, it should be close enough that there is no functional or cosmetic disability. Fractures into joints frequently lead to severe functional disability with only small displacement of the fracture fragments. This disability can be compounded by prolonged immobilization. Intra-articular fractures are therefore frequently dealt with operatively to diminish the degree of functional disability, whereas many diaphyseal and metaphyseal fractures can be treated conservatively.

Fractures of the Clavicle

Clavicle fractures usually occur after a direct fall on a shoulder. The clavicle is clinically separated into a medial third, middle third, and distal third with fractures occurring 5%, 85%, and 10%, respectively. Clavicle fractures, especially through the medial and middle thirds, are typically treated conservatively. This treatment involves a sling in the adult and possibly a sling and swathe in a child for 4 to 6 weeks. Fractures along the outer third at the acromioclavicular (AC) junction can lead to marked displacement because of

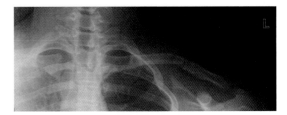

FIGURE 23.2.   Middle third clavicle fracture.

disruption of the ligamentous complexes and has a higher rate of nonunion and therefore may require fixation. Fractures of the clavicle can infrequently be associated with vascular and nerve injury, pneumothorax, skin compromise and nonunion. Open reduction and internal fixation may be performed with neurovascular injury, severe ipsilateral concomitant injuries, many distal third fractures, middle third fractures in select patients, those with deformity, or skin compromise and nonunion after attempted closed treatment (Fig. 23.2).

Fracture of the Scapula

Although they are uncommon injuries, the diagnosis of a scapular fracture should raise suspicion for other serious injuries. Because the scapula is well protected by a large posterior muscle mass and the thorax anteriorly, high energy would be required to create a fracture. Associated injuries have been quoted as occurring between 35% and 98% and may include additional ipsilateral fractures (clavicle, humeral shaft, shoulder dislocations), pneumothorax, and pulmonary contusion, and spine and neurovascular injuries. Most scapular fractures are treated nonoperatively, although the presence of those fractures should certainly raise the suspicion for other injuries.

Fractures of the Proximal Humerus

Fractures of the proximal humerus are seen commonly in the elderly and have a female-to-male ratio of 2:1 likely secondary to osteoporosis. Patients typically present splinting the involved extremity and will complain of severe shoulder pain and exhibit often severe diffuse edema, shoulder and upper arm ecchymosis and crepitus. Axillary nerve function should be evaluated by assessing sensation over the lateral aspect of the deltoid.

Fractures of the proximal humerus involving the surgical neck can be grouped into two general categories: impacted or displaced. Fractures in which the fragments have been driven together have an innate stability. This type of fracture can be treated conservatively with early immobilization in a sling and then various exercise programs in 2 to 3 weeks. The fractures that have displacement of the fragments tend to require operative treatment.

Fractures involving the anatomic neck are rare and notoriously difficult to treat with closed reduction. These fracture patterns likely require prosthetic replacement (hemiarthroplasty) in the elderly and attempts at open reduction internal fixation in younger patients. Fractures that involve the surgical neck and tuberosities of the proximal humerus are more common and have been subclassified by Neer into two-, three-, and four-part fractures as well as fracture dislocations. The parts include the greater and lesser tuberosities, humeral shaft, and humeral head. Those that involve displacement of the neck fracture and displacement of both tuberosities are treated by hemiarthroplasty. Fractures with displacement of the shaft and single tuberosity may be dealt with by open reduction and internal fixation. These same fractures, when associated with a dislocation, are often treated by hemiarthroplasty. The rationale has to do with the remaining blood supply to the humeral head fragment and the likelihood of survival of the humeral head. With displaced surgical neck fractures with displacement of both tuberosities or one tuberosity and the head dislocated, the likelihood that the nutrient blood supply has been disrupted is high.

In cases where the tuberosities are intact but the surgical neck fracture is displaced, the fracture can frequently be close reduced but may redisplace. Stabilization with some form of intermedullary rod or percutaneous wire fixation may be necessary.

Fracture of the Greater Tuberosity

Nondisplaced fractures of the greater tuberosity are treated similarly to stable or impacted fractures of the surgical neck. The arm is immobilized for a short time (2–3 weeks), and then rapid mobilization occurs. Displaced fractures of the greater tuberosity involve disruption of the rotator cuff in addition to the mechanical difficulties caused by displacement of the tuberosity. These injuries are generally dealt with operatively.

Fractures of the Humeral Shaft

Approximately 90% of humeral shaft fractures can be successfully treated conservatively. A considerable amount of angulation and up to 3 cm of bayonet apposition is acceptable with no residual functional or cosmetic compromise. They are managed with 3 to 4 weeks of immobilization in a coaptation splint followed by a period of another 3 weeks of limited motion often placed in a cast-brace. Full motion is initiated around the sixth week.

The structure most likely to be injured is the radial nerve. This is especially true of fractures at the junction of the middle and distal thirds. Controversy exists over the indications for surgical treatment of humeral shaft fractures. Patients who present for initial evaluation with an intact radial nerve but who then lose function of the radial nerve during fracture reduction are clearly in need of an open reduction and internal fixation with simultaneous exploration of the radial nerve. A relative indication may exist in patients who present with a radial nerve injury initially. These injuries most often prove to be a neuropraxia rather than nerve entrapment and function typically returns in 3 to 4 months. Further indications include polytrauma, vascular injury, open fracture, bilateral humeri fractures, nonunion, segmental fractures, "floating elbow" (midshaft humerus fractures with ipsilateral midshaft radius and ulnar fractures) injuries, and patients with pathologic fractures. Fractures of the humerus may be treated by open reduction internal fixation or intramedullary nailing depending on certain patient profiles.

Fractures of the Supracondylar Region of the Humerus

Fractures of the supracondylar region of the humerus tend to occur most commonly in children and the elderly. In both situations, they can be managed successfully conservatively for minimally displaced fractures or fractures in the elderly population with preexisting compromised function. For fractures that are either not acceptably reducible or present in a young adult population, occur with a vascular injury or open fractures, surgical management with open reduction and internal fixation with wires or plate and screws are the treatments of choice. In select elderly patients, a total elbow replacement may be indicated. Structures at risk for injury include the brachial vessels and the median and radial nerves. Frequent neurovascular examinations and evaluation for compartment syndrome are required.

Fractures of the Radial Head

Nondisplaced fractures of the radial head are treated with minimal immobilization for 7 to 10 days, followed by active range of motion exercises of the extremity. Fractures of the radial head with displaced fragments are treated by open reduction and internal fixation, excision of the fragment, or radial head replacement. Fractures of the radial neck are treated in a similar manner if only minimally displaced. Displaced fractures of the radial neck are treated with radial head excision or radial head replacement to permit recovery of full supination and pronation.

Fractures of the Olecranon

Displaced fractures of the olecranon represent an avulsion fracture of the triceps mechanism. As such, they require open reduction and internal fixation to reconstruct the muscular attachment. The most common technique involves tension band wiring of the displaced fracture, which permits immediate mobilization of the extremity, but other treatments include open reduction internal fixation with plate and screw fixation, intramedullary screw fixation, and excision. Fractures that are nondisplaced can be treated by conservative means in a long arm cast for approximately 3 weeks, as the triceps mechanism is intact. Care must be taken to mobilize these individuals early to prevent loss of function. Almost half of the patients have decreased range of motion most notably, lack of full extension.

Fractures of the Radial Shaft

Displaced fractures of the radial shaft in adults are treated by open reduction and internal fixation. Generally only severe open fractures lead to associated injury of the radial artery and median nerve. Nondisplaced fractures can be treated by casting.

Fractures of the Ulnar Shaft

Proximal ulnar fractures with associated radial head dislocation are referred to as Monteggia fractures. This fracture dislocation is dealt with by reduction of the radial head and plate-and-screw fixation of the ulna. It

rarely requires operative intervention at the radial head–capitellar joint, as the fracture generally reduces with ulnar reduction. Fractures of the ulnar shaft that are the result of a direct blow are commonly referred to as nightstick fractures. Most patients are young men involved in an assault. These fractures can be treated with minimal immobilization and early range of motion exercises of the extremity if it is only minimally displaced. Open reduction internal fixation is indicated if the fracture is displaced, the ulna is significantly angulated, or more than 50% displacement of the shaft occurs.

Fractures of the Radius and Ulna

Both bone fractures of the forearm are treated operatively in adult patients if there is any displacement whatsoever. Failure to do so leads to pronounced loss of supination and pronation or dysfunction at the distal radial–ulnar joint leading to posttraumatic arthritis.

Fractures of the Distal Radius

Many eponyms are attached to fractures of the distal radius. The most common is the Colles fracture, which involves fracture of the distal radius with dorsal displacement and angulation of the distal fragment. Classically, it is described as a small fracture of the ulnar styloid as well. A fracture that has displacement in the opposite direction is frequently referred to as a Smith's fracture. Fracture of the radial styloid is often referred to as a Chauffeur fracture as the scaphoid is driven into the radial styloid in a motor vehicle accident.

Distal radius fractures occur in the younger population as a result of high-energy trauma such as a fall from height or motor vehicle accident. In the elderly, distal radius fractures may occur from low-energy trauma such as a simple trip and fall on an outstretched hand. Careful neurovascular examinations should be performed, as distal radius fractures are frequently associated with median nerve injury. Treatment of this type of fracture depends on the age of the patient. The single major factor in determining treatment is the degree of intra-articular involvement. In an elderly population with a whole or primary extra-articular fracture, most of these fractures can be treated conservatively with closed reduction and application of a cast for 4 to 6 weeks.

In a younger population, this fracture represents a high-energy injury and has a high degree of associated intra-articular involvement. It has a poor prognosis unless restoration can be anatomic or near anatomic in nature. The primary mode of operative treatment at this time is open reduction internal fixation with various constructs including locking plates although other forms of treatment include application of external fixator and percutaneous pins.

Fractures of the Scaphoid

Fracture of the scaphoid is one of the most commonly missed injuries about the wrist. The injured individual may report having sprained the wrist some time ago, and initial radiographs may be completely unremarkable. Careful attention must be given to physical examination of these individuals, looking for pain on palpation of the anatomic snuffbox of the wrist. When a patient has pain in the anatomic snuffbox but no radiographic evidence of fracture, the patient is treated in a thumb spica cast or splint. After 2 weeks, the cast or splint is removed and the patient reevaluated—this may often include an additional x-ray, magnetic resonance imaging (MRI), bone scans, or computed tomography (CT) scan.

Nondisplaced fractures of the scaphoid recognized early and treated conservatively have an excellent prognosis and often heal uneventfully. Those that are missed, with treatment initiated late, have a much higher incidence of nonunion and frequently require surgical intervention (Fig. 23.3). Immobilization for a nondisplaced scaphoid fracture may be necessary for 10 to 12 weeks. The major vascular supply to the scaphoid enters distally hence the increased probability of nonunion with minimal fracture displacement. Displaced fractures of the scaphoid are probably best treated with either wire or screw fixation (Herbert screw). Fractures diagnosed late may require the above form of fixation, an additional bone graft, or both.

Fractures of the Pelvis

Fractures of the pelvis occur in two situations. They can involve relatively low-energy trauma, such as a slip and fall against the edge of a bathtub, or be the result of a high-speed trauma, such as a fall from a height, automobile–pedestrian encounters, crush injuries, or an automobile or motorcycle accident. Fractures that represent relatively low-energy household accidents occur frequently in the elderly. They present as fractures of the pubic symphysis, pubic rami, or ischium.

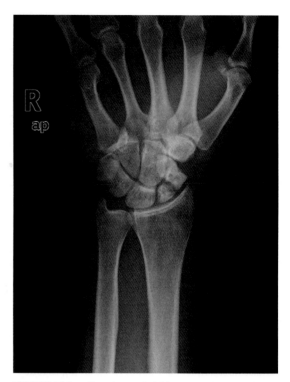

FIGURE 23.3. Chronic scaphoid fracture missed on initial presentation 1 year earlier.

These injuries are typically managed with observation, analgesia, and rapid mobilization of the patient.

High-energy pelvic fractures are grouped by the proposed mechanism of injury. Although no injury happens according to a rigid set of rules, where a force is exerted from a single direction, the concept of the mechanism of injury is helpful prognostically and therapeutically in managing pelvic fractures. The first of the three major mechanisms of injury is external rotation, commonly referred to as open-book injuries. Here the two wings of the pelvis rotate apart with the pelvis opening anteriorly. The second major mechanism of injury is lateral compression, where a force is applied to the lateral aspect of one side of the pelvis, driving the two sides of the pelvis together, as in a fall onto the lateral portion of the pelvis. The final mechanism of injury is a sheer fracture. This represents a vertical shearing force delivered to one side of the pelvis, translocating one side superiorly and posteriorly relative to the contralateral side. In the trauma setting, a combination of mechanisms is common.

For each mechanism of injury, there is a range, from relatively stable to unstable injuries. Several broad generalizations can be made. External rotation injuries tend to be at the more stable end of the spectrum relative to vertical shear injuries, which tend to be at the more unstable end of the spectrum. Disruption of the posterior elements, through the bone or ligamentous structures, is the key to bony stability and is an indicator of severity. Fractures that completely disrupt and posteriorly dislocate the structures about the sacrum lead to a much higher mortality rate than those that leave these structures intact.

The Young and Burgess pelvic classification scheme is the most commonly used and includes lateral compression, anteroposterior (AP) compression, vertical shear, and combined mechanisms (Fig. 23.4). Each category has multiple subtypes depending on severity of injury.

Unstable pelvic fractures are usually the result of high-energy trauma and can obviously be life threatening. These patients require a full trauma evaluation and cooperation of emergency department staff, trauma, and orthopaedic surgeons. A careful search for additional injuries and evaluation of hemodynamic status is imperative. The most common associated injuries include hemorrhage, thrombosis, neurological injury, and urogenital injuries. Often, application of pelvic binders and/or application of external fixators are required immediately to stabilize patients' hemodynamic status. Mortality from high-energy pelvic fractures has been reported to be between 10% and 50%. Closed head injury and hemorrhage are the most common causes of early death. Open pelvic fractures have reported mortality rates of 50% to 80%. Most trauma centers have specific treatment algorithms in place for high-energy pelvic fractures.

Acetabular Fractures

Fractures through the hip socket can occur with or without dislocation. The Letournel and Judet acetabular fracture classification system is most commonly used. This system classifies acetabular fractures on the basis of fracture patterns: posterior wall and column, anterior wall and column, transverse, T-shaped, and a combination of these. As with pelvic fractures, acetabular fractures are the result of high-energy trauma, and associated injuries are common. Unlike pelvic fractures, acetabular fractures are not typically treated emergently unless an open injury or irreducible dislocation is associated. Acetabular fractures that require operative intervention can be done so once the patient is adequately resuscitated.

Fractures that are essentially nondisplaced can be dealt with conservatively through skeletal traction and early range of motion of the joint. Fractures that have displaced to any significant degree must be dealt with operatively through relatively complex surgical approaches. The associated structure most likely injured is the sciatic nerve as it exits the sciatic notch and ranges from 2% to 6% in one series. Sciatic nerve palsies after acetabular fracture is estimated between 10% and 15%. Fractures of the acetabulum that involve the posterior column of the acetabulum have a higher incidence of injury to the sciatic nerve and the incidence of posttraumatic arthritis is estimated between 17% and 35%.

Hip Fractures

Fractures of the proximal femur are commonly referred to as hip fractures. There are more than 250,000 hip fractures/year in the United States, and this number is projected to double or triple by 2050. Hip fractures are more common in women by a factor of two to eight times. There are several major types of hip fractures; the most common classifications differentiate the fracture types anatomically. The first major classification is the femoral neck fracture, which occurs through the junction of the neck and head of the femur. The second major type is the intertrochanteric fracture, which occurs in the area between the greater and lesser trochanters. These fractures are frequently subgrouped into fractures of the base of the neck, intertrochanteric, and pertrochanteric (which extends beyond the lesser trochanter). For all intents and purposes, the management and prognosis are identical throughout the intertrochanteric region.

Fractures about the hip occur primarily in an elderly population and result from low-energy trauma such as a simple fall. When they occur in a younger population, they represent a high-energy injury.

Femoral Neck Fractures

The blood supply to the femoral head travels along the capsule of the hip through the region of the femoral neck and enters the head of the femur at the neck–head junction. As a result, fractures that occur through the femoral neck–head junction tend to disrupt the blood supply to the femoral head if displaced (Fig. 23.5). The most widely accepted classification system is referred to as the Garden classification of femoral neck fractures. A Garden 1 fracture is of the subcapital region and is impacted with mild valgus

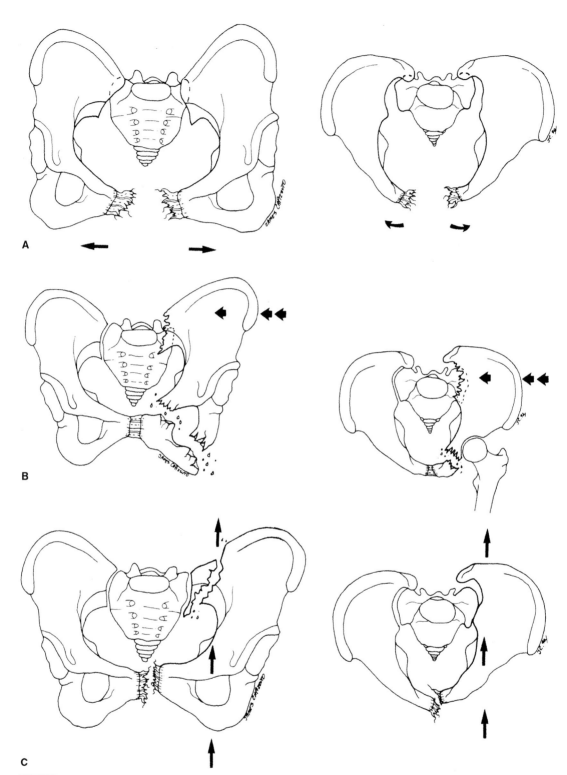

FIGURE 23.4. Fractures through the pelvis occur by three major mechanisms of injury. **A:** External rotation injury. **B:** Lateral compression injury. **C:** Vertical shear injury.

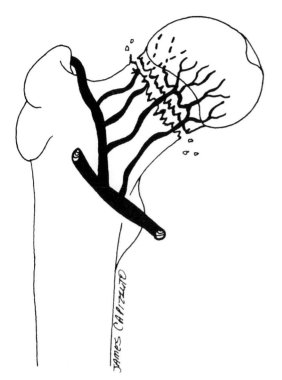

FIGURE 23.5. Vessels nourishing the femoral head enter at the neck–head junction. Displaced fractures in this region lead to disruption of the vasculature to the femoral head.

displacement, or it is an incomplete fracture. A Garden 2 fracture is complete but nondisplaced. A Garden 3 fracture is in varus, and a Garden 4 fracture is a fracture that is completely displaced from the femoral neck. Garden 1 and 2 are considered stable and 3 and 4 are considered unstable. Treatment depends on the degree of displacement (stable vs. unstable) and the physiologic age of the patient. In patients who have a nondisplaced or impacted valgus fracture or who have displaced fractures but are physiologically below the age of 65 (the cutoff is individual), the fracture is likely to be treated by cannulated screw fixation of the femoral head.

In individuals who are elderly with displaced fractures, the fracture is treated by prosthetic replacement—hemiarthroplasty. This practice decreases the incidence of a second operation to deal with a fracture that has not healed, has displaced, or has had the femoral head undergo avascular necrosis. It also allows rapid mobilization of the patient with full weight bearing and requires little cooperation on the part of the patient, which is especially useful in an elderly population with diminished mental capacity (Fig. 23.6).

Intertrochanteric Fractures

Intertrochanteric fractures require operative intervention. The major classifications of intertrochanteric fracture have to do with fracture stability (Fig. 23.7). The more stable the fracture pattern, the more likely the patient is to be able to bear weight on the fracture without difficulty after surgery. Most intertrochanteric fractures are currently treated by either a sliding screw-and-plate construct or a cephalomedullary device. The term "nailing a hip" stems from earlier days when large nail-like appliances were utilized. For today's treatment, a large screw is placed up into the proximal fragment and head of the femur, and a plate is placed over it, which allows sliding at the junction of the plate and screw. Newer devices involve intermedullary rods with transfixation screws or helical blades that go up into the head and neck. Early stabilization (<48 hours) for patients with stable medical comorbidities has shown a decrease in 1-year mortality. Many studies have shown that the 1-year mortality rate approaches 20% (Fig. 23.8).

Fractures of the Femoral Shaft

Fractures of the femoral shaft occur in the region between the lesser trochanter and the supracondylar region of the femur. These fractures, unless contraindicated, are treated operatively. Such repair allows for rapid mobilization and prevents the difficulties encountered with prolonged traction. Skeletal traction can be used successfully to treat these fractures when absolutely necessary, but the time and disability involved for the patient are much greater than if it is treated surgically.

Surgical treatment today involves placement of an intermedullary rod. Image intensifiers allow placement of these rods through "closed" techniques; that is, the surgical incision is made at a site distant to the fracture, in the region of the greater trochanter for an antegrade rod and the intercondylar notch for a retrograde nail. The rods are then placed over a guidewire after reaming the femoral canal.

Supracondylar Fractures of the Femur

Supracondylar fractures of the femur occur most commonly in elderly patients; in younger patients, they are the result of high-energy trauma. Although they also can be dealt with by skeletal traction, the common treatment involves plates and screws and recently utilizing submuscular locking plate designs.

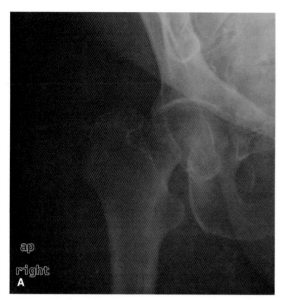

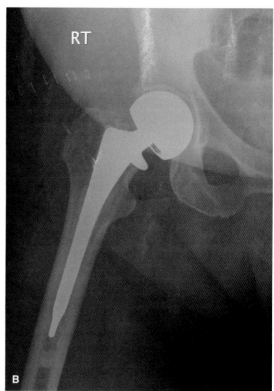

FIGURE 23.6.   Femoral neck fracture. **A:** Garden IV femoral neck fracture. **B:** After hemiarthroplasty.

This allows rapid mobilization of the joint and rapid return to normal activities for the patient. Fractures in this region can also involve individual condyles of the femur. This intra-articular fracture is treated by open reduction and internal fixation if there is any displacement.

Fractures of the Tibial Plateau

Fractures of the weight-bearing surface of the proximal tibia are common in all adult age groups. The more common plateau to be fractured is the lateral one, but isolated medial plateau fractures and bicondylar plateau fractures are seen. These fractures occur when the condyle of the femur drives down through the tibial plateau, splitting, or depressing the weight-bearing surface. Elevating the weight-bearing surface, maintaining its position with a bone graft, and fixing the fracture fragments with plates and screws or screws alone treat these fractures. Fractures that are less extensive are amenable to treatment through a combination of arthroscopic visualization of the fracture surface and percutaneous screw fixation of the fracture fragments.

Fractures of the Patella

Displaced fractures of the patella represent disruption of the quadriceps mechanism of the leg. Nondisplaced fractures can be treated with immobilization for a period of 6 to 12 weeks, but displaced fractures must be treated by open reduction and internal fixation. The preferred treatment involves some form of tension-band wiring, which allows early range of motion of the knee.

Fractures of the Tibial Shaft

Fractures of the tibial shaft are the most common fractured long bone. Nondisplaced fractures of the tibial shaft or fractures that can be reduced into acceptable alignment can be treated conservatively with a long leg cast. It is widely agreed that early weight bearing on this type of fracture leads to an improved union rate. Fractures that cannot be maintained in acceptable alignment and fractures that cause shortening of the tibial shaft are dealt with operatively. Treatment is most commonly an

FIGURE 23.7. Intertrochanteric features. **A:** Stable fracture. **B:** Unstable fracture.

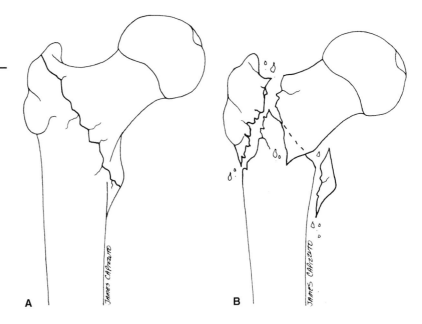

intramedullary nail placed through an incision distant from the fracture site. This "closed" intramedullary nail allows rapid return to normal activities. Fractures that are highly comminuted or demonstrate excessive shortening of the extremity require interlocking screws placed proximally and distally through the intramedullary nail to preserve position and length. It has been shown that intramedullary nail fixation increases union rates compared with closed treatment of displaced fractures (Fig. 23.9).

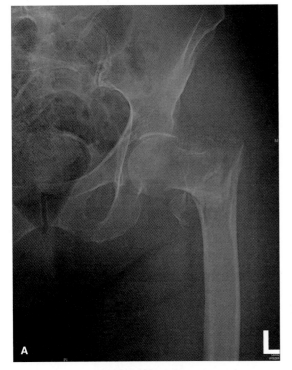

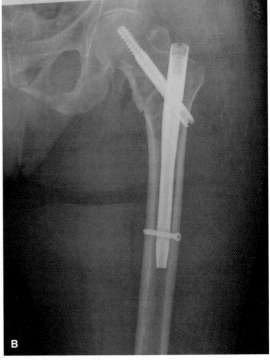

FIGURE 23.8. **A:** Intertrochanteric fracture. **B:** After cephalomedullary device placed.

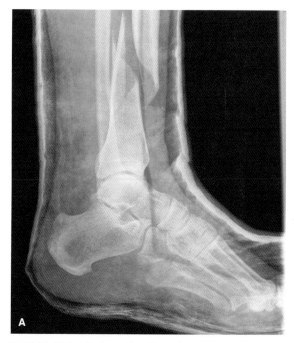
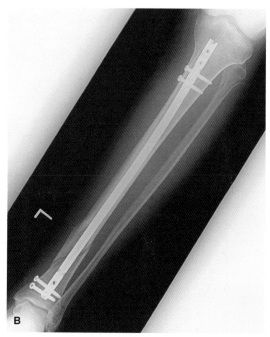

FIGURE 23.9. **A:** Lateral radiograph of a distal one-third tibial shaft fracture. **B:** Anteroposterior radiograph after intramedullary nail placed.

Fractures of the tibial shaft are the most common form of open fracture. Management of open tibial fractures is one of the most time-consuming and difficult elements of orthopaedic surgery. These fractures must be attended to at the time of injury with irrigation, debridement, and stabilization of the fracture. The modalities of stabilization are external fixation of the fracture and, more commonly in recent years, intramedullary fixation. External fixation represents construction of an exoskeleton with pins placed above and below the fracture site and rods of metallic or composite material placed between the pins to hold the position and length. Many reports have shown that intramedullary nailing leads to decreased secondary surgeries and an earlier return to weight bearing compared with external fixation.

The injured tibia with a high-grade open injury to the soft tissues has a high potential for infection and irrigation and debridement and fracture stabilization early. For this reason, although controversy still exists, type III open tibia fractures amenable to intramedullary nailing are done so unreamed. Reamed intramedullary nailing is performed for type I and II open fractures.

Ankle Fractures

Ankle fractures involve one malleolus (lateral or medial), two malleoli (bimalleolar fracture involving both lateral and medial), or three malleoli (a trimalleolar fracture involving the lateral, medial, and posterior malleoli). Displaced ankle fractures may also involve dislocation of the talus from underneath the tibia.

Unimalleolar fractures are lateral or medial malleolar fractures. The more common is the lateral malleolus involving an eversion injury of the ankle. These fractures, if not associated with secondary ligamentous damage to the opposite side of the ankle or the syndesmosis, can be treated conservatively in a short leg-walking cast.

If a bimalleolar fracture is essentially nondisplaced or it can be reduced to an acceptable position, it or bimalleolar equivalents (fractures of one malleolus with disruption of the ligaments on the opposite side) can be treated in a long leg cast. Displaced bimalleolar fractures are treated with open reduction and internal fixation involving plates and screws in the lateral malleoli and screws in the medial malleoli. Trimalleolar ankle fractures are uncommonly nondisplaced. These fractures are generally treated by open reduction and internal fixation, which allows early mobilization of the joint. The posterior malleolus can be difficult to get to, and small fractures of the posterior malleoli involving less than 25% of the articular surface are not generally fixed. Those involving 25% or more of the joint surface can undergo open reduction and internal fixation (Fig. 23.10).

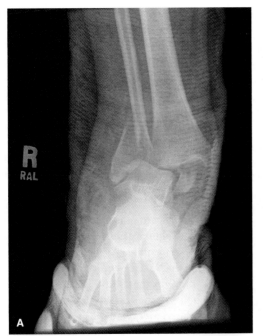

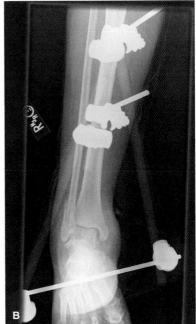

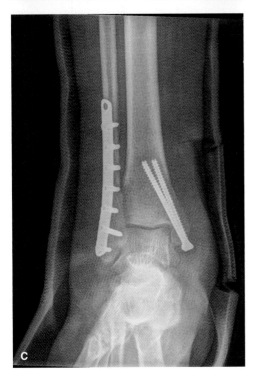

FIGURE 23.10.   Open ankle fracture dislocation. **A:** Anteroposterior radiograph after reduction. **B:** After application of external fixator
so that open wound care may be performed.
C: After definitive fixation.

Fractures of the Foot

Fractures of the midfoot and hindfoot occur with impact loading, such as a fall from a height, or violent twisting injuries. Fractures of the talar neck can be nondisplaced or displaced. Nondisplaced fractures that are truly anatomic have a reasonably good prognosis and can be treated conservatively. They are uncommon. Displaced fractures require open reduction and internal fixation. The higher the degree of initial displacement, the worse the prognosis.

In the past, fractures of the calcaneus were universally treated conservatively, with a uniformly mediocre to poor result for severe fractures. In recent years, more and more attempts are proving successful with open reduction and internal fixation of calcaneal fractures. Still, displaced calcaneal fractures, even with open reduction and internal fixation, can lead to a high degree of long-term disability for the patient.

Fractures of the Metatarsals

Fractures of the metatarsals can generally be treated conservatively. Multiple fractures or fractures grossly displaced can be treated with percutaneous pinning or open reduction and pin or screw fixation.

Fractures of Toes

Fractures of the toes with minimal displacement or those capable of being reduced are treated by taping the injured toe to an unaffected toe. Multiple phalangeal fractures or those grossly displaced may require pin fixation.

SPINAL FRACTURES

Evaluation of the polytraumatized patient for serious spinal injury represents one of the highest priorities when caring for these individuals. Any patient with severe facial or scalp lacerations should be suspected of having suffered a spinal injury. During early resuscitation and transportation efforts, care must be taken to immobilize the cervical spine, utilizing backboards, and in general treating the individual as if he or she has an unstable spinal injury until a thorough evaluation can take place. Of all the causes of death during the first year after a spinal injury, death en route to the hospital is by far the most significant, representing 90% of the total.

History taking should focus on the mechanism of injury—most often motor vehicle accidents, falls, or gunshot wounds—presence of transient motor or sensory loss, loss of consciousness, impairment secondary to drugs and alcohol, and severe facial and head trauma. The treating physician must be aware of spinal cord injury as a potential cause of hypotension secondary to loss of sympathetic tone. In contrast to hypovolemic shock, neurogenic shock, most common in cervical or upper thoracic injuries, is characterized by warm extremities and bradycardia, not tachycardia or diaphoresis.

Neurologic injuries can be classified as either complete or incomplete spinal cord injuries. Complete spinal cord injuries occur when there is no sensation or voluntary movement distal to the level of the injury. An incomplete spinal cord injury is defined as one in which some sensory or motor function is evident distal to the injury. In general, the greater the function present distal to the site of injury, the more rapid the recovery, and the greater the prognosis.

Orthopaedic management, although obviously concerned with the general condition of the patient and the neurologic state, also encompasses the concept of spinal stability regarding fractures. Fractures that include gross dislocations are clearly unstable, which present management difficulties in the neurologically compromised individual and potential for further injury in the neurologically noncompromised individual. The three-column theory of spinal stability has gained popularity in an effort to categorize the potential for instability of nondislocated fractures of the vertebrae, especially those referred to as burst fractures. These fractures tend to occur with axial loading and may well explode the vertebral body and posterior elements.

The bony spine is divided into three columns: anterior, middle, and posterior. The anterior column includes the anterior longitudinal ligament and the anterior half of the vertebral body. The middle column includes the posterior half of the vertebral body and the posterior longitudinal ligament. The posterior column is made up of the remaining structures in the posterior elements including pedicles, lamina, facet joints, and spinous processes. Fractures that completely disrupt two of the three columns are considered to be orthopaedically unstable. Management is discussed under specific regions of the spine (Fig. 23.11).

Fractures of the Cervical Spine

Treatment of cervical spine injuries primarily aims to realign the spine, prevent loss of function in the

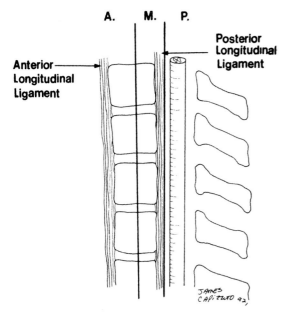

FIGURE 23.11. The spine is divided into three columns. The anterior column is the anterior longitudinal ligament and the anterior one-half of the disk and vertebral body. The middle column is the posterior one-half of the disk and vertebral body and the posterior longitudinal ligament. The posterior column is made up of the pedicles, lamina, facet joints, spinous processes, and interspinous ligaments.

spared tissue, and improve neurologic and functional recovery. Adequate radiographs of the cervical spine are essential for evaluation of injuries in this region. These include, at least, AP, lateral, and open-mouth odontoid views. Care must be taken that all vertebrae from C1 through the top of T1 are visualized. During initial evaluation, management consists at least of a rigid collar until the evaluation is completed.

Fractures of C1: Jefferson Fracture

Also called a burst fracture, a Jefferson fracture is characterized by two fractures in the posterior arch and two fractures in the anterior arch of the C1 ring. Relatively nondisplaced fractures are treated by collar immobilization for a 3-month period. For displaced fractures with involvement of the lateral masses displaced more than 7 mm past the articular surfaces of the axis, reduction should be performed with halo traction. Treatment consists of 3 to 6 weeks of

cervical traction followed by a halo vest for the remainder of the 3 months. Fortunately, because of the wide canal diameter in this region, cord injuries are uncommon.

Injuries to the transverse ligament can occur with C1 arch fractures. The normal atlantoaxial distance as visualized on a lateral view is less than 5 mm. If this distance is increased to more than 5 mm, it is indicative of atlantoaxial instability; and C1–2 wiring and fusion are required to prevent cord compression. Atlanto-occipital ligamentous disruption can also occur, and if the patient survives it, occiput—C2 fusion is indicated.

Odontoid Fractures

Fractures of the odontoid are best visualized through the open-mouth view. Nondisplaced fractures are, in general, managed by 3 months of halo immobilization. Fractures are generally divided into three types. Those involving the odontoid itself are classified as type 1; those involving the junction of the odontoid and the body of the axis are type 2; and those fracturing down through the body of the axis are type 3. If displacement of more than 5 mm occurs in these higher-type fractures, C1–2 posterior wiring and fusion are performed.

Fractures of C2: Hangman's Fracture

A fracture occurring through the posterior elements of C2, often consisting of bilateral pedicle fractures, is referred to as a hangman's fracture. These injuries are usually treated successfully with halo immobilization for several months. When associated with dislocation, the injuries may be irreducible and require open reduction, wiring, and fusion.

Fractures of Cervical Vertebrae C3 through C7

Because of the small diameter of the canal in the C3 to C7 region, neurologic injuries are often associated with fractures of these vertebrae. Fractures considered to be stable in this region can be treated successfully with immobilization. Unstable fractures in this area require reduction, stabilization, and fusion. This regimen often requires combined anterior decompression, anterior bone graft with a block of bone, and posterior instrumentation and fusion.

Facet Injuries

Facet injuries can be purely ligamentous disruptions with dislocation or can involve fractures. C5–6 is the most common site of dislocation. Dislocations with displacement of less than 25% of the vertebral body may well represent only single-facet dislocation, whereas larger displacements represent bilateral facet dislocations. Resulting in a positive outcome, open reduction and internal fixation of unilateral facet dislocation is recommended. If unilateral facet dislocation can be reduced in skull traction, then a halo vest may be used for 3 months, and stability may be obtained by spontaneous fusion. Significant facet injuries generally necessitate posterior instrumentation and single-level fusions.

Fractures of the Thoracic and Lumbar Spine

Anterior compression fractures occur with hyperflexion caused by abrupt deceleration, most often a result of a motor vehicle accident, falls, or athletic participation. Nonoperative treatment, including thoracolumbar spinal orthoses, hyperextension casting, lumbosacral corsets, Jewett braces, or hyperextension bracing, is the standard of care for vertebral compression fractures and some burst fractures. Injuries that involve more than 40% of the vertebral body and those to the middle column or the posterior elements are considered unstable, and operative treatment is indicated. Operative management involves posterior instrumentation and fusion.

Burst Fractures

Burst fractures occur with sudden deceleration injuries. On radiographic imaging, these fractures present with a loss of posterior vertebral body height and splaying of the pedicles. The concept of stability has been discussed previously. Unstable fractures must be managed operatively. The method for dealing with retropulsed fragments is controversial. Many fragments reduce with distraction. The need for immediate decompression of retropulsed fragments remains controversial.

Pathologic Fractures

Pathologic fractures of the spine can occur at any level. The most common causes are metastatic tumor, multiple myeloma, and osteoporosis. A pathologic fracture occurs when relatively minor trauma causes a significant structural abnormality within a bone. Fractures secondary to metastatic lesions, if stable, may be managed conservatively in conjunction with treatment directed at the tumor in that locale. If unstable, they may require fixation as described above.

Compression fractures in the elderly secondary to osteoporosis are managed with rest initially, followed by rapid mobilization as tolerated, analgesics, and at times braces (Fig. 23.12).

DISLOCATIONS

Acromioclavicular Joint Dislocation

Dislocations of the AC joints are also known as shoulder separations. The degree of displacement of the joint is a reflection of the severity of ligamentous disruption. AC injuries are divided into six categories and are best viewed by an A-P radiograph aimed 10 degrees cephalad and an axillary lateral radiograph as well. A grade I AC joint separation represents only a partial disruption of the ligamentous structures; there is still joint integrity, and the joint does not dislocate even under load. A grade II AC joint separation involves complete disruption of the AC ligaments with some integrity through the coracoclavicular ligaments. This joint is displaceable under load. A grade III AC separation involves complete disruption of both the AC ligaments and the coracoclavicular ligament complex, and the joint is dislocated even at rest. A grade IV injury occurs when the clavicle is dislocated posteriorly and pushes through the fascia of the trapezius muscle. In grade V injuries, the glenohumeral joint is severely displaced inferiorly. Finally, grade VI injuries entail the distal end of the clavicle becoming locked below the coracoid process.

Treatment of these injuries varies widely through the more severe grades. Grade I and II injuries are universally treated with a sling for about 2 to 4 weeks; grade III is more controversial, with some recommending nonoperative techniques and others recommending surgical intervention; grades IV to VI are treated with open reduction and internal fixation accompanying reconstruction of the coracoclavicular ligament.

Shoulder Dislocations

Dislocations of the glenohumeral joint can be anterior or posterior. Some individuals are classified as having multidirectional instability after numerous

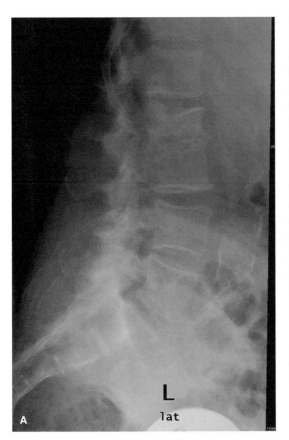
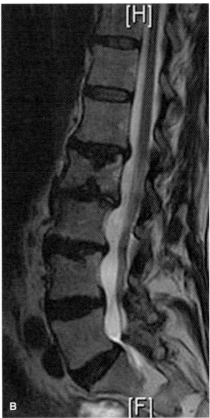

FIGURE 23.12.   Compression fracture. **A:** Lateral radiograph showing L2 compression fracture. **B:** Comparison MRI of same compression fracture.

dislocations. The most common is an anterior gleno-humeral dislocation (Fig. 23.13). In a younger age group, this is almost always accompanied by a Bankart lesion, which is a disruption of the fibrocartilaginous structure known as the labrum from the glenoid or bony socket of the shoulder joint. This relatively avascular structure may not heal back to the bony glenoid, which leads to a potential for redislocation with an appropriately applied force through the joint.

Elderly individuals may dislocate with low-energy trauma and in a higher percentage of cases may leave the labrum intact and simply tear through other soft tissue structures. This leads to a lower likelihood of redislocation.

After reduction of the dislocation, patients in all age groups are treated by immobilization. The shoulder is immobilized for 2 to 6 weeks, and then an exercise regimen is begun that slowly introduces the motions of abduction and external rotation. Individuals who have undergone multiple dislocations require

surgical reconstruction. A variety of procedures exist, many of which limit external rotation and abduction. Several of the more commonly performed procedures involve reconstruction or reattachment of the labral structures and capsule of the shoulder (Bankart procedure).

The structure most likely to be injured is the axillary nerve, which can lead to denervation of the deltoid and loss of sensation over the lateral aspect of the upper arm. Chronic dislocations in the elderly are sometimes recognized late, and attempts at closed reduction can have disastrous effects on the vascular structures of the axilla. These structures may be scarred and adherent to the shoulder capsule, and on attempts at reduction there are reports of rupture of the brachial artery.

Elbow Dislocations

Elbow dislocations can be anterior, posterior, medial, or lateral. The most common dislocation is posterior.

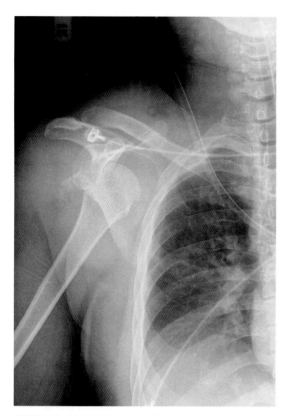

FIGURE 23.13. Anterior shoulder dislocation.

It represents a rather severe injury, with possible injury to associated vascular structures anteriorly and to the median and ulnar nerves. These injuries can often be managed with closed reduction and splint for several weeks and then mobilization of the elbow joint. After relocation and immobilization, treatment consists of active range of motion exercises. Occasionally, residual instability requires reconstruction of ligaments.

Wrist Dislocations

Dislocations about the wrist can occur through the carpals and distal radius or through the carpal bones themselves. The most common dislocations involve the scapholunate joint. This can involve a fracture of the scaphoid and is then known as a trans-scaphoid perilunate dislocation. Dislocations of the lunate itself can occur. Intercarpal ligamentous ruptures will heal if the bones to which they are normally attached are kept in their normal anatomic relationship. This may be accomplished by closed reduction of the intercarpal

dislocation. More often, open reduction, pin fixation, and surgical repair are necessary. Regardless of the particular type of dislocation, they frequently require surgical reconstruction, as the ligamentous disruption leads to long-term instability at the wrist if it is not reconstructed.

Hip Dislocations

Dislocations of the hip can be anterior or posterior. Posterior dislocations are far more common and are generally brought on by a blow to the knee in a flexed position. The classic position on dislocation is that of a shortened extremity held in a flexed, adducted, and internally rotated position. With anterior dislocations there is a shortened extremity in an externally rotated position. Posterior dislocations are associated with a significant incidence of injury to the sciatic nerve. They may be accompanied by fractures of the acetabulum or fractures of the femoral head (Pipkin fractures).

Treatment involves rapid closed reduction of the joint. If plain films and a CT scan reveal no evidence of any debris within the joint and no associated fractures, conservative management may be all that is necessary. If there are associated fractures, they may require open reduction and internal fixation. There is a significant incidence of debris within the joint with a fracture, which should be removed via irrigation and debridement of the joint.

Following reduction, treatment varies according to the injury. For soft tissue injuries with stable reduction, traction for a few days followed by exercises is standard. Full weight bearing may be achieved at 6 weeks. For an unstable reduction, treatment consists of immobilization in a spica cast or abduction brace for 4 to 6 weeks.

Knee Dislocations

Knee dislocations can be anterior, posterior, medial, lateral, rotatory, or a combination thereof. They are equally devastating and have a high incidence of associated injury to the popliteal vessels. After relocation of the knee, even in the face of normal pulses, an angiogram may be required to rule out an intimal tear of the artery. These dislocations are associated with devastating consequences on the function of the knee. A number of ligaments are disrupted depending on the direction of the dislocation. The patient may have disrupted the anterior cruciate, posterior cruciate, and medial and lateral collateral ligaments among others. Extensive reconstructive surgery is necessary to obtain adequate knee function.

Ankle Dislocations

Ankle dislocations occur most often in conjunction with fractures and have been discussed under ankle fractures.

Subtalar Dislocations

Also called peritalar dislocation, a subtalar dislocation occurs when both the talocalcaneal and talonavicular joints dislocate simultaneously. Dislocations of the hindfoot and midfoot around the talus occur with violent twisting injury. Medial dislocation caused by inversion is by far the most common type. They may be reduced closed, followed by immobilization in a short leg cast for 6 weeks, or may require open reduction and pin fixation. One fracture of this region that frequently requires open reduction and pin fixation is the Lisfranc fracture dislocation, which is a fracture dislocation of the metatarsals from the tarsals. A variety of patterns exist based on the direction of the four lateral digits and involvement of the base of the first metatarsal. This fracture dislocation must be reduced anatomically and held with pins or screws percutaneously, at least; frequently it requires open reduction and internal fixation.

SPORTS INJURIES

As the field of sports medicine expands, more and more injuries are being considered sporting injuries. Each sport or activity has an area of the musculoskeletal system that can be overtaxed or injured by that particular activity. The more common entities dealt with by sports medicine orthopaedic surgeons are discussed here.

Shoulder Injuries

Recurrent shoulder dislocation (see the section entitled Shoulder Dislocations, above) requires reconstruction in the active adult. As sophistication within the area of arthroscopic surgery of the shoulder has increased, a broader spectrum of abnormalities has been recognized. At the core of most of these entities is the glenoid labrum. Shoulder arthroscopy has allowed recognition and remedy of loose bodies within the shoulder joint, excision of labral tears that cause locking of the shoulder, diagnosis of shoulder subluxation in contrast to frank dislocation, and diagnosis of multidirectional instability. Although many of these entities can be dealt with directly through the arthroscope, some controversy still exists over reconstruction of shoulder dislocations.

A number of arthroscopic procedures exist for stabilization of the shoulder. The standard of comparison, however, remains an open reconstruction of the labrum and anterior capsule.

Knee Ligament Disruption

Advances in the field of sports medicine have led to an increased awareness of ligamentous injuries about the knee. Increased diagnostic acumen has led to a greater number of diagnoses of serious knee ligament abnormalities at an early stage. The ability to deal with them surgically has helped decrease the likelihood of crippling arthritic degeneration later in life. Disruption of anterior and posterior cruciate ligaments with associated medial collateral or lateral collateral ligament instabilities leads to an increase in abnormal motion within the knee. These abnormal motions result in torn menisci and early degenerative changes.

The most common entity causing substantial instability within the knee is rupture of the anterior cruciate ligament. This injury frequently has associated lateral side instability, which in the long term leads to degenerative changes within the knee. In the short term, it frequently prevents individuals from participating in sporting activities as they did in the past. The patient experiences a sense of the knee giving way during attempts to plant the extremity and pivot. Tests such as the Lachman test (a test for the ability to translocate the tibia anteriorly on the femur) and a "pivot shift" test, which recreates the giving-way episode, help diagnose the entity.

A number of procedures have been utilized to reconstruct an anterior cruciate ligament. Currently, the most promising procedures involve arthroscopic replacement of the deficient ligament with a substitute tendon graft. The most common grafts are autologous patellar tendon bone grafts and hamstring tendon grafts; allografts are also available and indicated in certain circumstances. These procedures, whether performed for substitution of an anterior cruciate or posterior cruciate ligament, although technically demanding, can lead to substantially improved performance.

Meniscal Injuries

Injuries to the menisci are due to acute trauma or the accumulation of trauma over time; commonly referred to as degenerative menisci. Tearing of the medial meniscus is more common than tearing of the lateral meniscus because it is attached to the entire periphery of the joint capsule. Clinical presentation of pain with flexion or extension beyond a certain point, inability to fully flex or fully extend the knee, pain over the joint line, swelling within the joint, and a history of trauma are indicative of a possible meniscal injury. MRI has helped confirm the diagnosis of injuries to the meniscus but is no substitute for a careful history and physical examination. Arthroscopic meniscal surgery with resection of the damaged portion of the meniscus and recontouring of the remaining menisci is the treatment of choice. Peripheral tears in select individuals can be effectively repaired.

ADULT ORTHOPAEDIC SURGERY: ARTHRITIS

Arthritis simply means inflammation of a joint. Two major categories of arthritis are recognized: those that are a result of a local phenomenon, such as posttraumatic arthritis or osteoarthritis (not primarily an inflammatory process, but rather a degenerative joint disease and those that are, in general, thought to be a manifestation of a more generalized or autoimmune phenomenon, such as rheumatoid arthritis or psoriatic arthritis. These major categories of arthritides can be distinguished by the patient's presentation. Rheumatoid-type arthritides tend to be polyarticular. They present with multiple joint involvement and generally all joints of the body are at risk. Osteoarthritis occurs commonly in a few joints and uncommonly in others. The weight-bearing joints of the hips and knees, small joints of the spine, and base of the thumb are common sites, whereas shoulders, ankles, and wrists are less common ones. In the major weight-bearing joints such as the hips or knees, rheumatoid arthritis presents radiographically as diffuse narrowing of the joint space with a reactive osteopenia. Osteoarthritic degeneration tends to be more pronounced through the weight-bearing surfaces and frequently has hypertropic (osteophyte formation) bony reaction.

When conservative management has failed in either type, surgical management is appropriate. The most commonly replaced joints for arthritic degeneration are the hips and knees. Shoulder replacements and elbow replacements are less commonly performed but function reasonably well, especially in patients with rheumatoid arthritis. Replacement of finger joints in rheumatoid arthritis also is successful. Replacement of wrist and ankle joints has been tried, but at present there are few well recognized functioning prostheses. An alternative treatment in these areas is arthrodesis, the creation of a bony union across a joint.

Both hip and knee prostheses have undergone substantial improvement in design over the last decade. Current prosthetic implants can be expected to function at a reasonably high performance level for many years depending on the age and general condition of the patient. The use of cement fixation of the prosthesis remains an area of controversy. Relatively sedentary patients in their late 70s and 80s who require total hip or total knee replacement can predictably undergo cemented joint replacement and feel confident that the joint will perform adequately for the remainder of their lives, barring uncommon complications such as infection. The cemented total joint replacement in this age group remains the standard by which all other methods must be judged (Fig. 23.14).

Individuals in their 50s who require total joint replacement, especially active individuals who have only single joint involvement, cannot expect a cemented total joint replacement to perform for the remainder of their lives. These implants fail at the bone–cement interface in a substantial percentage of cases. The advent of porous coated prostheses that allow, at least theoretically, a biologic interlock via bony ingrowth into the interstices of the prosthesis, in theory, offer longer performance. Early performance reports appear promising.

In today's orthopaedic practice, patients in their 50s or younger in most cases, if otherwise suitable, have uncemented prostheses placed. In many practices, those in their late seventies and above routinely have cemented prostheses, although this is not universally so. In between, the decisions are individualized on the basis of the patient's overall condition and the surgeon's general experience, whether to receive a cemented prosthesis, an uncemented prosthesis, or a hybrid (one component cemented and the other components not cemented).

In general, the performance level of hip and knee replacements, given today's technology, is good. The

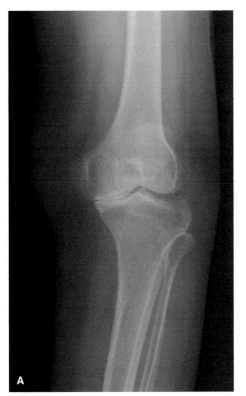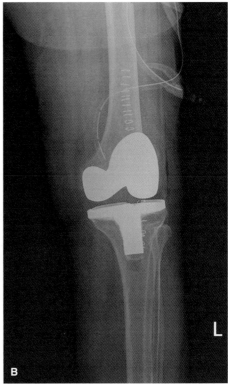

FIGURE 23.14.   **A:** Patient with significant knee osteoarthritis showing severe joint space narrowing. **B:** Postoperative total knee arthroplasty.

longevity, although affected by age and activity level, is acceptable.

SOFT TISSUE INFLAMMATION AND ABNORMALITIES

Almost any soft tissue structure in the body, be it ligament, tendon, or muscle, can be inflamed or irritated. This can lead to acute or chronic pain syndromes, loss of function, and possible rupture of a tendon or musculotendinous junction. Several problems mentioned here occur commonly, and their presentation and treatment are discussed.

Shoulder Impingement Syndrome

Repetitive overhead motion over a substantial period of time, such as occurs in tennis, pitching, or swimming, may affect the space between the humeral head and the coracoacromial arch (the acromion, coracoacromial ligament, and the coracoid process).

Impingement of this space causes microtrauma to the rotator cuff muscles, which results in inflammation, swelling, and pain and may continue on to partial or complete rotator cuff tears.

The term impingement syndrome arises from the fact that the space between the humerus and the acromion is a relatively fixed distance and that a number of structures including the rotator cuff, subacromial bursa, and biceps tendon all must glide within this space without difficulty. When inflammation begins within this region, the swelling within the soft tissue structures causes impingement on the bony undersurface of the acromion. Many structures have been implicated as the initiating cause, from a tight coracoacromial ligament in young muscular individuals to osteophyte formation underneath the acromion in the elderly. The problem may be simple inflammation of the biceps tendon or subacromial bursa or a mechanical defect into the rotator cuff.

Shoulder impingement syndrome is a descriptive term for a broad spectrum of painful problems about the shoulder. Into this category fall a variety of shoulder problems including bursitis, tendonitis, rotator cuff inflammation, and painful arc syndrome. The patient usually presents complaining of weeks to months of pain in and about the shoulder. The pain is most commonly anterior, although it can present as lateral, posterior, or even anterior deltoid insertion. The patient frequently denies any specific trauma that could have caused the pain. In many cases, the patient relates an activity or a trauma that seemed to start the problem, but this is not universal. Patients often complain that the pain is worse at night, awakens them from sleep, and forces them to rise early in the morning. They report that the pain is brought on within a reproducible arc of motion, which can be anywhere from just a few degrees of abduction to the extreme limits of abduction, external rotation, or forward flexion. The problem can be acute in nature, being present only a few days, or chronic, lasting many months.

Initial management of all of these entities is conservative, with anti-inflammatory drugs, either oral or locally injected, activity modification, and physical therapy. In addition, motion of the shoulder must be maintained to prevent adhesive capsulitis. For the cases that fail on prolonged conservative management (minimum of 3 months), resection of the underside of the acromion, by open means or arthroscopic technique, may be indicated or excision and repair of the damaged area of the rotator cuff (or both). However, this technique has become increasingly controversial as a recent randomized study of rotator cuff repair found no statistical difference between performing a subacromial decompression or not. Furthermore, a retrospective study of about 100 patients found that after a decade, decompression might not prevent progression from impingement to a tear.

Lateral Epicondylitis

Inflammation of the origin of the extensor tendons of the forearm is commonly referred to as tennis elbow. This inflammation, also called lateral epicondylitis, is an abnormality of the extensor origin. It may be brought on by repetitive activities, such as tennis or working on an assembly line, but in many cases it is idiopathic in origin.

Most of the patients are handled conservatively. Initial treatment may involve decreasing specific activities, wearing a tennis elbow band to decrease the force per unit area on the muscle, and a simple exercise regimen. If this treatment fails, oral anti-inflammatory drugs or, more commonly, steroids by injection may be administered. Most of the individuals have pain relief with this type of regimen, but some do not. In those individuals, especially those in whom the etiology is the performance of a repetitive task, release of the extensor origin may be required. Several procedures exist for this, most with an excellent outcome.

De Quervain Syndrome

Stenosing tenosynovitis of the first extensor compartment of the wrist is commonly referred to as De Quervain syndrome. Patients present with pain over the distal radial aspect of the wrist. They report pain with activities that require them to deviate the wrist ulnarly while adducting and flexing their thumb or that require twisting the wrist, such as opening a door or a jar. The presentation is frequently accompanied by a small nodule in this area. Initial treatment is conservative, with local injection, anti-inflammatory drugs, or splint. Surgery, consisting of release of the overlying retinaculum, is reserved for recalcitrant cases. But this elective surgery must be performed with caution as the sensory branch of the radial nerve runs directly over the first compartment.

Trochanteric Bursitis

Similar to individuals presenting with pain about the shoulder secondary to bursitis, inflammation of the abductor musculature about the hip is common. It is sometimes confused with sciatica, but these individuals are usually distinctly tender over the greater trochanter. Treatment, again, involves either nonsteroidal agents or local injection, with a high likelihood of improvement.

Pes Anserine Bursitis

Inflammation of the medial side of the knee is one of the more common soft tissue complaints seen in an orthopaedist's office. A variety of soft tissue inflammations are grouped under this term. Whether the inflammation is of a pes anserine tendon at its insertion, a small bursa underneath the medial collateral ligament, or the ligament itself is difficult to ascertain. Frequently, there is an underlying cause for the inflammation. Many individuals who suffer from it have early degenerative changes within the medial compartment of the knee. Treatment is conservative with rest, anti-inflammatory drugs, and possibly local injection.

Achilles Tendon

Inflammation or rupture of the Achilles tendon occurs most commonly during the third through fifth decades. Complete ruptures are often associated with unusual physical activity. The "weekend warrior" syndrome, in which a rather sedentary individual plays a high-demand sport on a weekend and suddenly feels a tearing sensation in the calf, is a common presentation. The patient presents with an inability to actively plantar-flex the foot; although dorsiflexion is present, pain may limit the excursion. Positioning the patient supine on a table with the knee flexed and the foot held in a neutral position while the calf is squeezed (Thompson test) leads to plantar flexion of the foot with an intact Achilles tendon. With a ruptured tendon, no movement of the foot occurs. This test is reliable for diagnosing complete rupture of the Achilles tendon.

Chronic inflammation of the Achilles tendon can present as soreness at the musculotendinous junction with a nodule forming in this area. It can lead to rupture with ordinary activities, such as stepping off a curb.

Treatment of a ruptured Achilles tendon, if diagnosed early in the active adult, remains controversial. Excellent results are reported with management in a plantar flexion cast if the diagnosis is made in a 24- to 48-hour period. Because performance athletes have shown slightly better results with operative treatment, it is unclear if there are any benefits from this type of treatment in the average individual. The choice for conservative versus operative management, however, remains one for the individual surgeon based on his or her expertise and experience.

In cases of chronic Achilles tendon ruptures, because the tendon ends have usually become frayed and shortened, techniques interpositional grafts are employed. Postoperatively, the course includes 6 weeks of non–weight bearing and 3 months in a cast.

Plantar Fasciitis

A painful heel is commonly referred to as a "heel spur." The tough plantar fascia of the foot can become inflamed at its origin. If calcification has occurred at this site, radiographs may show a spur at the anteroinferior aspect of the tuber of the calcaneus. The presence of the spur, however, is not necessary for the diagnosis, and many individuals are asymptomatic even when the spur can be seen.

Treatment overwhelmingly is conservative, with nonsteroidal drugs, heel pad appliances, or local injection. It is uncommon to treat this entity surgically.

Lower Back Pain

Abnormalities of the lower back account for more time lost from work, more compensation payouts, and more time in the orthopaedic surgeon's office than any other orthopaedic problem. In fact, studies show that more than 80% of people suffer from some form of lower back pain at some point in their lives. It may be a problem only a few days, or it may last as long as several months. Anatomically, it is not surprising that the spine is a source of anguish and knowledge of the anatomical composition of the spine is useful in understanding the pain. The spine is made up of a series of small joints, each of which is constrained by numerous ligaments. In addition, cartilaginous disks exist between the vertebral bodies in close association with numerous neurologic structures.

Fortunately for doctors and patients alike, most episodes of low back pain are self-limited. With rest, support, and education, the preponderance of patients are returned to normal activities in a relatively brief time. The individual who suffers from recurrent bouts, lower back pain that does not respond within a relatively short time, and of course those who have lower back pain associated with neurologic findings may have structural abnormalities that require surgical intervention.

The individual who presents with a history of only several days of back pain related to some traumatic incident (it may have been a mild incident) and who has improved and had no neurologic findings, no neurologic complaints, no radiation of pain to the leg indicative of a possible radiculopathy, and normal plain radiographs can be confidently managed conservatively. Those patients who do not fall into this type of presentation—those who complain of radicular symptoms, frequent recurrence, or specific reproduction of their symptoms with a particular activity—all warrant further workup. This workup may include a CT scan or more likely an MRI.

Recently, the intervertebral disc has been more recognized for being a pain generator. Essentially, the posterior portion of the annulus fibrosis is innervated by fibers from the dorsal root ganglion and irritation

TABLE 23.2

Lumbar Level	Motor Loss	Sensory Distribution
L2–3	Hip flexors	Anterior thigh
L3–4	Anterior tibialis, quadriceps	Medial lower leg
L4–5	Extensor digitorum longus, extensor hallucis longus	Lateral lower leg, dorsum of foot
L5–S1	Gastrocnemius, soleus complex	Posterior lower leg, plantar aspect of foot

of the nerve branch is thought to be responsible for axial back pain.

A *herniated nucleus pulposus*, or "slipped disk," classically represents a disruption of the hard outer ring of the disk (annulus fibrosis) with extrusion of the gelatinous nucleus pulposus of the disk and possibly fragments of the hard annulus. Classically, patients present with back pain and pain radiating down the leg below the knee into the leg and foot. They may present with weakness of motor function in the distal extremity and decreased sensation in a dermatomal distribution. Straight-leg raising produces pain radiating down the leg, and the patients in general are quite incapacitated. In the absence of hard neurologic findings, most individuals with a documented herniated disk on MRI, CT scan, or myelogram may well settle down conservatively. Those who present with a neurologic deficit and those who fail to improve after more than 1 month of activity modification may warrant surgical intervention for decompression of the nerve root.

Another common entity, seen primarily in elderly patients, is *spinal stenosis*. The classic presentation is that of pain in the buttocks radiating into the leg with exercise. The complaints may sound much like vascular claudication and, in fact, probably represent vascular claudication of the spine. Typically, the pain is reproducible with the same activity or distance walked each episode. Pain may also be brought on by standing erect for any period of time. One feature differentiating it from vascular claudication is that patients frequently report that to feel better they must sit down or bend forward and put their hands on their thighs. This flexed position increases room within the spinal canal for the neural elements, diminishing the symptoms. Neurogenic and vascular claudication may be difficult to distinguish from one another so cooperation among vascular and orthopaedic surgeons is important. Treatment of spinal stenosis is surgical decompression with possible instrumentation.

Some of the neurologic findings in lumbar disc disease may include motor and sensory loss in specific distributions as shown in the Table 23.2.

TUMORS

Whether a lesion is a primary bone tumor or a metastatic lesion, accurate description of the presentation usually yields a narrow differential diagnosis. Age and past medical history are particularly relevant to the differential diagnosis of bone tumors. The most frequent metastatic tumors of bone generally affecting patients older than 50 years arise from primary breast, prostate, lung, renal, and thyroid carcinomas. Multiple myeloma is the most frequent primary bone tumor and occurs with a peak incidence during the seventh decade. Osteosarcoma is the most frequent primary bone sarcoma and usually occurs during the second decade. Age coupled with a thorough history and some additional studies helps confirm the diagnosis. The size, location, and quality of the mass must be determined, and any tenderness near the mass, associated swelling, and quality of the skin overlying the mass must be recorded. Large tumor size, a high histological grade, and a deep mass within the extremity indicate a poor prognosis.

Most orthopaedic oncologists use the Enneking staging system for tumor classification, which grades tumors on the basis of their biological and histological qualities and their likelihood for metastasis. Stage I depicts a low-grade sarcoma with less than 25% chance of metastasis, stage II refers to a high-grade sarcoma with more than 25% chance of metastasis, and stage III is used to classify either a low- or high-grade sarcoma that has already metastasized. In the Enneking system, tumors are further classified as type A or type B depending on whether they are intracompartmental or extracompartmental, respectively. Type A tumors, anatomically bound by distinct boundaries, such as a fascial plane, tend to remain local and are more easily removed by a surgeon than are type B tumors. Although localization is an important indicator for a better prognosis, size may be even more important. Tumors larger than 5 cm are considered unfavorable.

Benign Bone Tumors

Bone Cysts

Simple bone cysts usually present in the first and second decade and occur about twice as often in boys as in girls. Primarily metaphyseal lesions in active individuals, they are recognized incidentally or when a fracture occurs. Current treatment recommendations suggest aspiration/injection with bone marrow or corticosteroids three to five times over the course of 2 to 3 months. Curettage and bone grafting may also be effective. Injections of demineralized bone matrix and autogenous bone marrow have yielded promising results, with a 20% recurrence rate (down from 30%–50% for curettage and grafting) and low morbidity.

Aneurysmal Bone Cyst

Aneurysmal bone cysts present during the second and third decades as rapidly expansile, locally aggressive lesions. They appear much as simple bone cysts. Other tumors may have an aneurysmal component so a biopsy with multiple samples is needed to rule out other possible tumors, such as chondromyxoid fibroma, giant cell tumor, and telangiectatic osteosarcoma. Treatment is curettage and bone grafting.

Nonossifying Fibroma

Seen during the first to third decades of life, most often in the lower extremities of children, nonossifying fibromas, which are cortical lesions, have a characteristic radiographic presentation. These are the most common benign tumors of bone and are usually diagnosed incidentally. They are well-circumscribed, eccentric cortical lesions in the metaphyseal region of long bones. No treatment is required.

Osteoid Osteoma

Osteoid osteoma, the most common benign osteoid-forming tumor, occurs primarily during the second decade. The patient usually complains of night pain frequently relieved by aspirin. More common in males than in females, osteoid osteoma is most frequently found in the proximal femur. It also occurs about the spine and may present as scoliosis with the convexity

toward the lesion. The classic radiograph shows a sclerotic lesion with a small radiolucent nidus centrally. Most cases can be treated symptomatically with nonsteroidal anti-inflammatory drugs or aspirin. If this fails, surgery may be needed. Treatment is intralesional resection and care must be taken not to remove too much of the surrounding sclerotic bone so as not to weaken the bone resulting in fracture. A less invasive strategy is CT-guided radiofrequency ablation used to cause tumor necrosis and results in similar outcomes to surgical resection.

Osteochondroma

Osteochondromas are also referred to as exostoses and are the second most common benign tumors of bone. These are primarily benign bony excrescences with cartilaginous caps that occur during the second and third decades of life. They may be either isolated lesions or part of a hereditary syndrome (multiple hereditary exostoses). To make the diagnosis of osteochondroma, there must be an associated cartilaginous cap on the bony base of the tumor. Malignant degeneration of the cartilaginous cap has been reported. Isolated exostoses are rare but are slightly more common in the hereditary multiple form of the disease. Individuals presenting with pain or other indications of rapid growth are best treated by excision of the lesion but otherwise, asymptomatic patients do not require surgery.

Benign/Aggressive Tumors of Bone

Giant Cell Tumor of Bone

Giant cell tumors are solitary, epiphyseal lesions of the bone, most commonly occurring in the distal femur. It presents during the third through fifth decades with a spectrum from low-grade to high-grade malignancy. Although uncommon, these tumors can metastasize to the lung, and rarely, may be fatal. Treatment of low-grade tumors involves curettage, often with an adjuvant such as argon beam coagulation, followed by a bone graft. Recurrences and more highly malignant tumors require wide excision and reconstruction as necessary with a bone graft.

Malignant Tumors of Bone

Classic Osteosarcoma

Most often occurring during the adolescent growth spurt, and more frequently in males than in females, classic osteosarcomas usually present during the second or third decade of life. The tumor is found in the metaphyseal portion of long bones and the distal femur is the most common site. Typically, patients complain of pain before a mass is noticeable. On radiograph, lytic destruction of the bone is evident, and the tumor eventually breaks into the subperiosteal space and then forms a Codman triangle (radiographic evidence of periosteal reaction) at the diaphyseal end of the tumor. The periosteal reaction may have the classic radial or sunburst pattern. Treatment with chemotherapy and surgical intervention yields a 5-year survival rate of 70%. For osteosarcoma in the extremities, the standard treatment is limb-sparing surgery with wide resection of the tumor. Some cases may require amputation. For cases with pulmonary metastases, multiple thoracotomies and chemotherapy have yielded a 5-year survival rate of 30%.

Multiple Myeloma

Multiple myeloma, the most common malignant bone tumor, usually presents after the fifth decade. The classic radiographic appearance is that of a lytic lesion without a sclerotic border that causes endosteal erosion, cortical expansion, or both. A classic diagnostic criterion is the presence of Bence Jones proteinuria with possible renal damage. Rarely are lesions found below the knee or elbow. Bone scans are considered less sensitive than the skeletal survey in this entity, as the scan may well be negative even with large lesions present on radiographs. With the new discovery that myeloma cells enhance osteoclast formation through the osteoprotegerin/ RANKL pathway, new treatment paradigms are aimed at inhibiting RANKL and subsequently decreasing osteolysis. Current treatment involves chemotherapy, use of cemented intramedullary nails and prosthetic devices following intralesional debridement, and radiation.

Ewing Sarcoma

Radiographically, Ewing sarcoma, most often presenting between the ages of 5 and 25 years, has an elongated permeative appearance on radiographs and frequently has abundant periosteal new bone formation. In 90% of the cases, a chromosomal abnormality has been found on chromosomes 11 and 22. The differential diagnosis includes metastatic neuroblastoma, infection, osteosarcoma, and lymphoma. The tumor destroys much of the cortical bone and eventually appears as a typical onionskin, multilaminated lesion. Ewing sarcoma is aggressive and treatment with multidrug chemotherapy yields a 5-year survival rate of 70%, but for patients with a nonlocalized form, the 5-year survival rate is 30%. Ewing sarcoma is radiosensitive so radiation over 5 weeks is used to treat local disease. Surgery has been investigated as a means for local control but remains a controversial treatment method.

PEDIATRICS

Fractures

Children are subject to most of the same fractures as adults. However, they have a more complex bony anatomy due to the presence of growth plates. The cartilaginous growth plates sandwiched between the metaphysis and epiphysis create a composite structure with different properties than those of adult bone. Although the higher metabolic activity of children's bone allows a greater percentage of bony remodeling after fracture, damage to the growth plate from fracture leads to deformities that are progressive rather than static, as in the adult. The Salter–Harris classification has been developed as a prognostic aid for dealing with fractures through the growth plate; the higher the classification, the more likely is physeal arrest to occur. More recently, Ogden extended the Salter–Harris classification to include periphyseal fractures; although not commonly used, they are included for completeness (Fig. 23.15).

Salter I Fractures

A Salter I fracture is a transverse fracture through the growth plate that in general is nondisplaced and frequently not visible on radiographs. It is therefore commonly diagnosed clinically. The prognosis for normal growth is excellent.

Salter II Fractures

A Salter II fracture occurs transversely through the growth plate at the same level as a Salter I but exits through the metaphysis before completely transversing the growth plate. These fractures may or may not be displaced and, although of a slightly higher severity than a Salter I fracture, with acceptable reduction carry a good prognosis, as the resting or germinal layer of the growth plate has remained unaffected.

Salter III Fracture

Salter III fractures involve a transverse fracture of the growth plate with exit across the germinal layer of the growth plate out through the epiphysis of the bone. Not only do these fractures involve the articular surface,

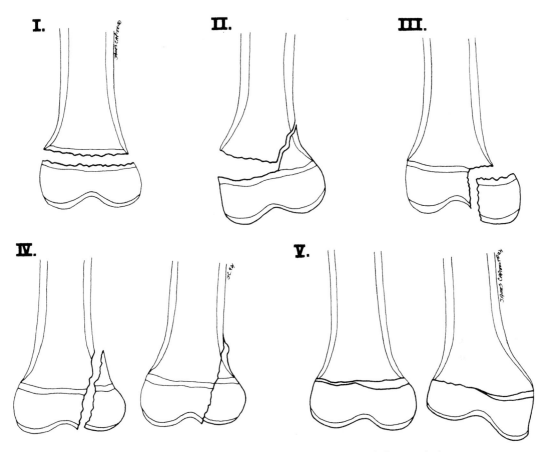

FIGURE 23.15.   Salter–Harris classification of fractures through the growth plate.

leading to a potential for functional abnormality, they also disturb the germinal layer. If sufficient area has been damaged, it can lead to cessation of growth of all or a portion of the growth plate, resulting in increased anatomic and functional deformity. Anatomic reduction and fixation without disrupting the physis are pivotal.

Salter IV Fracture

Salter IV fractures occur in line with the longitudinal axis of the bone. They cross the growth plate in a perpendicular manner and, as with Salter III fractures, affect the articular surface of the joint and germinal layer of the epiphyseal plate, and require anatomic reduction and fixation.

Salter V Fracture

Salter V fractures cause crush of the growth plate, greatly affecting the germinal layer. As such, they have high potential for growth abnormality and increasing deformity.

Ogden VI Fracture

An Ogden VI fracture is characterized as an injury to the perichondral ring at the edge of the physis. Since peripheral physeal bridges are common, the prognosis can vary case to case.

Ogden VII Fracture

Ogden VII fractures only involve the epiphysis and include osteochondral fractures and epiphyseal avulsions. Depending on the location of the fracture, the prognosis is variable.

Ogden VIII Fracture

Ogden VIII fractures are metaphyseal. Primary circulation to the area of the cartilage where remodeling cells lie is disrupted.

Ogden IX Fracture

An Ogden IX fracture is diaphyseal with a good prognosis. The periosteum is interrupted so union of the tibia/fibula or radius/ulna may occur if the respective periosteums cross.

Treatment

Salter I and II fractures, if they can be adequately reduced, can be maintained in a cast and treated conservatively. Salter III and IV fractures have the potential to be treated conservatively if completely nondisplaced. However, because of the potential for late displacement and the rapidity with which this type of fracture solidifies even when nondisplaced, many surgeons opt for pin fixation. Displaced fractures of this category require surgical intervention.

All of these fractures require close monitoring for growth abnormality. These growth abnormalities can be dealt with if there is local tethering of the growth plate through resection of the area of tethering. If an entire growth plate or the major portion of a growth plate has been affected, epiphysiodesis or obliteration of the growth plate in that extremity or the contralateral one (or both) may be necessary.

Long-standing limb length abnormalities may require surgery for limb elongation. A variety of external fixation devices are available that can lead to excellent results in skilled, competent hands.

Child Abuse

Child abuse prevails among many varying socioeconomic classes. Although potential for abuse, whether physical, psychological, or sexual, is always difficult to assess, the suspicion of child abuse carries a moral, ethical, and in many states legal obligation to report. There are no specific fractures or fracture patterns that are pathognomonic of child abuse, but there are situations that may be indicative. Paramount in suspected abuse is determining if the history given is plausible. Fractures of long bones in nonambulatory children, especially those with spiral patterns, are uncommon in situations other than child abuse. Although clearly some situations can cause this type of injury that are not child abuse, all too often the ultimate etiology is either some sort of physiologic abnormality or child abuse. The wrenching or twisting of an extremity is the source of this type of fracture.

A second presentation that is highly suspicious is multiple fractures of differing ages within a single individual. This, again, is either indicative of a physiologic abnormality or more commonly, of child abuse.

Treatment of abuse fractures usually consists of simple closed methods and almost all of the fractures heal or remodel rapidly.

Slipped Capital Femoral Epiphysis

Slipped capital femoral epiphysis usually occurs early in the adolescent years and is characterized as a hip disorder where the femoral head is displaced from the femoral neck. One of the primary causes of osteoarthritis in young adults, it affects both males and females and the patients are often overweight. Patients are usually in a growth spurt and complain of pain about the hip or knee (referred pain to the knee is often a source of misdiagnosis). When a patient in this age group complains of pain about the knee, a thorough examination and radiographs of the hips are a must. Slipped capital femoral epiphysis is a progressive disorder so early detection and treatment are crucial. Treatment involves maintaining the position of the femoral head with pins or screws until the femoral epiphyseal plate stops growing. A significant incidence of bilaterality exists, and caution must be exercised to observe the contralateral side.

QUESTIONS

Select one answer.

1. Early fracture stabilization of long bone and pelvic fractures in polytrauma patients reduces the risk of all of the following Except
   a. Sepsis
   b. Negative nitrogen balance
   c. ARDS
   d. Fat embolism
   e. Malunion or nonunion

2. Principles for managing high-grade complex open fractures include all of the following EXCEPT
   a. Intravenous antibiotics.
   b. Thorough irrigation and debridement.
   c. Cast immobilization.
   d. Meticulous soft tissue care.
   e. Careful assessment of compartment pressures.

3. The nerve most commonly injured in anterior shoulder dislocations is the
   a. Suprascapular nerve.
   b. Ulnar nerve.
   c. Median nerve.
   d. Axillary nerve.
   e. Long thoracic nerve.

4. Posterior dislocations of the hip most commonly injure which nerve?

a. Femoral nerve.
b. Obturator nerve.
c. Sciatic nerve.
d. Peroneal nerve.
e. Interosseous nerve.

5. Vascular compromise has been associated with all of the following injuries EXCEPT
   a. Clavicle fracture.
   b. Knee dislocation.
   c. Patella fracture.
   d. Sternoclavicular joint dislocation.
   e. Supracondylar fracture of the humerus.

6. Which of the following scenarios warrants operative exploration of the radial nerve after closed manipulation of a fracture of the shaft of the humerus?
   a. No radial nerve function at the time of the initial physical examination.
   b. No radial nerve function on presentation and without improvement after closed manipulation.
   c. Intact radial nerve function at presentation and after closed reduction, but no function at the initial office visit 1 week after the fracture.
   d. Intact radial nerve function on presentation but no function after closed reduction.
   e. Intact radial nerve function on presentation, after manipulation, and at subsequent office visits.

7. A 23-year-old male motorcyclist presents to the emergency department with bilateral closed femoral fractures. He is placed in bilateral traction and admitted. Twenty-four hours later, he is confused and tachypneic. The most likely diagnosis is
   a. Pulmonary embolism.
   b. Myocardial infarction.
   c. Fat embolism.
   d. Urinary tract infection.
   e. Stroke.

8. The most common primary bone malignancy is
   a. Osteosarcoma.
   b. Synovial sarcoma.
   c. Multiple myeloma.
   d. Malignant fibrous histiocytoma.
   e. Chondrosarcoma.

9. The position in which a patient with a posterior dislocation of the hip holds the affected extremity is
   a. Abducted, flexed, and externally rotated.
   b. Abducted, flexed, and internally rotated.
   c. Adducted, flexed, and internally rotated.
   d. Adducted, flexed, and externally rotated.
   e. Abducted, extended, and internally rotated.

10. Which of the following types of childhood Salter fractures of long bones is associated with the highest likelihood of subsequent growth arrest?
    a. Type I.
    b. Type II.
    c. Type III.
    d. Type IV.
    e. Type V.

11. The most important diagnostic test in an adolescent with knee pain and normal knee radiographs is
    a. Ipsilateral hip radiographs.
    b. Ipsilateral femur radiographs.
    c. AP pelvis.
    d. Bilateral hip radiographs.
    e. Ipsilateral tibia radiographs.

12. A young female patient presents with pain with an L5 radiculopathy and weakness of the extensor hallucis longus on the right. The level of the herniated disc most likely is
    a. L2–3.
    b. L3–4.
    c. L4–5.
    d. L5–S1.

13. An osteosarcoma of the distal femur that has been shown by MRI to have broken through into the surrounding muscle would be classified as a
    a. IB
    b. IIA
    c. IIB
    d. IIIB

14. The following regarding scapular fractures are true:
    a. Uncommon injuries.
    b. May be associated with additional ipsilateral fractures.

c. Are associated with pneumothorax, pulmonary contusions, and spine fractures.

d. Often treated nonoperatively.

e. All of the above.

15. All of the following are indications to surgically fix midshaft humerus fractures EXCEPT

a. Open fracture.

b. Polytrauma.

c. Young patient.

d. Segmental fracture.

e. Floating elbow.

16. All of the following regarding hip fractures are true EXCEPT

a. More common in women.

b. Often occur from low-energy trauma in the elderly.

c. Patients are able to bear weight as tolerated postoperatively with modern implants.

d. Is defined as a fracture of the proximal femur.

e. Later stabilization of the fracture has the same 1-year mortality as early fracture stabilization (<48 hours).

17. The following are true regarding intra-articular fractures:

a. Require surgical fixation if more than minimally displaced.

b. Have low morbidity.

c. Heal well with prolonged immobilization of the involved joint.

d. Patients can be weight bearing as tolerated immediately.

e. All of the above.

18. All of the following regarding knee dislocations are true EXCEPT

a. They are often undiagnosed an estimated 50% to 60% of the time.

b. Require amputation.

c. Are associated with multiple ligamentous disruption.

d. May be associated with peroneal nerve injury up to 25%.

e. Are a devastating injury.

19. A 13-month-old boy is seen in the emergency department with a complaint of redness and swelling of his right leg. The child appears in pain. He is not yet walking as per the parents, and they did not observe any trauma. He has a spiral fracture of his right femur on radiographs. You should

a. Indicate the child for surgery.

b. Apply a splint and instruct the parents to follow-up with an orthopaedic surgeon.

c. Perform a skeletal survey.

d. Obtain a more detailed account of the occurrence and consult orthopaedics and child services.

e. Apply a hip spica cast.

20. Patients diagnosed with slipped capital femoral epiphysis:

a. Are often obese.

b. Present with inability to ambulate and complain of knee pain.

c. May often have bilateral disease.

d. Usually treated surgically.

e. All of the above.

SELECTED REFERENCES

Bone LB, Johnson KD, Weigelt J, Scheinberg R. Early versus delayed stabilization of femoral fractures. A prospective randomized study. *J Bone Joint Surg Am* 1989;71(3):336–340.

Brundage SI, McGhan R, Jurkovich GJ, et al. Timing of femur fracture fixation: effect on outcome in patients with thoracic and head injuries. *J Trauma* 2002;52(2):299–307.

Canale ST, Beaty JH. *Campbell's operative orthopaedics*, 11th ed, Vol 1–3. Philadelphia, PA: Mosby Inc., 2008.

Denis F. The three column spine and its significance in the classification of acute thoracolumbar spinal injuries. *Spine* 1983;8:817.

Gustilo RB, Anderson JT. The prevention of infection in the treatment of one thousand and twenty-five open fractures of long bone. *J Bone Joint Surg Am* 1976;58:453–458.

Gustilo RB, Merkow RL, Templeman D. The management of open fractures. *J Bone Joint Surg Am* 1990;72:299–304.

Hoppenfeld S. *Physical examination of the spine and extremities*. Norwalk, CT: Appleton-Century-Crofts, 1976.

Joyce A, Martin MPH, Brady E, et al. Division of Vital Statistics. *National Vital Statistics Report.* CDC 2005;54(2).

Koval KJ, Zuckerman JD. *Handbook of fractures*, 2nd ed. Philadelphia, PA: Lippincott Williams & Wilkins, 2002.

Pape HC, Grimme K, Van Griensen M, et al. EPOFF Study Group. Impact of intramedullary instrumentation versus damage control for femoral fractures on immunoinflammatory parameters: prospective randomized analysis by the EPOFF Study Group. *J Trauma* 2003;55(1):7–11.

Patel RV, DeLong W Jr, Vresilovic EJ. Evaluation and treatment of spinal injuries in the patient with polytrauma. *Clin Orthop Relat Res* 2004;(422):43–54.

Scalea TM, Boswell SA, Scott JD, et al. External fixation as a bridge to intramedullary nailing for patients with multiple injuries and with femur fractures: damage control orthopaedics. *J Trauma* 2000;48(4).

Seibel R, LaDuca J, Hassett JM, et al. Blunt multiple trauma (ISS 36), femur traction, and the pulmonary failure-septic state. *Ann Surg* 1985;202(3):283–295.

Skinner HB. *Current diagnosis and treatment in orthopaedics*, 4th ed. New York: McGraw-Hill Companies, Inc., 2006.

Taeger G, Ruchholtz S, Waydhas C, et al. Damage control orthopaedics in patients with multiple injuries is effective, time saving, and safe. *J Trauma* 2005;59(2):409–416.

Selected Principles of Plastic Surgery

S elected principles of plastic surgery of interest to general surgeons and may be important components of a knowledge base expected of a practicing general surgeon. This chapter deals with various aspects of hand surgery, principles of wound healing and soft tissue coverage, and breast reconstruction.

HAND ANATOMY

Surface Anatomy

The surface anatomy of the hand is separated into a volar surface and a dorsal surface. The thenar musculature relates to the thumb and the hypothenar musculature to the little finger. Starting proximally, the joints of the fingers are called the metacarpophalangeal (MCP) joint, proximal interphalangeal (PIP) joint, and distal interphalangeal (DIP) joint.

Nerve Supply to the Hand

The median nerve innervates the finger flexors and is needed for thumb opposition and thumb abduction. Its sensory distribution is to the radial three and one-half digits (thumb, index, long, and radial half of the ring finger). Compression of the median nerve at the wrist is the cause of carpal tunnel syndrome.

The ulnar nerve supplies innervation to the intrinsic muscles of the hand (finger abduction) and facilitates wrist flexion. Sensory branches supply the dorsum of the ring and little fingers as well as the palmar aspect of the little and ulnar border of the ring finger. An injury to the ulnar nerve results in a claw hand.

The radial nerve supplies all of the extensor muscles of the hand and wrist. It has a dorsal sensory branch to the dorsum of the thumb, index, and long fingers. Radial nerve injury results in wrist drop.

Sensibility in the hand is best tested by moving two-point discrimination. Median intrinsic function is best demonstrated by thumb opposition (bringing the thumb out of the plane of the rest of the hand). Ulnar intrinsic muscles are tested by crossing the index and long fingers over each other or abducting and adducting the little finger. Motor function of the radial nerve can be tested by assessing wrist extension.

Tendons of the Hand

Muscles that power the hand are divided into extrinsic muscles (having their muscle bellies in the forearm and tendon insertion in the hand) and intrinsic muscles (having their origin and insertion within the hand). The extrinsic muscles include the long extensor tendons, which are arranged in six compartments on the dorsum of the wrist. They are essentially MCP joint extenders. The superficial flexor tendons function as PIP joint flexors, and the profundus tendons function as DIP joint flexors.

Intrinsic muscles include the thenar muscles, the lumbrical muscles, the interosseous muscles, and the hypothenar muscles. The MCP joints are flexed by the intrinsics. The lumbrical muscles have their origin from the profundus tendon and insertion into the dorsal expansion. They function to flex the MCP joint and extend the interphalangeal joint.

Sublimis function is tested by flexing the finger while blocking the motion of the fingers on each side of the finger being tested. The common profundus tendons are then blocked in extension. Profundus function is tested by blocking superficialis function by holding the middle phalanx extended.

Vascular Anatomy

The hand and fingers are supplied by a deep and a superficial vascular arch. The deep arch is the dominant arch. The ulnar artery is the dominant arterial supply to the hand in 80% of cases. Adequacy of hand circulation is checked by capillary refill in each fingertip and the Allen test. The Allen test is performed by occluding both the radial and ulnar arteries at the wrist. After flexion and extension of the fingers several times, each artery is released separately, and circulation is monitored by the return of capillary refill to all of the five digits.

FLEXOR TENDON INJURIES

As a general rule, flexor tendon repairs should be undertaken only when wound conditions are satisfactory. Ideally, repairs are performed within 1 week through a closed, healing, noninfected wound.

EXTENSOR TENDON INJURIES

Extensor tendon injuries at the level of the hand, wrist, and forearm are repaired end to end. Because of intertendinous junctura, such tendons are held in place and do not tend to retract. Late repairs of finger extensor tendons are possible several weeks after injury. The prognosis following repair of isolated extensor injuries is good. When they are associated with other injuries such as fractures of the metacarpals and digits, adhesions may develop.

Mallet Finger

A mallet finger may be a result of either an open or closed injury. Either a laceration of the dorsum of the DIP joint or forced flexion of an actively extended finger may result in loss of full extension of the distal joint. A closed injury with a large associated fracture (30% of the joint surface) may require reduction and fixation of the fracture. Open lacerations are sutured, including repair of the severed tendon. Following repairs, the fingers are splinted. Closed injuries without major fractures and late open injuries may be treated successfully by splinting in extension for a period of 6 weeks to 3 months. Untreated mallet fingers may result in swan-neck deformities, where the PIP joint is hyperextended and the DIP joint is held in flexion. Repairs of this deformity are complex.

Boutonnière or Buttonhole Deformity

The boutonnière deformity is a result of an open or closed injury to the extensor tendon over the middle phalanx or PIP joint. This injury allows the lateral bands to slip volar to the PIP joint axis. The extensor mechanism shifts proximally, resulting in DIP joint hyperextension and PIP joint flexion. Early injuries may be treated with prolonged periods of splinting in extension allowing the extensor tendons to heal via the formation of functional scar. Several techniques for secondary surgical repairs have been described, the simplest involving shortening of the functional scar and repair of the tendon.

INFECTIONS

All infections of the hand should be considered serious since delayed recognition and treatment may result in osteomyelitis, skin necrosis, and amputation. Infections in the hand tend to be "closed-space" infections with little room for collections of large quantities of purulence. In general, antibiotics play a supportive role to adequate surgical drainage and débridement. Prolonged rehabilitation therapy following an infection may be necessary to avoid sequelae such as hand dysfunction.

Bites to the Hand

- *Dog bites*—approximately 50% of dog bites become infected. The organisms involved are *Pasteurella multocida*, *Staphylococcus aureus*, and/or *Bacteroides*. The treatment of choice remains amoxicillin with clavulanate (AM/CL).
- *Cat bites* have a very high incidence of becoming infected (80%) and the wounds, therefore, are usually left open. The organisms involved are *P. multocida* or *S. aureus*. All cat bites get treated with AM/CL.
- *Human bites* frequently become infected. A multitude of organisms are often involved including *Eikenella corrodens*, *Bacteroides*, *Streptococcus viridians*, *S. epidermis*, *S. aureus*, and *Cornybacterium*. Human bites should not be closed primarily and require aggressive treatment with antibiotics. Early bites with no signs of infection are treated with AM/CL. Infected bites are treated with ampicillin + sulbactam, cefoxitin, or trimethoprim + sulfamethoxazole if the patient has a penicillin allergy.

Paronychia

A paronychia is an infection of the soft tissues around the fingernail. It is usually caused by *S. aureus*. Long-standing chronic paronychia is often fungal in origin. The tissue around the nail is usually red, swollen, and painful. Direct incision into the abscess proximal to the nail is often adequate to treat these infections. Rarely, it is necessary to raise a flap of skin overlying the proximal nail fold. When this is performed, one risks damaging the germinal matrix of the nail, which may result in a permanent nail deformity. Improperly treated paronychias may result in felons and osteomyelitis. In diabetics, paronychia and felons can be serious infections and hospital admission and intravenous antibiotics should be considered. Careful follow-up is mandatory.

Felon

Felons are pulp space infections of the digits, often caused by *S. aureus.* Tight septa attach the volar tip skin of the digits to the terminal phalanges, dividing the fat pad into multiple compartments. All felons require appropriate surgical drainage and intravenous antibiotics. Adequate drainage requires division of these septa to open all of the involved spaces. A popular incision is a subungual "hockey stick" type, extending from the anterodistal border of one side of the fingertip around to the proximal portion of the nail on the opposite side, with the incision carried down to the bone. Proper placement of the incision is critical to divide all of the septa and to avoid necrosis of the fat pad. Improperly treated felons can result in osteomyelitis of the distal phalanx.

Herpes Simplex Virus

Herpes simplex (herpetic whitlow) infections show signs of vesicle formation. They can be distinguished from other infections on the basis of a 24- to 72-hour prodromal period of burning pain. A diagnosis can be established with a Tzanck smear demonstrating multinucleated giant cells. Surgical treatment is generally contraindicated, and if performed can lead to a super infection. Most infections resolve spontaneously. Immunocompromised patients should be treated with acyclovir.

SEVERE INFECTIONS OF THE HAND

Suppurative Tenosynovitis

These are infections that spread along the flexor tendon sheath. A small quantity of purulence within the tendon sheath may present as a severe infections

because it is contained in a closed space. Kanavel's classic signs for the recognition of tenosynovitis are (a) swelling of the involved digit, (b) exquisite pain with passive extension, (c) tenderness elicited by palpation over the sheath, and (d) the patient maintaining the finger in slight flexion (to avoid extension). *S. aureus* is the most common causative organism, although mixed infections have become more common.

Treatment involves intravenous antibiotics and surgical drainage of the tendon sheath. Drainage with continuous irrigation has been used successfully. For neglected infections, wide drainage and excision of necrotic tissue is often necessary.

Superficial Lymphangitis

Following an abrasion or superficial puncture wound of the hand, a rapidly spreading superficial lymphangitis may develop in 24 to 48 hours. The hallmark of this is red streaking, extending from the point of injury linearly up the forearm and arm. Most infections are due to *S. aureus* or *Streptococcus.*

FINGERTIP INJURIES

For fingertip injuries, it is often best to consider the simplest method of closure. This frequently involves debridement and reattachment of the amputated tip skin as a full-thickness skin graft. Harvested skin from the hypothenar area, lateral border of the foot, or thigh may also be used. Grafts are applicable only in those settings where minimal exposed bone is present or when debridement of exposed bone may result in only minimal shortening of the involved digit. In the case of the thumb, length and sensibility are critical for function, and every effort should be made to preserve functional length.

In children, secondary healing should be considered in cases where skin is not available from amputated specimens. The final healed result often equals that of grafted digits and donor-site deformity is eliminated.

Crush injuries to the fingertip that result in subungual hematomas require removal of the nail plate for exploration of the nail bed. The disrupted nail bed must be repaired to ensure normal nail growth.

TRAUMATIC AMPUTATIONS

General indications for replantation are multiple digital amputations, thumb amputations, and single-digit amputations in young patients or those with special occupational requirements. Amputations of border digits (i.e., the index or little finger), a single digit in zone 2 of the hand (area where the superficialis tendon inserts into the finger, also known as "no mans land"), severe crush or contamination, and patients with medical illnesses that contraindicate surgical intervention are not candidates for replantation.

Proper handling of the amputated parts prior to transfer to replantation centers is critical if microvascular repairs are to be attempted. The amputated specimens should be transported with the patient even if deemed nonreplantable, because they can often be utilized for "spare parts" such as vein, skin, and nerve grafts. Amputated parts should be wrapped in saline soaked gauze and placed in a plastic bag. The plastic bag should be placed on an ice bath.

Because of the severe functional disability associated with major amputations, attempts should be made to replant these parts when feasible.

OTHER HAND DISORDERS

Volkmann Ischemic Contracture

Volkmann ischemic contracture is the result of a forearm compartment syndrome. On examination, patients have pain in the forearm with passive extension and a tense forearm with motor weakness and sensory deficits. Normal compartment pressures are 0 to 8 mm Hg. In the presence of a compartment syndrome, these pressures rise to 30 to 50 mm Hg.

The etiology of Volkmann-type injuries includes massive crush injuries, supercondylar fractures of the elbow, elbow dislocations, high-pressure injection injury, emboli, snake bites, and fractures of the radius or ulna. Muscle swelling and necrosis cause secondary fibrosis and contracture. The classic deformity is a flexion contracture of the wrist and all five digits. Claw hand deformity secondary to intrinsic muscle paralysis is present, as are median and ulnar nerve sensory deficits.

Prevention of the secondary deformities of Volkmann ischemic contracture requires adequate and expeditious fasciotomy. This often means decompression of the carpal tunnel, the volar forearm (both the superficial and deep compartments), the dorsal musculature, and the intrinsic muscles of the hand.

Carpal Tunnel Syndrome

The median nerve, along with the nine flexor tendons to the digits, passes through the carpal tunnel beneath the transverse carpal ligament at the wrist. Carpal tunnel syndrome is a compression neuropathy and may be associated with pregnancy, rheumatoid arthritis, wrist fractures, diabetes, thyroid disease, and chronic renal failure. Most cases are idiopathic.

Patients complain of numbness and tingling in the radial three and one-half digits (i.e., thumb, index, long, and radial border of the ring finger). Often the pain occurs at night and is relieved by dependency. In long-standing cases, there can be muscular atrophy with thenar muscle wasting. On examination, tapping over the wrist may produce an "electric shock" type of response over the median nerve (Tinel's sign). Symptoms are elicited when the wrist is held in flexion for 1 minute (Phalen's test). Nerve conduction studies and electromyography demonstrate slowing of nerve conduction and denervation activity in involved muscles.

In early cases with only sensory involvement, treatment with splinting and local injection of steroids may be satisfactory. Long-standing cases and those with motor involvement are treated surgically. An incision is made ulnar to the thenar crease in the palm. It may be continued onto the distal forearm for a short distance by an incision that crosses the wrist crease at a 60-degree angle. The nerve is identified in the proximal portion of the incision and protected as the transverse carpal ligament is opened from the wrist to the superficial palmar arch. The anterior epineurium is split until a normal fascicular pattern is noted pouting out of the nerve (external neurolysis). Internal dissection (internal neurolysis) is generally reserved for treatment failures.

Stenosing Tenosynovitis (Trigger Finger)

Any of the five digits may be involved in stenosing tenosynovitis. Snapping of the flexor tendon as it passes under the first annular pulley (A1 pulley) located proximal to the MCP joint is the early sign of the syndrome. Often the involved digit starts locking in flexion, as the thickened tendon catches under the pulley. The tendon may be painful to palpation at the MCP joint.

Treatment initially consists of steroid injection into the tendon sheath at the level of the involved pulley. If this fails, surgery is performed through a small transverse incision, usually located in the distal palmar crease. The A1 pulley is identified and divided.

De Quervain Syndrome

De Quervain syndrome is a nonspecific tenosynovitis involving the first dorsal wrist compartment tendons (abductor pollicis longus and extensor pollicis brevis).

Pain over the area of the radial styloid that may radiate up the arm and down to the thumb is present. The pain is elicited by active use of the thumb when grasping and may be reproduced when the thumb is grasped by the other digits, and the wrist is ulnar deviated (Finkelstein test).

Steroid injection and splinting are usually tried as the first therapeutic modality. If these fail, the first dorsal compartment is decompressed surgically. A transverse incision is made over the radial styloid, with care taken to avoid injury to the radial nerve sensory branches. A linear incision is made through the dorsal carpal ligament, and the tendons are freed from the compartment.

Glomus Tumors

Glomus tumors in the hand are characteristically found subungually. Most glomus tumors are associated with paroxysmal, severe, radiating pain. Subungual lesions may be exceptionally small and difficult to locate and may be visible only as a small area of salmon or bluish discoloration underneath the nail. The tumors are derivatives of the glomus body, a normal arteriovenous communication, and are benign lesions. They may be identified on magnetic resonance imaging.

These tumors require surgical excision. Attempts should be made to preserve the overlying nail bed during operative removal to minimize postoperative nail deformity.

Dupuytren Contracture

Dupuytren contracture is a proliferation and contracture of bands of the palmar aponeurosis between the skin and the flexor tendons. It occurs most frequently in the ring and little fingers. It begins as a nodule and progresses to include fibrous bands extending to the digits, pulling them into a flexed position. It is a slowly progressive process and is generally painless and nonulcerating. The condition affects only extension. The fibrous process closely involves the digital nerves.

Dupuytren contracture is generally thought to be hereditary and not occupational. The disease occurs in a male to female ratio of approximately 8:1. Patients with Dupuytren diathesis are diagnosed by (a) a strong family history, (b) early age of onset, (c) ectopic areas of involvement such as Peyronie disease of the penis and contractures of the toes, and (d) associated diseases such as epilepsy, alcoholism,

cirrhosis, pulmonary tuberculosis, and diabetes. The disease is often bilateral and associated with knuckle pads on the dorsum of the hand.

Initial management is conservative with stretching exercises. Operation is indicated when the patient is unable to flatten his or her hand on a tabletop. In patients without the diathesis, conservative surgery consisting of subtotal fasciectomy often suffices. A longitudinal incision is made over the band of contracture, and after careful identification and preservation of the digital neurovascular bundles, the involved tissue is excised. The incision is then closed with multiple Z-plasties.

Total fasciectomy is performed in patients with Dupuytren diathesis. The entire palmar aponeurosis is resected, including resection into the involved fingers. Skin grafts may be necessary for closure.

PRINCIPLES OF WOUND HEALING AND SOFT TISSUE COVERAGE

Wound Healing

There are three phases to wound healing: the inflammatory phase, the proliferative phase, and the remodeling phase.

Inflammatory Phase (2 to 3 Days)

Following an injury the inflammatory phase begins. This begins with vasoconstriction of surrounding vessels to achieve hemostasis followed by the formation of a platelet plug and the activation of the clotting cascade. Inflammatory cells migrate to the wound. At 24 hours, neutrophils are the predominant cell and help with removal of debris. Macrophages follow and peak within 2 to 3 days. Macrophages stimulate collagen formation.

Proliferative Phase (4 to 21 Days)

During this phase collagen synthesis, angiogenesis, and re-epithelialization occur, and granulation tissue begins to fill the wound. After 3 weeks of increasing collagen content, collagen formation and collagen breakdown equilibrate and the third phase of wound healing begins.

Remodeling Phase (Lasts up to 1 Year)

The remodeling phase is the least well-understood phase of wound healing. Type I collagen replaces type

III until it reaches a 4:1 ratio. Wound contraction occurs via fibroblast and myofibroblasts, and wound strength increases from 20% to 70% of unwounded skin.

Excessive Scar Formation: Keloid and Hypertrophic Scars

Keloid and hypertrophic scars are forms of abnormal scar formation. Keloid scars are much less common and affect mostly African American or Asian populations. They have an autosomal dominant genetic component. Histologically, keloid scars are found to contain thick collagen bundles and clinically extend beyond the border of a scar. Typically, keloid scars do not improve with time.

Hypertrophic scars often occur along flexor surfaces of the upper torso. They are more likely to cause contractures and can be distinguished from keloid scars by their tendency to stay within the boundaries of an original wound. They will sometimes regress spontaneously.

Both keloid and hypertrophic scars can be treated with steroids, silicone sheeting, or pressure garments. Severe keloids are often treated with direct excision and immediate external beam radiation.

Soft Tissue Coverage

The factors that dictate appropriate wound closure are the site of tissue loss, the presence of contamination or infection, the exposure of underlying vital structures, the need to perform pre- or postoperative radiation therapy, and the need to perform secondary procedures in the same operative field.

Free Skin Grafts

A skin graft is a segment of dermis and epidermis that has been completely separated from its blood supply and donor-site attachment before being transferred to another area of the body. Skin grafts are generally classified according to their thickness. Split-thickness skin grafts include the epidermis and part of the dermis. This graft is versatile and popular, and it is likely to survive on its recipient site. The donor site heals rapidly by re-epithelialization, and large amounts of donor material can be obtained with little morbidity. Its main disadvantage is that it undergoes a greater degree of soft tissue contracture; and, depending on its thickness, hair follicles and sebaceous glands may not be included in the graft.

Full-thickness skin grafts comprise the entire thickness of the skin, both the dermis and the epidermis. Because of its thickness, this type of graft is more difficult to harvest and is slower to revascularize. Although it undergoes less contracture and generally gives a superior cosmetic result, optimal conditions are required for a complete take.

Initial graft take is dependent on diffusion of nutrients from the recipient bed to the skin graft, a process known as imbibition. Vascular inoculation can be completed within 48 to 72 hours, with capillary blood flow and neovascularization. Factors leading to graft loss include fluid collections, hematomas or seromas between the graft and the graft bed, shearing forces between the graft and the graft bed, an improper recipient bed, or bacterial contamination of more than 10^5 bacteria per gram of tissue.

Soft Tissue Expansion

Skin, both dermis and epidermis, has the ability to contract and stretch. In soft tissue expansion, a deflated silastic balloon is placed underneath normal skin adjacent to an area that must be removed. Over a period of time, the balloon is inflated with saline injections, thereby stretching the skin over the balloon. Enough excess skin can be generated to allow coverage of adjacent defects.

During the course of soft tissue expansion, a number of changes can be expected. There is thickening and hyperplasia of the epidermis, with increased melanocytic activity. There is also thinning of the dermis with increased collagen synthesis. The adipose tissue is most sensitive to this process and shows compression, with either necrosis or some contour deformities that may be permanent. Muscle function is retained during soft tissue expansion, but there may be thinning and compression of the muscles. There is an enhancement of the vascularity to the overlying skin, which has been demonstrated by the increase in capillaries, arterioles, and venules. Finally, with respect to the dermal appendages, there seem to be no changes in hair follicles, sebaceous glands, sweat glands, sensory nerves, and end receptors.

Vacuum-Assisted Wound Closure (VAC)

Negative pressure wound systems have been an important recent advance in wound care. With this technique, acute traumatic and other wounds can be managed in a nonemergent manner, and surgery for permanent closure can be either avoided or planned for appropriately. A wound VAC changes the microenvironment of a wound by decreasing edema and removing debris through negative pressure. It is important to note that the wound VAC device is contraindicated in the presence of a malignancy, severe infection, or ischemic wounds.

Flaps

A flap is a unit of tissue transferred from a donor site to a recipient site while maintaining its blood supply. Flaps can be used in the following situations: (a) for reconstructing complex defects that will not have an adequate cosmetic result with simple closure or skin grafting, (b) for covering defects in densely scarred areas or areas of functional stress, (c) for covering exposed bone devoid of periosteum, (d) for covering tendons to achieve wound healing and preserve function, (e) for covering nerves, and (f) in areas where secondary surgical procedures may be necessary.

Flaps can be categorized by their tissue composition, method of movement, and vascularity.

1. *Tissue composition*: Flaps can be classified on the basis of their tissue composition.
   - *Fasciocutaneous flaps*: These flaps consist of skin and fascia. They are adaptable and may be used for local or free flaps.
   - *Musculocutaneous flaps*: These flaps contain skin, fascia, and muscle. They have a dominant blood supply or vascular pedicle and may be used as pedicled or free flaps. Muscle flaps are frequently utilized for pressure sores, head and neck cancer reconstruction, breast reconstruction, and reconstruction of irradiated wounds.
   - *Vascularized bone flaps*: These flaps include a portion of bone and are used to reconstruct bony defects often of the head and neck (i.e., mandibular reconstruction).
2. *Method of movement*: The method used to close or reconstruct a defect will depend on the complexity and size of the defect. Local or distant flaps can be used.
   - *Local flaps*: When the donor tissue is adjacent to a defect, the flap is described as a local flap. Examples of local flaps would be advancement flaps, rotation flaps, and z-plasty flaps.
   - *Distant flaps*: These flaps are utilized when the donor site is not adjacent to the defect. These flaps can be direct flaps where the donor tissue can be approximated into the defect. When this is not feasible, a free tissue transfer is needed. Tissue with an attached vascular pedicle (free flap) is

transferred to a distant site and an arterial and venous microsurgical anastomosis is performed to reconstitute blood supply to the donor tissue.
3. *Vascular supply*: Flaps can also be classified on the basis of their blood supply. They may be random, axial, reverse flow, or perforator flaps.
   - *Random flaps*: The blood supply to these flaps is based on the dermal and subdermal plexus and has no single dominant feeding vessel.
   - *Axial flaps*: These flaps contain a named direct cutaneous artery and vein and allow a longer pedicle for transfer.
   - *Reverse flow flaps*: In these flaps, the proximal blood vessel is divided, and blood flow to the flap is dependent on the distal vessels.
   - *Perforator flaps*: The blood supply to these flaps is supplied by isolated perforating vessels. These vessels may pass through or perforate between the deep tissues before they reach the flap. Often these flaps are used for distant coverage.

Breast Reconstruction Using Autologous Tissues

Following mastectomy, patients have many options for breast reconstruction. The two basic concepts available for breast reconstruction include the use of available tissue by placing tissue expanders and implants under existing skin and muscle or tissue adding techniques such as flaps.

An ever increasing variety of options are available for breast reconstruction using autologous tissue, including pedicled flaps and free flaps.

Pedicled Flaps

The latissimus dorsi flap is used in conjunction with an implant and can accomplish a single-stage reconstruction. It is a predictable flap with the thoracodorsal vessels as its dominant vascular pedicle. It can cause a significant donor site scar, and up to 50% of patients can develop a seroma.

TRAM (transverse rectus abdominous musculocutaneous) flaps can be used for both immediate and delayed reconstruction. It is a reliable pedicled flap with a predictable blood supply (superior epigastric vessels) that is easily harvested and provides excellent aesthetic results. It sacrifices the rectus abdominous muscle causing abdominal weakness and contour defects of the abdomen. Patients who have a significant smoking history or patients with obesity are at increased risk of fat necrosis or partial or total flap loss. Patients with abdominal scars are frequently not candidates for a TRAM flap.

Free Flaps

Free flaps require a microsurgical anastomosis for transfer of tissue. Examples include the free TRAM flap, DIEP (deep inferior epigastric perforator) flaps, gluteal flaps (GAP), and the lateral transverse thigh flap.

The DIEP flap uses the skin and subcutaneous tissue of the abdomen to create a new breast mound. No rectus muscle harvest is needed, and it uses perforator vessels as its blood supply. It requires meticulous dissection of the perforator vessels and microsurgical technique to create an anastomosis to the recipient vessels in the chest (usually to the internal mammary artery and vein).

This procedure requires advanced technical skills and increased operating time but has the advantage of less donor site morbidity, specifically less abdominal wall laxity and decreased hernia formation. Common risk factors for flap loss include obesity, smoking, diabetes, and previous scars.

QUESTIONS

Select one answer.

1. A 50-year-old female presents to the emergency department with a felon. She can flex and extend her finger without pain. What is the most appropriate treatment?
   a. IV antibiotics and hand elevation
   b. A hockey stick incision for drainage at the fingertip and IV antibiotics
   c. Warm soaks and IV antibiotics
   d. Close observation and acyclovir

2. A 32-year-old healthy pregnant female comes to your office complaining of tingling in her fingers and wrist pain. You expect the patient to have:
   a. A positive Tinel's sign—symptoms when her hands are held in flexion for 1 minute.
   b. A positive Tinel's sign—electric shock sensation when the wrist is tapped.
   c. A positive Phalen's sign—resolution of symptoms when her hand is held in flexion for 1 minute.
   d. A positive Phalen's sign—electric shock sensation when the wrist is tapped.

3. You are asked to evaluate a 16-year-old male with an abscess on the dorsum of his hand.

During the medical history interview he tells you that his cat bit him there 1 week ago. What is the most likely organism causing this infection?
   a. *Bacteroides*
   b. *Eikenella*
   c. *Streptococcus*
   d. *P. multocida*

4. Which finger is most crucial in a replant for the patient to have good hand function?
   a. Thumb
   b. Ring finger
   c. Index finger
   d. They are all equally important

5. What are the most common bacteria found in hand infections?
   a. *Bacteroides*
   b. *Pasteurella*
   c. *Staphylococcus.*
   d. *Eikenella.*

6. The patency of the radial and ulnar arteries and collateral circulation to the hand can be evaluated by:
   a. Finkelstein maneuver.
   b. Addison maneuver.
   c. Allen's test.
   d. Phalen's test.

7. Rupture of the extensor tendon at its insertion at the distal phalanx may result in:
   a. Mallet finger deformity.
   b. Swan-neck deformity.
   c. Both of the above.
   d. Neither of the above.

8. Two days following a puncture wound to the right ring finger a 45-year-old healthy male comes to the emergency department for care. His finger is swollen and flexed and he has severe pain with passive extension. Which statement is true?
   a. Examination is consistent with a felon and surgical drainage and antibiotics are indicated.
   b. Examination is consistent with acute suppurative tenosynovitis and surgical drainage and antibiotics are indicated.
   c. *S. viridians* is the most likely causative bacteria.

d. Intravenous antibiotics alone are adequate treatment.

9. Contraindications to replantation of amputated digits include:
   a. A thumb in a young patient.
   b. A thumb in a 20-year-old manual laborer.
   c. A complete amputation of the hand at the level of the wrist.
   d. A complete amputation of the index finger at the level of the proximal phalanx.
   e. A gunshot wound to the hand.

10. Dupuytren contracture:
    a. Occurs most frequently in the ring and little finger.

b. Is frequently thought to be a work-related condition.
c. Is frequently quite painful.
d. Prevents the patient from making a full fist.

SELECTED REFERENCES

Blondeel PN, Morris SF, eds. *Perforator flaps: anatomy, technique and clinical applications.* St. Louis, MO: Quality Medical, 2005.

Green DP. *Operative hand surgery.* New York: Churchill Livingstone, 2005.

Kaplan EB. *Functional and surgical anatomy of the hand,* 3rd ed. Philadelphia, PA: JB Lippincott, 1984.

Thorne CH, Beasley RW, eds. *Grabb and Smith's plastic surgery,* 6th ed. Philadelphia, PA: Lippincott Williams & Wilkins, 2007.

Urologic Surgery

T he general surgeon is often confronted with signs and symptoms that suggest pathologic processes involving the genitourinary system. During elective or emergency surgical procedures, unanticipated urologic conditions or problems may be encountered. Multiple trauma victims frequently present with gross or microscopic hematuria as the only manifestation of possible severe urinary tract injury. Accurate diagnosis and appropriate management in such situations require a fundamental knowledge of urologic conditions, surgical techniques, and available diagnostic tools. Such knowledge also helps minimize iatrogenic injury to genitourinary structures during unrelated general surgical procedures. This chapter reviews the more common urologic neoplasms and conditions, genitourinary injuries, and urologic emergencies. Clinical presentation, diagnosis, and treatment are emphasized.

RENAL MASSES

Cysts and Benign Tumors

Renal cysts are the most common mass lesions in the kidney, both clinically and at autopsy. Renal cysts are found in approximately 50% of individuals older than 50 years and are of no clinical significance except to be distinguished from malignancy. Ultrasonography, computed tomography (CT), and magnetic resonance imaging (MRI) are highly accurate in diagnosing benign renal cysts. Occasionally, however, the benign nature of complex cysts (i.e., cysts with thickened or irregular walls, inhomogeneous fluid, calcifications, loculations) can be determined by only surgical excision. Although most renal cysts are asymptomatic, they may cause hematuria, pain, abscess formation, or calyceal or renal pelvic obstruction.

Adult polycystic kidney disease (APKD) is an autosomal dominant condition with a high degree of pen-

etrance. Usually symptoms arise between the ages of 30 and 40. The most common initial symptom is pain in the lumbar region followed by hematuria. Liver cysts are found in approximately 30% of patients with APKD. APKD is also associated with a 10% to 20% incidence of cerebral aneurysm. Treatment, for the most part, is medical with regard to the associated progressive renal failure.

Angiomyolipoma (AML) is a benign clonal neoplasm consisting of varying amounts of mature adipose tissue, smooth muscle, and thick-walled vessels that can manifest clinically as pain, retroperitoneal hemorrhage, gross hematuria, or an abdominal mass. Bilateral or multiple AMLs are commonly associated with tuberous sclerosis (20% to 30%), a clinical syndrome classically characterized by mental retardation, epilepsy, and sebaceous adenomas of the face. Solitary renal hamartomas are most often found in women between the ages of 40 and 60. These tumors are most accurately diagnosed by CT scan or MRI, both of which clearly demonstrate the characteristic fat content. The management of AML is based on symptoms and size. An isolated asymptomatic AML less than 4 cm can be observed. Symptomatic lesions or lesions more than 4 cm can be treated initially by angiographic embolization. If embolization fails, surgical removal is necessary.

Renal cortical adenoma, usually an incidental radiographic or autopsy finding, is the most common benign parenchymal neoplasm. The diagnosis of renal adenoma remains controversial; many believe that all solid renal epithelium–derived masses are potentially malignant and should be treated as such. By definition, benign renal adenomas are less than 3 cm in diameter. These neoplasms have a propensity to grow and eventually metastasize once they are more than 3 cm; they should be extirpated in patients with a life expectancy of more than 10 years.

Oncocytomas represent 3% to 7% of all solid renal masses. They are often histologically indistinguishable from the eosinophilic or granular cell types of renal adenocarcinomas. The electron microscopic finding of cells packed with mitochondria is pathognomonic for oncocytoma. They are unfortunately indistinguishable from malignant renal neoplasms by radiographic imaging at this time. The accuracy of renal fine-needle aspiration or biopsy is compromised by difficulty in distinguishing oncocytoma from the granular forms of conventional renal cell carcinoma (RCC) or the eosinophilic variants of chromophobe or chromophilic RCC. Aggressive treatment is therefore recommended.

Other benign renal tumors, such as fibroma, lipoma, cholesteatoma, leiomyoma, and hemangioma, are exceedingly uncommon. Because radiologic techniques are often inconclusive for defining such tumors, surgical removal is generally necessary and results in partial or total nephrectomy.

Malignant Tumors

Renal cell carcinoma (clear cell adenocarcinoma) accounts for approximately 3% of adult malignancies, with a 2:1 male/female ratio usually presenting in the sixth to seventh decade. A higher incidence occurs in chronic hemodialysis patients, those with APKD, and those with von Hippel-Lindau disease, in which multiple and bilateral renal carcinomas are characteristic. The only generally accepted environmental risk factor for RCC is exposure to tobacco, although the relative associated risks have been modest, ranging from 1.4 to 2.5 compared with controls.

The classic clinical triad of pain, hematuria, and flank mass occurs in no more than 10% of cases as more cases are now found incidentally due to the frequency of radiographic imaging of the abdomen. Associated clinical disturbances include erythrocytosis caused by excessive erythropoietin production, hypercalcemia, hypertension, fever, and weight loss. Hepatic dysfunction in the absence of hepatic metastases occurs in up to 20% of cases.

A suspicion of renal tumor is often based on radiographic imaging usually a renal sonogram, CT scanning without and with intravenous (IV) contrast (the most sensitive diagnostic tool for renal carcinoma), or MRI.

Renal cell carcinomas spread by direct extension and by invasion into adjacent structures and regional lymphatics. The most common sites of distant spread are the lungs, liver, and bone. Approximately one-third of patients initially present with metastatic disease. Renal carcinoma has a characteristic propensity for extension and occasionally invasion into the renal vein or inferior vena cava in the form of a tumor thrombus. This thrombus may extend as far cephalad as the right atrium without invading the vessel wall(s). It is now widely accepted that patients with caval extension and tumor otherwise confined to the kidney are amenable to attempts at surgical cure. MRI has the capacity to demonstrate exquisitely the extent of tumor thrombus in the venous system. Involvement of regional lymph nodes, extension through Gerota's fascia, invasion into adjacent organs, and distant metastases portend a poor prognosis.

Radical nephrectomy, which includes en bloc removal of the kidney, the surrounding perirenal fat, and the ipsilateral adrenal gland, continues to serve as the only effective treatment for RCC and was traditionally considered optimal management for any suspicious renal mass. Renal parenchyma-sparing procedures such as partial nephrectomy or tumor enucleation with adequate margins were initially reserved for patients with a solitary kidney, synchronous bilateral RCCs, or a poorly functioning contralateral kidney. However, recent advances in our understanding of the biology of renal cancer as well as the importance of avoiding chronic renal insufficiency have expanded the indications for partial nephrectomy to include small tumors even in the setting of a normal contralateral kidney. Laparoscopy has also revolutionized the management of these tumors. Most centers of excellence routinely perform radical nephrectomy laparoscopically and reserve the open technique for tumors with renal vein or inferior vena caval extension. Some specialized centers are also performing laparoscopic partial nephrectomy generally considered to be the most challenging laparoscopic urologic procedure.

The results of treatment of metastatic RCC using chemotherapy or radiotherapy have generally been suboptimal. Although solitary metastatic lesions (e.g., bone, lung, and brain) are unusual with renal carcinomas and tumor otherwise confined to the kidney, these patients have 20% to 30% five-year survival after surgical removal of all tumor. Significant stabilization of disease or occasional partial regressions have resulted after treatment with vinblastine, Lomustine (CANO), percutaneous angioinfarction, progesterone, and interferon. Investigations with monoclonal antibodies and interleukin 2/LAK therapies have been promising.

Transitional cell carcinoma of the renal pelvis accounts for approximately 7% to 8% of renal tumors. An increased risk for the development of upper tract urothelial tumors is associated with Balkan nephropathy, analgesic abuse, and cigarette smoking. Squamous cell carcinoma of the upper tracts, though rare, is usually associated with chronic inflammation secondary to calculi, infection, or both. The treatment of choice for a localized transitional cell tumor of the renal pelvis is total nephroureterectomy with contiguous excision of a cuff of bladder mucosa.

Renal Mass Discovered at Surgery

The general surgeon occasionally discovers an unsuspected renal mass or congenital renal anomaly at operation. All renal masses should be palpated thoroughly without opening Gerota's fascia. Further exploration is not warranted; a well-planned workup can be performed postoperatively. Intraoperative puncture and aspiration of a renal mass should be confined to situations where a solid mass is highly suspected and is located in a region difficult to puncture via a percutaneous route. The importance of recognizing renal anomalies cannot be overstated. Ectopic, horseshoe, and pancake kidneys have been mistaken for pathologic processes and have been partially or completely excised.

PROSTATE

Prostate Carcinoma

Prostate cancer is the most common visceral malignancy in American men. Second only to cancer of the lung, it accounts for 14% of cancer deaths in men in the United States. The estimated lifetime risk of disease is 17.6% for whites and 20.6% for African Americans, with a lifetime risk of death of 2.8% and 4.7%, respectively. Prostate cancer is rarely diagnosed in men younger than 50 years, accounting for less than 0.1% of all patients. Peak incidence occurs between the ages of 70 and 74 years, with 85% diagnosed after the age of 65 years. With the advent of prostate-specific antigen (PSA) there has been a substantial shift to a diagnosis at a more favorable stage.

Approximately 75% to 80% of prostatic tumors are located in the periphery of the posterior region of the prostate and may be palpable by digital rectal examination (DRE). Any suspicious prostatic area should be biopsied usually under transrectal ultrasound (TRUS) guidance. The differential diagnosis of a prostatic nodule includes tuberculosis, granulomatous prostatitis, infarct, calculi, metastatic focus from another primary tumor, and postsurgical scarring. Management of prostatic carcinoma depends on the clinical stage of disease (Table 25.1).

A staging workup is indicated for patients with high risk of advanced disease usually based on initial PSA values. This usually consists of a bone scan (PSA more than 10) and a CT scan with IV contrast (PSA more than 20) as well as routine blood work. Although the specificity and sensitivity are relatively low, gross pelvic lymph node involvement can be initially evaluated by pelvic CT or MRI.

TABLE 25.1	**TNM Prostate Cancer Staging (AJCC 2002)**

TX: Primary tumor cannot be assessed
T0: No evidence of primary tumor
T1: Tumor not palpable or visible on imaging
  T1a: Tumor incidental histologic finding in 5% or less of resected tissue
  T1b: Tumor incidental histologic finding in more than 5% of resected tissue
  T1c: Tumor identified by needle biopsy (e.g., because of elevated PSA)
T2: Tumor confined within prostate
  T2a: Tumor involves 50% or less of one lobe
  T2b: Tumor involves more than 50% of one lobe but not both lobes
  T2c: Tumor involves both lobes
T3: Tumor extends through the prostate capsule
  T3a: Extracapsular extension (unilateral or bilateral)
  T3b: Tumor invades seminal vesicle(s)
T4: Tumor is fixed or invades adjacent structures other than seminal vesicles: bladder neck, external sphincter, rectum, levator muscles, and/or pelvic wall
Regional lymph nodes (N)
  NX: Regional lymph nodes were not assessed
  N0: No regional lymph node metastasis
  N1: Metastasis in regional lymph node(s)
Distant metastasis (M)*
  MX: Distant metastasis cannot be assessed (not evaluated by any modality)
  M0: No distant metastasis
  M1: Distant metastasis
  M1a: Nonregional lymph node(s)
  M1b: Bone(s)
  M1c: Other site(s) with or without bone disease

*outside of the pelvis

The DRE in conjunction with a PSA assay (a protease produced by the prostatic epithelium) is the accepted method for initially detecting prostate cancer. The likelihood of prostatic malignancy generally increases as the PSA titers rise. It should be noted that benign prostatic hyperplasia (BPH) can also cause elevated PSA levels (on the order of up to 0.33 ng/mL for every gram of BPH). PSA can also be elevated in the presence of inflammation, urinary retention, infarction, and prostatic manipulation (cystoscopy, catheterization, or biopsy). In two studies, a 4% to 9% positive biopsy rate was noted in men with normal PSA and DRE. The PSA assay is of greatest value when used as a comparative parameter over time (i.e., PSA velocity, doubling time) to assess success of treatment and rate of progression in patients being treated for prostate cancer.

Transrectal ultrasound is the definitive modality for measuring the size of the prostate or suspicious nodules and to detect extracapsular or seminal vesicle extension of cancer. TRUS is useful for detecting centrally or anteriorly situated foci of prostate cancer or suspicious areas. TRUS also allows accurate guidance for biopsies of suspicious or site-specific areas of the prostate. More than 95% of prostate cancers are adenocarcinomas. The remaining 4% to 5% are considered ductal carcinomas arising from the central portion of the gland. Histologically, they are transitional cell, mixed, or endometrioid carcinomas.

Prostate cancer often causes few, if any, specific symptoms. Prior to the advent of PSA, up to 75% of men with prostate cancer were initially diagnosed with metastatic disease-related symptoms: bone pain, weight loss, sciatica, lower extremity edema, anemia, and azotemia. Hematuria, occurring in fewer than 15% of prostate cancer patients, is more commonly associated with infection and obstruction. Many patients present with bladder outlet obstructive symptoms that are commonly caused by coexisting BPH.

Prostate cancer spreads by local extension and by lymphatic and hematogenous routes. Extension into the urethra, seminal vesicles, and trigone is common with advanced disease. One or both ureteral orifices may become obstructed by invasion. In decreasing order of frequency, the obturator, hypogastric, external iliac, presacral, and paraaortic nodes may become involved. Blood-borne metastases are most common to bone and invariably are osteoblastic. The pelvis, lumbar spine, femur, thoracic spine, and ribs are the most frequent sites of bone involvement. The most common visceral sites of metastasis are the lung and liver.

The appropriate therapy for patients with prostate cancer depends on the clinical stage of disease and the patient's life expectancy and general medical condition. Curative surgical procedures are indicated in patients with tumor clinically confined to the prostate gland, who have a life expectancy of more than 10 to 15 years, and who are medically stable. Pelvic lymphadenectomy may be performed in conjunction with (requiring frozen sections) or prior to definitive management.

Radical prostatectomy may be performed with an open, retropubic or perineal approach or with minimally invasive laparoscopic or robotic techniques. The most common complications are incontinence, impotence, rectal injury, and stricture at the vesicourethral anastomosis. A potency-sparing radical retropubic prostatectomy has gained wide acceptance. If the disease is organ confined, the nerve-sparing procedure is associated with an approximately 90% fifteen-year survival rate. The overall return-of-potency rate is approximately 65%. Definitive external beam radiotherapy can be performed on similarly staged patients who are at greater surgical risk or who decline surgery. The 1990s have seen a resurgence of interest in interstitial radioactive seed implantation therapy for prostate cancer (brachytherapy). Iridium-192, iodine-131, or palladium-103 seeds can be implanted by a transperineal approach using US guidance as an ambulatory procedure. Long-term follow-up is not yet available to assess its treatment efficacy compared to the more traditional external beam therapy. The 15-year survival rate of men with comparably staged disease who receive radiotherapy is on the order of 65% to 75%. Many patients with a shorter life expectancy (less than 10 years) and low-stage, low-grade disease do well without any therapy ("watchful waiting").

Normal prostatic cells and many populations of prostatic cancer cells are functionally dependent on androgen. The goal of hormonal therapy for prostate cancer is to eradicate or inhibit androgenic stimulation of the tumor. Bilateral orchiectomy (surgical castration), equally effective injectable luteinizing hormone-releasing hormone agonists (medical castration), and less effective oral estrogens (diethylstilbestrol) act to decrease the level of circulating testosterone. Complete androgen ablation can be accomplished by adding oral flutamide or nilutamide, each of which inhibits the production of adrenal androgenic metabolites in surgically or medically castrated men. Hormonal manipulation is indicated in patients with evidence of metastatic disease or progression of the primary disease, or in patients unsuitable for surgery or irradiation.

Benign Prostatic Hyperplasia

Benign prostatic hyperplasia is probably the most common neoplasm in men; it is an almost universal phenomenon of aging. BPH originates exclusively from the periurethral prostatic tissue. As this benign adenomatous neoplasm enlarges, the surrounding normal prostatic tissue becomes compressed, eventually forming a "surgical" capsule. With enlargement come prostatic urethral obstruction and its associated constellation of symptoms, often referred to as "prostatism." Obstructive symptoms include hesitancy, decreased force and caliber of the urinary stream, terminal or postvoid dribbling, a sense of incomplete emptying, and urinary retention. These problems must be considered separate from irritative voiding symptoms, such as dysuria, frequency, and urgency, that suggest infection or some other inflammatory process. Hematuria occurs much more commonly with BPH than with prostatic cancer.

The workup of a patient with suspected BPH includes urinalysis, urine culture, blood urea nitrogen and creatinine levels, PSA assay, acid phosphatase assay, uroflowmetry and often postvoid residual. Excretory urography or renal and pelvic sonography can document upper tract changes, the presence of bladder calculi, the degree of bladder emptying, and the presence of intravesical prostatic enlargement. Cystourethroscopy is essential for accurately assessing the entire lower urinary tract prior to considering surgical intervention.

Patients with mild symptoms and no significant abnormalities on routine investigation require reassurance and yearly follow-up. Patients with more severe symptoms or evidence of bladder or upper tract deterioration require pharmacologic or surgical intervention. Indications for surgical intervention include renal failure due to obstructive uropathy, persistent hematuria, recurrent urinary tract infections, significant urinary retention, bladder calculi, and bothersome symptoms unresponsive to medical therapy.

The objective of the various surgical approaches is to enucleate the adenomatous neoplasm from the surrounding compressed prostatic tissue, which is to remain. Generally, open prostatectomy is reserved for patients with glands weighing more than 75 g, depending on the individual surgeon. Suprapubic prostatectomy through a bladder incision is most appropriate when a large intravesical median lobe, bladder calculi,

or diverticula require removal or excision. Retropubic prostatectomy through a prostatic capsular incision is usually associated with less blood loss. Smaller glands can be resected via the transurethral route.

Transurethral resection of the prostate remains the gold standard of endoscopic prostate surgery. New and investigational endoscopic surgical approaches include transurethral incision of the prostate, transurethral laser incision of the prostate, laser ablation, vaporization, transurethral microwave hyperthermia, and endoscopic insertion of a metal alloy prostatic stent.

Noninvasive pharmacologic regimens have a role in the alleviation of symptoms related to BPH in appropriate patients. Terazosin (1 to 10 mg nightly) or doxazosin (1 to 8 mg nightly) are α-adrenergic antagonists, traditionally used as antihypertensives. They have a significant, measurable effect on relaxing the urethral internal sphincter mechanism, which includes the smooth muscle within the prostate and bladder neck. Numerous studies have consistently shown dose-dependent symptomatic improvement, improved urodynamic parameters, and limited side effects in men treated for symptomatic BPH. Finasteride, a 5-α-reductase inhibitor, inhibits the transformation of testosterone to the more active form, dihydrotestosterone, thereby effecting dihydrotestosterone-sensitive organs such as the prostate. Finasteride (5 mg daily) for a 4- to 6-month period decreases prostatic volume by an average of 20% and objectively alleviates symptoms in up to 50% of patients with acceptable and minimal side effects. It has been shown to reduce the risk of urinary retention.

BLADDER

Urothelial (transitional cell) carcinoma is the most common histologic type of bladder tumor (approximately 95%) in the United States and occurs three times more frequently in men than women. Proven and potential etiologic agents include industrial chemicals such as benzidine and 2-naphthylamine, artificial sweeteners, coffee, phenacetin, cyclophosphamide, and pelvic irradiation. Perhaps most importantly, cigarette smokers have a 4-fold increase in the incidence of bladder cancer. Most patients with transitional cell carcinoma initially present with superficial disease and usually do not progress to more invasive disease if followed up and treated appropriately. The likelihood of recurrence increases in patients with multiple tumors, high-grade lesions, and urothelial cell changes, such as severe atypia or carcinoma in situ

(CIS) in other areas of the bladder. Most of the patients with more aggressive, muscle-infiltrating tumors present de novo without a history of superficial disease.

The most common presenting sign or symptom of bladder cancer is painless microscopic or gross hematuria, occurring in approximately 85% of patients. Irritable bladder symptoms frequently occur in patients with invasive tumors or CIS. A routine workup consists of urine cytology, CT scan with IV contrast to determine the presence of upper urinary tract abnormalities, bimanual examination, and cystoscopy. After biopsies are done, the tumor may be resected, fulgurated, or ablated. Random bladder biopsy specimens are obtained to evaluate normal-appearing mucosa for urothelial atypia or CIS. Recurrent superficial tumors may be repeatedly resected, fulgurated, or ablated by laser. Intravesical instillation of Bacillus Calmette-Guérin (BCG) has become a standard method of treatment for recurrent superficial tumors and CIS in properly selected patients. BCG and instillation of mitomycin C, doxorubicin, or thiotepa can markedly reduce the frequency of recurrences or eradicate the disease. Muscle-invading and recurrent high-grade tumors or CIS require extirpative surgery. Partial cystectomy is rarely indicated, but can be considered in patients with isolated tumor in a bladder diverticulum, or patients who refuse total cystectomy. Patients with invasive disease and no evidence of metastatic spread require radical cystectomy with pelvic lymph node dissection. Recent evidence suggests that pelvic lymphadenectomy may be of both prognostic and therapeutic benefits. Preoperative radiation therapy for advanced disease has generally not been found to improve disease control significantly. Neoadjuvant, cisplatin-based chemotherapeutic regimens (e.g., methotrexate, vinblastine, doxorubicin, cisplatin [MVAC]) have been shown to improve overall survival in patients with advanced disease. Nerve-sparing procedures in conjunction with continent urinary diversion or ileal neobladder reconstruction have improved potency and postoperative quality of life in selected patients. Urethrectomy should be included in patients with a high potential for urethral recurrence, such as those with involvement of the trigone or prostatic urethra, or those with diffuse CIS.

Metastatic disease most commonly occurs in bone, lung, and liver. After radical cystectomy, 25% to 50% of patients with muscle-invading tumors develop metastatic disease within 3 to 5 years. Partial regression and control of the progression of metastatic disease have been achieved with various chemotherapeutic agents, most notably cisplatin-based regimens.

Although squamous cell carcinoma is the most common form of bladder cancer in schistosomiasis endemic areas, it represents only approximately 5% of bladder tumors. Chronic infection or inflammation, chronic foreign body irritation, and schistosomiasis are associated with the development of squamous cell carcinoma of the bladder. Radical cystectomy is the most effective form of treatment, with 5-year survival rate ranging from 15% to 50%. Adenocarcinoma represents fewer than 1% of bladder tumors and typically arises from the trigone or a urachal remnant at the bladder dome. Patients with a history of bladder extrophy have a higher incidence. Patients with a diagnosis of adenocarcinoma of the bladder should undergo colonoscopy to exclude a primary colonic malignancy.

Urinary diversion after cystectomy is performed with bowel anastomosis, either in the form of cutaneous diversion or with the creation of a neobladder. Post–urinary diversion patients have a 3% to 5% risk of postoperative bowel complications. Knowledge of the type of diversion is crucial to determining the proper treatment of bowel and urinary complications. The most common urinary diversion uses a loop of ileum to create a conduit to an external stoma. Common complications may include stomal stenosis, parastomal hernias, or electrolyte imbalance. Complications can also occur secondary to ureteral obstruction or reflux.

TESTICULAR NEOPLASMS

Testicular tumors are the most common solid tumors in men between the ages of 15 and 35 in the United States. Seminoma, the most common histologic type, rarely occurs below the age of 10. Yolk sac tumors predominate during infancy and childhood. More than 90% of primary testicular malignancies are germ cell tumors (GCTs) (seminoma, embryonal carcinoma, yolk sac tumor, teratoma, and choriocarcinoma). Simultaneous or metachronous bilateral testicular tumors occur in 2% to 3% of cases. Epidemiologic studies have calculated the risk of testicular cancer in cryptorchid patients to be 3 to 14 times the normal incidence. Among patients with a history of cryptorchidism and subsequent development of testis tumor, approximately 20% develop a malignancy in the contralateral descended testis.

Most patients present with a painless nodule, swelling, or altered consistency of the testis.

Approximately 10% of patients initially present with symptoms attributable to metastatic disease. Another 10% complain of a painful scrotal swelling that is frequently misdiagnosed and treated as epididymitis. Such patients should undergo exploration if no improvement occurs after 2 weeks of conservative management. Any patient presenting with new onset of scrotal swelling or a mass should undergo scrotal ultrasonography.

The most important initial therapy is prompt radical orchiectomy through an inguinal incision. Specific serum tumor markers measured prior to surgery and include α-fetoprotein produced by yolk sac cells, β-subunit of human chorionic gonadotropin (β-hCG) produced by syncytiotrophoblasts, and lactic acid dehydrogenase (LDH). Approximately 10% of patients with seminoma have an elevated β-hCG level; 90% of patients with nonseminomatous germ cell tumors (NSGCTs) have either α-fetoprotein or β-hCG elevation or both. Following orchiectomy, persistent elevation of tumor marker levels strongly suggests residual tumor. Unfortunately, up to 20% of patients with postorchiectomy normalization of tumor marker levels will develop metastatic disease.

The histology of the tumor and results of a metastatic workup determine subsequent management. Postorchiectomy evaluation consists of chest and abdominal CT scan, and tumor marker assays. Testicular tumors initially spread via the lymphatics in a predictable and stepwise manner. The primary lymphatic drainage of the right testis is to the interaortocaval nodes and right renal hilar region; the left testis drains into the paraaortic and left renal hilar areas.

In 2002, the American Joint Committee on Cancer (AJCC) published a consensus classification applicable to both seminoma and NSGCTs. The AJCC staging for germ cell tumors is distinct because a serum tumor marker category (S) is used to supplement the prognostic stages defined by anatomy alone. The staging of testicular tumors is outlined in Table 25.2.

Seminoma is exquisitely sensitive to radiation therapy. Postorchiectomy irradiation to the retroperitoneum and ipsilateral inguinopelvic regions (2,500 to 3,000 rad) in patients with seminoma can produce a cure in up to 99% of cases with a negative workup for metastatic disease. Stage IIA and IIB seminomas respond well to retroperitoneal irradiation. Stage IIC or III seminoma is treated with primary chemotherapy similar to that for nonseminomatous tumors.

TABLE 25.2	TNMS Testicular Cancer Staging (AJCC 2002)

Tis: Carcinoma in situ
TX: Primary tumor cannot be assessed
T0: No evidence of primary tumor
T1: Tumor has not spread beyond testicles, blood vessels, lymphatic vessels, or tunica vaginalis
T2: Tumor has spread to blood vessels, lymphatic vessels, or tunica vaginalis
T3: Tumor invades the spermatic cord
T4: Tumor invades the scrotum
NX: Regional lymph nodes cannot be assessed
N0: No metastasis to regional lymph nodes
N1: Lymph node mass 2 cm or less across; five or fewer nodes positive
N2: Lymph node mass between 3 and 5 cm across or metastasis to five or more lymph nodes, none more than 5 cm across
N3: Metastasis to at least one lymph node with the mass more than 5 cm across
MX: Distant metastasis cannot be assessed
M0: No distant metastasis (i.e., no spread to nonregional lymph nodes or other organs such as the lungs)
M1: Distant metastasis is present
M1a: Metastasis to distant lymph nodes or lung
M1b: Metastasis to organs such as the liver, brain, or bones
SX: Marker studies not performed
S0: Normal LDH, [beta]-hCG, and alpha-fetoprotein levels
S1: LDH level < 1.5 times the upper limit of normal; [beta]-hCG level < 5,000 mIU per mL (5,000 IU per L); alpha-fetoprotein level < 1000 ng per mL (1000 mcg per L)
S2: LDH level 1.5 to 10 times the upper limit of normal; [beta]-hCG level of 5000 to 50000 mIU per mL (5000 to 50000 IU per L); alpha-fetoprotein level of 1000 to 10000 ng per mL (1000 to 10000 mcg per L)
S3: LDH level > 10 times the upper limit of normal; [beta]-hCG level > 50000 mIU per mL (50000 IU per L); alpha-fetoprotein level > 10000 ng per mL (10000 mcg per L)

Retroperitoneal lymph node dissection is indicated in patients with NSGCTs with IIA or IB disease or patients with persistently elevated serum markers following orchiectomy. Patients with advanced disease should be treated with primary chemotherapy that may be followed by retroperitoneal lymph node dissection in selected cases. Extremely compliant patients with organ-confined, stage 1A or IB NSGCTs can be observed knowing that there is a 25% recurrence rate. These patients require an abdominal CT scan, chest radiography, and tumor markers every 3 months for the first 2 years followed by follow-up evaluations every 6 months for the next 3 years.

Combination chemotherapy with cisplatin, etoposide, and bleomycin (BEP) has remarkably improved overall and disease-free survival in patients with advanced metastatic testicular cancer. A cure rate of approximately 50% can be achieved in patients with NSGCT involving multiple organs (stage IIC or III). Choriocarcinoma, which accounts for 3% of testicular tumors, has the worst prognosis, as it usually presents with metastatic disease.

GENITOURINARY TRAUMA

Renal Trauma

A high index of suspicion and accurate assessment of traumatic renal injuries allow maximal renal salvage and minimization of complications from missed or delayed diagnosis. Approximately 5% to 10% of patients with penetrating abdominal trauma sustain renal injury. Conversely, 80% of patients with penetrating renal injuries have injuries to other intra-abdominal organs such as liver, colon, spleen, and stomach (in decreasing order of frequency). Renal injury should be considered in any patient who sustains blunt trauma to the abdomen, lower chest, or spine. Such injury is most commonly secondary to motor vehicle accidents, falls, or contact sports. Renal injury following minor blunt trauma is not uncommon in patients with preexisting hydronephrosis, renal tumor, renal cystic disease, or vascular malformation. Rapid deceleration can cause disruption of the ureteropelvic junction or vascular damage to the renal vessels. Penetrating renal injuries usually result from gunshot or stab wounds. Hematuria is the most common clinical sign of urinary system trauma; however, there is poor correlation between the degree of hematuria and the severity of injury.

Several large series have established criteria for the diagnosis and management of renal trauma. Radiographic evaluation, if feasible, is required for all patients with penetrating injuries to the abdomen with or without microscopic or gross hematuria. Radiographic imaging of the kidney has been found to be unnecessary in the adult patient with blunt trauma, stable blood pressure (over 90 mm Hg systolic), microscopic hematuria (fewer than five red blood cells/high-power field), and no clinical indication of flank trauma (e.g., lower rib or lumbar trans-

verse process fractures, flank bruises, seat-belt marks). All injured pediatric patients with any degree of hematuria must be assessed radiographically.

The increasing use of CT scans in stable trauma patients has essentially eliminated the need for IV pyelograms. Major trauma, such as deep renal laceration, avulsion/fracture, or vascular occlusion, is suggested by poor or nonvisualization of the kidney. Contrast CT scan can document differential perfusion of renal parenchyma. Invasive angiography is indicated only when CT scanning is unavailable or is necessary to evaluate some other injury. All blunt trauma patients with gross hematuria and patients with microscopic hematuria and signs of shock (systolic blood pressure less than 90 mm Hg at any time during evaluation and resuscitation) should undergo renal imaging, usually CT with IV contrast. All penetrating injuries with any degree of hematuria should be imaged. The American Association for the Surgery of Trauma Organ Injury Severity Scale for the Kidney is presented in Table 25.3.

Significant injuries (grade II and above) occur in approximately 5% of renal trauma cases. Ninety-eight percent of isolated blunt renal traumas can be managed nonoperatively. In the setting of a stable patient with penetrating trauma, an abdominal CT scan with contrast should be performed. Many patients with even high-grade injuries can be managed expectantly with close monitoring of vital sign, bed rest, and serial hematocrits. Delayed bleeding or expanding hematomas can often be managed with selective angioembolization, as renal exploration often leads to nephrectomy. If urinary extravasation is present, serial renal CT scans should be performed. If significant urinary leakage persists after 48 hours, a ureteral stent is indicated to prevent urinoma formation.

Persistent renal bleeding and expanding or pulsatile perirenal hematomas are indications for immediate surgical intervention. When associated with renal lacerations and urinary extravasation, nephrectomy is indicated, particularly when other intra-abdominal injuries are present. Restoration of renal function may be achieved in up to 80% of pedicle injuries if surgery is performed within 12 hours after the injury; success rates decline rapidly thereafter. Most arterial injuries are treated with autologous vein grafts. Use of synthetic grafts is discouraged because of possible contamination from other abdominal injuries. The mainstay of renal reconstruction includes complete renal exposure, debridement of

TABLE 25.3	The American Association for the Surgery of Trauma Organ Injury Severity Scale for the Kidney	

Grade	Type	Description
I	Contusion	Microscopic or gross hematuria, urologic studies normal
	Hematoma	Subcapsular, nonexpanding without parenchymal laceration
II	Hematoma	Nonexpanding perirenal hematoma confined to renal retroperitoneum
	Laceration	<1 cm parenchymal depth of renal cortex without urinary extravasation
III	Laceration	>1 cm parenchymal depth of renal cortex without collecting system rupture or urinary extravasation
IV	Laceration	Parenchymal laceration extending through renal cortex, medulla, and collecting system
	Vascular	Main renal artery or vein injury with contained hemorrhage
V	Laceration	Completely shattered kidney
	Vascular	Avulsion of renal hilum, devascularizing the kidney

nonfunctioning tissue, hemostasis, watertight closure of the collecting system, and closure of the parencymal defects. Parenchymal lacerations are closed with absorbable sutures and gelatin bolsters. When polar injuries cannot be reconstructed a partial nephrectomy should be performed and all nonviable tissue should be removed.

Occasionally, the general surgeon or urologist is confronted intraoperatively with an unexpected retroperitoneal hematoma. In the absence of life-threatening hemorrhage, intraoperative pyelogram should be done. This "one-shot" pyelogram is performed by administering 2 mL/kg IV contrast 10 minutes before abdominal flat plate imaging. The visualization of bilateral kidney function rules out significant pedicle injury. Further exploration is required only if gross urinary extravasation is demonstrated or parenchymal injury causing an expanding hematoma is present. When one or both kidneys are not functioning, immediate aortography is indicated. If the renal arteries are demonstrated to be patent, nonfunction is attributed to contusion or acute tubular necrosis. When a renal pedicle injury is identified, immediate repair may be attempted.

Ureteral Trauma

Optimal management of ureteral injury depends on early recognition, awareness of the presence of associated injuries, and the mechanism of injury. A missed ureteral injury frequently results in infection, fistula, or stricture formation. The ureter is fixed only at its junctions with the renal pelvis and bladder. Above the pelvic brim, the ureter is attached to the undersurface of the posterior peritoneum. Because the blood supply to the ureter is segmental and variable, dissection must therefore be performed outside the adventitial sheath. In a further attempt to avoid undue injury to the ureteral blood supply, the surgical approach to the ureter should be lateral above and anterior below the pelvic brim. A system for grading ureteral injury system is presented in Table 25.4.

TABLE 25.4	A System for Grading Ureteral Injury System	

Grade	Type	Description
I	Hematoma	Contusion or hematoma without devascularization
II	Laceration	<50% transection
III	Laceration	≥50% transection
IV	Laceration	Complete transection with <2 cm devascularization
V	Laceration	Avulsion with >2 cm devascularization

More than 95% of traumatic ureteral injuries are due to gunshot wounds. At least 10% of such patients have a normal urinalysis. Excretory urography delineates the injury in approximately 90% of cases. High-velocity injury to the ureter requires wide debridement because of the blast effect. One must assume a high-velocity injury if the bullet is not visible on radiographs and knowledge of the weapon is unavailable. When injury to an unsevered ureter is suspected, stenting the ureter and adequate Penrose drainage minimize delayed extravasation and allow healing to take place. More significant injuries may require excision and repair of the damaged segment. Rarely, severe deceleration injuries may cause avulsion of the ureter from the renal pelvis.

Proper management of associated injuries in patients with traumatic ureteral injuries is crucial to ureteral integrity. Pancreatic or duodenal injury must be drained away from the site of ureteral repair in conjunction with ureteral stenting and/or nephrostomy diversion. Stenting and nephrostomy drainage are also useful in patients with ureteral and large bowel injuries.

Failure to recognize intraoperative iatrogenic ureteral injuries will result in a significant increase in morbidity. Such injury most commonly occurs during abdominal hysterectomy, colon resection with surrounding inflammation, abdominoperineal resection, and aortic or iliac aneurysm resection. About one-third of injuries to the ureter occur during open surgery. The increase in laparoscopic procedures has lead to an increase in unrecognized intraoperative ureteral injuries. Preoperative contrast CT scan imaging is useful in any patient undergoing surgery in the retroperitoneal space. Improved visualization or palpation of the ureter can be achieved by initiating a diuresis with furosemide to produce a bolus of urine. Preoperative ureteral catheterization may assist in identification when an abnormal course is anticipated. Suspected ureteral injury may be easily confirmed or ruled out by IV administration of methylene blue or indigo carmine.

Iatrogenic ureteral injury may result from ligation, crushing, avulsion, devascularization, or transection. When a ureter is clamped or ligated, damage is minimal if the injury is recognized and treated immediately. A ureteral stent should be placed and left in place for 5 to 7 days. A partial transection of less than half the circumference of the ureter without vascular compromise can be repaired with simple sutures and drainage. With more severe degrees of transection or suspected vascular compromise, complete transection, debridement to healthy tissue, and ureteroureterostomy should be performed. Unfortunately, many iatrogenic injuries are not recognized until the postoperative period.

Early in the postoperative period, fever, ileus, flank pain, increased drainage, hematuria, or an abdominal mass may suggest ureteral injury. Contrast CT scan with delayed imaging (5 to 20 minutes) can accurately diagnose the injury in many cases. Blood urea nitrogen and creatinine assays in urinary drainage fluid show levels 20 to 30 times the normal serum values.

The following general principles are essential in the repair of ureteral injuries:

1. Successful repair requires a tension-free anastomosis.
2. Only absorbable suture material is used. Nonabsorbable sutures act as a nidus for calculus formation when placed in contact with urine.
3. Proximal urinary diversion (nephrostomy tube, intraureteral stent) in all but the most uncomplicated cases acts as a safety valve and can improve outcomes.
4. Adequate wound drainage is essential because extravasated urine can delay epithelialization and cause periureteral fibrosis and infection.

The choice of surgical repair depends on the location and extent of ureteral injury. Pyeloplasty techniques are used for ureteropelvic junction injuries. Ureteroureterostomy with opposing spatulated ends is adequate for upper and middle one-third injuries. A defect of up to 5 to 6 cm can sometimes be bridged without undue tension because of the inherent mobility of the ureter. A ureteral injury close to the bladder is usually amenable to ureteroneocystostomy (i.e., reimplantation). With more extensive injuries of the distal one-third, a psoas hitch or a Boari flap may be necessary to attain a tension-free anastomosis.

A variety of silastic or polyurethane nonmigrating (pigtail configurations on each end) internal ureteral stents are now available. These can be placed intraoperatively through the open wound/ureterotomy, with the proximal end coiled in the renal collecting system and the distal end in the bladder. Cystoscopic stent removal can be performed in 6 to 8 weeks in an office or outpatient setting.

Long ureteral defects are usually associated with high-velocity missile injuries with multiple-organ damage. In this setting, it is prudent to ligate the proximal ureter and insert a nephrostomy tube via a small renal pyelotomy incision through the dependent lower pole and exiting from a separate skin stab wound. If the kidney is also injured, nephrectomy is usually indicated. Ileal interposition or autotransplantation can be considered 3 to 6 months later.

Bladder Trauma

While an empty bladder is well protected by the bony pelvis, a full bladder is much more vulnerable to injury. The weakest part of the bladder and the most likely point of rupture is the superior portion, or dome, which is covered by peritoneum. In children more of the bladder lies in an intra-abdominal position and is more prone to intraperitoneal rupture. More than 90% of bladder injuries are secondary to blunt trauma and are often associated with pelvic fractures. Approximately 85% of patients with bladder injuries will have gross hematuria.

If a bladder injury is suspected, cystography with a postdrainage film is performed. If a urethral injury is also suspected, a urethrogram must be obtained prior to inserting a catheter. Retrograde urethrography should be performed first in any male patient with blood at the urethral meatus, scrotal or perineal hematoma, or abnormal position of the prostate on rectal examination. The bladder will generally remain intact with simple contusions. Extraperitoneal rupture is radiographically characterized by flamelike configurations of contrast. Intraperitoneal rupture results in extravasation of contrast into the peritoneal cavity, often outlining portions of bowel. When associated with pelvic fracture, the bladder often has a surrounding hematoma and will assume a teardrop shape on cystography.

Proper management of a bladder injury or rupture includes delineation of the extent of injury if possible, repair of the wall, adequate diversion of urine, and perivesical drainage. Intraperitoneal injuries should be explored routinely. Lacerations are closed in one to two layers using absorbable suture material. In male patients a 24F to 28F suprapubic cystostomy tube (e.g., Malecot catheter) is used to drain the bladder. In female patients a 24F to 26F urethral catheter is usually adequate for urinary drainage. Suprapubic or urethral catheters are removed at 7 to 10 days after cystography demonstrates the absence of extravasation. Extraperitoneal bladder injuries may be treated conservatively with a urethral catheter, particularly in the absence of other indications for surgical intervention.

Urethral Trauma

Urethral injuries are much more common in male patients because of the length and the fixation of the urethra to the pubic bone by the puboprostatic and suspensory ligaments. Injury to the anterior urethra, which extends from the urogenital diaphragm to the external meatus, usually results from straddle, penetrating, or crush injuries. Extravasation limited by Buck's fascia is confined to the penis. Extravasation limited by Colles' fascia, which is continuous with Scarpa's fascia, may extend into the abdominal and chest walls because of its peripheral attachments to the coracoclavicular fascia, the fascia lata of the thigh, and the triangular ligament posteriorly.

Anterior urethral injury often presents with blood at the urethral meatus and difficulty or inability to void. Retrograde urethrography is indicated for suspected injuries. Contrast material that is suitable for IV use should be used exclusively. Patients are encouraged not to void to prevent possible urinary extravasation. Penetrating injuries must be debrided. If conditions permit, primary repair may be performed; otherwise a suprapubic cystostomy tube may be placed and the repair may be delayed. Perineal extravasation of urine and blood secondary to blunt urethral trauma requires adequate local drainage. If the injury is minor, primary repair may be performed and an indwelling urethral catheter may be left in place for 10 days. Extensive urethral ruptures are more easily and effectively repaired after inflammation has subsided and initial suprapubic diversion is indicated.

Posterior urethral injuries are usually associated with pelvic fractures and occur in 5% to 10% of such patients. Although not always present, blood at the urethral meatus occurs frequently. Careful rectal examination may reveal a superiorly displaced urethral disruption at the level of the urogenital diaphragm. Initial urologic management is generally confined to suprapubic cystostomy placement, rather than an attempt at emergent primary repair of posterior urethral injuries. Restoration of urethral continuity by various reconstructive techniques is delayed for 3 to 4 months. The morbidity associated with both emergent and delayed repairs includes impotence, stricture formation, incontinence, and the need for additional urologic procedures.

RENAL CALCULUS DISEASE

Renal calculus disease is a common urologic condition that can be deceptive in its clinical presentation. Patients often present with complaints of severe flank or abdominal pain that may be associated with nausea, vomiting, and fever. Acute renal or ureteral colic may simulate acute cholecystitis, appendicitis, intestinal obstruction, pancreatitis, or ruptured abdominal aortic aneurysm. Findings highly suggestive of nephrolithiasis include costovertebral punch tenderness, absence of peritoneal signs, microscopic hematuria, or pyuria. Up to 90% of renal calculi are radiopaque and a plain abdominal radiograph will often confirm the diagnosis. Uric acid calculi are radiolucent; cystine and struvite (infection) stones are relatively nonopaque but are usually faintly visible. A noncontrast CT scan may be definitive in determining the size, density, and location of renal and ureteral calculi.

Approximately 70% to 75% of renal calculi are predominantly composed of calcium oxalate. The most common cause of calcium oxalate stone formation is intestinal hyperabsorption of calcium, often in conjunction with inadequate fluid intake. Less common causes include regional enteritis, short bowel syndrome, and bypass surgery for obesity. Primary hyperoxaluria is a rare congenital enzymatic defect in the metabolism of glyoxylic acid characterized by diffuse calcium oxalate deposition in the kidney and may lead to renal failure.

Numerous metabolic diseases are associated with calcium stone formation. Primary hyperparathyroidism accounts for 2% to 4% of renal calculi and most calcium phosphate (brushite) stones. Another cause of brushite stones is renal tubular acidosis, particularly the more common type II, proximal renal tubular acidosis. Cystinuria, a congenital defect in proximal tubule reabsorption of cystine, ornithine, lysine, and arginine (COLA), is manifested clinically only by cystine stone formation. Vitamin D intoxication, sarcoidosis, prolonged immobilization, medullary sponge kidney, metastatic or parathyroid hormone-producing neoplasms, milk alkali syndrome, and hyperthyroidism are all associated with calcium stone formation.

Uric acid calculus disease is related to a combination of hyperuricosuria, abnormally low urine pH, and inadequate fluid intake. Approximately 25% of patients having gout form renal calculi composed of or containing uric acid. Patients with gastrointestinal disorders such as ulcerative colitis and those requiring colostomy or ileostomy lose substantial amounts of bicarbonate and water through the intestinal tract. The kidneys respond by excreting more concentrated, acidic urine, an ideal environment for uric acid precipitation. A high incidence of uric acid stones occur in patients with gout, Lesch-Nyhan syndrome, in patients undergoing chemotherapy, and in patients with an unusually high-purine diet. The prevention of uric acid stone formation requires alkalinization of the urine with oral sodium bicarbonate when appropriate, allopurinol in patients with uric acid overproduction, and adequate hydration.

Persistent urinary tract infections caused by urease-producing (i.e., urea-splitting) organisms account for 5% to 10% of renal calculi. *Proteus mirabilis* is the most common bacterium associated with infection or struvite stones. These calculi are composed of magnesium ammonium phosphate admixed with smaller amounts of calcium phosphate and carbonate crystals. They are soft, relatively radiolucent calculi that often form casts of the renal collecting system and hence are termed "staghorn calculi." Antibiotic therapy is useful in the acutely septic patient or in the perioperative period.

The various surgical approaches to renal calculi are beyond the scope of this chapter. New techniques have been developed that markedly restrict the need for open surgery. Extracorporeal shock wave lithotripsy (ESWL) allows noninvasive stone disintegration by focusing shock waves at the stone through a water–skin interface under fluoroscopic or sonographic control. ESWL has an approximately 95% success rate in treating renal calculi less than 2 cm in diameter. Larger renal calculi (more than 3 cm) or staghorn calculi are routinely removed by initial percutaneous endoscopic debulking using an ultrasonic lithotrode, followed, if necessary, by ESWL of the remaining fragments. These techniques are associated with fewer major complications, shortened hospital stays, and more rapid return to normal daily activities when compared with open surgical procedures.

UROLOGIC EMERGENCIES

Renovascular Emergencies

Renal artery aneurysms represent approximately 1% of all arterial aneurysms. Seventy-five percent are noncalcified and prone to rupture, particularly during pregnancy. Although most renal artery aneurysms are asymptomatic, hypertension or hematuria can be present and pain or hemodynamic instability can occur with rupture. Fibromuscular dysplasia of the renal arteries with areas of aneurysmal dilatation is the most common etiology for renovascular hypertension in younger patients. Renal artery aneurysms that are greater than 2 cm in size, have intramural thrombus, or have associated occlusive disease should generally be treated. Endovascular techniques are widely used in the treatment of renovascular occlusive and aneurysmal disease. Open surgical techniques most commonly use aortorenal bypass with autogenous saphenous vein with or without resection of the associated aneurysm.

Embolic phenomena affecting the kidney represent 2% to 3% of all arterial emboli. Severe flank and lower back pain and hematuria are manifestations of renal ischemia or infarction. Lack of contrast enhancement on CT scanning should prompt urgent arteriography to establish the diagnosis and identify the location of the embolus. If more than 2 to 3 hours has elapsed from the time of embolization to diagnosis, embolectomy is usually unsuccessful in salvaging the kidney unless significant collateral flow is present. Heparinization must be started immediately to prevent further propagation of thrombus.

Testicular Torsion

Torsion of the spermatic cord obstructs the venous blood supply, causing edema, hemorrhage, and eventual obstruction of arterial blood flow. Torsion most commonly occurs during the second decade of life at or near puberty. Approximately 20% to 30% of cases are seen in men older than 20 years. Failure to intervene promptly results in irreversible testicular infarction. An acute scrotal condition in an adolescent or young man should be considered torsion unless proven otherwise. The differential diagnosis includes acute epididymitis, which is the most common cause of scrotal swelling and pain, acute orchitis, strangulated hernia, traumatic hematocele or hydrocele, and torsion of the appendix testis.

The clinical history and physical findings in patients with testicular torsion are, unfortunately, of limited value. A horizontal testicular lie, upward testicular retraction because of a shortened spermatic cord, and acute onset in the face of normal urinalysis strongly suggest torsion. Persistent pain on raising the testis (a negative Prehn's sign) is unreliable. Color Doppler sonography has been shown to be the most sensitive and specific study.

Torsion occurs within the tunica vaginalis (intravaginal) in the child and adult. The testis can be abnormally suspended in various forms of which the most common is described as a "bell clapper" configuration. In approximately two-thirds of cases the twist is from without inward (internal rotation). Approximately 50% to 60% of torsion cases have similar abnormalities of suspension on the opposite side. Extravaginal torsion occurs only during the neonatal period.

If torsion cannot be ruled out, expeditious scrotal exploration is performed. In the emergency room, manual detorsion can be attempted and, if successful, results in immediate relief of symptoms and converts

a surgical emergency to an elective procedure. Orchiectomy is not performed unless the testis is undeniably infarcted. Orchiopexy is performed by fixing the testes directly to the dartos muscle layer with at least two opposing nonabsorbable sutures. Contralateral orchiopexy is similarly performed to prevent future torsion.

Failure of the patient to seek early medical attention or misdiagnosis by the primary care physician results in orchiectomy in approximately 50% of cases. Testicular ischemic time of less than 12 hours is associated with at least a 90% salvage rate; infarction is almost certain after 24 hours of ischemia unless the torsion was intermittent. In general, higher testicular salvage rates can be achieved with a more aggressive approach to suspected torsion.

Priapism

Priapism is a prolonged, involuntary, usually painful erection unrelated to sexual stimulation. Unlike with a normal erection, the corpus spongiosum (i.e., glans penis and urethra) remains flaccid. With priapism, obstruction to corpus cavernosal venous outflow causes stagnation of blood, resulting in a viscous sludge that further impairs drainage. The most common conditions associated with priapism are sickle cell trait and disease (up to 89% of patients will experience an episode by the age 20) and leukemia. Other causes include amyloidosis, multiple myeloma, postdialysis state, and neurologic dysfunction as seen with spinal cord tumors, spinal cord shock, and paraplegia. Several drugs, such as phenothiazines, alcohol, cocaine, antihypertensives, and heparin, have been associated with priapism.

The goal of treatment is to establish adequate venous drainage of the corpora cavernosa and prevent permanent fibrosis and associated impotence. Treatment of the underlying cause, when known, often results in detumescence. Patients with sickle cell disease or trait are treated with oxygen, hydration, alkalinization, and transfusion. Leukemia patients require chemotherapy and splenic irradiation. Some patients respond to strong sedation. Ketamine, an anesthetic, has been successful in treating priapism and can be given in the operating room prior to definitive surgery.

Sequential intracorporal injections of dilute solutions of epinephrine or the safer phenylephrine may successfully detumesce a shorter-lasting (6 to 8 hours) priapism, sometimes in conjunction with intracorporeal irrigation with saline. This technique is most successful in patients with self-induced priapism secondary to therapeutic penile injections of papaverine with or without phentolamine for impotence.

When conservative measures fail, surgery in the form of a corpus cavernosa–spongiosa shunt (e.g., Winter procedure, formal window shunt) or corpus cavernosa–saphenous vein shunt is indicated. A Winter shunt procedure establishes bilateral fistulas between the glans penis and corpus cavernosa using a core biopsy needle. A formal cavernosa–spongiosa shunt entails approximation of opposing elliptical windows in the two structures at the level of the bulbous urethra through a perineoscrotal midline incision.

Infection

Severe acute pyelonephritis or acute focal or multifocal bacterial nephritis associated with an obstructive process requires prompt drainage by percutaneous nephrostomy or retrograde ureteral catheterization proximal to the obstruction. Simultaneous parenteral antibiotic therapy is imperative. Once the patient is afebrile and otherwise stable, the obstructing lesion can be corrected.

Scrotal gangrene is an uncommon but potentially fatal infectious process. It may be associated with urinary extravasation or other genitourinary disorders such as prostatitis, epididymitis, and traumatic scrotal or penile lacerations. Idiopathic, spontaneous scrotal gangrene, otherwise known as Fournier gangrene, accounts for approximately 50% of cases. Subcutaneous emphysema occurs in most cases. Treatment involves appropriate antibiotic coverage, colloid replacement, and prompt, aggressive debridement and drainage.

QUESTIONS

The following questions may have more than one answer.

1. The most common renal mass is a:
   a. Renal cell carcinoma.
   b. Adenoma.
   c. Benign cyst.
   d. Angiomyolipoma.
   e. Hemangioma.

2. During a routine right hemicolectomy, a right renal mass is noted. One should:
   a. Expose the mass and perform a wedge biopsy.
   b. Needle-aspirate the mass.
   c. Perform a nephrectomy.

   d. Palpate carefully and then work up postoperatively.
   e. Excise the mass with adequate margin.

3. Which of the following modalities is not useful for maximizing early detection of prostate cancer?
   a. Prostate-specific antigen.
   b. Prostatic acid phosphatase.
   c. Transrectal ultrasonography.
   d. Digital rectal examination.
   e. Clinical symptomatology.

4. BCG bladder instillations are useful in patients with:
   a. Solitary, superficial urothelial bladder carcinoma.
   b. Squamous cell carcinoma of the bladder.
   c. Superficial, recurrent urothelial bladder carcinoma.
   d. Carcinoma in situ.
   e. Recurrent urothelial bladder carcinoma with superficial muscle invasion.

5. What percentage of patients with stage I testicular carcinoma eventually progress without further treatment after radical orchiectomy?
   a. 10.
   b. 20.
   c. 30.
   d. 40.
   e. 50.

6. Symptoms and signs related to benign prostatic hyperplasia can be successfully treated pharmacologically.
   a. True.
   b. False.

7. Which testicular tumor has the worse prognosis?
   a. Seminoma.
   b. Embryonal carcinoma.
   c. Yolk sac tumor.
   d. Choriocarcinoma.
   e. Teratocarcinoma.

8. Which of the following parameters necessitate radiographic imaging of the urinary tract in the patient with blunt trauma?
   a. Adult patient.
   b. Microscopic hematuria.

c. Systolic blood pressure higher than 90 mm Hg.

d. Fracture of a lumbar transverse process.

e. History of renal cysts.

9. Proper ureteral repair after trauma requires all of the following except:

a. Tension-free anastomosis.

b. Adequate urinary diversion.

c. Adequate wound drainage.

d. Watertight closure.

e. Use of absorbable suture material.

10. Which of the following findings obviate the need for scrotal exploration in a patient with suspected testicular torsion?

a. Positive Prehn's sign.

b. Normal urinalysis.

c. Normal color Doppler ultrasound.

d. No history of scrotal trauma.

e. Shortened spermatic cord.

SELECTED REFERENCES

AUA Update Series. American Urological Association. www.auanet.org

Gillenwater JY, Grayhack JT, Howards SS, Mitchell ME, eds. *Adult and pediatric urology*, 4th ed. Philadelphia, PA: Lippincott Williams & Wilkins, 2002.

Hinman F Jr. *Atlas of urologic surgery*, 2nd ed. Philadelphia, PA: WB Saunders, 1998.

Tangho E, McAninch JW, eds. Smith's general urology (Lange Clinical Medicine), 17th ed. McGraw-Hill Professional, 2007.

Wein AJ, Kavoussi LR, Novick AC, Partin AW, Peters CA, eds. *Campbell– Walsh urology*, 9th ed. Elsevier, Inc., 2010

CHAPTER 26

Lillian Harvey Banchik

Nutrition in the Surgical Patient

INTRODUCTION

Malnutrition has become increasingly recognized as a cause of increased morbidity and mortality both in the inpatient and outpatient surgical population. The incidence of malnutrition ranges from 10% to more than 50% depending on geographic location, a patient's diagnoses, and treatments being undergone. Multifactorial in its etiology, malnutrition affects many, if not all, of the major organ systems. The ability to diagnose malnutrition and to plan the appropriate treatment both to prevent and correct its complications is an essential component in the management of the surgical patient.

Diagnosis

The Joint Commission on Accreditation of Healthcare Organization (JCAHO) mandates that all patients undergo some form of nutritional assessment within 24 hours of admission. This assessment can range from a screening questionnaire to a nutritionally targeted physical examination. Whatever form this assessment takes, it is important that both the patient's nutritional status and the correlation to the underlying disease state be determined.

Diet History

Diet history is one of the most easily obtained and, possibly, least accurate forms of nutritional assessment. Although a prospective diet diary may give a fairly accurate indication of nutritional intake, retrospective diet histories are fraught with inaccuracies. A skilled interviewer is required to elicit the necessary information from the patient. Factors such as early satiety, changes in taste and smell perception and exercise tolerance, and treatments may all affect nutritional intake but, occurring gradually, may not be per-

ceived by the patient who will report that their nutrient intake is "unchanged."

Physical Examination

Of all physical findings, the height and weight are the most easily obtainable objective measurements. Of more important than a single measurement is to determine if there has been any change from the patient's preillness usual weight. Changes of as little as 1% to 2% from the usual weight can be significant when they occur over a short time (Table 26.1). Body weight may also be elevated by fluid retention from intravenous or drug therapy giving a false sense of security that the patient is maintaining their usual weight.

Body mass index (BMI), the ratio of weight to height squared, has been used widely both as an indication of obesity and malnutrition (Table 26.2). Although there is normally a good correlation between BMI and total body fat, enough variations in body habitus exist to preclude its use as the sole indicator of either malnutrition or obesity.

Laboratory Assessments

Many attempts have been made to find the "Gold Standard" laboratory test, which will unequivocally determine the patient's nutritional status. Although many have been proposed over the years, each suffers from deficits, which preclude their use as a sole arbiter for nutritional status.

Nitrogen balance can be used to determine the adequacy of protein intake. A patient's protein intake is measured and the total nitrogen loss calculated (nitrogen balance = nitrogen intake − nitrogen loss). Although simple in theory, it suffers from many flaws; these include the difficulty in obtaining accurate measurements in the outpatient setting, acute and chronic alterations in renal function, as well as accurate

TABLE 26.1   Weight Loss

Time Period	Significant Weight Loss (%)	Severe Weight Loss (%)
1 week	1–2	>2
1 month	5	>5
3 months	7.5	>7.5
6 months	10	>10

measurement of the protein losses from other sources such as enterocutaneous fistulas.

Serum proteins such as albumin, prealbumin, and transferrin have also been investigated as markers of nutritional status. Although widely used as markers of nutritional status, these hepatic proteins more closely reflect the level of systemic inflammation in the patient. Acute inflammatory processes can decrease serum proteins by as much as 25% although patients who have simple starvation in the absence of inflammation may maintain near normal serum albumin and prealbumin levels. These hepatic proteins are therefore more useful as markers of acute inflammation rather than acute malnutrition.

Immune competence also is affected by malnutrition, and both delayed cutaneous hypersensitivity and total lymphocyte counts have been proposed as markers of nutritional status. Although potentially useful as a nutritional indicator in outpatients with uncomplicated malnutrition, acute inflammatory processes as well as immunosuppressive agents such as steroids may suppress immune function thus potentially suggesting the presence of malnutrition in a normally nourished patient.

As it can be seen above, no single test can be relied upon to give definitive results in the assessment of a patient's nutritional status. Accurate evaluation must rely on the combination of multiple factors including physical examination and laboratory studies.

Causes of Malnutrition

As noted above, malnutrition is a broad-based diagnosis, which does not give an indication of the etiology of the condition. The various etiologies of malnutrition can be broken into two major groups:

• Mechanical
• Metabolic

Mechanical Causes of Malnutrition

Mechanical causes of malnutrition are those which prevent nutrients from reaching the gastrointestinal (GI) tract in a form which can be absorbed (Table 26.3). In these cases, the small bowel is capable of absorbing nutrients normally, but the nutrients cannot reach that portion of the digestive tract. Correction of this type of malnutrition relies on the ability to determine the cause and the availability of treatment. In the case of upper digestive tract obstructions, bypass in the form of a percutaneous or surgically placed feeding tube is often possible and can allow for a temporary or permanent solution to the problem. The condition becomes more difficult to manage when the obstruction is in the small bowel. In many cases, feeding into the small bowel distal to the obstruction is not possible since

TABLE 26.2   BMI Interpretation

BMI wt (kg)/height^2 (m^2)	Interpretation
<16	Grade III malnutrition
16–16.9	Grade II malnutrition
17–18.4	Grade I malnutrition
18.5–25	Normal weight
25–30	Overweight
30–35	Obesity, grade I
35–40	Obesity, grade II
>40	Obesity, grade III

TABLE 26.3   Mechanical Causes of Malnutrition

Type	Example
Impaired chewing	Poor dentition
	Oral cavity surgery (e.g., partial glossectomy)
Impaired swallowing	Altered state of consciousness (e.g., sedation)
	Endotracheal intubation
Esophageal obstruction	Achalasia
	Tumor
Gastric outlet obstruction	Peptic ulcer disease
	Tumor
Small bowel obstruction (functional and mechanical)	Ileus
	Adhesions
	Tumor
Large bowel obstruction (functional and mechanical)	Tumor
	Acute diverticulitis pseudoobstruction

TABLE 26.4	Malabsorptive Causes of Malnutrition

Type	Example
Impaired gastric digestion	Postgastrectomy
Impaired pancreatic secretion	Post-Whipple procedure
Impaired small bowel absorption	Crohn disease
	Sprue
	Radiation enteritis
	Chemotherapy-induced enteritis

the nonobstructed small bowel is so distal that access at that point would lead to a functional short bowel syndrome. In these cases, definitive treatment would rely on the ability to bypass or resect the obstructed segment or, in the case of an external obstruction, relieve the obstruction.

Ileus presents as a functional bowel obstruction. Treatment of this relies on the correction of the cause of the ileus and, in many cases, enteral nutrition will not be possible until the ileus resolves.

Metabolic Causes of Malnutrition

Metabolic causes of malnutrition can either be of the type, which impairs intestinal absorption (Table 26.4) or systemic conditions, which alter nutrient metabolism (Table 26.5).

Treatment of these types of malnutrition relies heavily on the ability to correct the underlying metabolic abnormalities. For patients with malabsorption issues, treatments can range from increasing nutrient intake to compensate for the malabsorption to replacing missing pancreatic enzymes in the case of pancreatic insufficiency. In the case of hypermetabolic states or those with inefficient utilization of

TABLE 26.5	Metabolic Causes of Malnutrition

Type	Example
Hypermetabolic states	Sepsis
	Trauma
Unclear etiology	Cancer cachexia
	Cardiac cachexia

nutrients, provision of adequate nutrients may not be possible and the development of clinically significant malnutrition may be unavoidable.

Nutrient Requirements

Nutrients can be divided into two major categories: macronutrients and micronutrients:

Macronutrients are those which are required in large quantities. The three major macronutrients are the following:

- Protein
- Carbohydrates
- Fat

Micronutrients are those required in much smaller quantities and include items such as

- Electrolytes
- Trace elements that are nutrients, which comprise less than 0.1% of the total lean body mass. Examples include selenium or copper
- Vitamins

Protein

Protein is essential for life, indeed a specific form of malnutrition "kwashiorkor" will occur in the face of adequate caloric intake if protein intake is inadequate. It is also important to realize that, to the best of current knowledge, there are no storage forms of protein and that any loss of lean body mass may have detrimental effects on the patient.

Daily requirements for protein intake vary on the basis of the patient's clinical condition, but, in most adults, the minimal protein intake requirement is 1 g/kg/d. Conditions, which may require increased protein intake include those that increase protein losses (Table 26.6) and those that increase endogenous protein requirements (Table 26.7). More problematic are those conditions, which normally mandate a decrease in protein intake (i.e., hepatic failure or acute

TABLE 26.6	Causes of Increased Exogenous Protein Losses

Enterocutaneous fistula
Hemodialysis
Hemofiltration
Extensive burns

TABLE 26.7	Causes of Increased Endogenous Protein Requirements

Sepsis
Immediate postsolid organ transplantation
Pregnancy
Decubitus ulcerations

renal failure not on dialysis) but may occur in the setting of conditions, which have increased protein requirements such as sepsis or trauma. In these cases, the need for additional protein for healing needs to be balanced with the patient's ability to tolerate the byproducts of protein metabolism.

Providing adequate protein in the enterally fed patient relies on the ability to present the protein in a form, which may be absorbed by the GI tract. Although the overwhelming majority of proteins that enters the GI tract are in the form of intact protein, it is important to remember that the GI tract can only absorb protein in the form of amino acids and short chain (two to four amino acid) peptides. Pancreatic insufficiency, gastric bypass, or the alteration of gastric pH by proton pump inhibitors all can decrease the availability of active proteolytic enzymes and decrease the absorption of protein.

Carbohydrates

Carbohydrates represent the major nutrient in the usual diet representing anywhere from 45% to 65% of the daily caloric intake. Among the organ systems of the body, several, including the brain and red blood cells, are obligate carbohydrate metabolizers whereas others, such as muscle, utilize carbohydrates along with fats for energy. During overnight fasting, the liver produces carbohydrates to supply needed glucose at a rate, which approximates 2 mg/kg/min of total body mass; therefore, this rate appears to closely represent the basal carbohydrate requirements for patients at rest. It is important to realize that the only significant substrate for gluconeogenesis in human comes from protein. Although a minimal amount of glucose may be generated from the glycerol backbone of a triglyceride, the metabolism of fatty acids does not produce any substrate for gluconeogenesis. This is due to the fact that fatty acids are metabolized via the tricarboxylic acid (TCA) cycle and although oxaloacetic acid, a precursor of gluconeogenesis, is one step in this pathway, the two carbon fragments produced during

the breakdown of fatty acids to acetyl-CoA do not produce a net increase in oxaloacetic acid but rather supply the two carbon atoms, which are added to oxaloacetic acid in the first step of the TCA cycle to produce citrate and are then removed during later steps of the cycle. Since the goal of all nutritional therapy is to prevent breakdown of lean body mass while also supplying adequate nutrients to support healing, it should be apparent that supplying adequate carbohydrates to prevent protein breakdown for gluconeogenesis precursors is of paramount importance. What has become more apparent recently is that although adequate carbohydrate intake is important, control of hyperglycemia is also vital. In the past, keeping blood glucose levels of 180 or below was considered adequate control. It is now being realized that tighter control, in the range of 100 to 120 is necessary to prevent complications due to hyperglycemia. In a patient on parenteral nutrition (PN), this can be achieved by a combination of minimizing carbohydrate intake and either subcutaneous or intravenous insulin. In patients on enteral nutrition, this control may be more difficult to achieve since very often the patient's nutrition must be suspended for testing or treatment, and the danger of hypoglycemia must be balanced against the dangers of hyperglycemia.

Lipids

Lipids represent the third major nutrient in the normal diet. In actuality, lipids are a compound molecule consisting of up to three fatty acids attached to a backbone of glycerol. In humans only two of these fatty acids are considered essential, linoleic and linolenic. Lack of either or both of these acids in the food intake produces a condition known as essential fatty acid deficiency (EFAD) characterized by dry, scaly skin, thrombocytopenia, and anemia. Fortunately, the average diet contains more than adequate quantities of these fatty acids, and, in the normally fed adult, there is an adequate supply of these two acids stored in the adipose tissue to supply essential fatty acids for up to 1 month of starvation. These two facts combine to explain why EFAD was not seen in patients until the advent of total parenteral nutrition (TPN) when patients were fed a mixture of amino acids and dextrose without any lipids for weeks at a time. Prevention of EFAD in adults is easily accomplished by the provision of at least 2% of calories in the form of linoleic acid weekly. Presently any adult on a enteral diet will received more than this minimum amount whereas in patients receiving TPN, 500 mL of 20% lipid emulsion weekly will prevent

EFAD. Treatment of presumptive EFAD is equally easy and provision of 500 mL of 20% lipid emulsion weekly is all that is necessary to both treat and prevent recurrence of EFAD.

Vitamins

Vitamins are defined as organic substances not created endogenously by human, which are necessary for basic functions of life. Deficits in any of these substances produces a clinically recognizable syndrome, which may, potentially, be corrected by the repletion of the deficient vitamin. Only 13 vitamins have been clearly shown to be essential in adults. These can be divided into two broad groups:

- Fat soluble vitamins
  - Vitamin A
  - Vitamin D (steroid group)
  - Vitamin E
  - Vitamin K
- Water soluble vitamins
  - Vitamin B group
  - Vitamin C

Deficiency states for these vitamins have been clearly defined and are listed below (Table 26.8). Treatment of vitamin deficiency should be aimed at prevention; fortunately the nonvegetarian western diets, which include vitamin supplemented foods such as bread and milk normally supplies adequate

TABLE 26.8 Deficiency States of Vitamins

Vitamin	Deficiency State	Toxicity

A	Night blindness
	Anorexia
	Depressed helper
	  T-cell levels
		Acute—fatigue, bone and muscle pain
		Chronic—hepatic toxicity, pseudotumor
		  cerebri

B$_1$—Thiamin	Beriberi Lactic acidosis	None except in super high levels

B$_2$—Riboflavin	No specific symptoms
	  seen in isolated
	  deficiencies
		None

B$_3$—Niacin	Pellagra	Headache Vasodilatation
B$_6$—Pyridoxine	Dermatitis Anemia Stomatitis Glossitis	None
B$_{12}$—Cyanocobalamin	Pernicious anemia	None
Folate	Megaloblastic anemia	Seizures when given at 100 times RDA
Biotin	Anorexia Muscle pain Nausea and vomiting Depression and lethargy	None

Pantothenic acid	(Extremely rare and only
	  seen when metabolic
	  antagonists are given)
		None

C	Scurvy	Possible rebound scurvy when high-dose vitamin C is stopped
D	Metabolic bone disease	Symptomatic hypercalcemia Soft tissue calcification
E	Increased platelet aggregation Hemolytic anemia	Thrombocytopenia Hemorrhage Synthetic form may be hepatotoxic
K	Hemorrhage	

RDA, recommended dietary allowance.

amounts of all vitamins. Patients who are vegans may require folate supplementation to prevent deficiency states. Injectable multivitamins are available for patients who cannot consume an adequate enteral diet and will supply 100% of the recommended daily intake for all vitamins. It should be noted that as of 2000, the FDA mandated a change in the basic formulation of injectable vitamins with increases in the daily intake of vitamins C, thiamin, biotin, as well as, the addition of vitamin K to the formulation. This needs to be considered in patients who are receiving oral anticoagulation since upon discharge from the hospital, the cessation of parenteral vitamin K, will necessitate adjustment of anticoagulation.

Trace Elements

Trace elements are those minerals, which occur in quantities of less than 0.1% of total body mass. In patients on a normal enteral diet with adequate GI tract absorption, most deficiency states are extremely rare. Exceptions to this include iron, where deficiency can occur from excess blood loss, zinc deficiency in the elderly and alcohol abusing populations, and iodine deficiency in areas of iodine poor soil. Trace element toxicity is more common and is seen in patients with disorders of excretion such as renal failure. Most enteral diets supply adequate levels of trace elements and no supplementation is required. However, in patients receiving PN, deficiencies are prevented by the administration of parenteral "mixed trace elements" injections on a daily basis. Descriptions of deficiency and toxicity states for the most common trace elements are listed in Table 26.9. Treatment of deficiency is normally straightforward and consists of supplying the missing element. Toxicity is more

TABLE 26.9	**Descriptions of Deficiency and Toxicity States for the most Common Trace Elements**	
Trace Element	**Deficiency State**	**Toxicity**
Iron	Anemia	(Chronic overload) Cirrhosis Cardiomyopathy Pancreatic damage
Zinc	Nonspecific signs including Skin lesions Anorexia Diarrhea Altered taste and smell Impaired wound healing	Nausea and vomiting Dizziness Death
Copper	Hypochromic, microcytic anemia Leukopenia Hypercholesterolemia Abnormal EKG	Not seen in patients with normal hepatic function. In patients with hepatic dysfunction (e.g., Wilson disease, cirrhosis) may cause permanent liver damage.
Manganese	Infertility Congenital defects in bone and cartilage formation Ataxia Carbohydrate and lipid metabolism abnormalities	Severe CNS symptoms including Irritability Violence Hallucinations
Selenium	Keshan disease (endemic cardiomyopathy) Cardiomyopathy Skeletal muscle weakness	Nausea and vomiting Loss of hair and nails Tooth decay Peripheral neuropathy
Iodine	Hypothyroidism	Hyperthyroidism
Chromium	Weight loss Refractory hyperglycemia	None known

problematic and treatment can vary from chelating agents used in iron toxicity to dialysis.

Enteral Nutrition

Enteral nutrition is indicated in all patient requiring nutritional support of any type unless the GI tract is inaccessible or nonfunctional. It represents the physiologic means of nutritional support in that it supplies nutrients to the patient via the small intestine and these nutrients, with the exception of fats, are first presented to the liver for metabolic processing before being released to the rest of the body. This is in opposition to PN where the nutrients are given directly into the venous system without first passing through the liver. For enteral nutrition to be successful, several criteria must be met. These include the following:

• The ability to deliver nutrients to the small bowel in a form that may be absorbed.
• The ability to protect the airway from aspiration.
• The ability of the intestine to eliminate waste products.

Although enteral nutrition, in most cases, may be used to nourish the patient, success depends on adhering to the above criteria. The first criterion, the ability

to deliver nutrients in a form that may be absorbed, is the most complex. Problems ranging from poor dentition through exocrine insufficiency and various types of malabsorptive problems may require the selection of the appropriate diet as well the delivery of the diet to the appropriate part of the GI tract.

Various types of enteral diets are available to the clinician. This may be a source of confusion in selecting the optimal diet for use. The various classes of enteral diets as well as their indications and contraindications are listed below (Table 26.10). It is important to realize that there is often no benefit to going to a "designer" diet, such as an immune-enhancing diet where there is no clear clinical indication and that in some cases these diets may cause more problems than solving problems. Enteral nutrition in the form of "tube feeds" is normally ordered by a two-step calculation. First, the caloric and protein requirements are calculated and then the appropriate type of enteral nutrition is determined. It must be remembered that most "tube feeds" have a fixed protein calorie ratio, which cannot be significantly altered. In most cases, the next step is to determine what volume will be required to supply the needed calories. After this is determined, the amount of protein supplied by

TABLE 26.10   Enteral Diets

Type of Enteral Diet	Indications	Contraindications
Blenderized diets	Gastric feeding with intact GI tract that is patients with swallowing difficulties being fed by PEG	Lack of intact stomach
Fiber-containing formula	Promotion of normal intestinal function	Partial bowel obstruction
Semielemental diets	Increased availability of nutrients for absorption	None
Elemental diets	Short bowel syndrome Partial small bowel obstruction	None but may cause dumping syndrome if infused directly into the small bowel
Renal diet (i.e., low K, fluid restricted)	Acute or chronic renal failure	None when indicated
Diabetic diet (high in complex carbohydrates and relatively high in fats)	Diabetes	None when indicated
Pulmonary diet (high in fat and low in carbohydrates)	No clear evidence for their use	Inability to tolerate high fat content
Hepatic diet	No clear evidence for their use	None when indicated
Immune-enhancing diets	No clear evidence for their use	None

PEG, percutaneous endoscopic gastrostomy.

that quantity is determined. If they are both in an acceptable range, then the tube feed is ordered. If more protein is required, either the rate can be increased to supply the additional protein or a different formula with a higher protein to calorie ratio can be ordered.

Although enteral nutrition is the preferred means of nutritional support, many types of complications may occur with its use. These complications can include aspiration, diarrhea, and intestinal infarction.

Of these, aspiration is the most common and is a major contributor to increased morbidity and length of stay. The causes of aspiration can be multifactorial and include endotracheal intubation and intragastric feeding when in supine position. Most of the research into aspiration has been aimed at detecting early, subclinical, aspiration with the intent of preventing larger potentially life-threatening events. Unfortunately, the techniques developed including blue dye, tracheal glucose levels, and gastric residuals have not proven to be effective in either detecting or preventing aspiration. Several years ago the FDA stopped the use of blue dye after several reports of patient death. Gastric residuals have never been shown to be an accurate marker of gastric emptying nor of tolerance of intragastric feedings. The most effective method of preventing aspiration is feeding the patient in an upright position to at least 30 degrees or, preferably 45 degrees. If this is not possible, then feeding via a tube placed distal to the ligament of Treitz (not just post pyloric) has been shown to be effective in reducing the risk of aspiration.

Diarrhea from tube feeding can be multifactorial in origin. After ruling out infectious causes such as *Clostridium difficile* colitis, various other causes of malabsorption such as pancreatic insufficiency should be investigated. Treatment of diarrhea will depend on etiology. In many cases, the addition of soluble and insoluble fiber to a tube feeding, or changing to a fiber-containing formula is all that is required. In other cases, more radical changes such as going from bolus feedings to slow continuous feeding may be required. If the diarrhea persists and is refractory to treatment, then PN should be considered for adequate nutritional support.

Intestinal infarction is a rare but potentially lethal complication of enteral nutrition. Of unclear etiology it appears to be as a consequence of feeding the small intestine during times of relative ischemia. The presenting symptoms may be nonspecific and easily confused with an ileus, but failure to recognize the condition may lead to diffuse infarction of the intestine.

TABLE 26.11	Indications and Contraindications for Parenteral Nutrition

Indications for Parenteral Nutrition
Uncorrectable small bowel obstruction
Malabsorption not amenable to medical treatment
Hyperemesis gravidarum
Expected to be NPO for 7 or more days

Contraindications for Parenteral Nutrition
Functional, accessible GI tract
Patient with limited life expectancy expected to die before complications of malnutrition occur

---

Parenteral Nutrition

PN is indicated when the patient cannot tolerate enteral nutrition in amounts sufficient to provide adequate nutritional support. Specific criteria do exist as to when PN is most likely indicated as well as when it is contraindicated (Table 26.11). PN consists of concentrated solutions of dextrose and amino acids, with lipid either mixed in or infused separately. The osmolarity of these solutions, which can exceed 1400 mOsm/L require that they be infused into a large capacity vein such as the superior vena cava. Infusions of the solutions into a smaller vein, such as the subclavian, have been reported to cause occlusive thrombophlebitis of these veins.

Ordering of PN relies on the same principles as that for any other type of nutrition, but the specific orders will depend on the type of PN available in the institution. Fixed ratio PN can be ordered in a similar fashion to enteral nutrition. In some facilities, however, customized formulas are available. In this setting, the practitioner may order a formula with the specific amounts of protein, carbohydrates, lipids, and, to some extent, water desired. In either case, PN may be started at the desired rate as long as proper monitoring is in place. This monitoring is designed to prevent the major complications of PN; hyperglycemia and refeeding syndrome.

Hyperglycemia may occur even in patients who have no history of diabetes due to the large quantities of dextrose infused and the relative hyperglycemia induced by the underlying stress. In these cases, insulin can be added to PN to achieve adequate blood glucose control. Refeeding syndrome is the sudden drop in serum phosphorus, which may occur with the infusion of dextrose in patients who have been inadequately fed previously. Symptoms include muscular weakness especially of the respiratory muscles and may lead to respiratory failure. Prevention consists of careful monitoring of serum phosphorus levels and supplementation as required.

Conclusions

Malnutrition is a major cause of increased morbidity and length of hospital stay in hospitalized patients. The ability to adequately diagnose and treat malnutrition is of paramount import to today's clinicians. Careful attention to the patient's nutritional status and needs, and the adequate provision of nutrients can be a major step in the prevention of nutritional-related complications.

QUESTIONS

Select one answer.
  1. Which of the following represents a substrate for gluconeogenesis in humans?
     a. Fat
     b. Skeletal muscle
     c. Bone

  2. Indications for PN include
     a. Low-output fistula from Crohn disease
     b. Uncomplicated Whipple resection for pancreatic gastrinoma
     c. Chronic partial small bowel obstruction due to stage IV ovarian carcinoma

  3. Aspiration of gastric feeding can be effectively reduced by
     a. Elevating head of patient to at least thirty degrees
     b. Use of blue dye to detect aspiration
     c. Use of gastric residuals to evaluate tolerance of to tube feeding

SELECTED REFERENCES

Gottsclich MM, DeLegge MH, Mattox T, et al. *The ASPEN Nutrition Support Core Curriculum: a case based approach—the adult patient.* Silver Springs, MD: ASPEN, 2007 (self-published by the organization).

Rombeau JL, Caldwell MD. *Clinical nutrition. Enteral and tube feeding.* Vol 1. Philadelphia, PA: WB Saunders, 1984.

Rombeau JL, Caldwell MD. *Clinical nutrition. Parenteral nutrition.* Vol 2. Philadelphia, PA: WB Saunders, 1986.

Minimally Invasive Surgery

O f all the chapters in the new edition of this book, probably the one that needed to be revisited the most is Minimally Invasive Surgery (MIS). Since our last publication in 1999, the field had exploded to become an essential training part of every residency program. Many of the procedures have become the gold standard in the surgical field. It's an exciting time for MIS; the surge of robotic surgery, natural orifice transluminal endoscopic surgery (NOTES), and other modalities are transporting the field to different levels.

It was not until after 1986, following the development of a video computer chip that allowed the magnification and projection of images onto television screens, that the techniques of laparoscopic surgery truly became integrated into the discipline of general surgery. The first laparoscopic cholecystectomy (LC) on a human patient was performed in 1987 by the French physician Mouret. The rapid acceptance of the technique of laparoscopic surgery by the general population is unparalleled in surgical history. It has changed the field of general surgery more drastically and more rapidly than any other surgical milestone.

LAPAROSCOPIC CHOLECYSTECTOMY

LC was the procedure that launched the modern era of MIS. Since the first LC was performed by Mouret in 1987, the procedure experienced a rapid acceptance and has now become the standard of care. LC has become the first-line surgical treatment of calculous gallbladder disease and the benefits over open cholecystectomy are well known.

Indications

Symptomatic gallstones disease, which comprises only a small subset of individuals with gallstones, along with its complications, remains the primary indication for cholecystectomy.

In the early days of LC, the procedure was associated with a high risk of bile duct injuries. New studies have shown that now with the addition of laparoscopic training into residency programs, and the developments of better optics and instrumentation, this risk is now decreased, but it is still higher than that for open cholecystectomy in most hands.

Contraindications

Access to the intraperitoneal cavity and safe trocar placement becomes a significant issue in patients with previous abdominal surgeries. The increased rate of adhesions to the abdominal wall in this group of patients increase the risk of procedure-associated complications. Once the initial trocar is safely placed, the remaining trocars may be placed under direct vision and the approach may be safely attempted.

Cirrhotic patients, even those with a Child–Pugh score A or B, present a special challenge during LC. The increased risk of profuse bleeding from the liver bed during dissection precludes many well-trained surgeons from feeling comfortable during the procedure. Also, the risk of bleeding from a hypervascularized abdominal wall during trocar placement should be taken into consideration. LC can still be safely performed on this group of patients with careful patient selection and appropriate preoperative work-up.

LAPAROSCOPIC APPENDECTOMY

In many centers, laparoscopic appendectomy remains the preferred approach to both, perforated and nonperforated appendicitis. Multiple studies had shown that the incidence of long-term complications, such as partial small bowel obstruction (PSBO), is more related to the chosen surgical approach than to the presence of perforation. The laparoscopic approach carries a very small risk of further development of adhesive bowel obstruction. There is now ample documentation in the literature that laparoscopic appendectomy is at least equally safe as an open appendectomy. At the same time, further evidence suggests that the laparoscopic approach offers the advantage of a faster recovery, decreased length of stay (LOS), and decrease in hospital morbidity.

Indications

The indications for laparoscopic appendectomy remain the same as the indications for appendectomy. Laparoscopic appendectomy carries the advantage in cases where the diagnosis is equivocal and diagnostic uncertainty persists, and a wider, more thorough abdominal exploration might be necessary. In these cases, a diagnostic laparoscopy will help direct therapy (surgical or otherwise) appropriately.

In situations where a normal appendix is encountered during diagnostic laparoscopy, a thorough exploration of the intraperitoneal cavity should be performed. If no other intraperitoneal pathology is encountered, then an appendectomy should still be performed with further pathological examination.

LAPAROSCOPIC HERNIORRHAPHY

Laparoscopic repair of hernias are broadly divided into two main categories: incisional/ventral hernias and inguinal hernias. The principles of the repair remain the same as with open surgery; patients must be suitable operative candidates and the repairs should be tension free.

Ventral/Incisional Hernias

Open ventral herniorrhaphy has been based on the Rives—Stoppa retrorectus tension-free mesh repair, where a wide dissection of the posterior fascia is performed and the mesh then placed posteriorly and fixed to the abdominal wall fascia using full-thickness permanent sutures. Laparoscopic repair differs in that the mesh is placed within the peritoneal cavity and is at least partially secured to the fascia using tacks or staples.

Indications

All ventral/incisional hernias that meet the criteria for open repair may be approached laparoscopically. The laparoscopic approach allows clear visualization of the abdominal wall and discernment of the contents of the hernia sac.

Contraindications

There are no absolute contraindications to laparoscopic ventral herniorrhaphy; however, patients with multiple previous surgeries may present significant challenges to the less experienced surgeon. Other potential difficulties arise in patients with previous intra-abdominal mesh placement, active wound infections, and loss of significant abdominal domain. Patients who are unable to undergo general anesthesia are obviously excluded from laparoscopic intervention for the hernias.

Complications

The spectrum of complications from laparoscopic ventral/incisional hernia repair are the same as those of open repair, including bleeding, seroma formation, ileus, bowel injury, and recurrence.

Inguinal Hernia

There are two main approaches to the laparoscopic repair of inguinal hernias, the transabdominal preperitoneal (TAPP) approach and the total extraperitoneal (TEP) approach. In both procedures, the hernia defect is repaired from the posterior approach. Cooper's ligament and the pubis are exposed, the hernia is reduced, the cord structures skeletonized, and then mesh placed.

Indications

The laparoscopic approach to inguinal hernias has been advised for a subset of patients, namely those with bilateral hernias and recurrent hernias. The preperitoneal approach allows for broad visualization, thus facilitating bilateral repairs through one set of incisions. In addition, the view of the posterior wall allows identification of sites of recurrence and repair of the floor of the hernia without entering scar tissue from previous repair. The laparoscopic approach may also be utilized in incarcerated hernias, as the contents of the hernia sac may be identified, assessed, and reduced with relative ease.

Contraindications

Laparoscopic intervention should not be used when a patient is unable to tolerate general anesthesia, although some successful repairs have been reported under locoregional anesthesia. In addition, local or systemic infection precludes laparoscopic intervention as the potential for mesh infection is elevated.

DIAGNOSTIC LAPAROSCOPY

Diagnostic laparoscopy is indicated for the diagnosis of intra-abdominal pathology in patients presenting with symptoms not diagnosed by noninvasive modalities. It provides a minimally invasive approach to directly inspect the intra-abdominal organs. At the same time, biopsies and cultures can be obtained as part of the diagnostic work-up. Diagnostic laparoscopy not only facilitates the diagnosis of intra-abdominal disease but also makes therapeutic intervention possible.

Possible applications include the following:

1. Staging laparoscopy for cancer: Staging of intra-abdominal neoplastic processes can be adequately achieved, along with lymph node (LN) biopsy.
2. Diagnostic laparoscopy (DL) for acute abdominal pain, without evidence of peritonitis.
3. DL for diagnosis of chronic conditions, such as endometriosis, chronic pelvic pain, etc.
4. DL for trauma: Exploratory laparotomies in trauma patients with suspected intra-abdominal injuries are associated with a high negative laparotomy rate and significant procedure-related morbidity. Diagnostic laparoscopy has been proposed for trauma patients to prevent unnecessary exploratory laparotomies with their associated higher morbidity and cost. In addition, it can be used to assess for diaphragmatic perforation and intra-abdominal injuries in penetrating trauma of the chest.

Contraindications

1. Homodynamic instability (defined by most studies as systolic pressure of <90 mm Hg)
2. A clear indication for immediate celiotomy such as frank peritonitis, hemorrhagic shock, or evisceration
3. Known or obvious intra-abdominal injury
4. Posterior penetrating trauma with high likelihood of bowel injury
5. Limited laparoscopic expertise

Benefits

1. Reduction in the rate of negative and nontherapeutic laparotomies (with a subsequent decrease in hospitalization, morbidity, and cost after negative laparoscopy)
2. Accurate identification of diaphragmatic injury
3. Ability to provide therapeutic intervention

Diagnostic laparoscopy is technically feasible and can be applied safely in appropriately selected trauma patients. The procedure has been shown to effectively decrease the rate of negative laparotomies and minimize patient morbidity. It should be considered in hemodynamically stable blunt trauma patients with suspected intra-abdominal injury and equivocal findings on imaging studies or even in patients with negative studies but a high clinical likelihood for intra-abdominal injury.

BARIATRIC SURGERY

Bariatric surgery encompasses a number of procedures designed to assist in excess weight loss for patients with obesity. In 1991, a patient selection criterion was recommended in the National Institutes of Health (NIH) Consensus Development Conference Statement. Patients recommended were those with a BMI of 40 kg/m^2 or more or those with a BMI of 35 kg/m^2 or more with a minimum of one medical comorbidity related to obesity, a demonstrated low probability to be successful with nonsurgical weight loss measures, and demonstrated ability to participate and maintain follow-up on a long-term basis. In addition to the selection criteria proposed in the NIH guidelines, the American Society of Bariatric Surgeons requires preoperative psychological evaluation to assess patients' capacity for adequate informed consent. An endocrine work-up is also a prerequisite to rule out endocrine pathology as the source of the excess weight.

There are three main laparoscopic procedures performed for weight loss: the adjustable gastric band (AGB), the Roux-en-Y gastric bypass (RYGBP), and the biliopancreatic diversion (BPD). The AGB is a purely restrictive, reversible procedure where a synthetic plastic ring with an inflatable balloon is placed around the stomach. Balloon inflation restricts the internal diameter of the stomach and thus restricts how much food can be tolerated before feeling full. Advantages of the procedure include the limited dissection required, the avoidance of micronutrient deficiencies that can incur from bypassed intestines, and the relatively easy removal of the band. Band slippage and less weight loss than the other bariatric procedures remain the most common disadvantages.

The RYGBP is the most commonly performed procedure. It is a combined restrictive and malabsorptive procedure requiring stapling off the gastric body, creating a gastrojejunal anastomosis and then a jejunojejunal anastomosis to restore intestinal continuity. An average of 50% to 60% loss of excess body weight can be expected with this method.

Because of the extensive stapling and anastomoses, a number of potential complications can occur. The most common include strictures and ulcers of the gastrojejunal anastomosis, which frequently present with symptomatology of obstruction or intestinal bleeding. Patients will require endoscopy for diagnosis and treatment.

Leakage from the anastomosis is also a potential complication. It usually presents with tachycardia, fever, and abdominal pain. Diagnosis may be by clinical suspicion alone or via radiographic evidence obtained from an oral contrast study or computed tomography. Treatment is reexploration, repair of leakage site if identified, wide drainage of the surgical field, and extended broad-spectrum antibiotic coverage.

Additional complications to be aware of are internal herniation through defects created in performing the reconstruction (Petersen's hernia), dumping syndrome, biliary stasis, and nutrient deficiencies associated with bypassing the duodenum and proximal jejunum.

The BPD is primarily malabsorptive procedure. Two forms are in current use. The classic form consists of a hemigastrectomy with drainage to a roux limb that bypasses the duodenum, jejunum, and proximal ileum, thus leaving a 50 to 100 cm common absorptive channel of intestine at the terminal ileum. The modified form, designated as the biliopancreatic switch involves the formation of a gastric tube and division of the duodenum near the pylorus. The proximal duodenal stump is drained by the distal Roux limb, which bypasses the remaining small bowel.

The BPD results in the greatest loss of excess body weight of any bariatric procedure due to the extensive amount of small bowel bypassed; however, it also results in the most nutrient deficiencies due to the same mechanism. The risks of anastomotic leak and internal herniation are similar to those associated with the RYGBP.

A consensus has not yet been reached as to the indications for bariatric surgery in the pediatric population. Some opine that the procedures are too drastic an approach, while others feel that early intervention may prevent the psychological and physical sequelae associated with adolescent obesity.

Thoracic Surgery

MIS have also impacted the field of thoracic surgery. Procedures that in the past required sternotomies or thoracotomies are now easily performed through a minimally invasive approach. Video-assisted thoracoscopic surgery (VATS) is now the standard of care for procedures such as lung biopsies, lymph node biopsies, and pleurodesis, among others.

Even more extensive procedures, such as lobectomies or esophageal surgery, can also now be performed with the aid of VATS and small incisions. Multiple studies have shown that VATS greatly reduces the postoperative pain that is associated with thoracic procedures. At the same time, this decreases postoperative morbidity and complications and reduces hospital LOS.

SILS and NOTES

The development of single incision laparoscopic surgery (SILS) and NOTES continues the progression of laparoscopic surgery. Neither is currently mature enough to allow them to be considered standard of care but both promise exciting developments over the next several years.

QUESTIONS

1. Which of the following is not an indication for open cholecystectomy
   a. Poor pulmonary or cardiac reserve
   b. Third-trimester gestation
   c. Childs's class C liver disease
   d. Suspected gall bladder cancer
   e. Previous gastric bypass procedure

2. Which of the following regarding laparoscopic appendectomy is true
   a. It is contraindicated in the face of diffuse peritonitis
   b. It is less likely to result in post-operative small bowel obstruction
   c. It is contraindicated in the elderly or immune-compromised
   d. The conversion rate to open appendectomy is over 50%
   e. Compared to open approaches, the laparoscopic approach has a higher rate of hospital morbidity

3. Indications for intra-operative cholangiogram include which of the following
   a. Poor visualization of the anatomy
   b. Pre-operative jaundice
   c. Dilated common bile duct
   d. Biliary pancreatitis
   e. All the above

4. Laparoscopy for blunt abdominal trauma is contraindicated in which of the following scenarios
   a. Suspicion for pancreatic injury
   b. A positive FAST study
   c. Pneumoperitoneum
   d. Previous abdominal surgery
   e. Suspicion for a diaphragmatic injury

5. Which of the following approaches can be used to performed a minimally invasive inguinal hernia repair
   a. Totally extraperitoneal approach
   b. Intraperitoneal approach
   c. Transabdominal preperitoneal approach
   d. All the above

SELECTED REFERENCES

Guller U, Hervey S, Purves H, et al. Laparoscopic versus open appendectomy: outcomes comparison based on a large administrative database. *Ann Surg* 2004;239:43–52.

SAGES. Guidelines for diagnostic laparoscopy practice/clinical guidelines published on: 11/2007 by the Society of American Gastrointestinal and Endoscopic Surgeons (SAGES).

Spaner SJ, Warnock GL. A brief history of endoscopy, laparoscopy, and laparoscopic surgery. *J Laparoendosc Adv Surg Tech A* 1997;7(6):369–373.

Strasberg SM. Avoidance of biliary injury during laparoscopic cholecystectomy. *J Hepatobiliary Pancreat Surg* 2002;9(5): 543–547.

Tsao KJ, St Peter SD, Valusek PA, et al. Adhesive small bowel obstruction after appendectomy in children: comparison between the laparoscopic and open approach. *J Pediatr Surg* 2007;42(6):939–942.

CHAPTER 28

Prathiba Vemulapalli
Emmanuel Atta Agaba

Bariatric Surgery

INTRODUCTION

Morbid obesity is a growing worldwide epidemic. In the past two decades, the number of overweight individuals has skyrocketed to a staggering global number of one billion overweight adults. In the United States alone, 25% of the overweight population is morbidly obese, which accounts for nearly 12 million morbidly obese individuals. Morbid obesity is defined as being 100 lbs above ideal body weight. Portion control, consumption of a low-fat diet, and regular physical activity are behaviors that protect against obesity; however, it is becoming increasingly difficult to adopt and maintain these behaviors in our modern society. Morbid obesity has been shown to be associated with premature death and is the second leading cause of preventable death in the United States after tobacco use. Obesity alone has been estimated to cause 400,000 deaths annually in the United States. Elevated body mass index (BMI) values are also associated with a heightened risk for heart disease, hypertension (HTN), diabetes, hypercholesterolemia, sleep apnea, osteoarthritis, and gallbladder disease.

Medical therapy for morbid obesity has limited short- and long-term success. Randomized controlled trials employing lifestyle modifications or pharmacologic interventions for weight loss resulted in only approximately a 7 lbs loss that was maintained over a 2-year period. Diets that are low in fat or low in carbohydrates often yield weight loss that is insufficient to alter comorbid conditions that are secondary to obesity. In addition, diet therapy has only been shown to work long term in approximately 5% of those patients who have tried them. Simply put, 95% of overweight individuals who try diets will fail to loss any weight. Pharmacologic therapy also has poor results. The latest antiobesity agent, orlistat, has shown to produce a maximum weight loss of 9%

body weight at 1 year with weight regain usually within 12 to 18 months.

BODY MASS INDEX

In the 1940s, the Metropolitan Life Insurance Company constructed actuarial data to determine at what weight men and women lived the longest. These weights became known as ideal body weights. Today, clinicians recognize that these weights do not always accurately reflect patients' healthiest weights and therefore are not realistic goal weights. Therefore, the most widely used determination for healthy weights is BMI, a relation between height and weight. It is weight in kilograms/(height in meters)^2. A BMI between 20 and 25 kg/m^2 is considered normal weight. A BMI between 25 and 30 kg/m^2 is considered overweight. BMIs between 30 and 40 kg/m^2 are considered obese. A BMI greater than or equal to 40 kg/m^2 is considered morbidly obese. In addition, a BMI between 35 and 40 kg/m^2 is considered morbidly obese when associated with other medical problems such as diabetes, HTN, sleep apnea, and osteoarthritis, just to name a few.

THE BASICS OF HUNGER

A great deal of research has been done on obesity to try and identify hormonal and neural causes of overeating. The hunger center in the hypothalamus of the brain is tonically active and is inhibited by the satiety center only after eating. We now recognize that satiety centers in the brain interact with hormones released from the gastrointestinal (GI) tract and the vagus nerve to suppress the hunger center of the hypothalamus. The most well recognized of these hormones are ghrelin and leptin. Ghrelin is secreted from neuroendocrine cells of the gastric mucosa. It stimulates the hunger center and inhibits the satiety center. In addition, it exhibits prokinetic activity on the stomach. In the obese, the expression of ghrelin is blunted, they exhibit low levels. Some studies have shown that after gastric bypass ghrelin levels are suppressed but this has not been uniformly shown.

Leptin, the other GI hormone, works in concert but exactly opposite to ghrelin. In fact, when one hormone expression is up, the other is suppressed. Leptin is secreted from both adipocytes and the GI tract. It works to inhibit an individual's appetite peripherally via the vagus nerve and centrally by working directly on the hypothalamus. During starvation, for instance, leptin levels fall to stimulate hunger. In the obese, leptin levels are high, suggesting that there may be resistance to the end organ effect of this hormone in the obese.

CANDIDATES FOR SURGERY

Surgery has been proven to be the only effective long-term treatment of morbid obesity. A 1991 National Institutes of Health (NIH) consensus conference determined the most appropriate candidates for bariatric surgery. These guidelines are endorsed by the American Society of Metabolic and Bariatric Surgery (ASMBS), Society of Gastrointestinal and Endoscopic Surgeons (SAGES), American College of Surgeons (ACS), and most bariatric centers in the United States. Patients are eligible for bariatric surgery if they have a BMI between 35 and 40 kg/m^2 with significant comorbidities. These comorbidities are defined as sleep apnea, HTN, diabetes, asthma, congestive heart failure, severe reflux, and osteoarthritis. In addition, patients with a BMI of 40 kg/m^2 or greater without comorbidities qualify for surgery. All patients undergoing surgery, per the NIH consensus statement, must have attempted one or more weight loss programs in the past. Approximately 200,000 bariatric procedures are performed in the United States.

CONTRAINDICATIONS TO BARIATRIC SURGERY

Absolute contraindications to surgery are an untreated metabolic or endocrine disorder, a substance abuse problem, an untreated psychiatric disorder (most commonly major depression) or eating disorder (binge eating disorder), and women who desire to become pregnant in the next 18 months. Once patients are treated

for their major depression and binge eating and are on a stable dose of medication and therapy sessions, their candidacy can be reevaluated. Pregnancy 2 years after bariatric surgery is the recommended time course to avoid birth defects in the fetus and nutritional problems in both the mother and the fetus.

As surgeons have become more facile with the laparoscopic approach, medical problems, extremes of age, and history of prior surgeries are no longer by themselves considered contraindications to bariatric surgery. Each patient must be evaluated on a case-by-case basis.

HISTORY OF BARIATRIC SURGERY

Bariatric surgery is not a new concept. The first bariatric procedures were done in 1954 by Kremer, Linner et al., who preformed jejunoileal bypass. Bypasses of this nature grew out of favor because patients complained of uncontrollable diarrhea and suffered from severe malnutrition, dehydration, electrolyte imbalances, and even hepatic failure. Jejunoileal bypasses were abandoned until 1996, when Scopinaro revised them to a biliopancreatic diversion (BPD). BPD produces its weight loss effects mainly by malabsorption but also includes a small restrictive aspect created by a reduced stomach volume. The intestinal reconfiguration promotes malabsorption of fat and protein. Protein malnutrition is the most serious potential complication of BPD that may be associated with hypoalbuminemia, anemia, edema, asthenia, and alopecia. Treatment often requires hospitalization with hyperalimentation. The duodenal switch, first presented by Hess in 1992, is a modification of the BPD that reduces the severity of protein calorie malnutrition, decreases the incidence of dumping syndrome, and prevents ulcers.

At present, gastric bypass has become the gold standard of weight loss surgery. Mason and Ito in 1967 developed the principles of gastric bypass surgery after they noticed that females who had undergone partial gastrectomy for peptic ulcer disease were often underweight and had difficulty gaining weight.

Vertical banded gastroplasty (VBG), first reported in 1982 by Mason, grew in popularity with the advent of mechanical staplers. It was thought to be a safer alternative to gastric bypass. It was the first purely restrictive operation preformed for the treatment of obesity. A pouch is created on the lesser curvature of the stomach with a stapler and a polypropylene mesh band is placed around the pouch outlet. There are very few complications to this procedure since no anastomosis is created. Hess later described the first laparoscopic VBG. VBG has grown out of favor since patients regain all of their weight.

Another purely restrictive bariatric procedure is nonadjustable gastric banding. This procedure was first described in 1978 by Wilkinson who placed a 2-cm Marlex mesh around the upper part of the stomach, separating the stomach into a small upper pouch and the remainder of the stomach. This procedure failed secondary to pouch dilation causing poor weight loss. It was revised in 1983 by Kuzmak who used a 1-cm silicone band to encircle the stomach. This created a 13-mm stoma and a 30- to 50-mL proximal gastric pouch. The band was then modified by inserting an inflatable balloon to adjust the band and stoma size.

MODERN DAY BARIATRIC SURGERY

Since the advent of laparoscopy, there has been a steep patient demand for bariatric procedures. The mass media, Internet, U-tube, and pop culture have given patients the information and knowledge about bariatric procedures igniting its popularization with the public. In addition, the surgical community has altered its perception on bariatric surgery. Advanced laparoscopy is now a growing field among graduating surgical residents. With a minimally invasive approach, patients and many referring physicians have the incorrect perception that laparoscopic bariatric surgery is with minimal risk and is an easy solution to fight obesity. Bariatric surgery can be divided into restrictive procedures and malabsorptive procedures.

Restrictive Procedures

Restrictive procedures employ a small gastric pouch that limits caloric consumption and creates early satiety. The three main minimally invasive restrictive procedures used in the United States are the adjustable gastric band, sleeve gastrectomy, and VBG.

Vertical Banded Gastroplasty

VBG is considered a purely restrictive procedure. A silastic ring is placed around a pouch created in the lesser curvature of the stomach (Fig. 28.1). VBGs have a low complication rate and are not associated with any micronutrient deficiencies. However, patients are often unable to maintain weight loss after this procedure and failure rate approaches nearly 80% in long-term follow-up. Well-described complications of this

procedure can occur up to 40% of the time and include pouch dilation and stoma stenosis. The pouch can dilate with time or due to poor surgical technique. Once dilated, however, patients typically suffer from solid food intolerance with reflux esophagitis and vomiting. Weight gain has been reported with inadequately sized pouches. Weight gain occurs because patients indulge on high-calorie liquids and soft foods that easily pass through the restricted pouch. For all of the previous reasons, VBG has fallen out of favor.

Gastric Banding

Gastric banding is the least invasive of the restrictive weight loss procedures. In the late 1990s and early 2000s, laparoscopic adjustable gastric banding was the operation of choice in Europe and later popularized in the United States. The Lap-Band™ system was Food and Drug Administration (FDA) approved in the United States in 2001. In 2009, the Swedish band became FDA approved in the United States. The Lap-Band is a high pressure, high-resistance band while the Swedish band is a low-pressure, low-resistance band. Neither has shown improved rates of weight loss or lower erosion rates when compared in Europe or in the United States. In this operation, a gastric band is placed around the upper portion of the stomach to create a small pouch and stoma resistance without dividing the stomach or creating an anastomosis (Fig. 28.2). Theoretically, the band induces early satiety. The band can be adjusted or filled in the office with sterile normal saline via the port that is placed subcutaneously. The port is similar to a portacath and can be adjusted in the office or under fluoroscopic guidance. The port should only be accessed with a Huber needle. The total volume the Lap-Band can hold varies between 10 and 14 cc. The average patient will require five to six fills or approximately half the band inflated before satiety is felt.

Weight Loss Profile

O'Brien et al. studied 277 patients who underwent lap banding and found that after 1 year, the initial excess weight loss was 51%. Over time, this subset of patients was able to continue weight loss and at 4 years had an initial excess weight loss of 68.2%. In his study, O'Brien also found only a 3.6% weight loss failure rate associated with the band. Multiple other authors have failed to show similar results with the Lap-Band and have shown lower weight loss rates and higher failure rates. Several studies have compared the outcomes of gastric banding to bypass surgery. Tice et al. completed a systematic review comparing gastric

FIGURE 28.1. Vertical band gastroplasty. A circular window is made in the upper portion of the stomach and then the stomach size is narrowed by placing a vertical row of staples to create a small pouch. A snug band is then placed around the distal end of the pouch to regulate the outflow and transit time of ingested food.

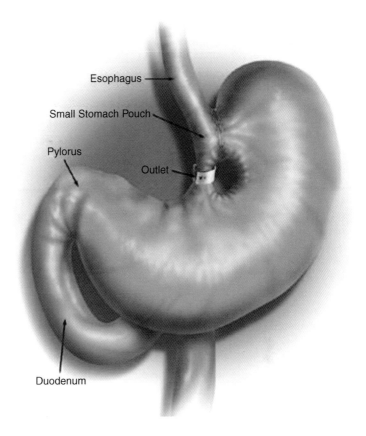

Esophagus

Small Stomach Pouch

Pylorus

Outlet

Duodenum

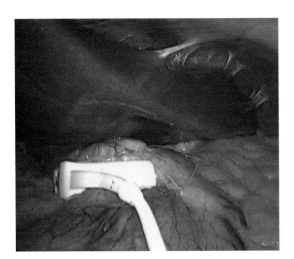

FIGURE 28.2. Intraoperative picture of the laparoscopic placement of a gastric band around the stomach. The adjustable band is placed around the proximal stomach to create a small pouch. The size of the pouch can be adjusted by either injecting or removing saline from the subcutaneous port. Because of the small gastric pouch, the patient will have early satiety and will remain to feel full because of the slow transit time caused by the adjustable gastric band.

banding and bypass and concluded that Roux-en-Y gastric bypass offered greater weight loss and improvements in obesity-related diseases. However, since gastric banding is a less invasive procedure with no staple line there may be a certain subset of patient that will benefit from this procedure.

Complications

Although rare, mortality does occur with the Lap-Band. Mortality with the band is 0.05%. Perforation is another rare complication that can occur during band placement (0.01%). Perforation occurs posteriorly on the stomach or esophagus. It is often unnoticed at the time of placement and is found on a postoperative upper gastrointestinal (UGI) series. Perforation often necessitates immediate removal followed by Graham patching if possible or wide local drainage. In case series, perforation has been treated in asymptomatic patients by leaving the band in place for several days as a mechanical Graham patch and then repeating the UGI. If no leak is seen, the band is removed and the patient needs no further treatment.

Esophageal dilation has also been seen in as many as 30% of band patients. It is unclear if this is solely due to stomal obstruction caused by tightening the band. If dilation of the distal third of the esophagus is seen, fluid placed in the band must be released and an endoscopy should be done for esophagitis.

Slippage. The most common band complications are anterior slippage of the band, which can occur 5% to 14% of the time. When placed the band should sit at a 45-degree angle on plain film. Stomach slips through the band anteriorly creating a large pouch above the band. Slippage often necessitates reoperation and repositioning of the band due to inadequate weight loss and satiety. In its most severe form, anterior stomach above the band can cause the band to lose its 45-degree angulation and become horizontal on plain film. Clinically, the slipped stomach above the band causes enough mechanical pressure on the band to make it appear flat on plain film. This can lead to obstruction of the stomach. When a patient starts vomiting despite all the fluid withdrawn from the band, this constitutes a relative emergency and the patient should be brought to the operating room (OR) for band repositioning before the obstruction progresses and causes gastric necrosis of the stomach above the band.

Erosion. Erosion is another potentially lethal complication of the band. It occurs about 1% of the time. The band over time erodes into the stomach often starting at the band buckle. Erosions often present as intermittent UGI bleeds, fevers, or port site wound infections. Erosions are best diagnosed on UGI series or endoscopy. On UGI series, the barium will track along or outline the band. On endoscopy, the endoscopist will see the white silicone plastic of the Lap-Band. If the patient is stable, asymptomatic, and able to maintain weight, erosions are best managed conservatively. Once the entire band erodes into the stomach as seen on endoscopy, then a combined laparoendoscopic approach is done to remove the band. If, however, the patient is symptomatic or fails to meet the above criteria, operative band removal with primary closure of the hole and Graham patching of the area with wide drainage is often the best approach.

Sleeve Gastrectomy

Sleeve gastrectomy is a restrictive procedure that eliminates the greater curvature of the stomach from the angle of His to approximately 4 cm from the pylorus (Fig. 28.3). The stomach is formed over a 32- to

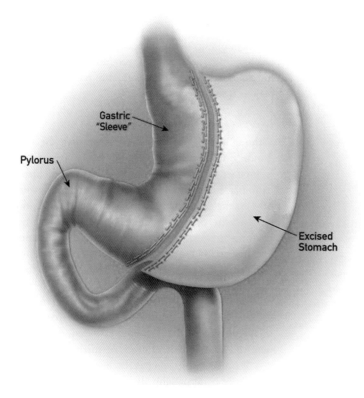

FIGURE 28.3. Sleeve gastrectomy. The elastic portion of the stomach is resected, leaving a narrow, tubular conduit for food. The gastric sleeve creates early satiety with a smaller amount of food.

Gastric "Sleeve"

Pylorus

Excised Stomach

46-French bougie to look like a banana. Sleeve gastrectomy was initially used as part of a two-staged weight loss procedure in the superobese patients who were felt to be too high risk for bypass or BPD. Currently, the sleeve is used as an independent weight loss procedure. Typically, laparoscopic Roux-en-Y gastric bypass (LRYGBP) or a BPD with duodenal switch can be used with the sleeve as a second stage if the weight loss is inadequate. The sleeve eliminates intestinal complications seen with the bypass, namely internal hernias that can be seen after significant weight loss. One of the relative contraindications to the sleeve is severe reflux, since the operation can symptomatically worsen these complaints.

Weight Loss Profile

Currently, 3- to 5-year data exist for the sleeve showing 60% excess weight loss at 2 years with maintenance of weight loss for 3 to 5 years. Studies of more than 5 years do not currently exist and no head-to-head comparisons of sleeve versus band versus bypass exist.

Complications

Leaks. Staple line leaks can occur with sleeve gastrectomies. The most common site is the angle of His. Staple line leaks after sleeves present the same as after gastric bypass. The symptoms are often vague but include postoperative tachycardia, tachypnea, as the early presenting symptoms. Leaks must be taken back to the OR for possible repair combined with wide drainage with nasogastric tube (NGT) and abdominal drains. In addition, it is advisable to place a jejunostomy feeding tube in patients so that they can be enterally feed and maintain adequate nutritional status until the leak heals. Wall stent placement over the leak can be tried; however, stent migration remains a problem.

Bleeding. The gastric staple line used to create a sleeve is long over a vascular organ; therefore, the tendency to bleed is high. Most bleeding can be treated with transfusion as staple line bleeding is often self-limiting. If bleeding persists, operative exploration may be necessary.

Obstruction. The gastric pouch along the lesser curvature can become narrowed in sleeves causing nausea and vomiting especially with solids. UGI with barium is the test of choice to diagnose a narrow channel. Endoscopic balloon dilation has been tried in these patients with varying success. Often it is difficult to dilate these patients for two reasons. The first is

because it is a long staple line that often needs dilation along its entire length. The second reason is because the staple lines are often zigzagged or crossing, making it difficult to achieve adequate dilation. If patients persist with obstruction, a jejunostomy tube for enteral feeds should be considered to stabilize nutritional status. After patients are nutritional optimized with j-tube feeds, the operation can be revised to a gastric bypass.

Laparoscopic Roux-En-Y Gastric Bypass

The laparoscopic approach for Roux-en-Y gastric bypass was first performed in 1993 by Wittgrove. In the year 2000, 20,000 LRYGBPs were preformed in the United States. Today that number is close to 200,000. It is considered the gold standard of obesity surgery and the most common procedure performed in the United States for morbid obesity (Fig. 28.4). It has malabsorptive components, but it primarily works by restricting the amount of food eaten. In this operation, a limb of intestine is connected to a very small stomach pouch. The remainder of the stomach and first segment of small intestine are excluded from the food channel (Fig. 28.5). The amount of bypassed intestine and the length of the Roux limb often vary with the degree of initial patient obesity. Patients with a BMI of less than 50 kg/m^2 often have a shorter limb of 100 to 125 cm, whereas patients with a BMI of more than 50 kg/m^2 have a slightly longer limb to augment a weight loss between 150 and 200 cm. After Roux-En-Y gastric bypass, patients feel early satiety and report enjoying healthy food options. It has been hypothesized that some of these feelings are due to altered levels of hormones such as ghrelin, gastric inhibitory peptide (GIP), glucagon-like peptide-1 (GLP-1), and peptide YY (PYY) that produce neural signals between the gastrointestinal tract and the hunger centers in the brain, triggering satiety. GLP-1, for instance, has been shown to increase about 10-fold after bypass in response to food intake. Comorbid conditions such as diabetes, HTN, dyslipidemia, and obstructive sleep apnea have resolved in large percentages of patients undergoing LRYGBP (see Table 28.1).

Weight Loss

After LRYGBP, the duration of active weight loss was for the first 18 to 24 months. Typically in this time frame patients lose between 60% and 80% of excess weight. Patients will have the greatest weight loss in the first 6 to 8 months after surgery by which time they will lose two-thirds of their total weight loss. In

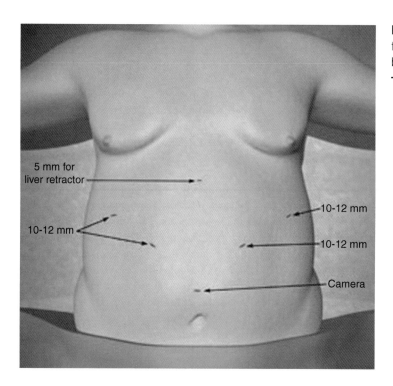

FIGURE 28.4. Typical port placement for a laparoscopic Roux-en-Y gastric bypass.

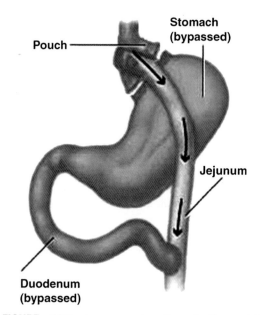

FIGURE 28.5. Laparoscopic Roux-En-Y gastric bypass. A small gastric pouch is created by stapling across the proximal portion of the stomach. The Roux limb is created by stapling across the jejunum approximately 50 to 60 cm distal to the pylorus of the stomach. The jejunum is then anastomosed to the gastric pouch forming the alimentary limb, which bypasses the stomach and duodenum.

the last 6 months, patients will often regain about 5% of their weight. However, in long-term follow-up studies, Roux-en-Y gastric bypass patients can have a significant weight regain after a 2-year period, if they have failed to make lasting lifestyle changes.

Complications

Laparoscopy revolutionized this surgery, decreasing pain, postoperative wound infections, postoperative hernias, and even decreased the incidence of pulmonary embolism (PE). Prior to laparoscopy, the incidence of wound infections and hernias occurred up to 30% of the time. Laparoscopy has decreased this incidence to 2%.

Leaks. Leak is still the most dreaded complication after LRYGBP. Leaks occur 1% to 4% of the time after surgery. They usually present in the first 2 to 5 days postoperatively. However, they can present in a delayed fashion during days 7 to 10. Leaks most often occur at the gastrojejunostomy but can also occur at the jejunojejunostomy. Mortality associated with a leak is about 22%. Just like leaks in other bariatric operations, patients can present with a multitude of symptoms including tachypnea, tachycardia, shortness of breath, vague abdominal pain, shoulder pain, and decreased urine output. Radiographically leaks can be

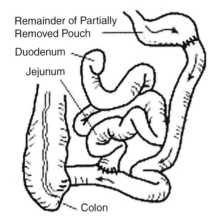

Remainder of Partially
Removed Pouch

Duodenum

Jejunum

Colon

FIGURE 28.6. Biliopancreatic diversion. Ingested food will travel through the small gastric pouch, which is anastomosed to 250 cm of distal small intestine. The duodenum and jejunum, carrying all the digestive enzymes is connected to the ileum, 50 cm proximal to the ileocecal valve. Digestion can only occur in the distal 50 cm of small intestine and therefore patients often suffer from severe malabsorption.

seen on UGI or computed tomography (CT) scans with Gastrografin contrast. However, if a leak is suspected going directly to the OR is the best course of action as it is both diagnostic and therapeutic. Management surrounding a leak is centered on closing the site of leak primarily if possible. If a site of leak cannot be clearly identified then wide drainage with an NGT and multiple abdominal drains is

advised. In addition, placement of a gastrostomy tube for initial decompression of the gastric remnant and later for enteral feeds is mandatory at the time of operation. If the leak persists long term and the patient is stable or a well-localized late leak presents, wall stent placement at the gastrojejunostomy can be considered. This is a relatively newer therapy for well-localized leaks that allows improved healing while allowing the patient to eat orally. Stent migration does remain a challenge.

Strictures. The gastrojejunostomy anastomosis should ideally be about 1 cm in diameter. This causes the relative outlet obstruction seen at the gastrojejunostomy and produces prolonged food satiety in postbypass patients. As this anastomosis heals, it can stricture down and cause nausea/vomiting and severe dysphagia to even liquids. Strictures are most likely to occur between 2 and 6 weeks postoperatively. Strictures occur up to 5% of the time after LRYGBP and are diagnosed endoscopically. They can be treated by a skilled endoscopist with balloon dilation. Patients who stricture will often restricture after initial dilation and need multiple dilations and should be surveyed for recurrence of this problem.

Marginal Ulcers. Ulceration at the gastrojejunostomy occurs 4% to 5% of the time. Marginal ulcers present as severe epigastric pain, worse with eating. The pain is so severe that it often prevents patients from eating. Endoscopy is used to make the diagnosis of an ulcer

TABLE 28.1	**Resolution of Medical Problems After Gastric Bypass Surgery**				
N **= 104** **1-year post-op**	**Number Prior to Surgery**	**% Worse**	**% No Change**	**% Improved**	**% Resolved**
Osteoarthritis	64	2	10	47	41
Hypercholesterimia	62	0	4	33	63
GERD	58	0	4	24	72
Hypertension	57	0	12	18	70
Sleep apnea	44	2	5	19	74
Hypertriglyceridemia	43	0	14	29	57
Peripheral edema	31	0	4	55	41
Stress incontinence	18	6	11	39	44
Asthma	18	6	12	69	13
Diabetes	18	0	0	18	82
Average		1.6%	7.6%	35.1%	55.7%
				90.8% Improved or Resolved	

in the jejunum at the gastrojejunal anastomosis. Treatment consists of a proton pump inhibitor orally combined with an agent to coat the mucosa such as sucralfate.

Patients have to be counseled on avoiding nonsteroidal anti-inflammatory drugs (NSAIDs), alcohol, or anti-inflammatory medications often used for osteoarthritis.

Gastrointestinal Hemorrhage. Postoperative bleeding can occur at the gastric staple lines secondary to the stomach's robust blood supply in 1% to 4% of patients. It may be in the form of intraluminal bleeding or intra-abdominal bleeding from fresh staple lines. This bleeding is often self-limiting and rarely requires operative intervention.

Regardless of whether the patient presents with hematemesis or melena in the immediate postoperative period, a UGI source should be considered first. Bleeding is often self-limiting and may require the patient to be transfused. Bleeding from the pouch or gastrojejunostomy can be diagnosed endoscopically. A skilled endoscopist can clip the area or heater probe the bleeding source. A trip to the OR is rarely required and should be reserved for the hemodynamically unstable patient. The goal of operative management is to evacuate clot and to oversew the site of bleeding. If not identifiable at the time of exploration, all staple lines should be oversewn. Finally, a gastrostomy tube should be placed in the remnant to decompress the distended bypassed stomach and to remove clots.

Hernias. Hernias can occur at incision sites as in any surgery. The incidence of incisional hernias in LRYGBP is less than 1%. However, internal hernias can cause postoperative small bowel obstructions 2% of the time in gastric bypass surgery. Unlike the previous complications, which occur relatively early in a patient's course, internal hernias usually occur later in a patient's course at least 6 months postoperatively. Internal hernias occur after significant weight loss has occurred and potential mesenteric spaces enlarge as mesenteric fat dissolves. The most common site of internal herniation in gastric bypass patients is the Petersen's hernia defect. This represents the space under the Roux limb of the gastric bypass. In retrocolic gastric bypass where the Roux limb is tunneled through the transverse mesocolon, this is often a small defect but can enlarge with time as the fat of the small bowel mesentery shrinks. In the antecolic bypass, this space is very large postoperatively

and can become larger as the small bowel mesentery thins. There are authors who have reported large closed-loop obstruction from internal hernias with small bowel necrosis in both antecolic and retrocolic patients. Internal hernias can also occur at the transverse mesocolic defect in retrocolic gastric bypass, when the mesenteric fat of the transverse colon thins out. The third site of herniation is the jejunojejunostomy defect. This is probably the rarest site of internal herniation in gastric bypass patients. Adhesive small bowel obstructions can also occur in these patients. However, it is rare since there is a paucity of adhesions caused by laparoscopy.

Small bowel obstruction can also occur in these patients without vomiting. These patients often present with left upper quadrant pain and increased liver function tests (LFTs) as their only symptom from a distended gastric remnant and a distended biliopancreatic limb. A closed-loop obstruction results often from an internal hernia involving the jejunojejunostomy. These patients should go directly to the OR because of the risk of bowel perforation and bowel necrosis.

Deep Venous Thrombosis/Pulmonary Embolism. The incidence of deep venous thrombosis (DVT) is as high as 2% in patients with a prior history of venous stasis disease. Despite this low incidence, PE is the leading cause of bariatric deaths. Patients undergoing gastric bypass are at increased risk for DVT not only in the immediate postoperative period, but also for a period up to 6 months postsurgery. Patients are often prophylaxed with heparin SQ or dalteparin (Fragmin), antiembolic stocking, and early ambulation in an effort to prevent DVT.

Inferior vena cava (IVC) filter placement is done selectively. There are no absolute recommendations for filter placement, but considerations include patients with a hypercoagulable state, a DVT that is present, a prior history of DVT or PE, and supersuperobese (BMI >60 kg/m²).

Malnutrition. Typically, the amount of small bowel bypassed is not enough to create micronutrient or protein malnourishment in the absence of any other mechanical or psychological problems.

Anemia and osteoporosis are common long-term deficiencies that may develop. Calcium and iron absorption occurs primarily in the duodenum, which after surgery is excluded from the oral pathway. Gastric bypass patients should be on long-term treatment with iron and calcium supplements. In addition, all patients should also be on multivitamins because of decreased vitamin intake that occurs as a byproduct of decreased food intake.

Malabsorptive Procedures

Biliopancreatic Diversion

BPD, first described by Scopinaro, has restrictive features but is primarily a malabsorptive procedure. A distal gastrectomy creates some restriction of ingested food. However, patients are able to eat up to a 60- to 100-cc meal after surgery. A state of malabsorption is created by diverting pancreatic secretions and bile that aid in digestion away from ingested food. The bowel is reconstructed so that the biliary limb is anastomosed approximately 50 cm from the ileocecal valve (Fig. 28.6). At this site, the digestive enzymes and the ingested food are able to mix, leaving 50 cm of small bowel for fat absorption. This leads to fat calorie malabsorption. Incomplete breakdown of food occurs due to the short segment of bowel in which ingested food and digestive enzymes are combined. In addition, malabsorption occurs because ingested food has contact with a decreased surface area of small bowel and therefore, less absorption of nutrients can take place. The anatomic reconstruction of small bowel is similar to LRYGBP except that the length of intestine in the common channel is substantially shorter, hence creating a state of malabsorption. In long-term follow-up studies, BPD patients kept excellent weight loss results after the initial 2 years. BPD has been shown to have the best long-lasting results in terms of weight loss and improvement in obesity-related morbidities. However, it is not commonly preformed in the United States because of the high leak rates associated with BPD and because of the severe nutritional issues that can arise including severe protein, fat, calorie malnutrition, and intractable diarrhea secondary to malabsorption.

Changes in Comorbidities

Massive weight loss significantly alters ones quality of life physically, mentally, and socially. Many medical conditions significantly improve or are completely resolved after moderate weight loss.

Diabetes Mellitus Type II

Weight loss can result in a normalization of fasting blood glucose in approximately 85% of patients and improved glucose control in the remainder. Weight loss improves insulin sensitivity and beta cell function.

Diabetic control for most patients occurs almost immediately, even prior to the 10% body weight loss. This has caused researchers to hypothesize that duodenal bypass of food is a central component to diabetes resolution.

Hypertension

HTN is closely associated with obesity. Weight loss offers an improvement in both systolic and diastolic blood pressure. After weight loss, blood pressure becomes more manageable and many patients no longer require antihypertensive therapy.

Dyslipidemia

Increased levels of triglyceride and decreased levels of high-density lipoproteins (HDLs) characterize the dyslipidemia of obesity. Dyslipidemia is associated with atherogenesis causing coronary artery disease and vascular events. Substantial weight loss leads to an improvement of the total cholesterol to HDL ratio.

Osteoarthritis

Patients with osteoarthritis often have done irreversible damage to knee, hip, and back joints. Bariatric surgery cannot reverse this damage. However, when surveyed 54% of patients who complained of severe osteoarthritis prior to surgery, noted improvement in ambulation with a decrease in arthritic pain post—weight loss.

QUESTIONS

Select one answer.

1. The optimal management of most postoperative leaks after gastric bypass is:
   a. NPO, hyperalimentation, IV antibiotics.
   b. UGI to determine site of leak and operate only if the site can be clearly identified.
   c. IV antibiotics, CT-guided pigtail placement near the gastrojejunostomy anastomosis, NGT placement.
   d. Operative exploration, endoscopic NGT placement, good drainage of anastomotic site, G tube placement, IV antibiotics.

2. All of the following are false EXCEPT:
   a. Ghrelin is secreted from adipocytes.
   b. Ghrelin is high in the obese.
   c. Leptin comes from the stomach.
   d. Leptin is high in the obese.
   e. PYY and GLP-1 decrease after gastric bypass.

3. The initial resuscitation of a postoperative bariatric patient with hypotension and suspected sepsis is:

   a. Transfuse blood, followed by vasopressors, usually dopamine at 5 mg/kg/min.

   b. Fluid bolus of 1,000 cc of crystalloid or colloid over 30 minutes.

   c. Elevate the foot of the bed and position left side down to increase venous return.

   d. Stat blood cultures, followed by blood transfusion, followed by broad spectrum antibiotics.

4. Two years after lap banding a patient presents to the emergency department with severe epigastric pain and nausea. The white blood cell (WBC) count is 20,000 and UGI shows a complete obstruction. Which of the following is true:

   a. Remove all fluid in the band, if the pain is not alleviated go to the OR to access the band and the pouch.

   b. Place the patient on IV antibiotics for a gastric erosion.

   c. Endoscope the patient to make sure that there is no erosion.

   d. Anterior slippages are rarely emergencies, remove the fluid and discharge the patient for follow-up with their bariatric surgeon.

5. Three months after LRYGBP a patient presents to the emergency department with hematemesis. The patient is on clopidogrel (Plavix) and acetylsalicylic acid (ASA) for cardiac stents. Which of the following is the most appropriate management of this patient:

   a. Transfuse as needed with blood and platelets and observe in the ICU.

   b. Endoscope the patient after stopping the ASA and Plavix.

   c. Endoscope the patient when stable to diagnose and treat a marginal ulcer.

   d. Empirically start the patient on proton pump inhibitors.

SELECTED REFERENCES

Ahroni JH, Montgomery KF, Watkins BM. Laparoscopic adjustable gastric banding: weight loss, co-morbidities, medication usage and quality of life at one year. *Obes Surg* 2005;15(5)641–647.

Allison DB, Fintaine KR, Manson JE, et al. Annual deaths attributable to obesity in the United States. *JAMA* 1999; 282:1530–1538.

Angrisani L, Lorenzo M, Borrelli V. Laparoscopic adjustable banding versus Roux-en-Y gastric bypass: 5 year results of a prospective randomized trial. *Obes Surg* 2007;(3)127–133.

Balsiger BM, Pogio JM, Mai J, et al. Ten and more years after vertical banded gastroplasty as a primary operation for morbid obesity. *J Gastrointest Surg* 2000;4:598–605.

Buchwald H. Overview of bariatric surgery. *J Am Coll Surg* 2002;194:367–375.

Centers for Disease Control, National Hospital Discharge Summary Survey, DHHS publication series 13 No 153;2001.

Chapman AE, Kiroff G, Game P. Laparoscopic adjustable gastric banding in the treatment of obesity: a systematic literature review. *Surgery* 2004;135(3)326–351.

Chopra M, Gallbraith S, Darnton-Hill I. A global response to a global problem: the epidemic of overnutrition. *Bull World Health Organ* 2002;80(12):952–958.

Chu CA, Gagner M, Quinn T, et al. Two-stage laparoscopic biliopancreatic diversion with duodenal switch: an alternative approach to super-super morbid obesity. *Surg Endosc* 2002; 16:S069.

DeMaria EJ, Sugarman HJ, Meador JG, et al. High failure rate after laparoscopic adjustable silicone gastric banding for treatment of morbid obesity. *Ann Surg* 2001;233:809–818.

Deviere J, Ojeda Valdes G, Cuevas Herrera L, et al. Safety, feasibility and weight loss after transoral gastroplasty: first human multicenter study. *Surg Endosc* 2008;22: 589–598.

Garcia JA, Martinez M, Elia M, et al. Obesity surgery results depending on technique performed: long term outcome. *Obes Surg* 2009;19:432–438.

Gastrointestinal surgery for severe obesity: National Institute of Health Consensus development Conference Statement. *Am J Clin Nutr* 1992;55(Suppl 2):S615–S619.

Gravente G, Araco A, Sorge R, et al. Wound infections in post bariatric patients undergoing body contouring abdominoplasty: the role of smoking. *Obes Surg* 2007;17:1325–1331.

Gusenoff JA, Messing S, O'Malley W, et al. Temporal and demographic factors influencing the desire for plastic surgery after gastric bypass surgery. *Plast Reconstr Surg* 2007; 6:2120–2126.

Hagen ME, Wagner OJ, Swain P, et al. Hybrid natural orifice transluminal endoscopic surgery (NOTES) for Roux-en-Y gastric bypass: an experimental surgical study in human cadavers. *Endoscopy* 2008;40(11):918–924.

Harvey A, Blackburn G, Apovian C, et al. Commonwealth of Massachusetts for patient safety and medical error reduction. Expert panel on weight loss surgery: executive report. *Obes Res* 2005;13:205–226.

Hedley AA, Ogden CL, Johnson CL, et al. Prevalence of overweight and obesity among US children, adolescents and adults 1999–2002. *JAMA* 2004;291:2847–2850.

Hess DW, Hess DS. Laparoscopic vertical banded gastroplasty with complete transaction of the staple line. *Obes Surg* 1994;4(1):44–46.

Hill JO, Peters JC. Environmental contributions to the obesity epidemic. *Science* 1998;280(5368):1371–1374.

Huang CK, Houng JY, Chiang CJ, et al. Single incision transabdominal laparoscopic Roux-en-Y gastric bypass: a first case report. *Obes Surg* 2009. Eprint.

Hubens G, Balliu L, Ruppert M, et al. Roux-en-Y gastric bypass procedure performed with the da Vinci robot system: is it worth it? *Surg Endosc* 2008;22(7):1690–1696.

Janosz N. Impact of surgical and nonsurgical weight loss on diabetes resolution and cardiovascular risk resolution. *Curr Diab Rep* 2009;9(3)223–228.

Kremer AJ, Linner JH, Nelson CH. An experimental evaluation of the nutritional importance of the proximal and distal small intestine. *Ann Surg* 1954;140(3):439–447.

Kurian M, Thompson B, Davidson B. *Weight loss surgery for dummies.* New York, NY: Wiley Publishing, 2005.

Kuzmak LL. Silicone gastric banding: a simple and effective operation for morbid obesity. *Contemp Surg* 1986;28:13–18.

Larsen M, Polat F, Stook FP, et al. Satisfaction and complications in post bariatric surgery abdominoplasty patients. *Acta Chir Plast* 2007;49(4):95–98.

Lee W-J, Yu P-J, Wang W. Gastrointestinal quality of life following laparoscopic vertical banded gastroplasty. *Obes Surg* 2002;12:819–824.

MacDonald KG Jr, Long SD, Swanson MS, et al. The gastric bypass operation reduces the progression and mortality of non-insulin dependent diabetes mellitus. *J Gastrointest Surg* 1997;1:213–220.

Mason EE. Vertical banded gastroplasty for obesity. *Arch Surg* 1982;117:701–706.

Matarasso A. Abdominoplasty: a system of classification and treatment for combined abdominoplasty and suction-assisted lipectomy. *Aesthetic Plast Surg* 1991;15: 111– 121.

Mitchell JE, Crosby RD, Ertelt TW, et al. The desire for body contouring surgery after bariatric surgery. *Obes Surg* 2008; 18:1308–1312.

Nguyen N, DeMaria E, Ikramuddin S, Hutter M. *The SAGES manual: a practical guide to bariatric surgery.* New York, NY: Springer, 2008.

Nguyen NT, Hinojosa MW, Smith BR, Reavis KM. Single laparoscopic incision transabdominal (SLIT) surgery-adjustable gastric banding: a novel minimally invasive surgical approach. *Obes Surg* 2008;18(12):1628–1631.

Nguyen NT, Longoria M, Gelfand DV, et al. Staged laparoscopic Roux-en-Y: a novel two-staged bariatric operation as an alternative in the super-obese with massively enlarged liver. *Obes Surg* 2005;15:1077–1081.

O'Brien PE, Brown WA, Smith A, et al. Prospective study of a laparoscopically placed, adjustable gastric band in the treatment of morbid obesity. *Br J Surg* 1999;86:113–118.

Pinkey JH, Sjostrom CD, Gale EA. Should surgeons treats diabetes in severely obese people? *Lancet* 2001;357: 1357–1359.

Pitombo C, Jones K, Higa K, Pareja JC. *Obesity surgery principles and practice.* New York, NY: McGraw-Hill, 2007.

Powell LH, Calvin JE III, Calvin JE, Jr. Effective obesity treatments. *Am Psychol* 2007;62:234–246.

Shermak MA, Chang D, Magnuson TH. An outcomes analysis of patients undergoing body contouring surgery after massive weight loss. *Plast Reconstr Surg* 2006;4:1026–1031.

Shermak MA, Chang D, Magnuson TH. Factors impacting thromboembolism after bariatric body contouring surgery. *Plast Reconstr Surg* 2007;5:1590–1596.

Song AY, Rubin JP, Thimas V, et al. Body image and quality of life in post massive weight loss body contouring patients. *Obesity* 2006;14:11626–11636.

Spector JA, Levine SM. Surgical Solutions to the problem of massive weight loss. *World J Gastroenterol* 2006;12: 6602–6607.

Strauch B, Herman C, Rhode C, et al. Mid-body contouring in the post bariatric surgery patient. *Plast Reconstr Surg* 2006; 17:2200–2211.

Sugarman H, Nguyen N. *Management of morbid obesity.* New York, NY: Taylor & Francis Group, 2006.

Tice JA, Karliner L, Walsh J, Peterson A, Feldman M. Gastric banding or bypass? A systematic review comparing the two most popular bariatric procedures. *Am J Med* 2008; 121 (10):885–893.

Weigle DS. Pharmacological therapy of obesity: past, present and future. *J Clin Endocrinol Metab* 2003;88:2462–2469.

Wilkinson LH. Reduction of gastric reservoir capacity. *Am J Clin Nutr* 1980;33(2):515–517.

CHAPTER 29

Alexandra Bastien

Principles of Anesthesia for the General Surgeon

A dvances in anesthetic techniques and monitoring, the development of new agents, and better perioperative monitoring have ensured that many more and increasingly complicated procedures can be safely performed on very ill patients. In contrast to 100 years ago, when approximately 25% of patients who received chloroform anesthesia had severe, often fatal dysrhythmias, mortality today from anesthesia is approximately 1 per 500,00 procedures.

Complications do arise, however, from interactions among anesthetic drugs, underlying disease, and surgical intervention. The most common problems include misplaced endotracheal tubes, pulmonary aspiration, hypotension, cardiac dysrhythmias, adverse drug effects, and machine failure. Improved preanesthetic preparation, discussion with the patient and family, and close and continuing communication with the surgical team can reduce mortality and morbidity to close to zero.

ASA PHYSICAL STATUS CLASSIFICATION SYSTEM

This was developed in 1940 by a committee of American Society of Anesthesiologist (ASA) to allow practitioners to compare outcomes within/out of their institutions based on specific criteria. It also alerts different practitioners as to the serious comorbid issues the patient may possess requiring sensitive medical management.

- P1: A normal healthy patient
- P2: A mild systemic disease
- P3: A severe systemic disease
- P4: A severe systemic disease that is a constant threat to life
- P5: A moribund patient that is not expected to survive without the operation

- P6: A declared brain-dead patient whose organs are being removed for donor purposes
- An E is added to the above criteria to indicate emergency surgery

PREOPERATIVE EVALUATION

Preparing a patient for surgery depends on a number of variables, including the type of surgery to be performed, anesthetic concerns such as the patient's comorbid diseases, family history, and position during surgery. Anesthesiologists may require specific laboratory evaluation or preoperative assessment and in some cases further specialist consultation to prepare a patient for surgery. While it is not possible to list all anesthetic concerns and appropriate preoperative evaluation, the following demonstrate the thought process involved and in some cases specific preoperative recommendations.

The ASA does not recommend routine laboratory testing for groups/individual patients. Further testing should be done when indicated. An 80-year-old man who jogs 5 miles a day routinely may not require extensive cardiac evaluation but a 16-year-old who gets chest pain and is short of breath at ambulating short distances may require further cardiac workup.

CARDIOVASCULAR SYSTEM

The most extensive and common workup done in the preoperative evaluation process is risk stratification of the cardiovascular system. When patients present with risk factors such as cholesterol, hypertension, obesity, diabetes mellitus, and family history along with signs and symptoms of further cardiovascular compromise, such as diminished exercise ability, the physician surgeon is encouraged to seek further workup/consultation to help with the perioperative management of his or her patient. The American Heart Association along with the American College of Cardiology and ASA have created an algorithm to guide the surgeon as to the necessary preoperative evaluation of the cardiac patient undergoing noncardiac surgery.

In this decade we have seen a rise in the treatment of coronary artery disease with medications and lifestyle changes as well as coronary artery bypass grafting; a significant increase in patients with coronary stents has resulted in a number of management decisions for patients undergoing noncardiac surgery with bare metal versus drug-eluting stents. Coronary stents placed after angioplasty to decrease narrowing of diseased arteries come with slow release (eluting) of drugs to block cellular proliferation of these stents. This prevents fibrosis, clotting and thus restenosis. Patients are usually on daily aspirin therapy as well as clopidogrel (Plavix) for 1 year. Extensive planning for nonemergent surgery has to be done to deal with the increased risk of bleeding and perioperative coronary thrombosis.

PULMONARY SYSTEM

Evaluation of the pulmonary system is critical to determine extent of pulmonary diseases that might impact the ability to oxygenate and ventilate the patient intraoperatively. History of dyspnea, cough, and/or extensive smoking should alert a practitioner for the need of further workup including but not limited to chest x-ray, arterial blood gas, and pulmonary function tests. Further pulmonary consults can provide aid to the anesthesiologist for management with bronchodilators, steroids etc, limitations of ventilatory support, as well as the need for postoperative support and pulmonary care.

Postoperative care can also be enhanced by known preoperative information on chronic obstructive pulmonary disease, CO_2 retainers, and pulmonary lesions. Spirometry information can be predictive of postoperative complications and increased mortality.

HEMATOLOGIC SYSTEM

Endocrine

Our patient population presents extensive clinical challenges, those accompanying the diabetic patient are particularly challenging to the anesthesiologist.

Attention to end-organ damage and vigilance toward metabolic derangements as well as increased risk for cardiovascular, cerebral, and renal insult are some of those specific challenges. Specific treatment protocols for the regulation of blood glucose levels have been established.

EXTENSIVE FAMILY/PERSONAL HISTORY

It is vital for any patient undergoing an anesthetic to provide details of previous anesthetic reactions in their personal or family history. Death from previous anesthetics, malignant hyperthermia (MH), prolong emergence, extensive unexplained neuromuscular blockade, incidence of postoperative nausea and vomiting (PONV), drug allergies, and holistic/herbal remedies all can contribute to an unstable if not fatal anesthetic.

OBESITY/OBSTRUCTIVE SLEEP APNEA

Social History

Smokers are at an increased risk for developing respiratory complications. Cessation of smoking for more than 6 weeks has been shown to decrease these risks. Changes in airway reactivity, mucociliary transport, and secretions all contribute to these risks. The number of pack years is directly proportional to measurable changes in airflow and closing capacity. Acute cessation of smoking 24 to 48 hours preoperatively can cause improved oxygen delivery to tissues. But this time period may cause increase airway reactivity. Full benefits of smoking cessation require 2 to 3 months.

NPO GUIDELINES

Intake of fatty foods, meat, diseases such as diabetes or trauma can prolong gastric emptying time and thereby increase the risk of pulmonary aspiration in patients requiring general anesthesia, regional anesthesia, or sedation. Both the amount and type of food ingested have to be considered when determining fasting periods. NPO guidelines are set for healthy patients undergoing elective surgery at all ages. Eight hours for a heavy fatty meal, six hours for a light meal, infant

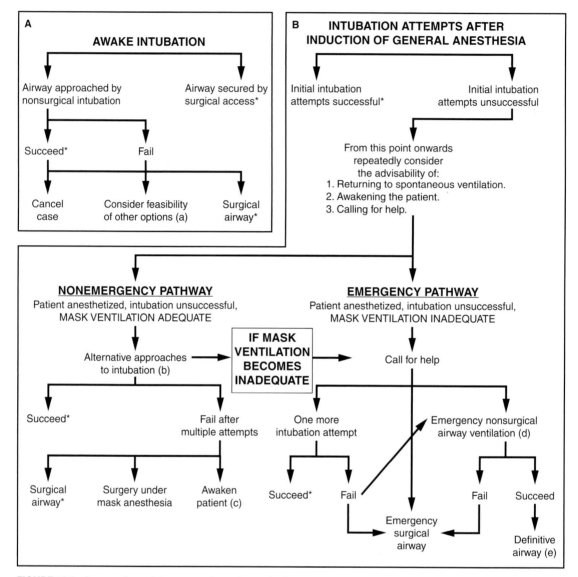

A

AWAKE INTUBATION

Airway approached by nonsurgical intubation

Airway secured by surgical access*

Succeed*   Fail

Cancel case   Consider feasibility of other options (a)   Surgical airway*

B   **INTUBATION ATTEMPTS AFTER INDUCTION OF GENERAL ANESTHESIA**

Initial intubation attempts successful*

Initial intubation attempts unsuccessful

From this point onwards repeatedly consider the advisability of:
1. Returning to spontaneous ventilation.
2. Awakening the patient.
3. Calling for help.

NONEMERGENCY PATHWAY
Patient anesthetized, intubation unsuccessful,
MASK VENTILATION ADEQUATE

EMERGENCY PATHWAY
Patient anesthetized, intubation unsuccessful,
MASK VENTILATION INADEQUATE

Alternative approaches to intubation (b) →

IF MASK VENTILATION BECOMES INADEQUATE

→ Call for help

Succeed*   Fail after multiple attempts

One more intubation attempt

Emergency nonsurgical airway ventilation (d)

Surgical airway*   Surgery under mask anesthesia   Awaken patient (c)

Succeed*   Fail

Fail   Succeed

Emergency surgical airway

Definitive airway (e)

FIGURE 29.1. A comparison of the commonly used anesthetic agents

formula. Four hours for breast milk, and two hours for clear liquids such as water, tea, black coffee, and juices with no pulp.

The use of preoperative gastric stimulants, pharmacologic blockade of gastric acid secretion, preoperative antacids and antiemetics may increase patient comfort, reduce adverse outcomes, improve patient satisfaction, utilization of resources, and decrease cost. These measures are to be determined for selective patients, some of whom are high risk for aspiration and should not be used routinely (Fig. 29.1).

ANESTHETIC AGENTS

Inhalation anesthetics (fluorinated hydrocarbons) (Table 29.1) are unique to anesthesiologists with the exception of nitrous oxide. The mechanism by which these agents produce anesthesia is still unknown. Theories suggesting critical volume causing expansion of the cell membrane and disrupting its matrix, or a specific receptor in which the inhaled anesthetics produce an effect, and alterations in neurotransmitter formation, release, or breakdown as well as others have been hypothesized but not proven.

TABLE 29.1	**Inhalational Anesthetics and Their Effects**					
	Isoflurane	**Halothane**	**Enflurane**	**Sevoflurane**	**Desflurane**	**Nitrous Oxide**
Cardiovascular	Decrease in BP, CO, SVR Reflex tachycardia	Arrhythmogenic with epinephrine HR no change	Same as isoflurane	Same as isoflurane	Same as isoflurane	Mild sympathomimetic effect on BP & CO
Pulmonary	Decreased PVR, CO_2 response, hypoxic response Increased RR	Same as isoflurane	Same as isoflurane	Same as isoflurane	Same as isoflurane	Increased PVR
Central nervous system	Decrease $CMRO_2$ Increase CBF, ICP	Same as isoflurane	Same as isoflurane Seizures	Same as isoflurane	Same as isoflurane	Same as isoflurane
Hepatic	Least organ toxic	Nephrotoxic Hepatotoxic	Nephrotoxic	Less organ toxic	Less organ toxic	DNA synthesis affected, B_{12} Neuropathy

BP, blood pressure; CO, cardiac output; SVR, systemic vascular resistance; HR, heart rate; PVR, pulmonary vascular resistance; $CMRO_2$, cerebral metabolic rate of oxygen; CBF, cerebral blood flow; ICP, intracranial pressure; RR, respiratory rate.

The equivalent steady-state plasma concentration of inhalation anesthetic agents is known as MAC. MAC is the minimum alveolar concentration necessary to respond to noxious stimuli at 1 atm.

Inhalation anesthetics have proven beneficial in the pediatric population where an IV may be avoided for induction. They are also cost-effective in maintaining a balanced anesthetic technique for most adult general anesthetic procedures. They do require a complex vaporizer apparatus to administer and exhaust.

IV ANESTHETICS

Ketamine

Ketamine is a phencyclidine derivative producing dissociative anesthesia on electroencephalography between the thalamic and limbic systems. It provides intense analgesia secondary to opioid receptor interaction. Increased secretory effects, seizures, and unpleasant visual, auditory sensations leading to emergence delirium are possible. Bronchodilation, cardiovascular sympathomimetic responses, and intense analgesia make it an ideal drug for burn patients.

Propofol

Diisopropylphenol is a lipid soluble anesthetic with a rapid onset and one of the most rapid awakening form

of anesthetic. This is secondary to its rapid metabolism and redistribution. Its low incidence of PONV along with the rapid onset and prompt recovery with minimal residual makes it ideal for short ambulatory procedures. Side effects include respiratory and cardiovascular depression, seizure activity, and pain on injection.

Etomidate

Etomidate is a carboxylated imidazole compound that produces one arm-brain time anesthesia (<30 seconds). Cardiovascular stability is a characteristic making this drug useful for patients with limited cardiovascular reserve who are euvolemic. Nausea and vomiting are common. Potential also exists to suppress adrenal cortical function after one dose for many hours. Other disadvantages include painful injection, involuntary skeletal muscle movement, and activation of seizure foci.

Dexmedetomidine

Dexmedetomidine, also known as Precedex, is a presynaptic α-2 agonist that reduces stress, decreases anxiety, and causes pain relief. It is currently approved by US Food and Drug Administration for use by critical care specialists and anesthesiologists. Patients can exhibit bradycardia and cardiac arrest if infused rapidly (vagotonic). Concerns such as withdrawal-like

TABLE 29.2	Amnestics (benzodiazepines)		
Diazepam (Valium)	$T_{1/2}$ 30 hr (active metabolites) Peak 1–2 min	Dose 1–2 mg	Antiseizure Sedative hypnotic
Midazolam (Versed)	$T_{1/2}$ 2.5 hr Peak 2–4 min	0.5–2 mg	Amnestic Sedative hypnotic
Lorazepam (Ativan)	$T_{1/2}$ 15 hr Peak 5–15 min	0.25 mg	Sedative hypnotic
Flumazenil (Reversed)	$T_{1/2}$ 2 hr Peak 5 min	0.2–1 mg	Reversal of respiratory and other benzodiazepine effects

symptoms, as in clonidine, can be seen clinically. In spontaneously ventilated patients respiratory drive may be maintained with stable cardiovascular responses. Redistribution is in 6 minutes while $T_{1/2}$ elimination is 2 hours. Metabolism is via the liver.

Barbiturates

Classes of drugs derived from barbituric acid with substitutions at C2 and C5 carbon atoms resulting in sedative hypnotic effects. At #5 substitutions branched chains have a greater hypnotic activity, whereas phenyl substitutions have greater anticonvulsant properties. The mechanism of action is by depressing the reticular activating system. These drugs have a rapid redistribution with long elimination half-lives because they are purely metabolized. They are extensively studied for the treatment of neurosurgical patients with increased intracranial pressures. They have a great potential for abuse. The excitatory activity produced by Methohexital makes it ideal for the treatment of depressed patients undergoing electroconvulsive therapy. Thiopental has been the neuroprotective drug of choice to induce anesthesia in patients with increased inductively coupled plasma.

Pentobarbital and thiopental infusions have been used to decrease cerebral metabolic rate of oxygen ($CMRO_2$) and produce an isoelectric electroencephalograph, effectively eliminating neuronal firing. Currently only hypothermia is reliable in reducing both electrical activity and slowing basal cellular functions of the brain.

AMNESTICS (BENZODIAZEPINES) (TABLE 29.2)

Mechanism of action: benzodiazepines attach to α-subunits of γ-aminobutyric acid (GABA) enhancing the chloride gating function of this inhibitory neurotransmitter. Other pharmacological characteristics of benzodiazepine include anterograde amnesia, anticonvulsant, depression of respiratory and cardiovascular system, as well as sedative hypnotic effects.

Local Anesthetics

Local anesthetics act by blocking the sodium upstroke of the neural conduction impulse thus resulting in reversible blockade. Local anesthetics are classified according to their metabolism. Amides are metabolized by the liver and esters by hydrolysis (Table 29.3).

Local anesthetics are weak bases chosen for characteristics such as onset (acid dissociation constant [Pka] can be affected by acidic environment), duration (protein binding), and potency (lipid solubility). Systemic toxicity due to low plasma concentration of local anesthetics results in to numbness of tongue and lips, higher levels of local anesthetics start to produce central nervous system symptoms such as restlessness and tinnitus. Even higher levels will produce slurred speech and skeletal muscle twitching eventually leading to tonic-clonic seizures. Cardiovascular toxicity requires higher plasma concentration of local anesthetics causing them to

TABLE 29.3	Local anesthetics and their metabolism
AMIDES (Liver Metab.)	**ESTERS (Pseudocholinesterase)**
Ropivacaine	Procaine
Bupivacaine	Chloroprocaine
Lidocaine	Tetracaine
Etidocainet	Cocaine
Mepivacaine	Benzocaine
Prilocaine	

serve as antidysrhythmics. Higher concentrations lead to conduction blockade. Selective cardiotoxicity of bupivacaine should elicit caution or avoidance in highly vascularized areas. Bupivacaine's high protein binding and lipid solubility results in slower release of the drug from myocardial tissues thus resulting in bradycardia or asystole.

REGIONAL ANALGESIA

Muscle Relaxants

In clinical practice muscle relaxants are used by anesthesiologists to facilitate airway management, provide optimal surgical working conditions, and ease mechanical ventilation. The choice depends on onset, duration, and side effect avoided. The neuromuscular blockers have a structural relationship to the endogenous neurotransmitter acetylcholine. They interrupt transmission of impulses at the neuromuscular junction. Depolarizing muscle relaxant (succinylcholine) attaches to the nicotinic cholinergic receptor and mimics the action of acetylcholine causing depolarization of the postjunctional membrane. Plasma cholinesterase produced by the liver hydrolyze the succinylcholine prior to arrival at the neuromuscular junction. Succinylcholine action at the neuromuscular junction is terminated by passive diffusion away from the nerve terminal. Plasma cholinesterase activity can be reduced by liver disease, drugs, or atypical plasma cholinesterase causing prolongation of neuromuscular blockade by succinylcholine. Eighty percent of normal plasma cholinesterase is inhibited by the local anesthetic dibucaine, whereas atypical plasma cholinesterase is inhibited by the amide local anesthetic dibucaine up to 20%.

Nondepolarizing neuromuscular blockers competitively inhibit nicotinic cholinergic receptors by not causing the receptors to depolarize. At larger doses some can even block the neuromuscular junction. This type of blockade is characterized by decreased twitch response, fade with train of four, post-titanic potentiation, potentiation by other nondepolarizers, and antagonism by anticholinesterases.

Anticholinesterases inhibit the enzyme acetylcholinesterase (true cholinesterase), normally responsible for hydrolysis of acetylcholine. Along with anticholinergics to counter the effects of preganglionic anticholinesterase activity, anticholinesterases are effective in reversible inhibition, forming carbamyl esters or irreversibly inactivation by organophosphates.

Postoperative Nausea and Vomiting

Nausea is the subjective unpleasant sensation associated with the urge to vomit. Vomiting is forceful expulsion of gastric contents from the mouth (Fig. 29.2).

Twenty to thirty percent of patients experience PONV with many persisting for as long as 5 days postoperatively. PONV is a major factor limiting early discharge of ambulatory surgery patients. It is the leading cause of unanticipated hospital admissions after surgery. The medical consequences of PONV include patient discomfort, wound dehiscence, hematoma, aspiration, as well as increased cost. Factors affecting incidence of PONV include history of PONV or motion sickness, age, gender, obesity, anxiety, gynecologic, laparoscopic, eye, and ENT procedures.

Pain/Analgesics

Options for postoperative pain management are dependent on many factors: type of surgery, previous experiences, prior therapy, extensive medical conditions as well as the risk/benefit ratio of the available techniques. Perioperative techniques for pain management include principal component analysis with systemic opioids, epidural or intrathecal opioid analgesia, and regional techniques. Multimodal techniques for pain management with differing mechanism of action provide superior coverage with reduced adverse effects.

Narcotics

Meperidine, morphine, fentanyl, Sue Alfent Remi, and naloxone.

MONITORS

Anesthetic monitors are not specific to the anesthesiologists only. These monitoring standards are recommended to all practitioners engaging in deep sedation techniques as well. Although in emergency situations appropriate life-saving measures take precedence if monitoring is not possible.

The following standards apply when conducting anesthetic management:

The ability to monitor oxygenation to ensure adequate oxygenation of blood and tissues during a

Proposed Etiology(ies) of PONV

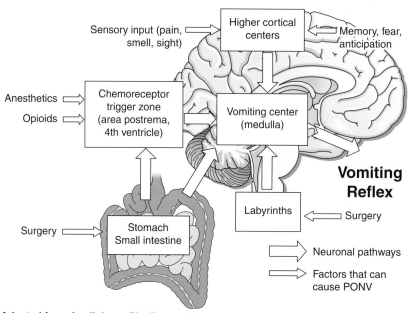

Adapted from Amdipharm Plc, Essex, UK, 2004. Available at:
http://www.nauseaandvomiting.co.uk/NAVRES001-3-PONV.htm. **Accessed October 2005.**

FIGURE 29.2. Proposed etiologies of PONV

procedure. Methods include assessing the patient's color and use of qualitative measuring devices such as pulse oxymetry. Anesthesiologists use devices to measure inspired oxygen concentration in the anesthetic breathing system with additional alarm apparatuses to alert them if the inspired concentration of gases has fallen.

The ability to monitor adequate ventilation. Methods include body plethysmography, auscultation, and quantitative measurement of end tidal carbon dioxide concentrations.

Upon intubation of the trachea it is strongly encouraged that carbon dioxide measurements aid in determining correct initial placement of the endotracheal tube. Alarming devices that determine disconnects are based on threshold levels of end tidal carbon dioxide not achieved.

The ability to monitor evidence of hemodynamic stability/lability. Methods include continuous electrocardiogram monitoring, and assessment of blood pressure and heart rate. Monitoring this aspect of the patient ensures adequate circulatory function of the major organ systems.

A means of measuring the patient's body temperature should be available. Intended changes in a patient's body temperature should be measured in cases of extended anesthetics and intentional hypothermia, as well as high-risk patients with endocrine abnormalities or extremes of age.

The most important standard is having a qualified anesthesiologist present throughout the procedure because changes in a patient's status require vigilance and directed care.

MALIGNANT HYPERTHERMIA

Hotline: 1–800–644–9737

Malignant hyperthermia is a hypermetabolic disorder in which increased levels of intracellular calcium cause activation of metabolic pathways resulting in a high mortality clinical syndrome if untreated. The incidence of this disorder is approximately 1 per 50,000 adult anesthetics and can vary in different regions. It is described as autosomal dominant, multifactorial with variable penetrance.

The caffeine-halothane contracture test (CHCT) is the gold standard for diagnosing MH. Patients with MH elicit contractures from their muscle biopsies at low levels of trigger agents caffeine and halothane. Molecular genetic testing is less expensive and less invasive and can be used for family members of patients diagnosed with MH. This testing is very specific if positive but not highly sensitive (25%–30%).

Signs of MH include masseter spasm after succinylcholine, limb muscle rigidity, hyperthermia, increased end-tidal CO_2 ($ETCO_2$), tachycardia, and tachypnea. Patient will then develop acidosis, myoglobinuria, hyperkalemia, and increased creatine kinase levels.

Acute-phase treatment of MH patients requires stopping offending agents such as flourocarbon inhalation agents and succinylcholine. Also terminating nonemergent surgery if possible. Oxygenating with 100% oxygen while getting help is important since diluting the treatment drug dantrolene, which comes in 20 mg powder using 60 mL of sterile water, is required. A dose of dantrolene, 2.5 to 10 mg/kg can reverse signs of MH. Dantrolene acts by decreasing the release of calcium from the sarcoplasmic reticulum by decreasing the mobility of the calcium across cell membranes.

Other acute-phase treatment of MH includes treating metabolic acidosis with bicarbonate, cooling the patient if the core temperature rises above 39°C, and treating dysrhythmias with antidysrhythmics other than calcium channel blockers that may cause cardiac arrest. Treating hyperkalemia with insulin, glucose, bicarbonate, hyperventilation, and calcium.

Following the patient in acute care to continue dantrolene, prevent myoglobin precipitation in renal tubules that would cause acute tubular necrosis. Control metabolic signs such as acidosis, coagulation disorders, electrolyte abnormalities, and hyperthermia.

QUESTIONS

Select one answer.
1. A 35-year-old man with well-controlled diabetes would be considered an ASA classification of:
   a. P1: A normal healthy patient.
   b. P2: A mild systemic disease.
   c. P3: A severe systemic disease.
   d. P4: Incapacitated.
   e. P5: A moribund.

2. Triggering agents for malignant hyperthermia include:
   a. All inhalation agents.
   b. Succinylcholine.
   c. Benzodiazepines.
   d. Potassium salts.

3. Recommendations for reducing the risk of pulmonary aspiration include:
   a. Particulate antacids.
   b. Infant formula for more than 4 hours.
   c. High gastric volume.
   d. High pH.

4. True statements concerning flumazenil include:
   a. It reverses the effects of some opioids.
   b. It reverses only the respiratory and amnestic effects of benzodiazepines.
   c. It is a benzodiazepine antagonist.
   d. It has a relatively long half-life (prevents resedation by benzodiazepines).

SELECTED REFERENCES

ASA Task Force on Preoperative Fasting. Practice guidelines for preoperative fasting and the use of pharmacologic agents to reduce the risk of pulmonary aspiration: application in healthy patients undergoing elective procedures. *Anesthesiology* 90:896, 1999.

Bailey PL, Egan TD, Stanley TH: Intravenous opioid anesthetics. *Anesthesia*, 5th edi. Miller RD, Ed. Churchill Livingstone Inc, Philadelphia, 2000, p. 273.

Clinical Anesthesia, 6th edition. Barash PG, Cullen BF, Stoelting RK, Cahalan, M, Eds. Lippincott Williams & Wilkins, Philadelphia, 2009.

Eagle KA, Berger PB, Calkins H, et al: ACC/AHA Guideline Update for Perioperative Cardiovascular Evaluation for Noncardiac Surgery—Executive Summary. Circulation 105:1257–1267, 2002.

Rosenberg H, Antognini JF, Muldoon S: Testing for malignant hyperthermia. *Anesthesiology* 96: 232–237, 2002.

Stoelting's Anesthesia and Co-existing Disease: Expert Consult: Online and Print. Hines RL, Marschall K. Philadelphia, Churchill Livingstone, 2008.

CHAPTER 30

Marcia E. Epstein
Angela C. Kim
Taynet T. Febles
Maria Amodio-Groton

Surgical Infections and Principles of Antibiotic Use

INTRODUCTION

Surgical infections are defined as infections that require operative management (such as appendicitis, empyema, necrotizing fasciitis) or infections that are complications of surgical procedures (such as postoperative wound infections). In this chapter, we discuss host and pathogen risk factors that predispose to infection as well as review specific infections and the currently available antimicrobial agents.

RISK FACTORS FOR INFECTION: HOST AND PATHOGEN

Immune Status

Protection against antimicrobial invasion depends on the combination of a general, nonspecific defense system (skin, mucous membranes, complement, etc), an innate immunity, and a highly adaptive and specified defense system. The first two lines of defense involve surveillance and engulfment of invading pathogens by phagocytic cells, namely polymorphonuclear neutrophils, macrophages, and dendritic cells. In addition, serum proteins called complement, once activated, play a role in direct bacterial killing. They also facilitate engulfment of microbes as well as attract leukocytes to sites of infection. Acquired or adaptive immunity includes B-cell lymphocytes that produce antibodies responsible for neutralizing invading microorganisms, activating complement, and opsonizing pathogens, enabling the phagocytes to engulf them. T-cell lymphocytes are part of the cell-mediated immune system and are important in intracellular bacterial, viral, mycobacterial, and fungal infections. As survival between both solid organ and bone marrow transplant recipients improves, we will encounter more patients with surgical issues who present with more subacute and occult signs and symptoms of infection as a result of immunosuppression from the underlying disease itself and the antirejection medications. Some frequently used agents include corticosteroids, the calcineurin inhibitors (cyclosporine and tacrolimus), mycophenolate mofetil, azathioprine, and sirolimus. Microbiologically, this patient population is more at risk for fungal infections, mycobacterial infections, and infections by intracellular pathogens (including viruses). In addition, diabetes, chronic kidney disease, liver disease, malnutrition, and alcoholism all negatively affect the immune system.

In addition to producing opsonizing antibody, the spleen helps in the clearance of encapsulated bacteria. Functionally, asplenic or surgically splenectomized patients are at risk for post-splenectomy sepsis in which rapid deterioration occurs especially with encapsulated bacteria. When possible, immunization should be given 2 weeks prior to elective splenectomy. Trauma-related splenectomies tend to be performed on an emergent basis; therefore, immunizations should occur after 2 weeks, leaving postoperative recovery time to elapse. Twenty-three-valent unconjugated capsular pneumococcal polysaccharide vaccine or heptavalent-conjugated pneumococcal vaccine, conjugated Hib polysaccharide, and quadrivalent nonconjugated polysaccharide meningococcal vaccine should be administered in the same time frame.

Local Factors

Commensal bacteria that live in the mucous membranes that line the gastrointestinal (GI) tract protect against more virulent and invasive bacteria. Disruption by perforation or loss of integrity of this barrier by other means allows for invasion to occur. Exposure to antibiotics (including those received for surgical prophylaxis) causes selective pressure toward fungal and more resistant microorganisms, allowing them to dominate. Parenteral nutrition predisposes to bacterial and fungal infections, especially *Candida* species. Other reasons for increased risk include predisposition to thrombosis (and therefore infection); the population requiring total parenteral nutrition tends to be sicker, malnourished, and inherently more at risk for infection. A prolonged duration of catheter placement for total parenteral nutrition increases risk of infection.

Antibiotic efficacy depends a great deal on local host factors. For example, the presence of foreign materials (urinary catheters, central venous catheters (CVCs), prosthetic heart valves, pacemakers, central nervous system shunts, orthopedic hardware) serves as a potential nidus toward formation of biofilms. Biofilms made up of a glycocalyx and embedded bacteria are extremely difficult to eradicate solely with antibiotics and often require surgical removal of the foreign body. In addition, impaired vascular supply negatively impacts wound healing and limits the effectiveness of antimicrobial therapy. Another local factor that can increase the rate of infection is shaving. If hair removal is necessary, clippers or depilatories are recommended in lieu of shaving.

Mechanisms of Microbial Pathogenicity

For a microorganism to cause infection, it must be able to overcome the host's natural defenses against disease. The two general mechanisms are methods to increase invasiveness and toxin production.

The integrity of the mucosal surfaces functions as a barrier to microbial invasion. *Bordetella pertussis* paralyzes the ciliary clearance function of the respiratory tract, facilitating colonization of this organism. *Pseudomonas aeruginosa* and *Staphylococcus epidermidis* form biofilm, whereas *Escherichia coli* produces an extracellular matrix that shields the bacteria from the host's immune system. Certain bacteria are able to resist phagocytic ingestion by forming a capsule that surrounds the cell wall (*Streptococcus pneumoniae, Haemophilus influenzae, Klebsiella pneumoniae*). Bacteria require a receptor and a ligand to adhere to a eukaryotic cell or tissue surface. The ligand, also called an adhesion, is the part of the bacterial cell surface that usually interacts with the host cell receptor. Certain *E coli* strains have adhesions called pili or fimbriae that promote urinary tract colonization and invasion. These "P" fimbriae have been shown to bind specifically to uroepithelial cells. It is well established that certain infections predispose to others. For example,

influenza infection predisposes to bacterial pneumonia. This occurs because the influenza virus destroys the mucosa, exposing basement membrane proteins, allowing bacteria to bind. In addition, influenza neuraminidase may degrade sialic acid in the lung, exposing receptors for bacteria and increasing adherence.

Microorganisms may use other strategies to evade the immune surveillance system. Pathogens may coat themselves with host proteins (such as *Treponema pallidum*). Other pathogens cause the host cells to signal incorrectly, leading to dysregulation of host's defenses (eg, *Yersinia*, *Mycobacterium*, and *Bordetella*) by inducing the host to produce anti-inflammatory cytokines. Several bacterial pathogens are able to survive and replicate within host cells after invasion. *Coxiella burnetii* is able to survive in the phagolysosomal vacuoles despite their low pH. *Mycobacteria* spp, *Salmonella*, and *Chlamydia* are able to survive in non-lysosomal vacuoles. Many viruses use antigenic variation and intracellular invasion to avoid host defenses.

Some bacteria contain cell-wall components that function as toxins, and other bacteria secrete toxins. Bacterial lipopolysaccharide (endotoxin) is embedded in the outer membrane of gram-negative bacteria. The toxic portion of the lipopolysaccharide, lipid A, causes the release of many host proinflammatory cytokines, triggering the induction of septic shock, the complement, and the coagulation cascade. Gram-positive bacteria do not contain endotoxin but contain peptidoglycan and teichoic acids that can also trigger a similar inflammatory response. Released toxins, or exotoxins, are usually enzymes and categorized by different systems. One major type of toxin is A-B toxins. These toxins have two subunits—the A subunit (which possesses the enzymatic activity) and the B subunit (which has the binding domain), for example, cholera toxin, diphtheria toxin, and pertussis toxin. Proteolytic toxins are another category of toxins that break down host proteins, such as the elastase and protease of *P aeruginosa*. Membrane-disrupting toxins found in several gram-negative bacterial species form pores in host cell membranes, resulting in cell lysis.

SPECIFIC INFECTIONS

Urinary Tract Infections

Urinary tract infections (UTIs) are the most common nosocomial infections in hospitals and nursing homes. In hospitals, 80% of nosocomial UTIs are associated with instrumentation of the urinary tract.

In hospitals, UTIs account for up to 40% of nosocomial infections. It is believed that a large number of UTIs could be avoided by proper management of the indwelling urinary catheters. Even with the adaptation of the closed method of urinary drainage, more than 20% of patients will become infected. This is particularly true for patients with advanced age, debilitation, or in the postpartum state. Even a single brief catheterization is associated with a 1% to 5% risk of infection.

Microorganisms gain access to the urinary tract via several routes. They can be introduced through the meatus or the distal urethra with the insertion of the catheter. Fortunately, healthy individuals are usually able to eliminate these microorganisms that were introduced by voiding or by the protective mucosa of the bladder. Microorganisms can also be introduced by traveling along the outside of the catheter or along the internal lumen of the catheter from the collection bag or the catheter–drainage tube junction. The use of a closed drainage system has significantly lowered the rate of UTIs, suggesting that this was a common pathway for microorganisms to enter the bladder.

According to the CDC guidelines, urinary catheterization should be limited to patients (a) to bypass a urinary-tract obstruction, (b) to allow bladder emptying in patients with a neurogenic bladder or urinary retention, (c) for recovery from urological surgical procedures, and (d) for accurate monitoring of urinary output in a critical-care setting. It should not be used as a replacement for nursing care in the incontinent patient or for diagnostic testing when the patient is able to void voluntarily.

Condom catheterization can be used in men with no outlet obstruction, but requires meticulous care and has been associated with skin maceration or phimosis. In the confused patient, manipulation of the drainage system has been associated with an increased risk of UTIs. It is not clear whether the suprapubic catheter offers an advantage with regard to infection control. Another alternative often offered to certain groups (spinal cord injury patients, patients with bladder-emptying dysfunction, etc) is intermittent catheterization, although no well-controlled clinical trials compare the risk of infection.

Special catheters that minimize development of biofilm formation can decrease and/or delay the onset of catheter-associated bacteriuria, and theoretically lower the risk of catheter-associated UTIs. A recent review of trials with either nitrofurazone-coated silicone catheters or silver alloy (either latex- or silicone-based) catheters concluded that they can prevent or delay the development of catheter-associated bacteriuria in selected hospitalized patients. However, this effect varied by several variables, and it is not clear how this impacted on the overall morbidity, mortality, and cost in caring for the patient.

Acidification of the urine also decreases rates of UTI. Normally higher urea concentration and osmolality in the urine (and therefore lower pH) serve an antibacterial function. pH also affects how certain antimicrobials function. Methenamine and nitrofurantoin are more effective when the urinary pH is lower; methenamine activity results in the release of formaldehyde when the urinary pH is below 5.5. Aminoglycosides are actually more effective in alkaline urine. Strategies to acidify the urine include administration of ascorbic acid or methionine. This process may precipitate urate or oxalate stones. Patients with renal insufficiency may be unable to eliminate the acid load and can become systemically acidotic if this strategy is used. Dietary restrictions of foods that alkalinize urine (milk, fruit juices [except cranberry juice], and sodium bicarbonate) are also useful. Cranberry juice has been shown to reduce bacteriuria and recurrent UTIs in women by 15% to 20% compared with placebo. The reason for this is not because of change in urinary pH, but rather the inhibition of bacterial adherence to the urinary tract epithelium.

Nosocomial Pneumonia

Pneumonia is the second most common cause of nosocomial infection. When it occurs postoperatively, mortality can be as high as 18%. According to the American thoracic society (ATS) guidelines, hospital-acquired pneumonia occurs 48 hours or more after admission whereas ventilator-associated pneumonia occurs more than 48–72 hours after endotracheal intubation.

Risk factors for nosocomial pneumonia can be divided into three categories: patient-, surgery-, and care-related factors. Patient-related factors include age, general health, obesity, underlying lung disease, diabetes mellitus, renal insufficiency, immunocompromised states, and level of consciousness (increased risk of aspiration with diminished consciousness). The type and anatomic location of surgery may influence the risk of nosocomial pneumonia. Incisions that approach the diaphragm, particularly of the upper abdomen and thorax, increase the risk of postoperative pulmonary complications. Other risk factors include the duration of nasogastric/orogastric tube or endotracheal intubation, frequency of ventilator tubing change (every

24 hours instead of 48 hours), frequency of endotracheal suctioning, and patient position (ie, elevation of head of bed to decrease aspiration).

Signs and symptoms of nosocomial pneumonia include a new or increase production of sputum, fever, leukocytosis, tachypnea, and decreased PaO_2 with radiographic evidence of new or worsening pulmonary infiltrates. Common pathogens include aerobic gram-negative bacilli, such as *P aeruginosa, E coli, K pneumoniae*, and *Acinetobacter* spp and gram-positive cocci (including methicillin-resistant *Staphylococcus aureus* [MRSA]). Treatment is often empiric and should cover the most common nosocomial pathogens based on local antibiograms. Important preventative measures include early extubation, ambulation, adequate pain control to prevent splinting, avoidance or early removal nasogastric/orogastric tube, proper positioning of patient to minimize the risk of aspiration, chest physical therapy, and incentive spirometry.

Catheter-Related Bloodstream Infections

Catheters, including CVCs, peripheral venous, and arterial catheters, establish vascular access; however, they place patients at risk for catheter-related bloodstream infections (CRBSIs). Regular evaluation, proper insertion techniques (sterile barrier precautions), and skin preparation with 2% chlorhexidine solution help decrease rates of infection.

Peripheral venous catheters, although more frequently used, rarely result in bloodstream infections but may cause phlebitis related to prolonged use. In comparison, CVCs account for approximately 90% of all CRBSIs. This increased risk is associated with prolonged use, frequency of manipulation, type of catheter, and patient comorbidities; however, studies have shown no benefit in changing central lines on a particular schedule.

The most common pathogens cultured are coagulase-negative staphylococci, *S aureus*, aerobic gram-negative bacilli, and *Candida albicans*. Laboratory diagnosis relies on a minimum of two sets of blood cultures (at least one percutaneously). According to the infectious disease society of America (IDSA) guidelines, a documented nontunneled CVC-related bacteremia or fungemia should be followed by prompt catheter removal. Treatment of potential tunneled CVC-related infection depends on clinician evaluation of the severity of illness. Empiric antimicrobials for suspected CRBSI depend on the patient population and severity of illness. Vancomycin covers the most common pathogens (ie, coagulase-negative staphylococci, *S aureus*, and MRSA) and therefore should be initiated pending culture results. In critically ill or immunocompromised patients, additional coverage for enteric gram-negative bacilli, *Pseudomonas* spp, and *Candida* spp should be considered.

C difficile–Associated Diarrhea

Clostridium difficile–associated disease is increasing in incidence and severity and is becoming more difficult to treat. Recent reports of a more virulent and possibly more resistant strain of *C difficile* in the United States have heightened awareness of this disease. *C difficile* is a gram-positive, spore-forming, anaerobic bacillus. It can be present in the stool as an asymptomatic colonizer or can cause disease ranging from diarrhea to pseudomembranous colitis, toxic megacolon, intestinal perforation, and/or death. Toxin A, an enterotoxin, causes secretion of fluid into the colon, and toxin B, a cytotoxin, causes cell damage in the lining of the colon. A third toxin, binary toxin, is sometimes present, although its clinical role is unclear.

The increased severity of *C difficile* is in part related to the spread of a hypervirulent strain (BI/NAP1) that overproduces toxins A and B and produces an additional binary toxin. Toxin production by these strains can be 16- to 23-fold greater than that of other strains. This strain also demonstrates hypersporulation. Traditional risk factors for *C difficile* include antimicrobial exposure, age greater than 65 years, severe underlying illness, GI surgery or manipulation, and prolonged hospital stay. Additional associated risk factors include use of a proton pump inhibitor, although there is conflicting data about this factor.

Treatment of *C difficile* starts with discontinuation of the inciting antibiotic and initiation of oral antimicrobial therapy, usually oral metronidazole for mild disease or oral vancomycin for more severe disease. Fidaxomicin was recently approved by the FDA for the treatment of *C difficile*. It was equally effective as vancomycin in the treatment of *C difficile* but had the added benefit of sustained clinical response in some patients. If the patient is unable to take oral medications, then intraluminal (intracolonic) vancomycin with or without IV metronidazole is suggested. Disease can progress despite appropriate therapy; therefore, patients should be followed closely for signs of toxic megacolon, peritonitis, or sepsis, at which point surgery may be considered.

Many alternative therapies have been explored, but none has proven to be more effective than metronidazole or oral vancomycin. Additional strategies against *Clostridium difficile*–associated disease include treatment of recurrent disease with pulsed or tapering doses of vancomycin or addition of probiotics such as *Saccharomyces boulardii* or *Lactobacillus* with or without IV immunoglobulins. Antiperistaltic agents are contraindicated and narcotics should be avoided. Appropriate infection control measures should be instituted to prevent the spread of this disease. Washing hands with soap and water is more effective than alcohol-based hand sanitizers in killing *C difficile* spores.

Surgical-Site Infections

Rates of surgical-site infections (SSIs) vary on type of wound and local and host factors. The risk of SSI is in part related to classification of the wound as clean, clean-contaminated, contaminated, or dirty-infected. Each is associated with increasing rates of infection. Topical antiseptics and prophylactic antibiotics help decrease superficial flora and contamination of the surgical field. The guidelines also recommend preoperative treatment of infections at remote body sites to reduce the risk of wound infections. Other risk factors for SSI include the presence of foreign bodies, blood clots, seromas, and devitalized tissues. Ischemia to a wound can result in a rise in bacterial load and subsequent increased risk of infection. Common causes of wound infection include *S aureus*, coagulase-negative staphylococci, enterococci, enterobacteriaceae and *P aeruginosa*, and usually result from contamination of the wound by the patient's own flora. Those colonized with *S aureus* in the nares are at increased risk of postoperative wound infection. For deeper infections, also called organ or space SSI, polymicrobial infections are commonly seen, possibly with more resistant flora. Typically, infections originating from the proximal GI tract may involve gram-positive and gram-negative aerobic and facultative organisms. Distal small-bowel perforations usually are caused by gram-negative facultative and aerobic organisms. Large-bowel–associated infections are caused by facultative and obligate anaerobic organisms. In addition to enterobacteriaceae, other examples include *P aeruginosa*, MRSA, or yeast.

There are several measures that the surgeon should take to help protect against SSI. One such measure is administration of antibiotic prophylaxis (Table 30.1). This is suggested for all GI, obstetrical, gynecologic, oropharyngeal, vascular, and open heart procedures. Prophylactic antibiotics are also recommended for neurosurgical procedures, joint replacements, vascular prosthesis, and craniotomy, where the risk of infection is low but the consequences would be tremendous. The prophylactic antimicrobial agent should be administered within 60 minutes prior to the procedure. Exceptions include vancomycin and fluoroquinolones, which should be infused up to 120 minutes prior to the first incision. Prolonged prophylactic antibiotics are not recommended except for cardiothoracic procedures, where antibiotics may be given up to 72 hours after the procedure.

Other important measures include tight glucose control in diabetic patients, avoiding shaving, and delayed primary closure for heavily contaminated wounds.

Skin and Soft Tissue Infections

MRSA

There is growing concern about MRSA infections in the community. These strains differ somewhat from the hospital-acquired strains. Many of the community-acquired MRSA (CA-MRSA) infections carry a novel genetic element, staphylococcal cassette chromosome (SCC-mec) type IV that includes the *mecA* gene. *MecA* encodes a penicillin binding protein, PBP2a, which has a very low affinity for penicillin and other β-lactam antibiotics. Many of these strains do not carry as many antibiotic-resistant genes as hospital-acquired MRSA strains. They do tend to carry the Panton-Valentine leukocidin toxin that appears to be associated with furunculosis and severe hemorrhagic pneumonia, but is rarely responsible for osteomyelitis or endocarditis.

Treatment of CA-MRSA infections relies heavily on surgical debridement. Most CA-MRSA strains are susceptible to trimethoprim-sulfamethoxazole and tetracyclines and their derivatives. Up to 50% of CA-MRSA strains have inducible or constitutive resistance to clindamycin. Several new antibiotics are active against CA-MRSA, including quinupristin/dalfopristin, linezolid, daptomycin, and tigecycline. Other potentially active investigational agents on the horizon include ceftobiprole (a cephalosporin with activity against MRSA), telavancin, dalbavancin, and oritavancin.

Burn-Related Infections

Burns are particularly prone to infectious complications for various reasons. Burns compromise the natural barrier to block entry of microbes. The necrotic

TABLE 30.1	Antimicrobial Prophylaxis for Surgery		

Nature of Operation	Common Pathogens	Recommended Antimicrobials	Adult Dosage before Surgery[a]
Cardiac	*Staphylococcus aureus, S. epidermidis*	Cefazolin or cefuroxime OR vancomycin[c]	1–2 g IV[b] 1.5 g IV[b] 1 g IV[b]
Gastrointestinal			
Esophageal, gastroduodenal	Enteric gram-negative bacilli, gram-positive cocci	*High risk[d] only:* cefazolin[g]	1–2 g IV
Billiary tract	Enteric gram-negative bacilli, enterococci, clostridia	*High risk[e] only:* cefazolin[g]	1–2 g IV
Colorectal	Enteric gram-negative bacilli, anaerobes, enterococci	*Oral:* neomycin + erythromycin base[f] OR metronidazole[f] *Parenteral:* cefoxitin[g] OR cefazolin + metronidazole[g] OR ampicillin/sulbactam	1–2 g IV 1–2 g IV 0.5 g IV 3 g IV
Appendectomy, non-perforated[h]	Enteric gram-negative bacilli, anaerobes, enterococci	Cefoxitin[g] OR cefazolin + metronidazole[g] OR ampicillin/sulbactam[g]	1–2 g IV 1–2 g IV 0.5 g IV 3 g IV
Genitourinary	Enteric gram-negative bacilli, enterococci	*High risk[i] only:* ciprofloxacin	500 mg PO or 400 mg IV
Gynecologic and Obstetric			
Vaginal, abdominal or laparoscopic hysterectomy	Enteric gram-negative bacilli, anaerobes, Gp B strep, enterococci	Cefoxitin[g] or cefazolin[g] OR ampicillin/sulbactam[g]	1–2 g IV 3 g IV
Cesarean section	Same as for hysterectomy	Cefazolin[g]	1–2 g IV after cord clamping
Abortion	Same as for hysterectomy	*First trimester, high risk[j]:* aqueous penicillin G OR doxycycline *Second trimester:* cefazolin[g]	2 mill units IV 300 mg PO[k] 1–2 g IV
Head and Neck Surgery			
Incisions through oral or pharyngeal mucosa	Anaerobes, enteric gram-negative bacilli, *S. aureus*	Clindamycin + gentamicin OR cefazolin	600–900 mg IV 1.5 mg/kg IV 1–2 g IV
Neurosurgery	*S. aureus, S. epidermidis*	Cefazolin OR vancomycin[c]	1–2 g IV 1 g IV
Ophthalmic	*S. epidermidis, S. aureus,* streptococci, enteric gram-negative bacilli, *Pseudomonas spp.*	Gentamicin, tobramycin, ciprofloxacin, gatfloxacin levofloxacin, maxifloxacin, ofloxacin or neomycin-gramicidin-polymyxin B cetazolin	multiple drops topically over 2 to 24 hours 100 mg subconjunctivally

(continued)

TABLE 30.1	Antimicrobial Prophylaxis for Surgery (*Continued*)		
Nature of Operation	**Common Pathogens**	**Recommended Antimicrobials**	**Adult Dosage before Surgery**[a]
Orthopedic	*S. aureus, S. epidermidis*	Cefazolin[f]	1–2 g IV
		or cefuroxime[f]	1.5 g IV
		OR vancomycin[c,l]	1 g IV
Thoracic (Non-Cardiac)	*S. aureus, S. epidermidis,* streptococci, enteric gram-negative bacilli	Cefazolin or cefuroxime	1–2 g IV 1.5 g IV
		OR vancomycin[c]	1 g IV
Vascular			
Arterial surgery involving a prosthesis, the abdominal aorta, or a groin incision	*S. aureus, S. epidermidis,* enteric gram-negative bacilli	Cefazolin	1–2 g IV
		OR vancomycin[c]	1 g IV
Lower extremity amputation for ischemia	*S. aureus, S. epidermidis,* enteric gram-negative bacilli, clostridia	Cefazolin	1–2 g IV
		OR vancomycin[c]	1 g IV

[a]Parenteral prophylactic antimicrobials can be given as a single IV dose begun 60 minutes or less before the operation. For prolonged operations (>4 hours), or those with major blood loss, additional intraoperative doses should be given at intervals 1–2 times the half-life of the drug for the duration of the procedure in patients with normal renal function. If vancomycin or a fluoroquinolone is used, the infusion should be started 60–120 minutes before the initial incision in order to minimize the possibility of an infusion reaction close to the time of induction of anesthesia and to have adequate tissue levels at the time of incision.

[b]Some consultants recommend an additional dose when patients are removed from bypass during open-heart surgery.

[c]Vancomycin is used in hospitals in which methicillin-resistant *S. aureus* and *S. epidermidis* are a frequent cause of postoperative wound inflection, for patients previously colonized with MRSA, or for those who are allergic to penicillins or cephalosporins. Rapid IV administration may cause hypotension, which could be especially dangerous during induction of anesthesia. Even when the drug is given over 60 minutes, hypotension may occur; treatment with diphenhydramine (Benadryl and others) and further slowing of the infusion rate may may be helpful. Some experts would give 15 mg/kg of vancomycin to patients weighing more than 75 kg, up to a maximum of 1.5 g, with a slower infusion rate (90 minutes for 1.5 g). To provide coverage against gram-negative bacteria, most Medical Letter consultants would also include cefazolin or cefuroxime in the prophylaxis regimen for patients not allergic to cephalosporins; ciprofloxacin, levofloxacin, gentamicin, or aztreonam, each one in combination with vancomycin, can be used in patients who cannot tolerate a cephalosporin.

[d]Morbid obesity, esophageal obstruction, decreased gastric acidity or gastrointestinal motility.

[e]Age >70 years, acute cholecystitis, non-functioning gall bladder, obstructive jaundice or common duct stones.

[f]After appropriate diet and catharsis, 1 g of neomycin plus 1 g of erythromycin at 1 PM, 2 PM and 11 PM or 2 g of neomycin plus 2 g of metronidazole at 7 PM and 11 PM the day before an 8 AM operation.

[g]For patients allergic to penicillins and cephalosporins, clindamycin with either gentamicin, ciprofloxacin, levofloxacin or aztreonam is a reasonable alternative.

[h]For a ruptured viscus, therapy is often continued for about five days. Ruptured viscus in postoperative setting (dehiscence) requires antibacterials to include coverage of nosocomial pathogens.

[i]Urine culture positive or unavailable, preoperative catheter, transrectal prostatic biopsy, placement of prosthetic material.

[j]Patients with previous pelvic inflammatory disease, previous gonorrhea or multiple sex partners.

[k]Divided into 100 mg one hour before the abortion and 200 mg one half hour after.

[l]If a tourniquet is to be used in the procedure, the entire dose of antibiotic must be infused prior to its inflation.

Recommendations for Surgical Prophylaxis. Reprinted with Permission from the *Medical Letter*. 2008.

material serves as a good medium in which bacteria can multiply; nonspecific humoral and cellular immune functions are also depressed by thermal injury.

Prophylactic antibiotics are not usually given to the inpatient burn patient. Instead, frequent inspection of the burn and the surrounding tissue is advocated. Effective topical agents, such as silver nitrate, have decreased the incidence of partial thickness wounds to full thickness wounds by local infection. Aggressive debridement of necrotic tissue is still required and closure of the wound with allograft is important. Silver nitrate necessitates use of an occlusive dressing and also discolors the wound, making evaluation more difficult. Other topical agents include mafenide acetate and silver sulfadiazine. In diagnosing a burn wound infection, surface cultures are of only limited value, mostly helpful in determining with what the patient is colonized. Biopsy with culture of the wound with quantitative cultures is the most useful in determining the status of the wound.

Animal Bites

Pets are the most common cause of bites. Dog bites occur more commonly; however, cat bites are more prone to infection due to their longer, sharper teeth that may produce deeper puncture wounds. Stray and wild animals, such as skunks, raccoons, and bats, also bite thousands of people each year. Snakebites occur mainly in the southwestern United States.

Bites by a wild animal or an unknown pet should prompt notification of animal control authorities while attempting to keep the animal within view in order for capture. The authorities can then determine if the animal needs to be impounded and checked for rabies. Any animal whose rabies vaccination status is unknown should be captured and quarantined, and if the patient might have been exposed to rabies, the patient should start the vaccination series immediately.

Approximately 4.7 million Americans are bitten by animals annually, and bites account for approximately 1% of all emergency department visits. An appropriate history should be obtained, and the nature of the bite, if it was provoked or not, and whether patient is at risk for rabies need to be determined. It is important to know if the victim is pregnant or immunocompromised, is up to date on vaccinations, has had a splenectomy or mastectomy recently, or has underlying liver disease. Wounds should be cultured. Usually wounds are not closed except in certain cases. Moderate-to-severe wounds should be prophylaxed with antibiotics.

Rabid bats have been reported in the 49 continental states. Raccoons, skunks, and foxes are the terrestrial carnivores most often infected with rabies in the United States. All bites by such wildlife should be considered as possible exposures to the rabies virus. Rodents are not reservoirs of the rabies virus. Small rodents (eg, squirrels, chipmunks, rats, mice, hamsters, guinea pigs, and gerbils) and lagomorphs (including rabbits and hares) are rarely infected with rabies and have not been known to transmit rabies to humans. Woodchucks account for 93% of infected rodents.

The management of a bite wound should always include a thorough cleaning with a 20% soap solution. Irrigation with a virucidal agent such as povidone–iodine is advisable. A tetanus shot should be given, if indicated. The clinician then must decide whether to administer passive and active immunization for rabies. If rabies is suspected, then rabies immune globulin should be administered at the same time as the first dose of the five-dose series of rabies vaccine. As much as possible of the human rabies immune globulin (HRIG) should be infiltrated in the wound area and the rest elsewhere. The rabies vaccine should be administered on the day of exposure and then on days 3, 7, 14, and 28. If possible, the vaccine should be administered in the deltoid muscle.

Necrotizing Fasciitis

Necrotizing fasciitis is a surgical emergency defined as a deep-seated soft tissue infection of the subcutaneous tissue that spreads rapidly along the fascial planes. Difficult to diagnose, it can lead to septic shock, limb amputation, and death, if early surgical intervention is not obtained. Type I necrotizing fasciitis is a polymicrobial infection consisting of mixed aerobic and anaerobic species. It occurs in patients with diabetes, in those with peripheral vascular disease, after surgical procedures, and in immunocompromised hosts. Type II is monomicrobial, usually with group A *Streptococcus* isolated alone or in combination with *S aureus*. This type of necrotizing fasciitis can occur in patients with a history of blunt trauma or penetrating injury, surgery, muscle injury, burns, childbirth, chickenpox, or with a history of nonsteroidal anti-inflammatory agents or IV drug use. Type II may occur in either immunocompromised or immunocompetent patients of any age.

Clinical features include fever, local tense edema, erythema, pain disproportionate to physical findings, blisters/bullae, crepitus, cutaneous anesthesia, and subcutaneous gas. Initially, skin appears hot, erythematous, and shiny, and is very tender. Then skin becomes grayish, leading to cutaneous bullae and necrosis. Progression may lead to compartment syndrome, necessitating emergency fasciotomy. Extremities, particularly the legs, are most affected, but necrotizing fasciitis can affect any part of the body including the abdominal wall, postoperative wounds, and the perineum (Fournier's gangrene—it should be suspected in diabetic male patients with scrotal pain and erythema and should prompt emergency urologic evaluation). Although nonspecific, leukocytosis, elevated liver enzymes and serum creatinine, and creatinine phosphokinase can be seen. Imaging (computed tomography [CT] and magnetic resonance imaging) may be helpful but delays diagnosis. Diagnosis depends on surgical intervention; lack of resistance along the fascial planes suggests necrotizing fasciitis.

Early surgical debridement is critical and antimicrobial therapy (with activity against gram-positive,

Clostridium spp and mixed aerobic/anaerobic organisms) is supportive. Monotherapy with β-lactams or carbapenems are acceptable regimens. Multidrug regimens have also been described. If MRSA is suspected, vancomycin, daptomycin, or linezolid should be included. Addition of clindamycin is advocated in those with clostridial and streptococcal infections, as it may help by inhibiting toxin production. Hyperbaric oxygen and IVIG use remains controversial.

Liver Abscess

Hepatic abscesses, either pyogenic or ametic, are the most common cause of all visceral abscesses. Potential sources include biliary disease (cholangitis, cholecystitis), hematogenous spread (endocarditis, pyelonephritis), and portal system/venous drainage from the GI tract (diverticulitis, pancreatitis, appendicitis, perforated peptic ulcers, amebic colitis, colon cancer, or post colon surgery). Associated risk factor are diabetes, history of malignancy (pancreatic or hepatobiliary), liver transplantation, geographic location (*Klebsiella* hepatic abscesses in East Asia), and post trauma. Approximately 20% of liver abscesses are cryptogenic. Hepatosplenic candidiasis occurs in immunocompromised hosts after recovery from prolonged neutropenia and presents with fever, elevated alkaline phosphatase, and multiple hepatosplenic lesions on radiographic imaging. Treatment includes a prolonged course of antifungal therapy.

Pyogenic Liver Abscess

Pyogenic liver abscesses (PLAs), which account for 13% of all intra-abdominal abscesses, typically affect individuals in their fifth and sixth decades of life. The most common source is biliary tract disease, and PLAs are usually polymicrobial, including mixed facultative and anaerobic species. Typical associated pathogens are the enterobacteriaceae (particularly *E coli* and *K pneumoniae*), *Streptococcus* spp, *Enterococcus* spp, and anaerobic pathogens (*Bacteroides* spp and *Fusobacterium* spp). Isolation of *S aureus* suggests hematogenous seeding. PLA more often occurs in the right hepatic lobe. Increased size and greater hepatic blood flow may explain this occurrence. Patients present with fever, nausea, vomiting, weight loss, malaise, right upper quadrant pain, and (rarely) jaundice. Nonspecific laboratory findings are a leukocytosis, elevated alkaline phosphatase, anemia, and hypoalbuminemia. Blood cultures are positive in up to 50% of cases. Diagnosis is based on radiographic imaging and culture. The most useful diagnostic test is culture of aspirated material by CT or ultrasound-guided percutaneous

drainage. Surgical drainage is recommended in patients with failed percutaneous drainage; multiple, loculated collections; obstruction of drainage catheter; or when diagnosis remains unclear. Empiric broad-spectrum antimicrobial therapy should be initiated once PLA is suspected or confirmed. Antimicrobial therapy can then be more targeted once the pathogens have been identified and susceptibility data become available. A typical course of therapy is IV antibiotics for the first 2 weeks followed by oral therapy for a total of 4 to 6 weeks.

Amebic Liver Abscess

Amebic liver abscess (ALA) is caused by invasive *Entamoeba histolytica* infection seen in immigrants and travelers of endemic areas. Infection occurs after ingestion of cysts of fecally contaminated water and food. Patients with ALA are 7 to 10 times more likely to be adult men younger than 50 years. A solitary abscess in the right lobe of the liver is seen in up to 80% of cases of ALA. ALA can present many years after exposure to an endemic area. Often, patients have right upper quadrant pain, fever, and referred right shoulder pain. Antibody to *E histolytica* is detectable in 85% to 95% of all patients with ALA as early as 1 week after infection and persists for many years after exposure. Other nonspecific laboratory abnormalities that can be seen are an elevated alkaline phosphatase, leukocytosis, and hepatic transaminitis. Needle aspiration should only be considered if (a) there is no response to initial therapy, (b) there is an increased risk of impending rupture, or (c) necessary to rule out a pyogenic abscess. The aspirated material is classically described as an anchovy-paste-like fluid. Differential diagnosis includes echinococcal cysts, which is a rarely fatal disease but is associated with complications including rupture leading to peritonitis and anaphylactic shock after attempted drainage. Serology helps differentiate it from ALA. Treatment of ALA consists of tissue agents followed by luminal agents. The most commonly used tissue agent is metronidazole for 10 days. Luminal agents used are paromomycin, iodoquinol, and diloxanide furoate.

Cholecystitis

Acute Cholecystitis

Acute cholecystitis is as an acute inflammation of the gallbladder caused by obstruction of the cystic duct, and is most commonly caused by gallstones. Risk factors include obesity, female gender, age, fatty diet, pregnancy, gastric surgery, and hemolytic disorders (such as sickle cell disease or hereditary spherocytosis).

Patients typically complain of nausea, vomiting, fever, and right upper quadrant and/or epigastric pain that may radiate to the right shoulder. A positive "Murphy's sign," right upper quadrant tenderness on palpation, may be present. Ultrasound should show possible gallstones, gallbladder wall thickening, edema, and pericholecystic fluid, and the patient may also express a positive sonographic Murphy's sign. If the diagnosis remains unclear after sonography, a hepatobiliary iminodiacetic acid scan should be performed. Although, acute cholecystitis is initially a sterile inflammation, a secondary infection may occur leading to necrosis, gangrene, and emphysematous cholecystitis. Timing of cholecystectomy remains controversial; however, most experts recommend early cholecystectomy. Early cholecystectomy (within the first week) by either laparotomy or laparoscopically is preferred over delayed surgery, which is associated with increased risk of recurrent or continued symptoms. In high-risk patients, percutaneous transhepatic cholecystostomy should be considered. Empiric therapy should cover the enteric flora. β-Lactam antibiotics, third- or fourth-generation cephalosporins, carbapenems, monobactams, or fluoroquinolones are all acceptable options. Addition of an anaerobic agent should be considered.

Acalculous Cholecystitis

In up to 15% of cases, acute cholecystitis presents as an acute necroinflammatory process in the absence of gallstones. Risk factors include immunocompromised status (HIV, diabetes, childbirth, critical illness—sepsis/hypotension, mechanical ventilation, total parental nutrition), major trauma, burns, multiple transfusions, surgery, drug induced (ceftriaxone—biliary sludge associated with ceftriaxone has been described), and vasculitis. These predisposing factors can lead to gallbladder ischemia and bile stasis, resulting in an increased concentration of bile salts. Acalculous cholecystitis should be considered in any critically ill patient with unexplained fever, abdominal pain, and leukocytosis. Diagnostic, complications, and treatment options are similar to those for calculus cholecystitis.

Emphysematous Cholecystitis

Emphysematous cholecystitis occurs in approximately 1% of all cases of acute cholecystitis and is typically seen in diabetic men older than 50 years and is a life-threatening variant of acute cholecystitis. It is caused by gas-forming pathogens in the gallbladder wall, lumen, and adjacent tissues. The signs and symptoms are similar to those of acute cholecystitis. Rarely, crepi-

tus of the abdominal wall can be seen. Imaging (ultrasound and CT scan) showing gas around the gallbladder is diagnostic. A normal plain abdominal film does not exclude the diagnosis. Emergency cholecystectomy and antibiotic therapy are imperative as morbidity and mortality remain high. The risk of perforation is five times greater compared with patients with acute cholecystitis, along with a 10-fold increased risk of mortality. Organisms isolated include *Clostridium* spp, *E coli*, *S aureus*, *Streptococcus* spp, *Pseudomonas* spp, and *Klebsiella* spp. Broad-spectrum antimicrobials should be started immediately, covering the most common pathogens, including *Clostridium* spp, and adjusted accordingly based on culture susceptibilities.

Cholangitis

Cholangitis, or inflammation of the biliary ducts, can be divided into several types including acute (ascending) primary sclerosing cholangitis, cholangitis, oriental or recurrent cholangitis, and acquired immunodeficiency syndrome (AIDS-related sclerosing cholangitis). This section will focus on acute (ascending) cholangitis, which is inflammation of the bile ducts caused by an infected, usually obstructed, biliary system, and bile stasis, which can lead to increased intraluminal pressure and bacteremia. Bacteria enter the biliary system hematogenously via the portal venous system or ascend from the intestinal tract specifically the duodenum. Obstruction occurs secondary to biliary stones, strictures, masses, and rarely, parasites (ie, *Clonorchis* spp, *Ascaris* spp, or *Echinococcus* spp).

Two clinical syndromes described are Charcot's triad and Reynold's pentad. Charcot's triad is right upper quadrant pain, fever, and jaundice. Reynold's pentad is Charcot's triad with mental status changes and shock. It is associated with increased morbidity and mortality. Laboratory findings are often nonspecific, however, elevated liver function tests, hyperbilirubinemia and leukocytosis are often seen. Diagnosis can be made by ultrasound, CT scan and magnetic resonance cholangiopancreatography, and by more invasive tests including endoscopic ultrasound and endoscopic retrograde cholangiopancreatography. Blood cultures should be obtained in any patient with suspected acute cholangitis. Bacteremia is seen in 21 to 83% of patients.

Drainage is accomplished percutaneously, endoscopically, or surgically. Choice of intervention depends on the clinical situation. Up to 90% of cultures taken from the bile (including stones and blocked biliary stents) are positive. Broad-spectrum antibiotics should be started immediately. Empiric therapy should include coverage against enteric gram-negative pathogens. Most common organisms recovered are *Enterobacter* spp, *Klebsiella* spp, *E coli*, and enterococcus spp. Once an organism has been identified, empiric antimicrobial treatment can be narrowed accordingly.

Peritonitis

Peritonitis is a diffuse or localized inflammatory process affecting the peritoneal lining. It can be categorized as primary, secondary, or tertiary. The presence of an indwelling catheter such as a peritoneal dialysis catheter or peritoneal drain may also lead to peritonitis.

Primary Peritonitis

Primary peritonitis is also known as spontaneous bacterial peritonitis (SBP) and occurs in patients with cirrhosis, ascites, and portal hypertension with no obvious source of intra-abdominal abnormalities/infections. Prevalence in hospitalized cirrhotic patients with ascites is 10% to 30%. Cirrhosis accounts for up to 25% of adults with SBP. Other risk factors include metastatic malignancy, chronic hepatitis, and congestive heart failure.

Patients may present with fever, abdominal pain, or nonspecific findings such as fatigue and encephalopathy. SBP should be included in the differential diagnosis in any patient with known cirrhosis and ascites with these symptoms. An elevated ascitic fluid polymorphonuclear leukocyte count (≥ 250 cells/mm^3) with a positive ascitic fluid culture is diagnostic. SBP is typically a monomicrobial infection. *E coli* is the most frequently isolated pathogen, followed by *K pneumoniae*, *S pneumoniae*, and enterococci. *S aureus* is infrequently seen. If anaerobes are recovered, an alternative diagnosis of secondary peritonitis from spillage of an intra-abdominal viscus should be considered. Empiric treatment should commence once SBP is suspected. Once culture results are available, therapy should be narrowed accordingly.

Secondary Peritonitis

Secondary peritonitis is generally caused by spillage of GI or genitourinary microorganisms into the peritoneal cavity. Most common causes are a ruptured appendix, perforated peptic ulcer, diverticulitis, cholecystitis, bowel trauma, perforated viscus, or ruptured intra-abdominal abscess. It is usually a mixed infection of aerobic and anaerobic species. Peritonitis secondary to a perforated viscus requires surgical intervention and antimicrobial therapy. The initial therapy for secondary peritonitis should cover the most common enteric organisms, gram-negative organisms, enterobacteriaceae, *S pneumoniae*, enterococci, and anaerobes (*B fragilis*). Other pathogens occasionally found are *Mycobacterium tuberculosis*, *S aureus*, and *Neisseria gonorrhoeae*.

Tertiary Peritonitis

Tertiary peritonitis refers to persistent intra-abdominal infection after initial surgical and antimicrobial therapy of secondary bacterial peritonitis. Patients may develop septic shock and multiorgan failure. Typically coagulase-negative *staphylococci* are most commonly isolated. Multiple drug-resistant pathogens, including enterococci, *Pseudomonas*, *Candida* spp, and *Enterobacter* spp, can be isolated peritoneal exudates.

Peritonitis Associated with Peritoneal Dialysis

Peritonitis is considered a major complication of peritoneal dialysis and is the primary reason for patients changing from peritoneal dialysis to hemodialysis. Clinically, patients may present with fever, abdominal pain, and cloudy abdominal fluid. A high index of suspicion should be maintained in any patient with vague symptoms on peritoneal dialysis. A thorough physical examination should include careful inspection of the catheter to rule out an exit-site or tunnel infection. Patients should meet two of the following three criteria: (a) a Gram stain demonstrating microorganisms or a positive culture of the dialysis effluent, (b) a dialysate white blood cell count higher than 100/mm^3 with at least 50% neutrophils, and (c) peritoneal signs or symptoms. The most common pathogens identified are *S epidermidis* and *S aureus*, followed by gram-negative bacteria; the remaining isolates are largely accounted for by fungi, anaerobes, and mycobacteria. If polymicrobial organisms are found in Gram stain and culture, bowel perforation and surgical evaluation should be considered. Either systemic or intraperitoneal antibiotic therapy can be given. If there is no clinical improvement, then catheter removal is warranted. According to the International Society for Peritoneal Dialysis guidelines, indications for catheter removal for peritoneal dialysis-related infections are refractory, relapsing, or fungal peritonitis and refractory exit-site/tunnel infection. Empiric antimicrobial treatment should cover gram-positive and gram-negative organisms and be adjusted accordingly.

Diverticulitis

Diverticulosis is defined as outpouchings, or diverticula, of the mucosa and submucosa through the muscularis propria of the colonic wall. Diets high in refined carbohydrates and little dietary fiber may result in decreased bowel transit time and increased intraluminal pressure. Therefore, diverticulosis is most commonly seen in Western and industrialized societies. Diverticular disease accounts for approximately 130,000 hospitalizations per year in the United States. Diverticulosis is most commonly seen in patients older than 50 years and is present in more than 80% of patients older than 85 years. Ninety percent of cases occur in the sigmoid and descending colon. Right-sided diverticulitis is more commonly seen in Asia.

Diverticulitis is inflammation and infection of the bowel. Complicated diverticulitis refers to the presence of a free intra-abdominal perforation, peritonitis, bowel obstruction, an abscess, fistula (most commonly colovesical fistulas 50% to 65%), bleeding, and strictures (as a result of repeated attacks). The most common manifestation of complicated diverticulitis is a pericolic abscess. The overall mortality in this group is between 20% and 30%. Mortality from purulent peritonitis and fecal peritonitis is approximately 13% and 43%, respectively, according to the Hinchey classification of diverticular perforations. Overall, approximately 20% of patients with diverticulitis require surgical treatment. Most patients present with left lower quadrant pain, nausea, diarrhea, fever, and leukocytosis. A CT scan is the imaging of choice in assessing a patient with suspected diverticulitis, helps in diagnosis of complicated diverticulitis, and guides in percutaneous drainage.

Surgical mortality can be as high as 5%. The primary goal of a surgical intervention is to remove the septic focus and restore bowel continuity while minimizing morbidity and mortality. Surgery has generally been advised after a first attack of complicated diverticulitis or after two or more episodes of uncomplicated diverticulitis. The choice of antibiotics should be based on the most common pathogens, which are principally gram-negative rods and anaerobes (particularly enterobacteriaceae and *B fragilis*) and adjusted based on culture results.

Pancreatitis

Acute pancreatitis associated with necrosis, a severe form of pancreatitis, is associated with increased mortality, particularly once infected. Pancreatic necrosis is defined by ≥1 area of focal or diffuse nonviable pancreatic parenchyma and identified radiographically by the absence of contrast enhancement. As more necrosis is present, the higher the risk of infection. Prophylactic treatment with imipenem/cilastatin is recommended for the prevention of infection. Most cases of infection with necrotizing pancreatitis will occur within 3 weeks. Infection is detected by Gram staining and culture of pancreatic tissue. Once infection is established, surgical intervention is usually required in conjunction with targeted antimicrobial therapy. A pancreatic pseudocyst (a walled off collection of pancreatic fluids) may occur ≥4 weeks after the onset of acute pancreatitis. Close observation over time may result in spontaneous recovery; however, persistent or worsening symptoms may require intervention such as transmural drainage either percutaneously or endoscopically, or more aggressive surgical internal drainage or cystectomy.

Septic Joint/Prosthetic Joint

Acute bacterial arthritis is usually monoarticular, and untreated or delayed therapy may lead to significant joint destruction. Infection usually begins after hematogenous seeding. Risk is increased in rheumatoid arthritis patients as well as previously diseased or prosthetic joints. Infection may also occur by penetration injury, trauma, surgery, or from a contiguous focus. *S aureus* accounts for most cases of septic joint. This is followed by *Streptococcus* and gram-negative bacteria such as *E coli*, *Proteus mirabilis*, *Klebsiella* spp, and *P aeruginosa*. Among younger, sexually active patients, *N gonorrhoeae* may be the cause of septic arthritis, in some cases. Some bacteria are epidemiologically linked to certain hosts, for example, *Salmonella* spp arthritis in sickle cell disease patients and *Pasteurella multocida* and *Capnocytophaga* spp causing septic joints associated with cat and dog bites. Joint aspiration or arthrocentesis aids in establishment of infection with cell count, protein, lactate dehydrogenase, glucose and crystal examination, Gram stain, and culture. A reactive arthritis may also present with an acutely inflamed joint in the setting of infection elsewhere; cultures should be negative. Early joint drainage and repeated aspirations along with targeted IV antimicrobial therapy are required. Late prosthetic joint infections often require removal of the prosthetic for curative treatment.

Transfusion-Related Infections

According to the American Red Cross, in 2001, 4.9 million patients received blood transfusions. The safety of the blood supply is an ongoing concern. The estimated risk of transfusion-transmitted diseases remains quite low but is not negligible. The first description of transfusion-associated HIV infection occurred in late 1982. Blood banks started screening for high-risk behavior in donors, resulting in an impressive decrease in transfusion-related HIV. In March 1985, HIV antibody testing was implemented. An additional test for antibodies to HIV type 2 was then added. In late 1995, blood banks started testing for p24 antigen. The estimated risk of transfusion-related HIV is now felt to be approximately 1 per 200,000 to 2 per 2,000,000.

Other viruses possibly transmitted include hepatitis A (1/1,000,000), hepatitis B (1/30,000 to 1/250,000), hepatitis C (1/30,000 to 1/150,000), human T-cell leukemia virus I/II (HTLV-I/II; 1/250,000 to 1/2,000,000), and parvovirus B19 (1/10,000). In 2002, when West Nile virus became endemic in the United States, there were 23 confirmed cases of transfusion-transmitted disease and seven related deaths. This is an example of an emerging pathogen agent that could threaten the blood supply. New nucleic acid technology was adapted for the detection of the virus and the risk is small. The prevalence of cytomegalovirus (CMV) seropositivity among blood donors ranges from 35% to 50%. Prevention of transfusion-transmitted CMV infection in high-risk patients can be effectively done with prestorage leukodepletion. High-risk individuals should receive CMV-seronegative blood components. Other potential transfusion-transmitted viruses include hepatitis E, hepatitis G, Epstein-Barr virus, human herpesvirus-6, human herpesvirus-8, torque teno virus, SEN virus, Creutzfeldt-Jakob disease (CJD), and variant CJD. Potential transfusion-associated parasitic infections include malaria, *Babesia*, *Trypanosoma cruzi*, and toxoplasmosis. Bacterial pathogens include coagulase-negative *Staphylococcus*, *Yersinia*, *Serratia*, *Brucella*, *Salmonella*, *Borrelia burgdorferi*, and the agents of Rocky Mountain Spotted Fever and ehrlichiosis. Platelets are more prone to bacterial infections than other components of blood because they are stored at room temperature for up to 5 days, whereas other blood supplies are refrigerated or frozen.

ANTIMICROBIAL AGENTS

The term "antibiotics" was introduced in the mid-20th century with the introduction of sulfonamides in the 1930s; however, penicillin and streptomycin in the mid-1940s marked when the antimicrobial era really began.

Significant advances in development of novel classes of antimicrobials as well as safety and ease of administration of antimicrobials have occurred since then.

In selecting an appropriate antimicrobial agent, one must focus on the site of infection, the host, renal and hepatic functions, and the susceptibility of the organism(s). Antimicrobials are used for prophylaxis, although they should be administered for a short period of time. This section focuses on β-lactams, which include penicillins, cephalosporins, monobactams, carbapenems, fluoroquinolones, aminoglycosides, vancomycin, metronidazole, and newer agents such as linezolid, daptomycin, and tigecycline. All antimicrobial agents have been associated with *C difficile*, including vancomycin.

Beta-Lactams (β-Lactams)

The β-lactams are bactericidal agents that inhibit bacterial cell wall synthesis of susceptible bacteria. Neurotoxicity is a known potential adverse effect associated with penicillins and cephalosporins in patients with renal impairment without dosage adjustment.

Penicillins

Although naturally occurring penicillins are still available, the penicillinase-resistant penicillins and broad-spectrum penicillins with β-lactamase inhibitors are often the most used agents. Penicillinase-resistant penicillins (eg, nafcillin, oxacillin, and dicloxacillin) are used in the treatment of infections caused by susceptible penicillinase-producing staphylococci (methicillin-sensitive *S aureus*, MSSA). The combination of penicillins and β-lactamase inhibitors has a wide spectrum of activity against gram-positive and gram-negative aerobic and anaerobic bacteria including *Staphylococcus* spp (not MRSA), *Haemophilus* spp, *Neisseria* spp, and *Bacteroides* spp. These agents include the aminopenicillins (amoxicillin/clavulanic acid, ampicillin/sulbactam), carboxypenicillin (ticarcillin/clavulanic acid), and ureidopenicillin (piperacillin/tazobactam). All penicillins may cause hypersensitivity reactions including anaphylaxis. The non–type 1 hypersensitivity skin reactions often associated with penicillins include a maculopapular, bullous, urticarial, and eczematoid rash. The most common adverse events are GI, which include nausea, diarrhea, constipation, vomiting, dyspepsia, and a black hairy tongue. Others include acute interstitial nephritis and central nervous system toxicity (headache, dizziness). An important drug interaction is penicillins combined with nonsteroidal anti-inflammatory agents, which are highly protein bound and can displace penicillins and inhibit renal excretion of penicillins. Penicillins taken with oral contraceptives decrease efficacy of the contraceptives and lead to an increased incidence of breakthrough bleeding. Probenecid will inhibit the renal tubular secretion of penicillins. This interaction can be exploited to increase blood levels of the penicillin agent when necessary. Allopurinol may increase the risk of rash to ampicillin if taken together.

Cephalosporins

There are currently five generations of cephalosporins. Ceftaroline was recently approved for the treament of cSSTI (complicated skin and soft tissue infections) including those with MRSA. *Enterococcus* spp, and *Listeria* spp. First-generation cephalosporins, including cefazolin and cephalexin, can be used in the treatment of MSSA and gram-negative infections due to *Proteus* spp, *E coli*, and *Klebsiella* spp. Cefazolin is frequently used for surgical prophylaxis. Cephamycins, second-generation cephalosporins including cefoxitin, are active against gram-positive aerobes and anaerobes. The third-generation cephalosporins, such as ceftriaxone and ceftazidime, are prescribed in the treatment of complicated and nosocomial infections. Cefepime, a fourth-generation cephalosporin, is highly resistant to hydrolysis by most β-lactamases and exhibits rapid penetration into gram-negative bacteria. It is commonly used in the treatment of *Pseudomonas* and nosocomial infections. The most common adverse events of cephalosporins include GI (diarrhea, nausea, and vomiting) and hypersensitivity reactions. Ceftriaxone has been associated with causing biliary sludge and pseudocholethiasis. The cross-allergenicity between penicillins and cephalosporins can vary from 1% to 15%. Patients with a history of anaphylaxis to penicillin should be carefully evaluated and possibly desensitized prior to receiving cephalosporins.

Carbapenems

Carbapenems are broad-spectrum antimicrobial agents with activity against gram-positive and gram-negative aerobes and anaerobes. Like penicillins and cephalosporins, they are bactericidal and inhibit cell wall synthesis. Currently, there are four carbapenems available: imipenem/cilastatin, meropenem, ertapenem, and doripenem. All carbapenems are excreted in the urine. Imipenem is available as a combination with cilastatin because imipenem is rapidly degraded by renal

proximal tubule dipeptidases and cilastatin is a dihydropeptidase inhibitor. The advantage of the carbapenems is coverage against strains of gram-negative bacteria that are often resistant to penicillins and cephalosporins. Some hospital-acquired pathogens have developed resistance to carbapenems. They are all approved for the treatment of complicated intra-abdominal infections, including appendicitis and peritonitis. Ertapenem has limited activity against *Pseudomonas* and *Acinetobacter* spp. The advantage of ertapenem is its long half-life that allows for once-daily dosing. It is also indicated for prophylaxis of SSI following elective colorectal surgery. No carbapenem is active against MRSA. The most common adverse reactions are GI (diarrhea, nausea, and vomiting). Carbapenems are contraindicated in patients with anaphylactic reaction to penicillins and seizures and other central nervous system (CNS) adverse events have been reported during treatment. Drug interactions include probenecid, which inhibits renal excretion and increases serum levels of carbapenems. Meropenem may reduce the serum levels of valproic acid to subtherapeutic levels; an alternative antiepileptic agent is recommended.

Aztreonam

Aztreonam is a monobactam antibiotic with activity limited to aerobic, gram-negative organisms. It is often used in patients with a history of severe allergy to β-lactams. It is administered IV and has been used in the treatment of intra-abdominal infections including peritonitis. Although generally well tolerated, adverse events include rash, GI (diarrhea, nausea, and vomiting), and injection-site reactions. Often, aztreonam is administered in combination with aminoglycosides, because it has been shown to be synergistic or additive in vitro. The combination of aztreonam and β-lactams has been shown to be additive or antagonistic; therefore, caution is recommended when combining these agents.

Aminoglycosides

In spite of the availability of many new antimicrobial agents and the progressive development of resistance, aminoglycosides remain very useful agents. They are effective against aerobic, gram-negative bacteria. They have in vitro activity against gram-positive organisms, but should not be used as monotherapy. Amikacin is often effective for the treatment of infections caused by gram-negative bacteria that are resistant to gentamicin and tobramycin. The most common adverse events still include renal and ototoxicity. Dosing of aminoglycosides should be based on renal function, ideal body weight, and serum aminoglycoside concentrations. Once-daily dosing of aminoglycosides is often used in patients with creatinine clearances greater than 70 mL/min. Current data suggest this dosing regimen is equally effective and less toxic than conventional dosing.

Vancomycin

Vancomycin is a tricyclic glycopeptide originally approved for use in the mid-1950s. Owing to early reports of ototoxicity and concern over the purity of the product, it was commonly referred to as "Mississippi Mud" and not well used until the early 1980s with the increased incidence of MRSA and *C difficile*–associated diarrhea.

It is now the most widely used agent for the treatment of gram-positive infections. The most serious adverse events associated with vancomycin include ototoxicity and nephrotoxicity. Ototoxicity and nephrotoxicity are likely to occur in patients with renal impairment, receiving high doses and/or for prolonged periods, and those who receive concomitant nephrotoxic agents. "Red-man" or "red-neck syndrome" has also been associated with rapid infusion of vancomycin. The anaphylactoid reaction is characterized by a sudden decrease in blood pressure, which can be severe, accompanied with flushing and either a maculopapular or an erythematous rash in the face, neck, and upper extremities. Slowing down on the rate of infusion with or without pretreatment with antihistamines may benefit. Other adverse events include leukopenia, eosinophilia, and thrombocytopenia, usually occurring after 7 days of therapy. Oral vancomycin is approved for the treatment of *C difficile* and is not systemically absorbed or useful for other infections. With the increased use of both IV and oral vancomycin, acquired vancomycin resistance has occurred with enterococci and rarely with *S aureus*.

Daptomycin

Daptomycin is a cyclic lipopeptide that is rapidly bactericidal. It is active against gram-positive aerobic and anaerobic organisms in vitro. It has no activity against gram-negative organisms. On the basis of safety and efficacy data, daptomycin is approved for the treatment of complicated skin and skin structure infections and bacteremia, including right-sided endocarditis, caused by MSSA- and MRSA-resistant isolates. Daptomycin should not be used for the treatment of pneumonia. Daptomycin is administered by IV infusion once daily for patient with creatinine clearances ≥30 mL/min. Increases in serum creatine phosphokinase values reported as adverse events occurred in 2.8% and 6.7% of patients treated with daptomycin for complicated skin and skin structure infections and *S aureus* bacteremia, respectively. Dosing daptomycin more frequently than once daily is associated with an increased risk of creatine phosphokinase elevations. Because data are limited on the coadministration of daptomycin with HMG-CoA reductase inhibitors (drugs that may cause myopathy), temporarily stopping use of HMG-CoA reductase inhibitors among patients receiving daptomycin should be considered. No reports of skeletal myopathy occurred when healthy individuals received simvastatin and daptomycin concurrently.

Linezolid

Linezolid is a synthetic oxazolidinone agent and is bacteriostatic. The mechanism of action is by inhibiting protein synthesis. It has a broad spectrum of activity against gram-positive organisms but no activity against gram-negative bacteria. Linezolid is available in both intravenous and oral preparation. Owing to rapid absorption (100% bioavailability), the oral and IV dosing are similar. Adverse effects include myelosuppression such as anemia, leukopenia, pancytopenia, and thrombocytopenia, which occur in patients receiving greater than 2 weeks of therapy. Vitamin B6 may not be effective in treating or preventing the hematologic toxicities. Other toxicities include optic and/or peripheral neuropathy and lactic acidosis. These toxicities were seen after prolonged linezolid therapy (more than 4 weeks). Linezolid is a mild monoamine oxidase inhibitor. Linezolid should not be used in patients taking any medicinal product that inhibits monoamine oxidases A or B (eg, phenelzine, isocarboxazid) or within 2 weeks of taking any such medicinal product and is not approved and should not be used for the treatment of patients with CRBSIs or catheter-site infections. Cases of serotonin syndrome (fever, agitation, mental status changes, tremors) associated with coadministration of linezolid and selective serotonin receptor inhibitors have been reported.

Tigecycline

Tigecycline is a glycylcycline agent structurally related to minocycline, a tetracycline. It is an expanded, broad-spectrum agent with activity against gram-positive, gram-negative, and anaerobic pathogens. It has no activity against *Pseudomonas* spp and *Proteus* spp. It is a bacteriostatic agent whose mechanism of action is inhibition of protein synthesis and is currently approved for the treatment of complicated skin and intra-abdominal infections.

Serum concentrations of tigecycline are low. It is rapidly and extensively distributed from the bloodstream to the tissue. The most common adverse event is dose-related nausea and vomiting, which occur up to 30% of patients. Prolonging the infusion does not improve the nausea and vomiting. Like other tetracyclines, tigecycline should not be used in children and pregnant women due to it causing tooth discoloration. Tigecycline can increase hepatic enzymes and bilirubin. No major drug interactions were noted.

Fluoroquinolones

The original quinolones were effective in the treatment of UTIs. With the modification of the quinolones by adding a fluoride atom, the newer fluoroquinolones have a wider clinical use and a broader spectrum of antibacterial activity against gram-positive, gram-negative, and some anaerobes (moxifloxacin). Although a number of fluoroquinolones are available in the market, several were removed due to adverse events. Currently, the agents available in the U.S. market include norfloxacin, ofloxacin, ciprofloxacin, levofloxacin, moxifloxacin, and gemifloxacin. Fluoroquinolones act by inhibiting two distinct targets in the bacterial cell wall, DNA gyrase and topoisomerase IV. They are bactericidal and overall well tolerated. They have been used widely for the treatment of infections including intra-abdominal infections. The excellent bioavailability of these agents allows for oral dosing to replace parenteral administration. The most common adverse events include GI effects such as nausea, diarrhea, vomiting, and abdominal pain. CNS side effects include headache, dizziness, insomnia, hallucinations, tremors, and (rarely) seizures. All fluoroquinolones have been shown to produce cartilage damage in immature animals. There is an US Food and Drug Administration–issued black box warning of tendonitis and tendon rupture in patients receiving fluoroquinolones. The fluoroquinolones may also prolong the QT interval and should be avoided in patients with known QT prolongation. Fluoroquinolone-associated hypoglycemia and hyperglycemia have been reported in patients with underlying diabetes. Concurrent use of antacids containing magnesium, aluminum, or calcium, as well as iron and zinc, results in a decrease in serum and urine concentration of oral fluoroquinolones; therefore, these agents should be taken either 2 hours before or 6 hours after taking a fluoroquinolone. Both fluoroquinolones and nonsteroidal anti-inflammatory agents inhibit GABA receptors in the CNS; concurrent use may cause CNS toxicity. Other drug interactions include warfarin, antiarrhythmic agents, and hypoglycemic agents.

Metronidazole

Metronidazole is a synthetic antibacterial and antiprotozoal agent administered by IV and orally and is currently used for the treatment of anaerobic bacterial infections. Metronidazole has no activity against aerobes. Its oral bioavailability is 100%. The most frequent adverse events of oral metronidazole include nausea, diarrhea, and metallic taste in the mouth. IV administration has been associated with thrombophlebitis. Long-term use of metronidazole has been associated with furry black tongue and peripheral neuropathy. The most significant drug interaction with metronidazole includes concomitant administration of alcohol, which can lead to a "disulfiram" -like reaction including flushing, headache, nausea, vomiting, and tachycardia. Avoid alcohol for at least 48 hours.

Clindamycin

Clindamycin is a semisynthetic lincosamide antibiotic. It is active against gram-positive organisms and anaerobes. It inhibits bacterial protein synthesis by a similar mechanism of action as erythromycin. In vitro, it is both bactericidal and bacteriostatic. Although clindamycin is primarily used in the treatment of anaerobic and gram-positive infections, it is also used as adjunct therapy to inhibit toxin production. It is available in both oral and IV preparations. The oral bioavailability is 90%. Clindamycin is not inactivated by gastric acidity. The most serious adverse effect of clindamycin is *C difficile*–associated diarrhea and colitis. Another common adverse effect is rash. Clindamycin is often used in the treatment of resistant gram-positive infections. Laboratory testing (D test) can determine if the strain is susceptible to clindamycin.

NONINFECTIOUS CAUSES OF FEVER

Not all fevers are caused by infections. A thorough history and physical examination is essential to understanding why patients have fever. Postoperatively, many patients, whether due to sedation or pain syndromes, do not take deep, full breaths and thus risk atelectasis. In addition, hospitalized and postoperative patients are not as mobile and, as a result, are at increased risk of deep venous thrombophlebitis with or without propagation to pulmonary embolism. Several medications are known to cause fevers. Anticonvulsants (carbamazepine, phenytoin, phenobarbital, primidone), antibiotics (β-lactams, quinolones), and allopurinol are a few examples. Neuroleptic malignant syndrome may occur after exposure to psychotropic medications such as haloperidol. Malignant hyperthermia, although rare, can be life threatening. It occurs after exposure to anesthetic agents. Inflammation at peripheral IV catheter sites without frank suppuration can also cause fevers. IV infusions of some commonly used medications are associated with chemical phlebitis, including, but not limited to vancomycin, amiodarone, and nafcillin. Crystal diseases, such as gout and pseudogout, frequently occur in hospitalized patients. Metabolic disorders, such as thyroid diseases, Addison's disease, and pheochromocytomas, can cause fevers. Other causes for noninfectious fever include pancreatitis, underlying malignancies, collagen vascular diseases, and Kikuchi's disease.

QUESTIONS

Select one answer.

1. A 45-year-old man from India is being evaluated preoperatively for hernia repair. CXR was taken as part of the preoperative testing. A lung nodule is noted. A CT of chest is then performed for further evaluation that shows an old granuloma in the RUL and partial liver views reveal a solitary liver abscess in the right hepatic lobe. He is asymptomatic with normal liver function tests. Aspiration of the lesion showed 35 cc of thick fluid with 47 WBC/HPF and 50 RBC/HPF and no organisms on Gram stain.

   The next most appropriate step should be
   a. send serology for *Entamoeba histolytica*.
   b. start paromomycin.
   c. start piperacillin-tazobactam.
   d. start mebendazole.
   e. start INH, rifampin, ethambutol, pyrazinamide.

2. A 60-year-old woman with hypertension was taking care of a feral cat that became pregnant. The cat became more aggressive and bit the woman when she was leaving out the food. Animal control personnel were contacted and succeeded at capturing the cat. The following day, the woman developed swelling of the right wrist and hand as well as erythema and fever.

   What should the next step be?
   a. rabies immunoglobulin.
   b. amoxicillin/clavulanic acid.
   c. Treat for Cat-scratch disease.
   d. Euthanize the cat.
   e. Cefazolin.

3. A 72-year-old woman with hypothyroidism, diabetes mellitus, and osteoporosis fell and sustained a right intertrochanteric hip fracture. She was taken for open reduction and internal fixation (ORIF) of the hip the following day. Perioperative prophylactic cefazolin was administered for 24 hours. Postoperative day 3, she had a loose bowel movement. The following day, she has fever to 102°F, leukocytosis of 23,400 WBC/HPF and 10% bandemia. Blood pressure is stable. Blood and urine cultures are sent. CXR showed right lower lobe atelectasis. What is the most appropriate treatment?
   a. Start empiric intravenous vancomycin.
   b. Encourage incentive spirometer use.
   c. Begin lactobacillus.
   d. Observe off antibiotics while awaiting cultures.
   e. Begin oral vancomycin.

4. A 23-year-old man was involved in a motor vehicle accident. On arrival to the emergency department, he became hypotensive. A CT of the abdomen showed a lacerated spleen. He was emergently taken to the operating room for splenectomy. There are no major complications and he is ready for discharge. In addition to educating him about his increased risk of infection especially with encapsulated bacteria, what steps should you take to minimize the risk?
   a. Prophylactic penicillin daily.
   b. Pneumovax, hib, and meningococcal vaccines every 5 years.

c. Pneumovax, hib, and meningococcal vaccines once.

d. Pneumovax every 5 years; hib and meningo-coccal vaccines once.

e. Pneumovax every 5 years; hib and meningo-coccal vaccines every 10 years.

5. A 43-year-old woman with irritable bowel syndrome was in her usual state of health until approximately 2 months ago. She complained of intermittent abdominal pain with nausea, vomiting, and diarrhea. No fever. Last night her pain became more severe and she presented to the emergency department with fever 103.5° F with rigors. In the emergency department, she had rigors and sclera icterus. Direct bilirubin 2.4, alkaline phosphatase 400, WBC 18,500, AST 20, and ALT 21. Ultrasound revealed a common bile duct stone.

What is the next step?

a. Antibiotics and urgent surgical biliary decompression.

b. Antibiotics and endoscopic biliary decompression.

c. Antibiotics and percutaneous transhepatic biliary decompression.

d. Antibiotics, surgical decompression, and cholecystectomy.

6. A 35-year-old woman underwent laparoscopic resection of a perforated appendix. The patient was given ciprofloxacin and metronidazole perioperatively. The patient returned 1 week later with fever, chills, and abdominal pain. CT of the abdomen revealed a collection in the right lower quadrant. The fluid was aspirated and 200 cc of purulent fluid was obtained. Cultures revealed a pan-sensitive *E faecium* and *E coli*.

Which of the following antibiotic regimens should be initiated?

a. cefotetan.

b. ceftriaxone/metronidazole.

c. daptomycin.

d. aztreonam/clindamycin.

e. ampicillin/sulbactam.

SELECTED REFERENCES

Blajchman MA, Vamvak EC. The continuing risk of transfusion-transmitted infections. *N Engl J Med* 2006;355(13):1303–1305.

Bratzler DW, Houck PM. Antimicrobial prophylaxis for surgery: an advisory statement from the National Surgical Infection Prevention Program. *Clin Infect Dis* 2004;38: 1705–1715.

Howdieshell TR, Heffernan D, Dipiro JT; Therapeutic Agents Committee of the Surgical Infection Society. Surgical Infection Society guidelines for vaccination after traumatic injury. *Surg Infect* 2006;7(3):275–303.

Jacobs DO. Clinical practice: diverticulitis. *N Engl J Med* 2007;357(20):2057–2066.

Levine DP. Vancomycin: a history. *Clin Infect Dis* 2006;42 (suppl 1):S5–S12.

McEachern R, Campbell GD. Hospital-acquired pneumonia: epidemiology, etiology, and treatment. *Infect Dis Clin North Am* 1998;12:761–779.

O'Grady NP, Alexander M, Dellinger EP, et al. Guidelines for the prevention of intravascular catheter-related infections. *MMWR Recomm Rep* 2002;51(RR-10):1–29.

Owens RC, Donskey CJ, Gaynes RP, et al. Antimicrobial associated risk factors for *Clostridium difficile* infection. *Clin Infect Dis* 2008;46(suppl 1):S19–S31.

Saint S, Kowalski CP, Kaufman SR, et al. Preventing hospital-acquired urinary tract infection in the United States: a National Study. *Clin Infect Dis* 2008;46:243–250.

Sunenshine RH, McDonald LC. *Clostridium difficile*-associated disease: new challenges from and established pathogen. *Cleve Clin J Med* 2006;73(2):187–197.

ANSWER KEY

CHAPTER 1
1. c	4. a	7. e
2. c	5. b	8. a
3. c	6. d	9. c

CHAPTER 2
1. c	5. c	9. b
2. d	6. a	10. e
3. e	7. e	
4. d	8. e	

CHAPTER 3
1. a	5. c	9. c
2. b	6. d	10. c
3. c	7. a	
4. c	8. b	

CHAPTER 4
1. d	5. b	9. e
2. a	6. e	10. d
3. d	7. a	
4. c	8. d	

CHAPTER 5
1. e	5. c	9. b
2. d	6. e	10. c
3. d	7. a	
4. d	8. e	

CHAPTER 6
1. c	5. c	9. e
2. b	6. c	10. a
3. e	7. c	
4. e	8. c	

CHAPTER 7
1. d	5. d	9. a
2. e	6. c	10. c
3. e	7. b	
4. e	8. d	

CHAPTER 8
1. e	3. a	5. a
2. b	4. e	

CHAPTER 9
1. b	5. d	9. b
2. a	6. b	10. c
3. c	7. d	
4. d	8. e	

CHAPTER 10
1. a, b, c	5. c	9. d
2. b	6. a, b, c	10. c
3. d	7. e	11. e
4. b	8. b	12. a

CHAPTER 11
1. c	5. a	9. a
2. c	6. b	10. c
3. b	7. c	11. a
4. b	8. c	12. d

CHAPTER 12
1. true	8. false	15. true
2. false	9. true	16. true
3. false	10. true	17. false
4. false	11. true	18. true
5. false	12. false	19. true
6. true	13. true	
7. true	14. true	

CHAPTER 13
1. c	5. c	9. a
2. c	6. e	10. e
3. c	7. b	
4. a	8. a	

CHAPTER 14
1. d	5. c	9. e
2. e	6. d	10. d
3. d	7. a	
4. c	8. b	

CHAPTER 15
1. e	6. c	8. a-false, b-true, c-true, d-false
2. c	7. a-iii; b-i, iv; c-ii, v; d-ii, v; e-i, iv	
3. d		9. e
4. e		10. d
5. a		

CHAPTER 16

Thyroid	4. b	2. d
Disease	5. c	3. b
1. b	Parathyroid	4. b
2. b	Disease	5. d
3. a	1. a	

CHAPTER 17

1. a	5. c	9. c
2. c	6. c	10. a
3. b	7. d	
4. b	8. e	

CHAPTER 18

Head and neck	4. b	2. c
cancer:	5. b	3. d
1. c	Salivary gland	4. b
2. b	disease	5. b
3. b	1. c	

CHAPTER 19

1. b	5. a	9. c
2. d	6. b	10. a
3. d	7. c	
4. c	8. c	

CHAPTER 20

1. b	3. c	5. e
2. e	4. b	

CHAPTER 21

1. b	5. c	9. b
2. c	6. b	10. c
3. d	7. a	
4. a	8. b	

CHAPTER 22

1. d	6. b	11. False
2. d	7. c	12. True
3. d	8. c	13. True
4. b	9. False	14. True
5. c	10. False	15. True

CHAPTER 23

1. c	8. a	15. b
2. e	9. c	16. e
3. d	10. e	17. e
4. c	11. d	18. b
5. b	12. c	19. c
6. b	13. c	20. b
7. a	14. d	

CHAPTER 24

1. b	5. c	9. d
2. b	6. c	10. a
3. d	7. c	
4. a	8. b	

CHAPTER 25

1. c	5. c	9. d
2. d	6. a	10. c
3. b	7. d	
4. a,c,d	8. d	

CHAPTER 26

1. b	2. c	3. a

CHAPTER 27

1. e	3. e	5. d
2. b	4. c	

CHAPTER 28

1. d	3. d	5. a
2. d	4. a	

CHAPTER 29

1. b	3. d	4. c
2. b		

CHAPTER 30

1. a	3. e	5. b
2. b	4. d	6. e

INDEX

Note: Page locators followed by f and t indicates figure and table respectively.

A

Abdominal aortic aneurysms, 83–86
  and coincidental malignancy, 86
  diagnosis of, 83
  EVAR in, role of, 84
  horseshoe kidney and, 85–86
  inflammatory, 85
  and related complication, 85
  ruptured, 84, 85
  treatment of, 83–85
Abdominal compartment syndrome, 286, 287
Abdominal trauma
  blunt
    criteria for evaluation of, 193t
    CT scanning for, 193, 194t
    DPL for evaluation of, 192, 193, 193t, 194t
    ultrasound for, use of, 193, 194t
  penetrating, 195–196
Abdominoperineal resection (APR), 46
Acetabular fractures, 341
Acetazolamide, 327
Acetylcholine receptors, 267
Acetylcysteine (Mucomyst), 173
Achalasia, 3–4
Achilles tendon, 357
Acid–base balance, 300–301
Acid clearing test, 2
Acid perfusion test, 2
Acinic cell carcinoma, 257
Acral lentiginous melanoma (ALM), 124–125
Acromegaly, 326
Acromioclavicular (AC) joint, 337
  joint dislocation, 350
Activated Protein C (APC), 287
Acute axillosubclavian venous thrombosis, 265
Acute cholecystitis, 58
Acute lung injury (ALI), 291
Acute renal failure (ARF), 289, 303–304
Acute respiratory distress syndrome (ARDS), 291
Acute subdural hematomas (ASDHs), 313–314, 314f, 315f
Acute tubular necrosis (ATN), 303
Addison's disease, 245
Adenocarcinomas
  of appendix, 41
  of esophagus, 8
  gastric, 17

of pancreas, 69–70
of small bowel, 32
Adenoid cystic carcinomas, 256–257, 269
Adenomatous polyposis syndrome, 45
Adenosine triphosphate (ATP), 285
Adjustable gastric band (AGB), 401
Adjuvant chemotherapy, 119, 253. *See also* Head and neck squamous cell carcinoma (HNSCC)
Adjuvant therapy, in breast cancer, 106–107
Adrenal glands
  anatomy and embryology of, 240
  surgical considerations, 245
Adrenal insufficiency, 245
  cause of, 245
Adrenal medullary tumors, 244–245
Adrenocortical tumors
  adrenocortical carcinoma, 243
  adrenogenital syndrome, 243
  aldosteronoma, 241–243
  Cushing's syndrome, 240–241
  incidentaloma, 243–244
  metastatic disease, 243
Adrenocorticotropic hormone (ACTH), 240, 288
Adrenogenital syndrome, 243
Adult polycystic kidney disease (APKD), 375
Adult respiratory distress syndrome (ARDS), 297–298, 334
  mortality causes in, 297
Advanced Trauma Life Support (ATLS), 286
Afferent loop syndrome, 15–16
Air enema, 175
Airway, assessment of, 185
Airway pressure release ventilation (APRV), 290
Albumin, 287
Aldosterone, 293
Aldosteronoma, 241–243
Alkalosis, 300
Alkylating agents, for cancer treatment, 116, 117t
Alkyl sulfonates, 117t
Allen test, 367
AlloDerm, 283
Amebic liver abscess (ALA), 432
American Association of Clinical Endocrinologists, 231
American Board of Surgery, 285
American Burn Association Fact Sheet, 276
American College of Surgeon's, 286
American Joint Commission, on cancer staging system, 114, 114t

American Joint Committee on Cancer (AJCC), 247
American Society of Anesthesiologist (ASA), 416
  physical status classification system by, 416
American Thyroid Association (ATA), 227
Aminoglycosides, 437–438
Amputation, in lower extremity arterial occlusive disease, 77
Anaerobic glycolysis, 285
Anal cancer, 50–51
Anal fissure, 50
Anal melanomas, 51
Anaphylactic shock, 286
Anaplastic astrocytoma, 325
Anaplastic thyroid carcinoma, 228–229
Anesthesia, 416
  benzodiazepines for, 420, 420t
  inhalation anesthetics in, 418–419, 419t
  IV anesthetics in, 419–420
    barbiturates, 420
    dexmedetomidine, 419–420
    etomidate, 419
    ketamine, 419
    propofol, 419
  local, 420–421, 420t
  monitoring during, 421–422
  and NPO guidelines, 417–418
  preoperative evaluation in, 416, 418f
    cardiovascular system, 416–417
    family/personal history in, 417
    hematologic system, 417
    pulmonary system, 417
    and social history, 417
  regional, 421
Aneurysms, 83–86
  abdominal aortic, 83–86
  infected, 86
  peripheral, 86
  visceral, 86
Angioaccess surgery, 88
Angiomyolipoma (AML), 375
Animal bites, 431
Ankle/brachial index (ABI), 75
Ankle dislocations, 353
Ankle fractures, 346, 347f
  bimalleolar, 346
  trimalleolar, 346
  unimalleolar, 346
Anorectal diseases, 49–51
Anterior cord syndrome, 320. *See also* Spinal cord injury
Anthracycline antibiotics, 117t
Antiandrogens, 118t